"Podiatry is that profession of the health sciences which deals with the examination, diagnosis, treatment, and prevention of diseases, conditions, and malfunctions affecting the human foot and its related or governing structures, by employment of medical, surgical, or other means."

AMERICAN PODIATRY ASSOCIATION*
House of Delegates, 1977

* Now the American Podiatric Medical Association

YALE'S PODIATRIC MEDICINE
Third Edition

JEFFREY F. YALE, D.P.M., F.A.C.F.S.

Diplomate, American Board of Podiatric Surgery
Diplomate, American Board of Podiatric Orthopedics
Fellow, American College of Foot Surgeons
President and Fellow, American Academy of Podiatric Sports Medicine
Chairman, Podiatry Section, Department of Surgery, Griffin Hospital, Derby, Connecticut
Chairman, Podiatric Medicine Section, National Board of Podiatric Medical Examiners
Past President, Connecticut Board of Examiners in Podiatry
Associate Clinical Professor, University of Osteopathic Medicine and Health Sciences, College of Podiatric Medicine and Surgery, Des Moines, Iowa
Director of Yale Podiatry Group, Ansonia, Connecticut
Consultant, Podiatric Section, Surgical Service, Veterans Administration Medical Center, West Haven, Connecticut
Author, Firm Footings for the Athlete—1981
Co-Author, The Arthritic Foot and Related Connective Tissue Disorders—1984

SANS TACHE

WILLIAMS & WILKINS
Baltimore • London • Los Angeles • Sydney

Editor: Jonathan W. Pine, Jr.
Associate Editor: Carol Eckhart
Copy Editor: Gail Chalew
Design: JoAnne Janowiak
Illustration Planning: Lorraine Wrzosek
Production: Anne G. Seitz

Accurate indications, adverse reactions, and dosage schedules for drugs are provided in this book, but it is possible that they may change. The reader is urged to review the package information data of the manufacturers of the medications mentioned.

Printed in the United States of America

First Edition, 1974
Second Edition, 1980

Library of Congress Cataloging in Publication Data

Main entry under title:

Yale, Jeffrey F.
Yale's Podiatric medicine.

Rev. ed. of: Podiatric medicine / Irving Yale.
2nd ed. c1980.
Includes index.
1. Podiatry. I. Yale, Jeffrey F. II. Title.
III. Title: Podiatric medicine [DNLM: 1. Foot
Dermatoses. 2. Foot Diseases. WE 890 Y27p]
RD563.Y33 1986 617'.585 85-22541
ISBN 0-683-09319-3

Printed at the Waverly Press, Inc.
87 88 89 90 10 9 8 7 6 5 4 3 2 1

In loving memory
of Irving Yale,
devoted husband,
father, author
and teacher.

Preface to the Third Edition

It has often been said that most people have difficulty differentiating the forest from the trees in their daily lives. Those who dare to take the far-sighted approach to everyday problems while being careful to attend to the problem at hand are often ridiculed and placed under suspicion. History tells us that instant gratification or cure without an appreciation of the past and an educated expectation of the future is rarely of lasting benefit.

This third edition of *Podiatric Medicine* is intended to provide an overview of podiatric medicine and surgery and to be a clinical text with application to the daily practice of podiatric medicine; it is designed to be both a standard medical text and a daily reference source for practitioners. The reader's ability to assimilate its didactic content and then obtain the essential clinical experience necessary to "relieve the painful foot" will determine the significance of this text.

Each chapter focuses on both the science and the art of podiatric medicine and surgery. Chapters on sports medicine, surgery, and trauma have been added to this edition. Other chapters have been completely revised and expanded to include areas on nutrition, pharmacology, physical therapy and treatment. Hundreds of specific references are cited at the end of each chapter. Additionally, the reader is referred to approximately 1,000 additional sources of information at the end of each chapter.

Family practitioners, orthopedic and general surgeons, dermatologists, physiatrists, physical therapists and others will find this text useful for reference in their daily practice.

Writing this book has been a labor of love associated with a great deal of personal joy for me.

JEFFREY F. YALE, DPM, FACFS

Preface to the First Edition

Podiatric educators have recognized the need for a textbook which provides insight into the general day-to-day practice of podiatry. The emphasis on graduate training for special areas of practice has all but dwarfed the 90% of the fine work that podiatrists perform in the everyday practice of their profession. *Podiatric Medicine* is written for the student and for the doctor who will find it a useful reference for reviewing, diagnosing and treating podiatric problems. Other medical disciplines and governmental and insurance agencies as well as the community at large will find this text a factual and inclusive approach to the general practice of podiatry and will recognize the tremendous importance of the podiatry profession as a major provider of health services to the community. The text is based on the author's extensive personal experience as a teacher, consultant, and practicing podiatrist with a critical review of podiatric and medical literature.

The reader will note that there are two different type faces used in the text corresponding as nearly as possible to the divisions of the text itself: diagnosis and treatment. The standard type is used for discussions and descriptive material. The "plain" or "*sans serif*" type is used for discussions of treatments for the various conditions described.

The chapters on podiatric equipment illustrate the need for specialized training for doctors of podiatry. Likewise, the instruments used in podiatry can best be manipulated by the specialized and skilled hand of the Doctor of Podiatric Medicine. The development of many new therapeutic modalities attest to the close liaison between foot doctors and industry in providing specialized instruments of high quality for the patient's good.

One has only to view the many and varied materials being used in the treatment of foot disorders to appreciate the degree of diversified knowledge that the podiatrist needs to practice his profession. Supplies range from pharmaceutical chemicals, dressings, adherents, rubber compounds, plaster, leather, a variety of plastics and countless other materials limited only by the resourcefulness of the operator and his staff.

The practical value of this text to the profession will depend on its everyday use by the doctor in general practice. Here the podiatrist will find a review of podiatric equipment, materials and instruments so necessary to his successful practice. Practical information is included on the clinical considerations, diagnosis, pathology and treatment of the great majority of common foot disorders. Despite the author's reputation as a diagnostician and foot radiologist, this book treats the radiograph as another tool in the overall armamentarium of the podiatrist. The reader is referred to the specialized texts in foot radiology. Surgery, foot orthopedics, podopediatrics and podogeriatrics are discussed only as they relate to the everyday practice of podiatry by the progressive podiatrist in his well-equipped operatory. This text places the common foot disorders in proper perspective as they relate to systemic disturbances.

It has been a joy to add this text to the other fine books written by podiatrists. It is my fond hope that others will be stimulated to contribute to the literature of Podiatric Medicine in the not too distant future.

IRVING F. YALE, DPM, ED.D. (HON.)

Acknowledgments

Doctors, educators and others contributed to the success and enabled the completion of this third edition of *Podiatric Medicine*. The following people lent their time and expertise in producing this outstanding text.

Without the understanding, love and support of my children, Brian and Andrew, first with the completion of *The Arthritic Foot and Related Connective Tissue Disorders* Williams & Wilkins, 1984, and now with the publication of the third Edition of *Podiatric Medicine*, this text would never have been written.

To the able office staff of the Yale Podiatry Group, P.C. under the direction of our office manager, Elizabeth Maciecki, and to Claire Gagne, medical assistant, for her untiring help with typing, my heartfelt thanks.

The faith, encouragement and affection of Lenore Bernsley were invaluable.

Thanks are extended to Robert Matusz, D.P.M. for his encouragement and helpful input.

The efforts of Louise Tortora, D.P.M., A.A.C.F.S. and John Zervos, D.P.M. in page proof reading and reference correlation, respectively, were greatly appreciated.

Bruce Backer, D.P.M., A.A.C.F.S. did an outstanding job with the index preparation.

Many thanks to Paula Monahan and Linda Sill for their untiring work typing the final manuscript for this text.

Appreciation is extended to Jeffrey M. Robbins, D.P.M., F.A.C.F.S., Associate Professor, Podiatric Medicine and Director of Clinical Education and Research at the Ohio College of Podiatric Medicine for his contributions to the nutrition section; to Stuart Snyder, D.P.M., Contributor, Pharmacology Section, Clinical Handbook of Podiatric Medicine, Second Edition, Ohio College of Podiatric Medicine and to Ronald Banta, D.P.M., F.A.C.F.S. for his contributions to the bicycling section.

Many of the observations, conclusions and treatment techniques contained in this text are a result of the combination of over 60 years of practice by Irving Yale, D.P.M. (40 years) and Jeffrey F. Yale, D.P.M. (20 years). Thank you Dad!

The sincere and professional guidance of Jonathan W. Pine, Jr., Editor, Carol Eckhart, Associate Editor, Anne G. Seitz, Book Production Sponsor, Gail Chalew, Copyeditor and their able staff at Williams & Wilkins has made this project sail a smooth course to completion. My appreciation and warm thanks for a job well done.

The effort and contributions of hundreds of podiatric physicians and surgeons, researchers and educators, have enabled this text to be published. With deep admiration and respect I salute and thank you all.

Jeffrey F. Yale

Contents

1

The Podiatric Operatory and Medical Emergencies

Podiatric Equipment

The most essential pieces of equipment in a podiatrist's practice are the podiatry chair, operating light and the podiatrist's stool. Patients must be seated comfortably with their extremities at a height convenient to the doctor. They should be at rest mentally and physically in order to derive maximum relief from the treatment by their foot doctor. Rotter et al. (1) present an empirical study of typical interaction profiles of podiatric patient care satisfaction. Overall findings indicate the satisfaction among podiatric patients was high.

The Podiatrist's Chair (Fig. 1.1)

The podiatrist's chair must have marked maneuverability. It should go up and down to allow for easy seating and egress by children, the elderly and the disabled. The movement of the chair should be simple, and an electrically powered chair is desirable. A toe's touch or simple touch by a finger to a switch should carry the chair into a position suitable for proper examination and treatment.

Operating Lights

Podiatric operating lights vary for specific purposes. The first and most necessary requirement for general practice is that the lighting be adequate and cool. Lights must have proper reflection from divergent angles to cover the operative field. A surgical light may be a mobile floor model, or it may be suspended from the ceiling or attached to a wall. Shadows should be kept to a minimum and the infrared rays filtered out. Regular operating lights may be incandescent or fluorescent. Some lights consist of both a 60-watt incandescent and a 22-watt fluorescent bulb. Most of these lights move with the slightest touch and are attached to wall brackets. Other lights are totally fluorescent using two standard T815-watt fluorescent bulbs.

The Podiatrist's Stool

The podiatrist's stool may or may not be used by all podiatrists. Some practitioners prefer to stand while working. However, the majority of practitioners sit while treating feet. A quality operator's stool is important if the foot doctor expects to have many productive years free of postural problems. The chair should be on sturdy rollers. The seat should be flexible for adjustment to leg length. The backrest must be adjustable to height and flexible enough to yield to back pressure. Seat padding should be comfortable and thick enough to protect the coccyx from repeated trauma. Upholstery may match the rest of the office furniture.

Podiatric Drills

A high-speed podiatric cord drill for treatment of a multitude of foot and nail problems is a necessary piece of equipment. Most offices have two or more cord drills. It may be mobile or attached to the

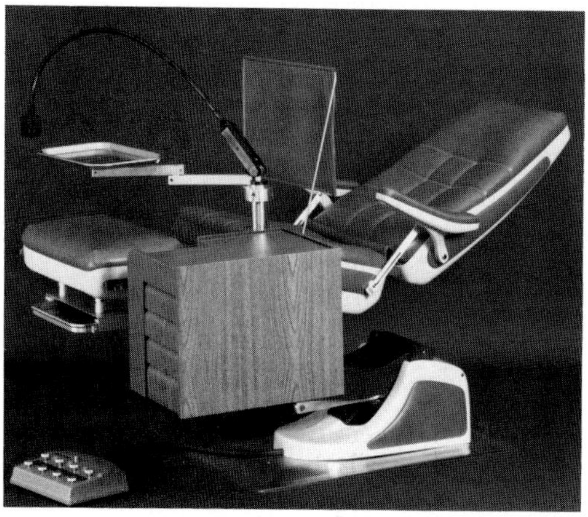

Figure 1.1. Dexta organizer chair with light, instrument and debris tray, swivel arms and instrument table.

wall or a cabinet. Its arm must be flexible enough to move about the affected part with ease. One-tenth horsepower is typical for a podiatric cord drill. The handpiece is precision constructed, and the drill is controlled by a foot rheostat. High-speed air- or nitrogen-powered drills are free of vibration and are most efficient for bone work and nail problems. Hand drills are available for use on house or hospital calls.

The minimum specifications for cord drills used by podiatrists are 14,000 rpm idle speed. High-speed drills at 100,000 or more rpm for bone work are available for specialized needs. The Zimmer, ultrahigh-speed air drill and the Stryker equipment operated by nitrogen gas pressure are especially applicable to podiatry. Also useful is the Beaver-Pedo high-torque (1000 GM–cm) portable electric handpiece system with ultralow variable speed (300–7400 rpm). The system provides a quick disconnect, autoclavable, foot-controlled reduction handpiece.

The high-speed drill, when controlled, is less traumatizing and minimizes postoperative pain and edema (2, 3). Jenkinson (4) used ultrasound waves for painless debridement of the nail bed and nail groove. The unit used is similar to current dental equipment with interchangeable inserts. When the machine is turned on, the tip of the insert moves back and forth 25,000 times a second in a 1/1000-inch stroke.

X-ray and Dark Room Equipment

X-ray equipment must be manufactured in accordance with radiation protection specifications of the Radiation Protection Section of the Bureau of Radiological Health. The x-ray machine head should be counterbalanced and maneuverable to within inches of the floor. It should be 100% protected and have a small, fine focal spot and built-in filter to minimize the soft rays. Exacting collimation is essential for good results and proper protection from secondary radiation.

Several x-ray machines are available for podiatric use. The X-Cel x-ray model P-700/AC has an adjustable lighted collimator that is continuously variable from closed position to 14 inches × 14 inches at 28 inches SID (Fig. 1.2). The Lixiscope is a light-weight, hand-held x-ray imaging device used to evaluate potential fractures, arthritic conditions, bone chips and spurs and to locate foreign bodies. An intraoperative aid, operative exposure levels are so low that it is reportedly unnecessary to use lead aprons or other shielding devices. However, it is of the utmost importance to utilize proper safety precautions when using any radiologic equipment.

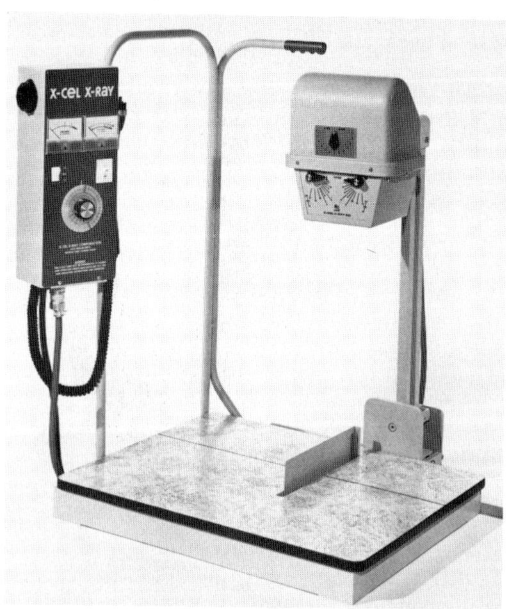

Figure 1.2. X-Cel X-Ray Floor Model Collimator and low base.

Min X-ray, Inc. (5) offers wall-mounted, stationary and mobile podiatric x-ray units. Features include full-field, light-beam collimation with central beam indicator, a collimator light that stays on during exposure, 0.8 mm focal spot and full- or half-film exposure collimating.

Dark room equipment may be standard medical equipment for the podiatrist. A 2½-gallon developing tank is desirable for the busy office. A variety of film sizes, screens, cassettes and film holders are necessary equipment for all offices. Screen film is used with cassettes or film holders. The film must be compatible with calcium tungstate and blue-emitting rare earth screens. Nonscreen (monopak) direct exposure film is individually packaged. The 10- × 12-inch nonscreen film has proven to be the most useful size for full-foot radiographs. Intensifying screens decrease exposure time and may be necessary to cut down radiation exposure without sacrificing quality. The use of automatic developing, fixing and drying equipment saves considerable office time. It allows auxiliary staff to perform other duties in the office and provides the doctor with a completely processed radiograph in about 90 sec. The Philips 810 XL Automatic X-ray Film Processor with bulit-in programmed replenisher accommodates 5-inch × 7-inch and 8-inch × 10-inch film (Fig. 1.3). Freund (6) describes the use of the Radiographic Visual Bisector for determining the bisection of skeletal structures seen on radiographs with speed, ease and accuracy.

Newer technologies are available to facilitate the podiatrist's task of diagnosis. Tomography (sectional radiography) eliminates unwanted shadows from the x-ray film. This technique is helpful in diagnosing tarsal coalitions, talar trochlear lesions, subtalar lesions and other foot pathology that is difficult to differentiate.

Computerized tomography (CT) scans are superior to two-plane x-ray and conventional tomography. Although quite expensive, a CT scan provides higher density resolution in discerning anatomical pathology. Osteomyelitis, fracture repair, bone tumors, soft tissue lesions and anatomy can be visualized.

Nuclear magnetic resonance (NMR), a nonionizing radiation imaging technique,

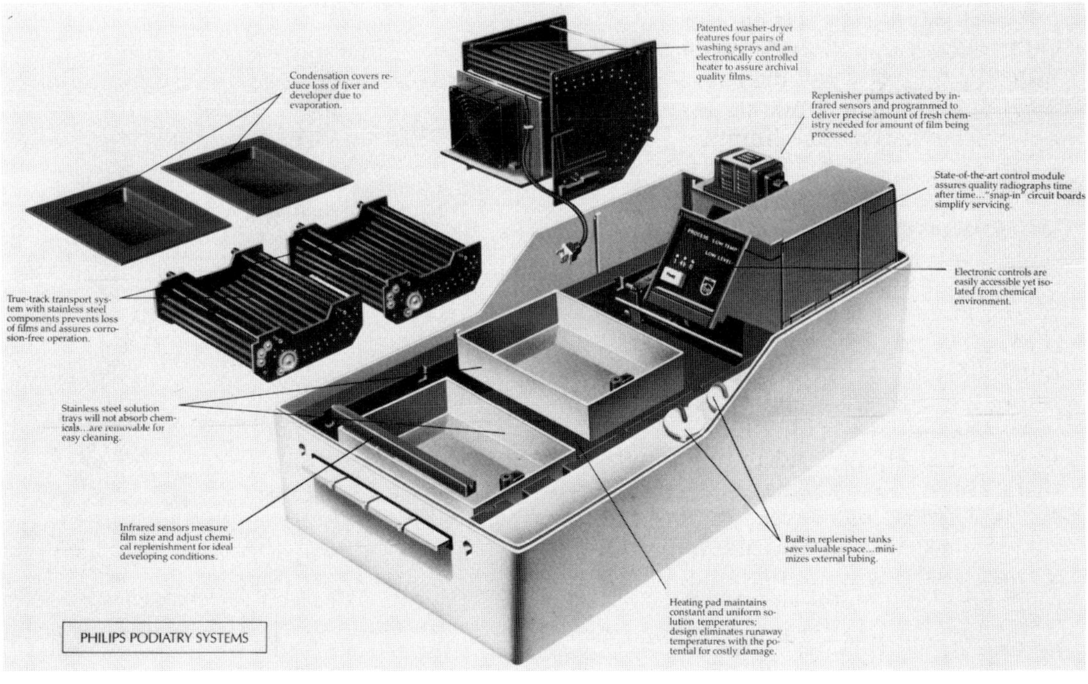

Figure 1.3. Philips 810 XL Automatic X-Ray Film Processor.

is becoming diagnostically more useful as its technology improves. Because images are produced relative to their water content, differentiation of normal versus diseased tissues is possible. This feature adds a new dimension in diagnosing foot pathology that does not affect the anatomy of the foot, such as metabolic and biochemical tissue changes, tissue density and blood vessel flow disorders.

Other Diagnostic and Therapeutic Equipment

For a modern, well-equipped office, the podiatrist should have available FCC, U/L approved ultrasound units; short wave generators that can be used for such surgery as electrodesiccation, fulgeration, coagulation and section; Hyfrecator, Electrocator and Bove units to destroy pathological tissue; and low-voltage multiple wave generators for muscle stimulation, testing and rehabilitation. Low-voltage generators also provide currents for iontophoresis and destruction of pathological tissue by electrolysis. Many doctors also find extensive use for hydrotherapy, ultraviolet irradiation and paraffin baths.

The Horwitron—Variometer is an electrodiagnostic and treatment device used for neuromuscular dysfunction. Evaluations made with this instrument determine the reflex tone of the neuromuscular mechanism. Treatment is based on accurate diagnosis and uses a ballistic impulse. Because of the reduced current (1⁄100 of the usual current) and the rapid ballistic-type impulse, the sensory nerve endings can be bypassed to influence only the motor end-plates.

Precision measuring equipment, such as forefoot devices, the Martins Goniometer, the tractograph and a protractor are essential for evaluating the degree of functional and structural alterations and establishing the necessary amount of correction (Fig. 1.4). At every chair clinical diagnostic equipment should include a lesion-measuring device, a tuning fork with brush and needle, a small flashlight for eye reactions to light and a tape measure. A skin thermometer and sphygmomanometer are helpful for proper evaluation of peripheral vascular disease.

Despite the value of good judgment and the need for the development of acute touch sensitivity, visual acuity and palpation, it often becomes necessary to corroborate findings by the use of electromechanical devices, such as thermocouples, plethysmographs and Doppler flow meters.

The Doppler provides a sound quality and recording readout mechanism that enables the clinician either to substantiate clinical findings or to learn more about

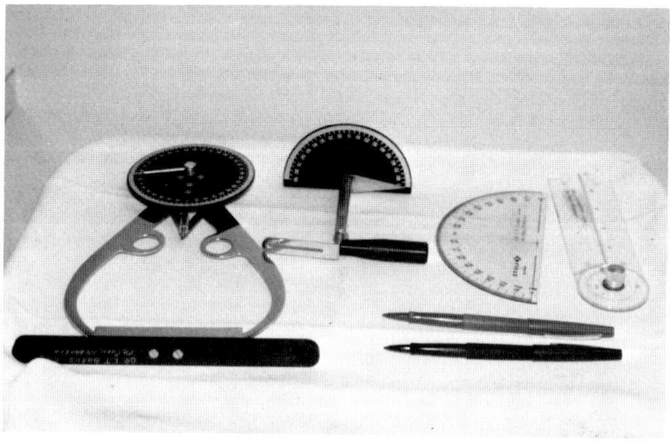

Figure 1.4. The basic instruments are laid out for the reader's inspection. On the left is the goniometer; next the forefoot varus measuring device; third, the large protractor, next the tractograph and last, but not least, the black and red marking pens for ease in distinguishing the inversion and eversion lines from each other. (Courtesy of Burns Podiatric Laboratory.)

the patency and status of arterial and venous circulation.

The Doppler utilizes a piezoelectric transmitter that produces an ultrasound beam penetrating the skin to the blood vessels. A suitable gel is used as a transmitting agent on the skin. A hand-held transmitting probe is applied over the site of the vessels, resulting in a back scattering of ultrasound waves commensurate with the change of frequency and proportional to the velocity of blood flow. The resultant sound and/or wave pattern created is recorded. Experience enables the podiatrist to evaluate the systolic and diastolic impulses heard or recorded in normal and abnormal circulatory functions. Occlusion or stenotic recordings are noted when the systolic sounds are feeble and the diastolic waves are lost distal to the pathology. The examiner should listen for sounds in the common and superficial femoral, popliteal, posterior tibial and dorsalis pedis arteries.

Time and space do not permit the exploration of technique and interpretation of abnormal findings. However, the reader is expected to know about the available equipment and that proper training and experience are necessary in order to understand the results of audible sound and wave recordings being produced.

The Podiatric Laboratory

A well-equipped podiatric office has two types of laboratories. One should be equipped for physiological testing of blood samples and urine. It should have such equipment as a microscope, test tubes, culture media, pipettes, counting chambers, a hemoglobinometer, reagents and the necessary sophisticated electronic devices. The other laboratory should be equipped to construct foot orthoses and devices for patients requiring additional support, correction, balancing, or protection. The orthotic laboratory requires stocks of leather, rubber and plastics capable of being skived by special knives and a basic grind-wheel for shaping and correcting orthoses to fit the feet. A trained technician should be capable of preparing plaster casts and constructing most orthotic devices under the doctor's supervision.

No office is complete without a grinder for its orthopaedic laboratory. The most popular unit is the Sani-Grinder, which provides a quiet, efficient vacuum action for dust collection, replaceable abrasive sleeves, a grinding drum and stone and taper chucks for buffing.

Maintenance of Sterile Supplies and Office Aids

Sterilizers are an essential part of podiatric equipment. Despite the disposable materials and syringes available today, no office can function without an autoclave. Surgical packs, instruments, suture removal kits, linens and a host of other specialized supplies are autoclaved. The inside dimensions of the autoclave should be large enough to handle essential supplies and instruments. Steam under pressure units should be of finest quality to ensure many years of use. The Soloman tray (7) is a light-weight cold sterilization instrument tray with carrying handle. There are separate instrument compartments for cold sterilization. Drainage of solutions is accomplished without tray removal.

Cabinets used to house supplies and instruments may be built-in and designed to match the decor of the office. Special wall cabinets are desirable to allow for easy maintenance of floors.

The Locke Sani-Tray is an indispensable heavy gauge stainless steel and aluminum tray that fits under the foot rest of most podiatric chairs. This tray provides a simple, clean method for capturing debris and excrescences removed from the foot during podiatric treatment. It eliminates the old-fashioned stigmatized floor pan, protects the operator's clothing and generally enhances the professional environment of the modern podiatric office.

Office management systems, whether computerized or not, are an integral part of the smooth-functioning podiatric medical practice. Individual practice style and preference determine the type of management. Solo, partnership, independent contractor, and group practice approaches require different management techniques and approach. Automated computerized office management systems (8) are available. Other systems (9) may provide multiple stations, patient statements, insurance forms, record and chart maintenance, statistical analysis of business and professional activities, word processor integration and records security.

The well-equipped podiatric office is surgically oriented. As in every specialized field, the operator is a responsible practitioner of the healing arts and recognizes the limitations and scope of practice. One of the foot specialist's responsibilities is to maintain sterile packs and available autoclaved surgical instruments for emergency and daily use in the practice of the podiatric profession. The surgical instruments, their basic features and use, are discussed below.

Instruments Used in the Practice of Podiatry

The highly specialized practice of podiatry requires special instruments for the successful treatment of podiatric problems. Many instruments are the exclusive product of the imagination and creativity of the podiatrist. Other instruments, which were orginally developed by other specialists for their specific needs, have been adapted by podiatrists for treatment of unusual foot disorders.

Because most instruments are of the cutting variety, beginning students develop the touch and ability to handle instruments skillfully and proficiently. With quality stainless steel surgical hand instruments, the podiatrist becomes a great respecter of the tissues that are treated. The student and doctor alike are cautioned about the purchase of inferior instruments. They must use only the finest instruments in an effort to provide the quality service so intimately associated with the practice of podiatry. The skilled operator can actually feel the tissue through the instrument (Figs. 1.5 to 1.8).

Operative instruments for the treatment of skin excrescences, such as helomas, tylomas and nails, may be classified as chisels, knives, special feature instruments and tissue forceps.

Chisels

Chisels come in small, medium or large sizes, depending on the width of the blade. Chisel blade size may be $\frac{1}{16}$, $\frac{1}{4}$, $\frac{3}{8}$, $\frac{1}{2}$ or $\frac{5}{8}$ inches; a variety of other sizes are available on a special order basis. The edge of the blade may be slightly curved or straight. The straight blade is generally angled to varying degrees for the purpose of easier handling of tissues by the podiatrist.

Replaceable curved or oblique chisel blades are convenient to use. Many foot specialists perfer finest quality stainless steel and replaceable chisel blades. Blade instruments must be sharpened often if sharp and safe instruments are to be available for regular daily use.

The handles of both chisels and knives are either octagonal, rounded or flat in shape. They may taper, and their surface may be irregular or smooth. Many instrument handles are constructed of stainless steel, aluminum or other metallic alloys.

Knives

Knives are either straight or curved back. Blades may be small, medium, large or extra heavy. The blades may also be replaceable with suitable handles, with the usual advantage of having a sharp blade available. The typical knife is a surgical scalpel. They are available in different sizes.

One popular instrument called a golf stick has the multiple features of being angled like a chisel, rounded like a regular scalpel knife blade and variable in size to serve a variety of purposes in treatment. As one would suspect, its blade shape is similar to that of a golf club head. The golf stick is commonly used to debride calluses.

The podiatrist regularly uses the instruments discussed above and must learn to master them by repeated use under controlled conditions in training clinics. Often the operator feels more comfortable with one type of instrument than with others and can adapt it for use in a variety of conditions. The use of instruments for specific operative problems is discussed below; however, the practical application of the theory of clinical practice depends on the experience acquired in an academic clinical environment.

Special Feature Instruments

Special feature instruments can be defined as those instruments scientifically designed to be used for specific types of pathology. A useful instrument is a soft corn spoon knife that is either round, oval, slightly curved or angular. A special feature corn chisel may have an oblique edge with a sharp point for special applications. Nucleus knives have a special construction for removal of small hyperkeratotic lesions. They come in a variety of sizes and shapes and require special handling techniques for successful use in practice. The Poddi Burr System is an alternative to sharp debridement in the palliative care of the patient with helomas and tylomas. The system includes an easy grip, varispeed motor and four tungsten carbide burrs.

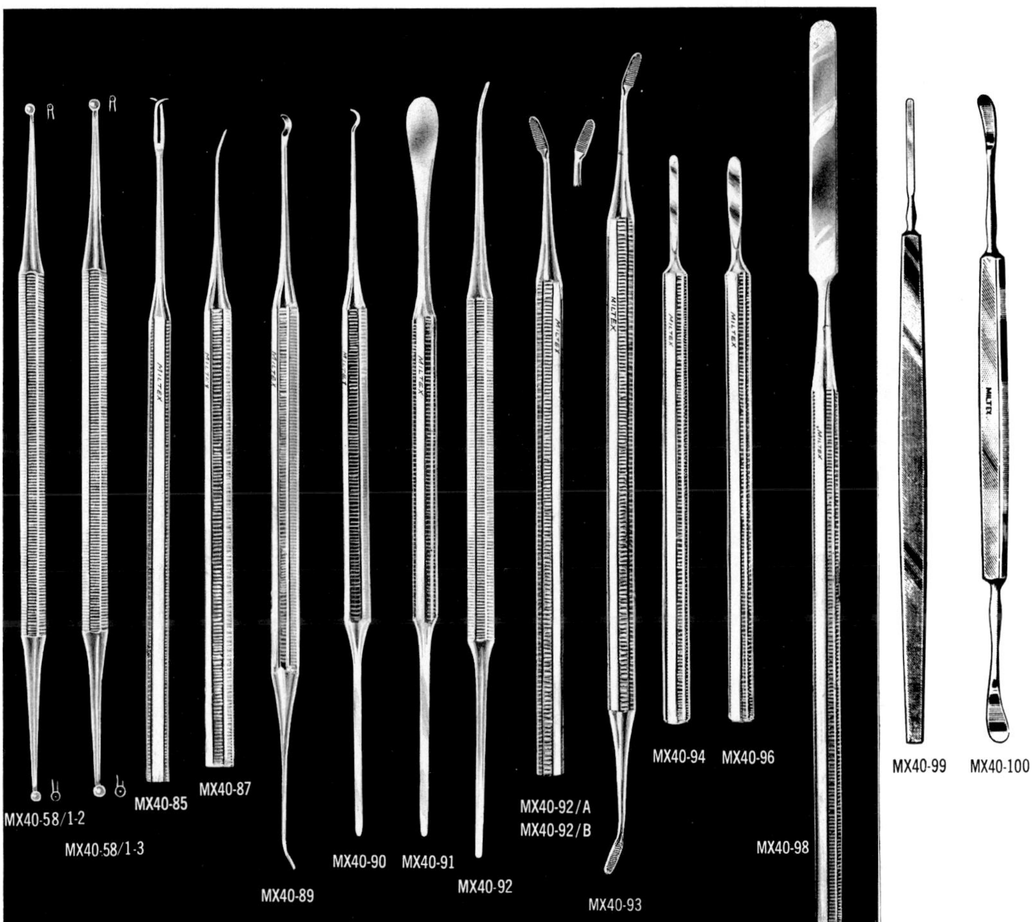

Figure 1.5. Podiatry hand instruments. MX40–58/1–2: double end curette excavator w/hole 1.5 and 2 mm.; MX40–58/1–3: double end curette excavator w/hole 1.5 and 2.5 mm.; MX40–85: fixator for lifting and holding tissue; MX40–87: probe stainless steel; MX40–89: probe and excavator, double ended; MX40–90: excavator and packer, double ended; MX40–91: spatula and packer, double ended; MX40–92: probe and packer, double ended; MX40–92/A: nail or bone rasp, angular, file inside; MX40–92/B: nail or bone rasp, angular, file outside; MX40–93: double ended nail or bone rasp, angular, file inside and outside; MX40–94: Locke elevator, narrow blade; MX40–96: Locke elevator, wide blade; MX40–98: flexible spatula, 2 × ¼ in.; MX40–99: Dix spud, half round; MX40–100: green spatula, double ended. (Courtesy of Miltex Instrument Corp.)

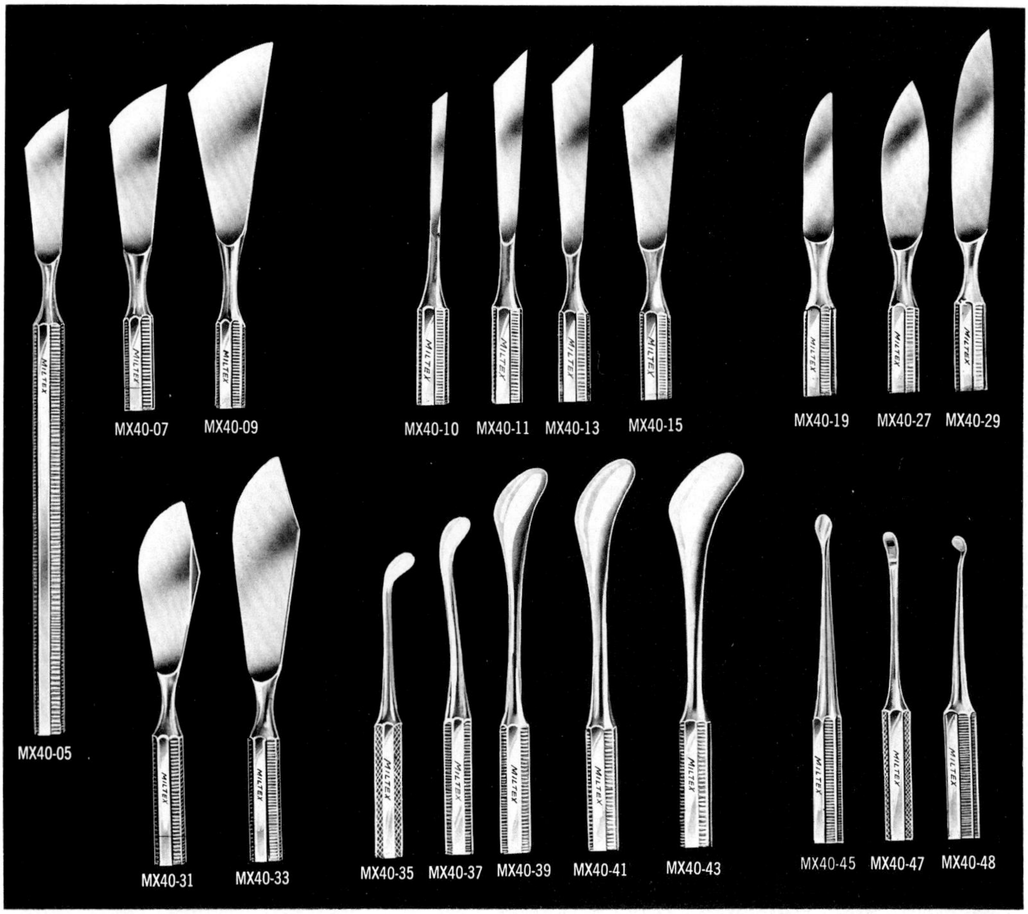

Figure 1.6. Podiatry hand instruments. MX40–05, MX40–07, MX40–09, MX40–10, MX40–11, MX40–13, MX40–15: chisels used for reduction of hyperkeratosis; MX40–19, MX40–27, MX40–29, MX40–31, MX40–33: scalpels used for surgical incisions and removal of excrescences; MX40–35, MX40–37, MX40–39, MX40–41, MX40–43: golf-stick shaped cutting instruments; MX40–45, MX40–47, MX40–48: curettes. (Courtesy of Miltex Instrument Corp.)

Tissue Forceps

Flat jaw and angle jawed forceps have a variety of uses in the treatment of tyloma, heloma, and nail pathology. The handles on these forceps vary enough to enable the operator to select an instrument that feels most comfortable.

Instrument Use

The clinical use of instruments is described in this section. Holding an instrument is a technique in itself. The movement of the fingers and wrists varies with the instrument being used, the location of the lesion and the assist from the opposite hand. Manual dexterity is developed with frequent use of a variety of instruments. Scullion (10) provides instrument usage documentation, including the theory, prehension and technique of painlessly debriding hyperkeratoses and enucleating heloma. These techniques have been employed by podiatrists for over 100 years. Firm skin tension, balancing of the instrument, wrist flexibility, sideward blade movement and debriding in an ordered fashion are stressed.

Chisels

A chisel may be used for the debriding of helomas and tylomas (Fig. 1.9). As a

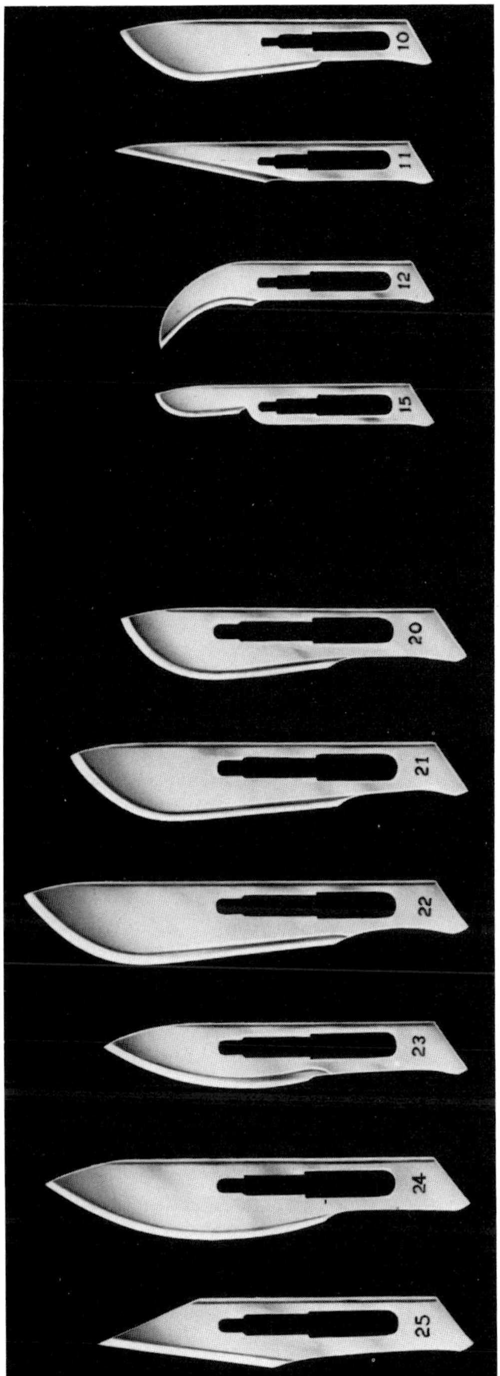

Figure 1.7. Scalpel blades. Note the variety of scalpel blade shapes. No. 25 suitable for straight incisions of even depth; nos. 10, 15, 20, 21, 22, 23 and 24 ideal for plantar tylomas. May also be used for surgical incisions and subcutaneous dissections. No. 12 is desirable for snap tenotomy and no. 11 for deep incisions of abscess to facilitate drainage. Nos. 10, 11, 12 and 15 fit B-P Handles nos. 3, 3L, 3LA, 5, 7 and 9. Nos. 20, 21, 22, 23, 24 and 25 fit B-P Handles nos. 4, 4L and 6. (Courtesy of Brad-Parker.)

rule, smaller-sized chisels are used on heloma and larger ones on plantar tyloma. In the treatment of a heloma on a toe, the proper chisel is selected and held between the thumb and forefinger; it rests on the third finger as in holding a pencil. The finger motions used to reduce a heloma consist of multiple forward and angled thrusts from the distal end of the heloma backward toward the toe base. The fourth and fifth fingers provide some stability by resting on the unaffected part of the foot. The fingers of the opposite hand maintain a taut skin on the affected toe. They form a steady base of support for the instrument-wielding hand.

If the heloma is complicated by deep centers of horny tissue, these are removed by dissection with a nucleus knife. The nucleus knife is held in the same hand position as the chisel. The blade is placed at the periphery of the nucleus, and with a downward and lateral force a circumscribed incision is made about the lesion. By a forward and lateral push and slight twirl between the fingers, a line of demarcation is made about the lesion, and it is gently separated from the surrounding

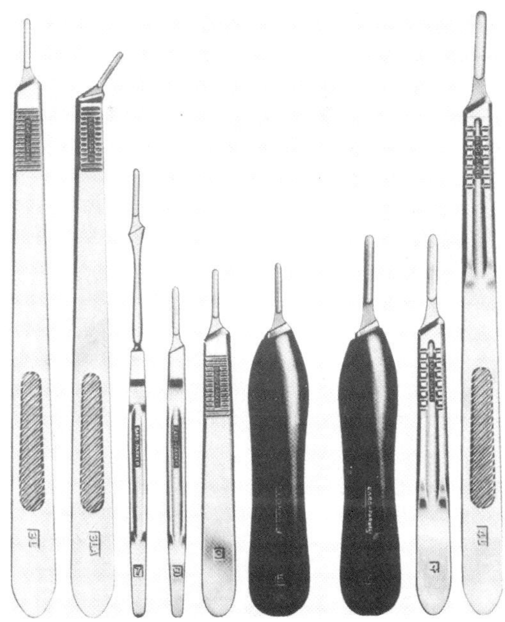

Figure 1.8. Scalpel handles. Design suitable for handling and deft instrumentation in surgical treatment of most foot disorders. (Courtesy of Bard-Parker.)

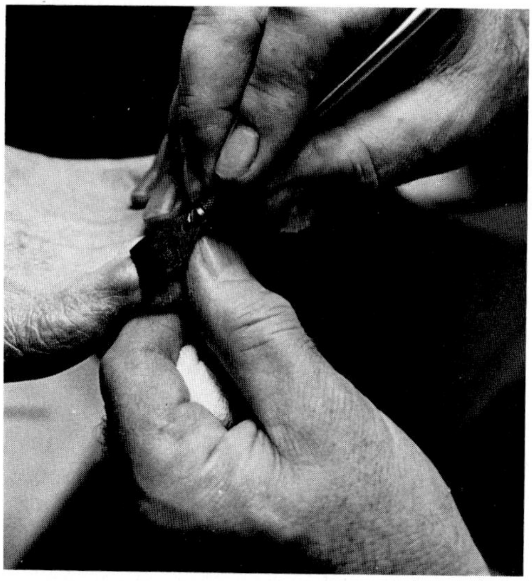

Figure 1.9. Use of heloma chisel. Observe position of fingers of the left hand grasping the toe and holding skin taut. Note position of instrument and fingers of right hand holding the instrument and resting on the dorsum of the foot for leverage.

tissue. Often the operator uses a tissue forceps in his or her left hand to grasp the pathological tissue while cutting it away with an instrument in the right hand.

The same type of chisel may be used to reduce tylomas. The choice of size and angle of the blade is left to the doctor's experience. Usually a wider chisel is chosen than the one used for helomas. The instrument is held in the same fashion as a pencil for tylomas overlying the hallux joint or fifth metatarophalangeal joint. However, plantar tylomas may be reduced by chisel as described below.

The chisel is held between the thumb and second and third fingers at its neck, with the handle resting between the fourth and fifth fingers. A semicircular motion is used that is effective in reduction of the excrescence. The third, fourth and fifth fingers may act as a fulcrum either separately or together.

Knives

Most of the knives used are scalpels (Fig. 1.10). They are held and used in the same fashion as the chisel on a tyloma. In the hands of the skilled podiatrist, the scalpel-type blade is most effective when used in reduction of tylomas. The point of the scalpel can be used to enucleate deep lesions.

The soft corn spoon looks somewhat like a miniature spoon with sharp edges. It is used as a spoon with excavation-like motions. The stroke on the heloma molle is a pushing and semicircular cutting action.

Tissue Forceps

Standard instruments used in treating skin lesions and nails are essential parts of the armamentarium for all podiatrists. Tissue forceps or nippers resemble small surgical nail clippers (Fig. 1.11). They may have convex or straight edges. They can be used for excising skin lesions and nails. In the hands of the skilled operator, tissue forceps can excise helomas and tylomas. The convex blade is generally useful for this purpose. However, the straight edge blade, which is easier to control, can be used for excising superficial and deep hyperkeratoses, as well as incurvated nail borders.

Curettes

Curettes are used extensively for removal of verrucas, poromas and callused nail grooves (Fig. 1.12). Curettes are sharp and measure from 1 to 2.5 mm in diameter. The most popular use is in curettage of

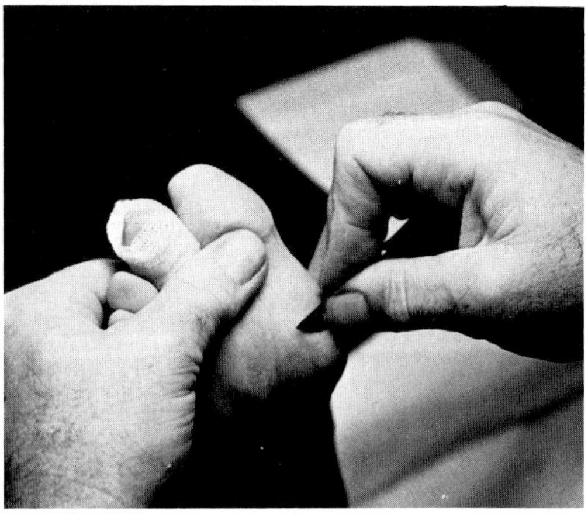

Figure 1.10. Use of tyloma scalpel. Position of left thumb holds skin taut while the right hand holding the scalpel rests its third, fourth and fifth fingers on the foot proper for leverage.

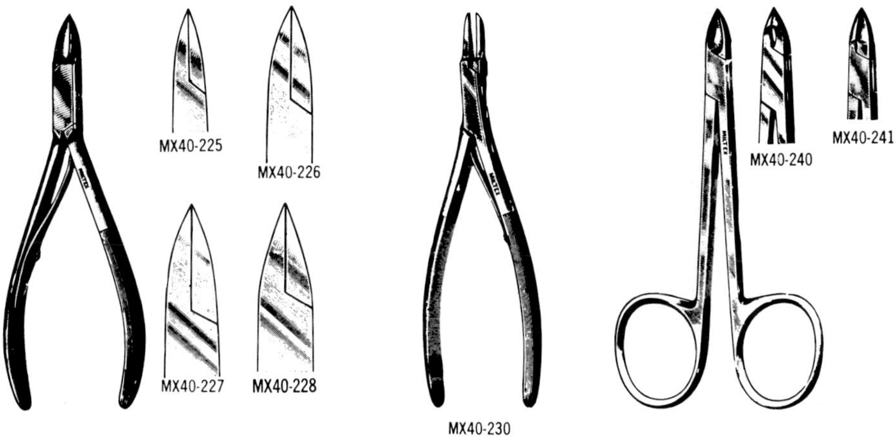

Figure 1.11. Tissue forceps and nail splitters. (Courtesy of Miltex Instrument Corp.)

nail margins and nail grooves. In curettage of nail grooves, the rounded section of the curette is carefully placed on the viable skin while the scooping motion of the sharp margins is directed into the free nail margins or keratosis in the nail groove. The motion is from the proximal end of the nail forward to distal. Verrucas and poromas are removed by sharp curettage under local anesthesia.

Nail Splitters

Nail splitters have straight and angled blades (Fig. 1.13). They must be kept sharp to be effective. The skillful use of the nail splitter requires a fine instrument, a feel for the type of tissue being cut and broad experience in treating nail diseases. The action from the distal to the proximal end of the nail plate is a pushing motion. Some nail splitters are in forceps form.

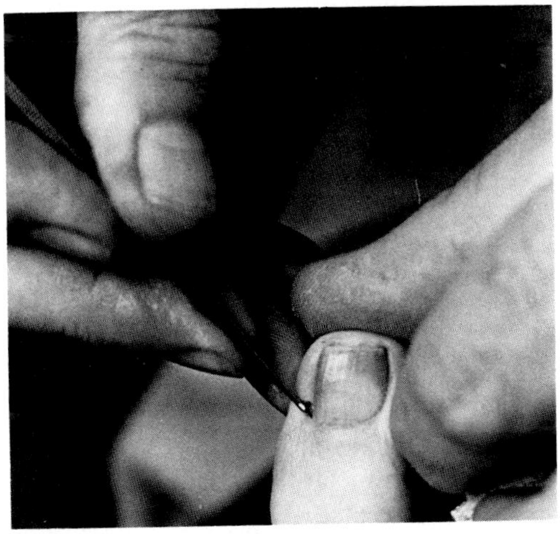

Figure 1.12. Curettage hallux nail. Note position of fingers holding hallux steady. Observe the position of the curette with the sharp concave surface cutting the margin of the nail and the smooth convexity of the curette moving along the skin margin in the nail groove.

Excavators, nail probes and soft tissue probes of many sizes, together with a miscellaneous group of specially designed instruments, are necessary for the scientific practice of podiatry.

Scissors, Dressing Forceps and Related Instruments

Surgical scissors have a variety of uses. The blades may be curved or straight, short or long, heavy or thin, straight-edged or serrated. Some scissors are used for cutting bandages, materials, skin, eponychial tissue and nails; others are designed for removal of sutures. Different types of scissors are used for sharp and blunt dissection. Some have serrated edges for cutting felt materials.

Cutting adhesive tape is an art that all podiatrists must master. In order to have a firm grip on the scissors and thus ensure maneuverability, place the thumb in one opening of the handle and the fourth finger in the other. The second and third fingers assist the fourth finger and are flexed over the handle for additional leverage. Adhesive tape should be cut with the "sticky" side facing upward.

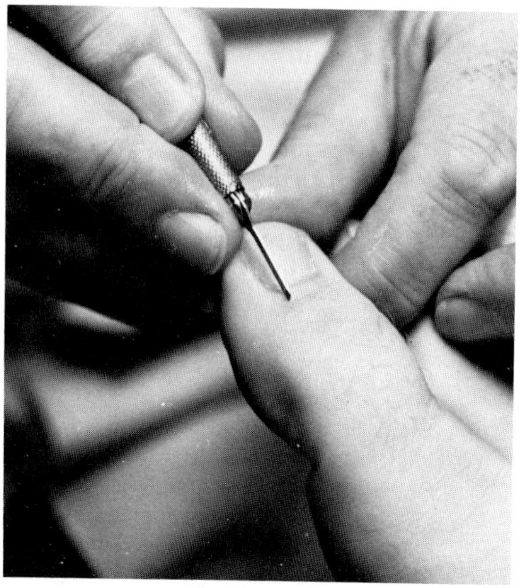

Figure 1.13. Nail being split in preparation for corrective surgery.

Splinter forceps have a variety of points for grasping foreign bodies.

The Hosch Derm-A-Brade is a surgical instrument used for the office debridement of helomas, tylomas, and other hyperkeratoses. It consists of two separate cutting blades especially designed for skin and nails, respectively. The Derm-A-Brade attaches to a cord drill or air drill and is used on the dry skin. Its action is much like a scalpel blade, and its use is easily mastered by the skilled podiatrist.

Dressing forceps and a variety of thumb forceps for grasping tissue are interesting in design. Ends may be serrated, pointed, mouse tooth or sharp. Forceps are used for skin grasping and also for surgical grasping of subcutaneous tissue for mobilization, dissection and retraction.

Mosquito forceps and Kelly forceps may be straight or curved. They are used for clamping bleeding vessels for hemostasis. Forceps help the operator in sterile instrument suturing. Tissues can be grasped and gently moved with the deft use of hemostats.

Suturing Instruments

There are several types of needle holders and their use in suturing depends on the discrimination of the operator. The Olsen-Hegar holder is a combination needle holder and scissor blade. Other popular models are the Mayo-Hegar and the Mathieu.

Clamps and Retractors

Backhaus and Jones towel clamps are necessary for an orderly and neat draping of the operative field. Working in a small field, the podiatric surgeon may use the 3½-inch clamp to advantage.

Retractors come in a variety of types and sizes. Senn retractors have three sharp prongs or three blunt prongs, and a blunt blade end. Some retractors have two prongs, and others have rigid or flexible necks. All of the above-mentioned retractors can only be used with an extra pair of hands, thus, of course, requiring an assistant who has scrubbed. Because an assistant may not be available for most office surgery, the operator will find useful the self-retaining retractors that can be applied by the surgeon alone. Proper exposure of the field when operating alone can be achieved by use of the Weitlaner, Alm and Miltex retractors. These retractors are self-retaining and meet the rigid specifications for good exposure. They are available in different sizes.

Locke developed a versatile bone clamp for foot surgery designed to grasp firmly a phalanx, metatarsal or sesamoid (Fig. 1.14). A wide variety of uses have been found for this clamp that causes minimal tissue damage.

Bone-Cutting Forceps, Rasps and Related Instruments

Bone-cutting forceps and rongeurs are straight or angled to suit the requirements of the operative procedure. The purchase of these instruments should be based on the necessary size and the practicality of the jaw shape for podiatric procedures. Bizarre designs are unnecessary. Special feature instruments adapted for specific bone lesions are highly desirable and necessary to extensive bone surgery.

Freed (12) designed a much-needed instrument for clamping sesamoids during hallux valgus procedures.

Bone files or rasps have attained greater acceptance and are being used in techniques for removal of exostoses and os-

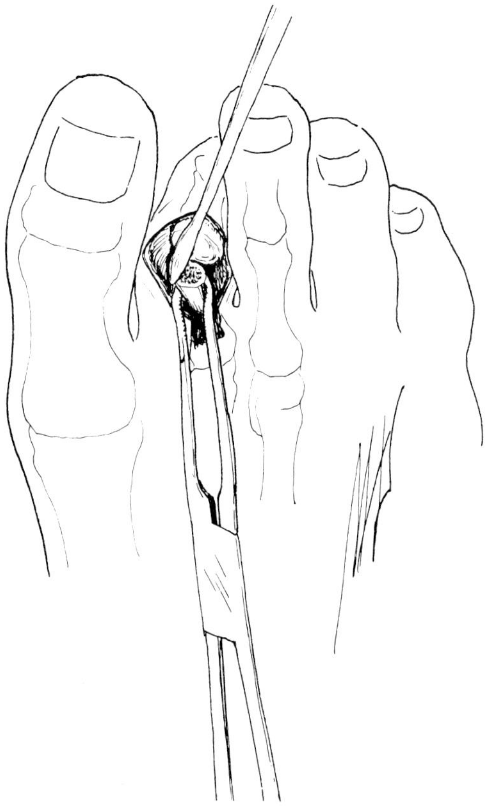

Figure 1.14. Locke clamp.

teophytic alterations on foot joints. Bone files may be fine or coarse and small, medium or large in size (Fig. 1.15). Bone chisels, saws, osteotomes, elevators and mallets are necessary instruments in the operatory of the podiatric surgeon. Their use is subsequently described in various operative procedures. Electronically controlled rasps are being used with greater frequency in minor foot surgery.

Kaplan and Cornfield (13) described a micropneumatic surgical instrument operated by a small, powerful pneumatic motor at speeds up to 35,000 rpm. They conclude that the use of such an instrument saves time, mimizes trauma, diminishes postoperative pain and provides excellent results in bone surgery. The rotary handpiece may use over 30 burrs and drills. A microreciprocating or oscillating saw is also available (Fig. 1.16).

Forceps are podiatrically designed to grasp and clamp sesamoids and phalanges. Other forceps for grasping sponges are necessary instruments in all operatories.

Kurzwell (14) developed a unique instrument that retracts the extensor tendon and dorsal soft tissue and elevates the head of the proximal phalanx, and is used in hammertoe surgery.

Cast spreaders and cutters may be used in the everyday practice of podiatry. Stryker or other electric cast cutters are a necessary adjunct to a busy general podiatric medical practice.

Podiatric Drills and Attachments

Electric drills are an absolute necessity for the proper practice of podiatry. Hand

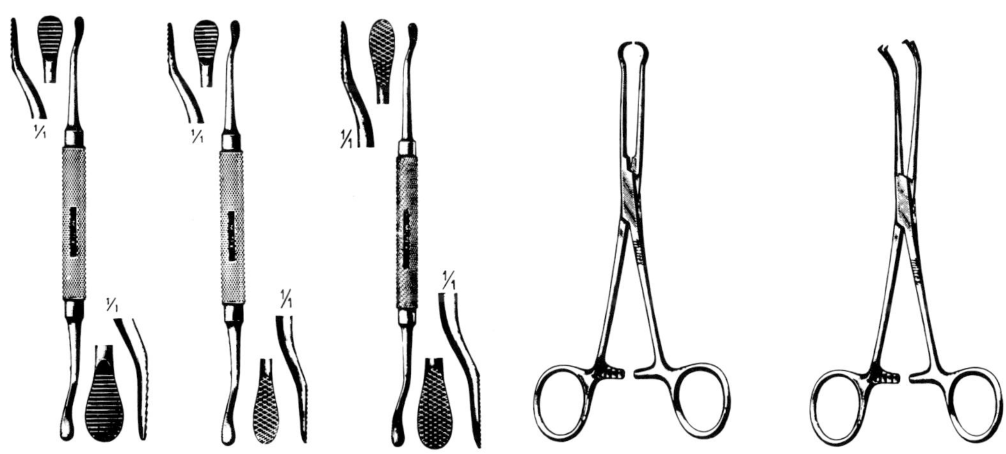

Figure 1.15. Bone instruments. (Courtesy of Miltex Instrument Corp.)

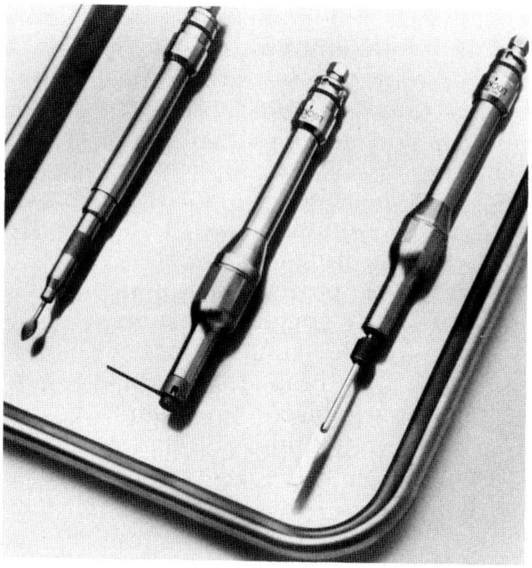

Figure 1.16. Stryker® nitrogen powered oscillating, reciprocating, and rotatory micro instrument hand pieces.

drills are used on house calls by many podiatrists and have their limitations. However, each operatory in the podiatrist's suite must have a high-speed electric cord drill for the treatment of hyperkeratoses and hypertrophied nails of whatever etiology. The drill should perform at about 14,000 rpm.

The cord drill appears to be the best type for reduction of vibrations. The revolutions are governed by a foot rheostat capable of increasing or reducing speed. A new concept in drills is a handpiece driven by air at low speed and high torque (Fig. 1.17). It can be used instead of conventional chisels, bone rasps or rongeurs. This light-weight handpiece relieves fatigue and improves tactile sensation. It weighs 4½ oz. and operates at speeds of 0–8000 rpm forward and reverse at 50 to 60 lb of pressure. The attachments can be autoclaved.

Many shapes and styles of burrs constructed of a variety of materials are needed for podiatric practice (Fig. 1.18). Burrs are made of stainless steel, diamond dust and sand finishes. They may be coarse or fine and are shaped for a variety of purposes. They can be pointed, sharp, broad and narrow.

Vacuum evacuation systems serve to protect both doctor and patient from airborne contaminants such as mycotic nail dust. A control system with a two-motor vacuum unit with a 140-inch lift is preferable.

Laser Technology

The medical use of the laser (light amplification by Stimulated Emission of Radiation) has been greatly refined since the first laser device was developed by Maiman in 1961. The laser is absorbed by tissue which causes a localized increase in temperature with resultant vaporization. The wave length and power (energy) of the laser emission versus tissue absorption of the beam determines its effectiveness as a surgical tool.

The four types of laser used in the United States in medical practice are: CO_2, neodymium:YAG, argon and ruby. Other lasers use zinc, cadmium, phosphorus, helium and cold. The neodymium:YAG and argon types are used only in the coagulation mode and are not practical for use in podiatric surgery. The ruby laser is used with fiber optics and is also not practical for use in podiatric procedures. The CO_2 laser uses carbon dioxide, nitrogen, and helium as its medium for production of energy.

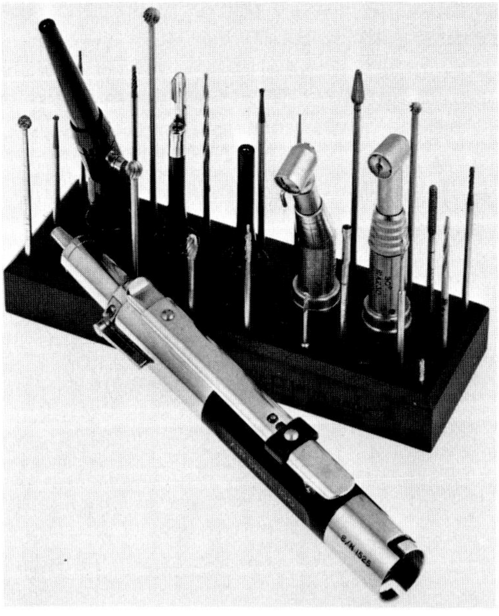

Figure 1.17. Air drill 100 with attachments and burrs. (Courtesy of Zimmer-Hall Inc.)

With both a cutting and coagulating capability, as well as a continuous or pulsed mode with power in excess of 300W and spot sizes from 0.1–2.0 mm, the CO_2 laser is the most useful type to the podiatrist. Almost all of the CO_2 laser beam is abosrbed by water in tissue, with negligible scattering coefficient. The zone of cellular damage varies from 0.3–0.5 mm. The CO_2 laser is ideal for making fine, millimeter-wide incisions and removing tissue. When defocused, the laser can be used for coagulation of small vessels or sterilization of mycotic nail beds.

Podiatric surgical applications include ablation of benign and malignant skin lesions, scars, and keloids; toenail matrix procedures; and Morton's neuroma and amputation neuroma excision. It is essential to take a biopsy specimen of the lesion prior to destruction by the laser. Future laser application will more than likely include bone-cutting capability.

Laser safety procedures include use of eye protective goggles or eyeglasses; a focusing guide, such as helium-neon light; a vacuum through water smoke evacuation system; blackened, poorly reflective instruments; and an operator's face mask. Draping with damp or wet towels and exclusion of combustible anesthetic gases or topical refrigerants from the area of the laser help prevent fire or explosion.

Syringes and Related Equipment

A variety of syringes and needle sizes are essential to the proper practice of podiatry. Syringes used for aspiration, injection of medication at varying levels of tissue and equipment for local anesthesia must be readily available (Fig. 1.19). Presterilized needles, syringes, and combinations of needle length and gauge are a necessary adjunct to other modalities.

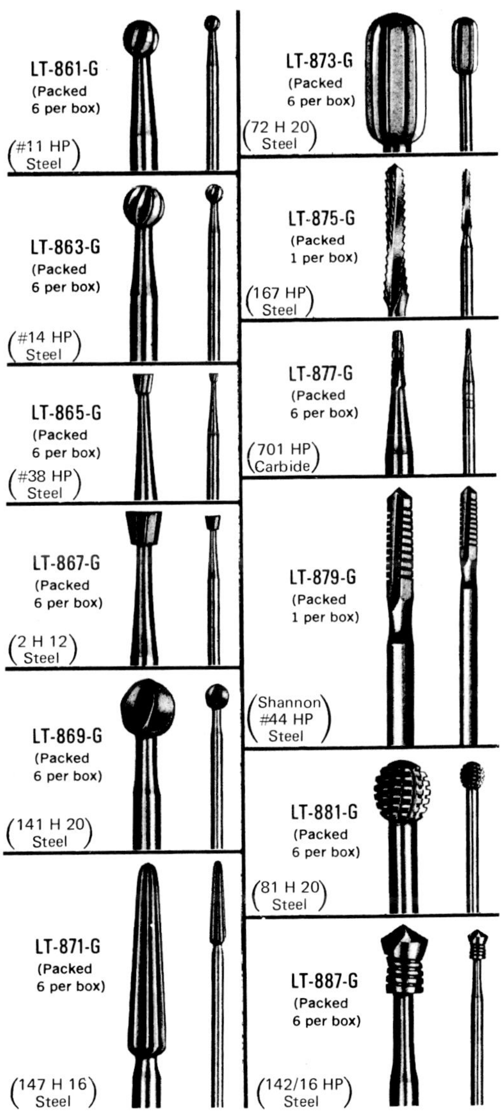

Figure 1.18. Burrs used in podiatry. Uses are as follows. LT–861–G: distal exostoses, tyloma medial of great toe, brushing or erasure technique; LT–863–G: distal exostoses, tyloma medial of great toe, bunionectomy—ambulatory procedure, brushing or erasure technique; LT–865–G: nail surgery, Perrone matrix erasure; LT–867–G: nail surgery, Perrone matrix erasure; LT–869–G: tyloma medial of great toe, bunionectomy—ambulatory procedure, heel spur, brushing or erasure technique; LT–871–G: capsular elevation or smoothing large bones; LT–873–G: reducing large bones, smoothing large bones; LT–875–G: hallux valgus, sectioning technique, gross removal technique, tailor's bunion; LT–877–G: sectioning—small bones; LT–879–G: heloma durum and molle, tailor's bunion, tibial sesamoid reduction, hallux valgus—brushing technique, hallux valgus—erasure technique, hallux valgus—sectioning, hallux valgus—gross removal; LT–881–G: reducing large bones, smoothing large bones, heloma durum and molle; LT–887–G: heel spur. (Pictures courtesy of Weber Co. Burrs available from Miltex Instrument Co. [Miltex stock numbers noted]).

Kaplan and Weinstock (15) described the use of hypospray injector as a precise instrument for administering medication and local anesthesia to a variety of sites on the foot. Their report was based on a study of 100 surgical patients, and they conclude that this method of delivering local anesthesia has some distinct advantages over using a needle in selected areas.

In a later paper, Kaplan and Weinstock (16) demonstrated the diffusion of injectable material by the high-powered spray, hypospray, using a solution of Hypaque mixed equally with lidocaine. They concluded that this method produced less pain than an ordinary injection, with the exception of the metatarsal area and toes. Bleeding was minimal. If not properly presented, the noise of injection was objectionable to some patients. There were no serious side effects.

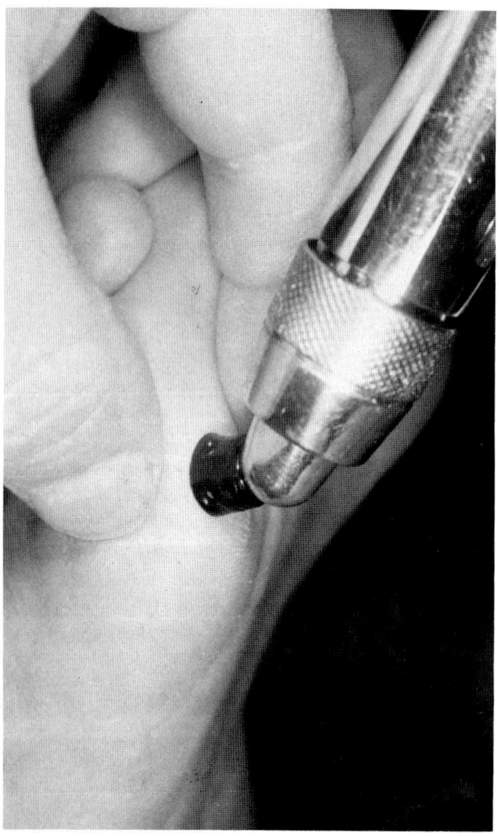

Figure 1.19. Intralesional jet spray of sclerosing agent into verruca. Penetration 4 to 6 mm in depth to deposit 0.1 ml of medication. (Courtesy of RK Locke, DPM.)

Materials and Their Usage in Podiatric Medicine

A representative group of materials used in podiatric practice are listed as follows:

1. Drugs—including anesthetics and other injectables
2. Dressings
   a. Gauze, cotton bandages
   b. Adhesive
   c. Plaster
   d. Rubber
   e. Special—watertight latex socks
3. Felt and similar materials
   a. Moleskin—thin, medium or heavy
   b. Cotton and wool felt—variety of densities and thicknesses
4. Rubber, foam, polyurethane, cork, styrene and combinations with rubber
5. Celastic—colloid cellulose acetate in a fabric base
6. Leather—various gauges for orthosis construction
7. Plastic, thermoplastics, acrylics, polyethylene
8. Latex—natural and synthetic
9. Chemicals
   a. Solvents
   b. Rubber cement
   c. Pharmaceuticals
   d. Skin adherants
10. Plaster of paris
11. Suture material
12. Antiseptic, germicidal solutions for cold sterilization

Podiatric Pads, Shields and Orthoses

There are many professional pads and shields that are prefabricated for use by discriminating foot specialists. They include hammertoe correctors, shields and protectors. They prove useful when stocked in a variety of sizes, shapes and densities. Precut or fabricated adhesive-backed moleskin, foam, sponge or felt pads in many sizes and shapes for heloma dura, heloma molle, tyloma and hallux joint pathology are used extensively as time-savers. Sling pads made of foam or felt in many sizes and densities are available for use over pressure areas. Combinations of foam covered by a closely knit material and other specially shaped removable pads are available for specific problems.

Dallek (17), in an illustrated catalogue, describes pads for a variety of uses, such as toe separators; toe sling pads; half-moon pads; duck pads for helomas between the fourth and fifth toes; oval pads; sling bunion pads; tailor's bunion pads; diamond-shaped, kidney-shaped, criss-cross, T-sling, bell sling, combination anterior and longitudinal pads; C-shaped, U-shaped and dancer pads. These pads are available commercially and can be of value in selected cases.

Overlapping toes and hammertoes may be treated and maintained in correct position by the prefabricated and adjustable Budin toe splint. These splints are especially useful where there is no joint disease or ankylosis and only soft tissues are involved. The Detroit Dynamic Toe Splint® may be used for dynamic postoperative flexion and/or adduction of the great toe after first metatarsophalangeal joint surgery.

A wide variety of accessories are prefabricated for the busy podiatrist who desires to construct his or her own prosthetic devices. Molded rubber heel wedges, longitudinal, metatarsal raises and special feature pads are useful in shoe therapy.

Molded cork inlays are often used as a base for construction of definitive orthoses. Several leather shells with low, medium and high flanges, dual flanges and extensions may be purchased for use as a base for corrective or accommodative removeable orthoses. Sponge rubber, acrylic, leather, cork, Celastic, aluminum, steel or steel-spring longitudinal raises are available as prefabricated orthotic materials.

Foot orthoses constructed from these materials may be a flexible or semirigid to rigid device and may have a low or medium to high raise. The laboratory assistant follows the doctor's orders for the type of raise and material to be used to construct an orthosis for each particular case. Selection of the proper orthosis requires considerable forethought and study for best results.

Should the patient require surgical intervention or biomechanical correction by the podiatrist, it is obvious that more sophisticated techniques, materials and equipment are necessary. Internal medication may be necessary to relieve pain, prevent infection and relax tissues.

There is no attempt to describe such techniques and materials in this chapter. The reader should refer to the specific disorders discussed in this book for a more sophisticated discussion of their treatment. The creative use of materials will depend on the clinical experience, laboratory skill and personal aptitude of the podiatrist and staff.

The author has attempted in this chapter to give the student and the doctor an appreciation of the importance to a profession of high-quality materials. No profession can improve without the cooperation of the allied sciences and the contributions of material engineers. The materials necessary for the practice of podiatric medicine are the product of painstaking research into their intelligent application.

Suture Materials

The general practitioner in podiatry must have a well-equipped operatory for emergency needs. Surgical packs, a variety of suturing materials and needles are essential. Small atraumatic cutting needles are recommended.

The necessary basic sutures are as follows:

- 2–0, 3–0, 4–0 Dexon or Vicryl for subcutaneous closure, capsule or small tendon repair
- 4–0, 5–0 monofilament stainless steel for plantar skin
- 2–0, 3–0, 4–0 monofilament nylon ethibond or ticron for tendon repair
- 4–0, 5–0 monofilament nylon for dorsal, medial, and lateral skin

Medical Emergencies

Psychogenic Syncope

Cerebral hypoxia (fainting) occurs with peripheral vasodilation due to single or multiple stimuli. Occasional lowering of the blood pressure may stimulate dizziness, cold sweat and pallor, with resultant loss of consciousness. It is essential to have smelling salts and oxygen available for immediate use. Application of cold compresses to the head is also helpful. With a weak, slow pulse, the doctor must evaluate the need for vasopressor medication. Often a clap or loud noise stimulates more rapid pulse and arouses the patient from loss of consciousness. Legs should be elevated with the patient supine.

Allergic Reaction—Anaphylaxis

Drug sensitivity with its alarming symptoms is an ever-present problem that may be avoided by taking a good history that often discloses previous reactions to drugs. Toxic reactions to local anesthetics include central nervous system (CNS) stimulation, CNS depression, cardiovascular or peripheral vessel collapse and allergic reaction. These toxic reactions may be sequelae to overdosage, rapid systemic absorption, inappropriate intravenous injection or overt allergen-antigen allergic reaction. The patient generally flushes from vasodilation. Itching, edema, dyspnea and anaphylactic shock are not uncommon.

A tourniquet proximal to the injection site slows down absorption. In addition, antihistamines, vasopressors and respiratory dilators are necessary supplies in the well-equipped office. One milliliter of epinephrine 1:1,000 injected into the injection site slows down absorption of the offending medication. Oxygen should be administered, and care should be taken to provide for adequate egress of vomitus. One-half milliliter of 1:1,000 epinephrine injected subcutaneously is helpful. Cardiac massage and artificial respiration are essential in the presence of cardiac arrest. Injections of 50 mg diphenhydramine hydrochloride (Benadryl) intramuscularly assist in slowing the release of histamine.

In allergic reactions, the medication used depends on the severity of the reaction. Symptoms vary from simple cutaneous wheals and itching to severe angioneurotic edema leading to laryngeal spasms and anaphylactic shock. Such antihistamines as Benadryl may be sufficient to relieve skin reactions. If severe, epinephrine 1:1,000 and Solu-Cortef may be used. If laryngeal edmea occurs, the patient develops a crowing-like sound that is unmistakable. In this case, epinephrine plus oxygen and possibly a cricothyrotomy or tracheotomy may be lifesaving. Patients suffering respiratory infections, colds, bronchitis or oral herpes may readily develop laryngeal spasm.

In respiratory asthmatic-like reactions to allergens, the patient is treated by maintaining an airway and by the injection of theophylline ethylenediamine (Aminophylline). Anaphylactic shock manifests as a circulatory collapse due to peripheral vasodilation, increased capillary permeability and marked bronchospasm. Lifesaving measures are necessary, such as an intravenous injection of 0.5 ml of 1:1,000 epinephrine. A tourniquet is placed proximal to the site of the antigen entrance in the extremity. Oxygen is administered early. The office staff should call an ambulance for emergency transport to the hospital.

Cerebral Vascular Accident (CVA)

In the presence of occlusion of the blood supply to the brain by thrombosis, embolism or cerebral hemorrhage, there may be a sudden loss of consciousness. Pulse, blood pressure and respiration are noted along with neurological deficits. With intracranial pressure the pupil is dilated on the affected side. Supporting respiration through clearing of the airways and use of oxygen is helpful. Good judgment is most important at this time, and the patient should be transferred to a hospital for more definitive treatment if necessary.

Adrenal Crisis

Patients on massive steroid therapy may become hypotensive when in crisis. Adrenocorticotropic hormone (ACTH) may be diminished and should be supplemented by injections of hydrocortisone sodium succinate. Lidocaine hydrochloride is metabolized and destroyed in the liver, thus providing additional damage to a patient with liver disorder, such as cirrhosis.

Hypertensive Crisis

The use of epinephrine in an anesthetic may cause a rise in blood pressure. Patients with a history of cardiac disease and hypertension must be carefully evaluated. It is essential to check the pulse rate and respiration as well as blood pressure, in all patients requiring local anesthesia. Diazepam (Valium) may serve as a sedative and tranquilizer in the hypertensive patient. Oxygen should be administered to a patient in hypertensive crisis.

Central Nervous System Stimulation

In the presence of a CNS disorder due to a stimulative anesthetic or other medication, the blood pressure may become elevated, the pulse may be rapid and muscles may twitch. Convulsions with serious sequelae may result. Respirations are generally shallow and rapid with hypoxia. The doctor must provide an adequate airway and administer oxygen.

Central Nervous System Depression

In CNS depression, the pulse is weak and rapid, blood pressure is lowered and respirations are slow. It is necessary to maintain the vital functions by patient reassurance, opening airways, providing oxygen and using intravenous vasopressors, such as ephedrine sulfate or methoxamine hydrochloride (Vasoxyl). These drugs must be used carefully so as to maintain an equilibrium of response.

Cardiovascular Collapse

Cardiovascular collapse with myocardial failure is characterized by low blood pressure, slow pulse and often nausea. The patient is placed in a Trendelenberg position of 5–10°. The treatment is to maintain an airway, provide oxygen and administer ephedrine sulfate. Atropine sulfate is used to increase the pulse rate when a parasympathetic blocking agent is necessary.

Vasovagal Shock

A bradycardia, hypotension, nausea and vomiting may occur in vasovagal shock, secondary to fear, anxiety or sudden severe pain. Skin is pallid and extremities are cool. A calm and reassuring staff is absolutely necessary. Atropine sulfate or ephedrine is generally helpful.

Diabetic Crisis

The diabetic patient may be allowed small amounts of liquid up to 3 hours before surgery. If the diabetic patient feels faint and becomes disoriented the podiatrist should administer orange juice or some food containing sugar. Hypoglycemic crisis with loss of consciousness is treated with 25–50 cc of 50% glucose solution intravenously. If the patient has a low blood sugar, a positive response will ensue. Insulin should be administered only in a controlled hospital setting subsequent to a hyperglycemic reaction.

The author's office maintains an emergency kit (Doctors Emergency Kit Healthfirst Corp. Edmonds, Washington), for treatment of severe physiological alterations. Office staff members are given periodic instruction in cardiopulmonary resuscitation (CPR). CPR should be mandatory for all personnel, including secretaries, aides, nurses, physical therapists and other professionals.

Drug Reactions

In a comprehensive clinical study of muscle relaxants, Owens (19) concludes that "anxiety often exacerbates the pain of muscular pathology." He notes that the antianxiety drugs preferred in his study in order of clinical effectiveness are "(1) benzodiazepines, (2) meprobamate, (3) phenobarbital." Owens cautions the practitioner concerning the relationship of periodic anxiety attacks and life experiences. He advocates a change in environment and careful dosages for relief of the anxiety and pain.

Cadwallader (20) stresses the need for doctors to be thoroughly knowledgeable of the action of drugs. He notes that "a large number of adverse drug reactions are being caused by drug interactions." "Drug interactions" he states, "occur when the effects of one drug are modified by the prior or concurrent administration of another drug." Cadwallader cautions against the use of drugs at their "near toxic levels" and the use of multiple prescription and over-the-counter drugs. Podiatrists, as specialists, must be aware of the type and dosage of medication being prescribed by other specialists.

The podiatrist must be fully aware of all drugs the patient is taking during a given period of time. Consultation with the patient's internist, pharmacist and all other prescribers may be necessary before prescribing new drugs.

Interactions of drugs take place at different levels of body physiology, such as during absorption and transport of drugs.

Due to enzymal activity, an increase or decrease in certain drug actions may have to be compensated for. A good route to follow in adjusting to microsomal enzyme activity that has increased the metabolism of a drug is to increase the dosage or decrease time intervals for medicating. If the opposite is true—that is, if the metabolism of a drug has been decreased due to other drugs competing for the same enzymes—the dosage should be decreased or the dosage time lengthened (21) Cutie and Cutie note that drugs interact in the presence of interference with drug absorption, drug distribution, biotransformation and drug excretion.

Drug biotransformation must be considered carefully in the administration of drugs. Many drugs undergoing metabolism may be chemically altered, resulting in an activity foreign to that for which they were prescribed. Biotransformation generally takes place in the liver, but may occur in the renal epithelium, blood plasma and the intestinal mucosa (21).

Hospital Emergencies

Many podiatrists are on staff at small, rural, understaffed hospitals. In the event of trauma and in an emergency situation, the podiatrist in a rural area may have to serve as a member of a team of primary physicians. Every minute is important, and his or her judgment may assist other specialists in saving life and limb. The following rules are essential to good medical practice in an emergency, before transfer of a seriously injured patient to a larger facility.

1. Careful examination and good complete records are essential; note the levels of consciousness and extent of head and neck injuries.
2. A neurological and vascular examination must be properly performed and evaluated.
3. The need for skull and neck radiographs should be discussed with the responsible physicians following trauma. In a stressful situation, these radiographs may easily be neglected.
4. Limit immediate narcotics or sedatives until one is sure that the patient is not unconscious or semicomatose.
5. Restore airways by endotracheal intubation if the patient has blood or vomitus in his or her mouth and is having respiratory difficulties.
6. In the presence of multiple injuries to the chest or abdomen and if the patient is hypotensive, respiratory support and fluid replacement are essential to raising the blood pressure and restoring blood.
7. Blood should be typed and crossmatched.
8. Urinary catheterization and urinalysis may be lifesaving.
9. Blood counts, hematocrit, blood gases, and electrolyte determinations should be routine procedure in severe trauma.
10. Oral fluids should not be ordered until the patient is stabilized and all emergency measures completed.
11. The primary physician should be encouraged to examine the chest and abdomen clinically and by radiograph. An abdominal tap may be another necessary lifesaving technique. Pneumo/hemothorax must be evaluated early; aspiration may be indicated along with other respiratory assistance.
12. In the presence of pelvic injury, hematuria should lead to the need for fluid replacement or retrograde pyelogram x-ray studies.
13. Minor wounds can await suturing in the presence of shock or loss of consciousness.

It is the responsibility of all doctors ministering to the traumatized patient to concern themselves with the serious life-threatening problems. Removal of the patient to a larger, well-staffed facility is not indicated until the patient is stabilized. Too many patients expire en route if the primary physician, in an overworked state, fails to provide the necessary emergency measures. The podiatrist can be of immeasurable help in emergency situations.

Shmock (22) cited the major causes of preventable medical incidents as

1. inadequate communication with the patient
2. incomplete medical records or failure to document pertinent information
3. systems failures (equipment resources)
4. poor medical judgment

Tetanus Prophylaxis

Bennet (23) emphasizes the need for careful cleansing and debridement of foot wounds. He states that active immunity is preferred over passive immunity. If passive immunity is absolute, tetanus human immune globulin is preferred over equine or bovine antitoxins.

If the podiatric patient has received a tetanus booster within the last year, most authorities consider immunization to be adequate. A tetanus-prone wound in a patient who has not been immunized within the last 10 years requires injection of 0.5 cc of toxoid plus 250 units of TIGH (tetanus immune globulin human) (24). If an infection is present or anticipated, the podiatrist must consider the use of prophylactic or therapeutic antibiotics based on sensitivity bacterial tests. Use of oxytetracycline or penicillin G should be considered if the patient is sensitive to equine antitoxin. If history and sensitivity tests do not indicate sensitivity, equine antitoxin may be given in a dose of 3,000 to 5,000 units. The seriousness of determining the patient's sensitivity must be emphasized because the TIGH may not be available. The disease is far more lethal than the sensitivity to and possible anaphylaxis from equine antitoxin.

References

1. Rotter D, et al.: Podiatrist—patient interaction during routine podiatry visits. *J Am Podiatry Assoc* 74:553–558, 1984.
2. Mâhrle D: Ultra high speed airdrill: A new instrument in podiatric surgery. *J Am Podiatry Assoc* 56:217, 1966.
3. Berman A, Gartland J: Metatarsal osteotomy for the correction of adduction of the forepart of the foot in children. *J Bone Joint Surg* 53A:498–506, 1971.
4. Jenkinson EO: Sound seen source of safe surgery. *Interview Podiatry News* 8:1–2, 1970.
5. Min X-ray Inc, 1732 Central St., Evanston, IL 60201.
6. Freund PA: Radiographic visual bisector. A new measuring device. *J Am Podiatry Assoc* 74:565–569, 1984.
7. Soloman SN, Davis RH: The Soloman tray. *J Am Podiatry Assoc* 73:525, 1983.
8. P.R.N., 6839 Riverdale Rd., Riverdale, MD, 20737.
9. Sage Practice Management System, 900 E. 8th Ave., King of Prussia, PA, 19406.
10. Scullion PF: Dermatologic review: Scalpel technique in removing heloma and hyperkeratosis. *J Foot Surg* 23:344–349, 1984.
11. Locke RK: Bone clamp for forefoot surgery. *J Am Podiatry Assoc* 56:368–370, 1966.
12. Freed JB: Sesamoidectomy clamp. *J Am Podiatry Assoc* 56:371–372, 1966.
13. Kaplan EG, Cornfield A: Micropneumatic surgical instruments and their application to podiatric surgery. *J Foot Surg* 8:11–30, 1969.
14. Kurzwell M: A new instrument for digital surgery. *J Am Podiatry Assoc* 51:274–275, 1961.
15. Kaplan EG, Weinstock R: Local anesthesia of the foot using jet injection. *J Am Podiatry Assoc* 57:370–373, 1967.
16. Kaplan EG, Weinstock R: Corticosteroid instillation by jet spray and check of penetration. *J Am Podiatry Assoc* 57:409–411, 1967b.
17. Dallek A: Podiatric Time Savers (brochure). Bronx, NY, 1971.
18. Bartolomei FJ, McCarthy DJ: Anaphylaxis: Mechanisms, manifestations, and management. *J Foot Surg* 23:485–488, 1984.
19. Owens RE: The clinical use of central depressant muscle relaxants and tranquilizers in musculoskeletal disorders. *J Am Podiatry Assoc* 66:671–681, 1976.
20. Cadwallader DE: Drug interactions: Some dangers of multiple drug use. *J Am Podiatry Assoc* 65:972–978, 1975.
21. Cutie MR, Cutie AJ: Podiatry drug reactions. *J Am Podiatry Assoc* 68:157–166, 1978.
22. Schmock CL: Quality patient care through risk management. *J Legal Med Pract* 1977.
23. Bennet I: Current concepts in tetanus prophylaxis. *J Am Podiatry Assoc* 67:259–263, 1977.
24. Graziano TA, Snider DW, Steinberg RI: Crush and avulsion injuries of the foot: Their evaluation and management. *J Foot Surg* 23:445–450, 1984.

Suggested Readings

Boyce-Smith, G: Common office emergencies. ACFS Scientific Seminar. Las Vegas, NE, 1984.

Boyce-Smith, G: Common respiratory emergencies in the perioperative period. ACFS Scientific Seminar. Las Vegas, NE, 1984.

Fruth R: Anaphylaxis and drug reactions: Guidelines for detection and care. *Heart Lung* 9:662, 1980.

Mueller TJ, Carlson BA, Lindy MP: The use of the carbon dioxide surgical laser for the treatment of verrucae. *J Am Podiatry Assoc* 70:136–141, 1980.

Perrone MA: *Podiatric Nail and Bone Surgery.* Canton, OH, The Webber Dental Manufacturing Co, 1972.

Sartoris DJ, Feingold ML, Resnick D: Axial computed tomographic anatomy of the foot. Part I: Hind Foot. *J Foot Surg* 24:392–412, 1985.

Sartoris DJ, Feingold ML, Resnick D: Axial computed tomographic anatomy of the foot. Part II: Midfoot. *J Foot Surg* 24:413–430, 1985.

Sartoris DJ, Feingold ML, Resnick D: Axial computed tomographic anatomy of the foot. Part III: Forefoot. *J Foot Surg* 25:19–38, 1986.

Schwartzentraub P: Drugs of choice: Possible emergency situations during podiatric office surgery. *J Am Podiatry Assoc* 64:854–861, 1974.

Shehadi WH: Contrast media adverse reactions. Occurrence, recurrence, and distribution patterns. *Radiology* 143:11, 1982.

Tipton PE: Chronic pulmonary problems. *J Am Podiatry Assoc* 66:850–853, 1976.

Wittenberg M: Reactions to injected drugs and their emergency care. *J Am Podiatry Assoc* 48:516–522, 1958.

2

History, Physical Examination and Nutrition

The practice of podiatric medicine is unlimited in scope. Foot pathology is often related to pathology found in other anatomical areas affecting different and often multiple body systems. A major factor involved in the diagnosis and treatment of foot disorders is a thorough understanding of podiatric biomechanics. The podiatric physician is the only professional uniquely educated and trained to treat the majority of foot disorders. It is important to appreciate that *routine foot care* does not exist. Multiple etiologies, pathologies, and treatments dictate an individual approach to each patient.

The foot is inseparable from the ankle and its related or governing structures. One cannot treat one without treating the other. Every available means of examination, diagnostic test and treatment modality should be utilized.

The podiatrist achieves a desired result in treating a specific condition by accurate diagnosis of the problem. The treatment of symptoms alone may provide temporary emergency care, but should only be a vehicle for establishing patient rapport until a diagnosis is made.

An inadequate diagnosis may result from too hurried an examination or failure to take a complete history of the case. Insufficient diagnostic equipment or the examiner's lack of knowledge and experience in interpreting the subjective and objective findings are other obstacles to establishing an accurate diagnosis.

It is necessary to understand the practical basis for taking a case history because of its importance to an accurate diagnosis. A reliable history depends upon the intelligent cooperation of the patient. If the patient cannot understand why the foot doctor must take a thorough history when treating the patient's feet, the patient must be shown the relationship between general health and foot health. Unfortunately, the average patient has been indoctrinated with the philosophy of "remove your clothes but keep your socks or stockings on."

The patient requires sympathetic kindness and understanding in history taking, as well as in therapy. Every move and facial expression indicates to the patient your attitude toward his or her case. There is nothing more important in successful treatment than having the patient's confidence. The patient gains confidence through the initial contact with the doctor.

Patients know more than the examiner does about their symptoms. Let them relate their troubles to you. Talking about their problems may help relieve their anxiety. The examiner should keep his or her eyes, ears and mind open for vital points of the patient's medical history. If the examiner asks too many questions, patients' responses may confuse interpretation of the main complaint.

Many doctors attempt to use a history form in directing questions to patients, but patients who are worried about their particular symptoms may be unable to give the necessary information in a logical and organized way. Skillfully guiding patients' discussion about themselves and their symptoms will bring the best results. The examiner must keep the loquacious patient on the subject, encourage the reticent person to say more and put the nervous individual at ease.

When the diagnosis is obvious, it should be supported by objective findings and then treated accordingly. If a patient complains of pain in certain joints of the feet, especially on arising in the morning, and has similar pain in the hands, knee or back, an investigation is in order to rule out other complicating factors; but simple complaints of pain in a fifth toe that presents a heloma do not necessarily require elaborate blood studies and sophisticated laboratory examinations.

Taking and Interpreting the General History

Adequate records require that the name, address and telephone number of all patients be kept. It is also desirable to maintain a record of who referred a patient to you. Whether the patient came to your office through personal, social, business or political affiliations or whether he or she was sent by a former patient or another doctor may make a difference in your new relationship and with the community you serve. Confidence is so important in patient-podiatrist relationships that this point of referral cannot be overlooked in asking questions for the history. Usually, a patient referred by another patient, a colleague or physician already has the necessary confidence.

A patient's address may alert you to environmental influences as a factor in diagnosis, and racial origins and hereditary factors are often revealed by the patient's family name. Knowing whether he or she lives near the river or close to a swamp where it is damp, near a rat-infested dump, in a tenement or in a more desirable locale often assists in interpreting the patient's symptoms.

Age

Ailments affecting the human body are in many instances related to the age of the individual (Figs. 2.1 and 2.2). Remember that children have wonderful imaginations and enjoy mimicry. Women about menopausal age may be exceptionally nervous and irritable. Circulatory involvement would be unlikely in a child, yet injuries to epiphyses are common in children and are not seen in adults. Rickets, of course, is a childhood disease and can be suspected in young children. Venereal disease is commonly acquired in the second and third decades of life.

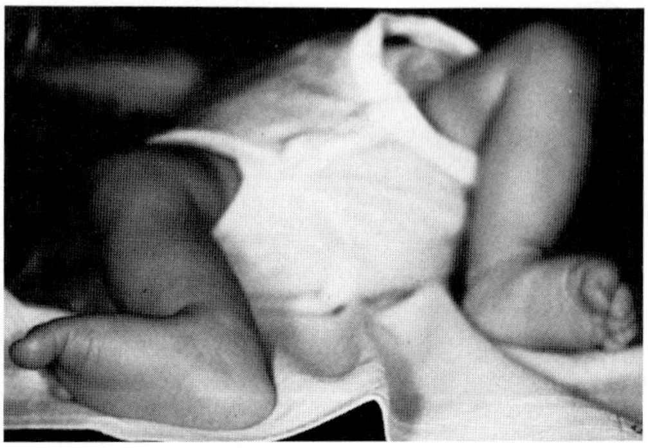

Figure 2.1. Double diapers capable of causing external rotation of limbs.

One must refrain from making a snap diagnosis with age as the only basis, however, because many conditions affecting adults with certain characteristic symptoms may be manifested entirely differently in childhood. Dietary deficiencies in children may cause certain skin and bone involvements. Eczematous lesions may be characteristic of the individual's age.

Kravitz and Boehm (1) note that normal children begin to flex their extremities rhythmically within the first 6 months of life. In an older child such symptoms may

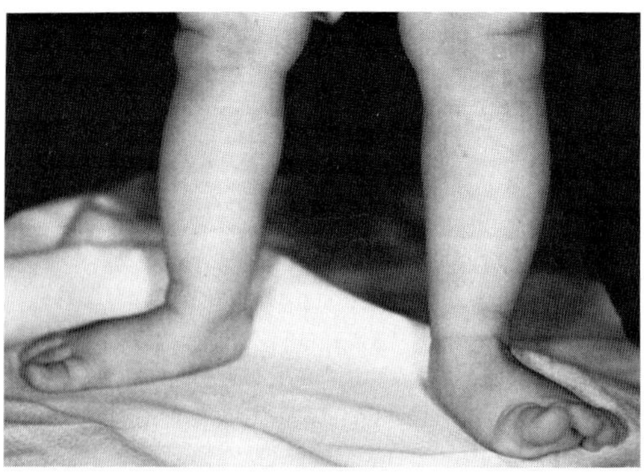

Figure 2.2. Pes planovalgus aggravated by double diapers and resultant external femoral rotation.

suggest a neuromuscular disorder. Gessell and Ilg (2) note that children between the ages of 6 and 7 years remove their shoes when coming into the house after school or periods of play. This behavior pattern must not be seen as a sign of discomfort or foot pathology. Yet one may suspect a neurosis, ill-fitting shoes or definite foot pathology when an adult has difficulty wearing shoes.

Tuberculosis is more common in childhood, although it may manifest at any age. Infectious diseases, congenital malformations and many injuries that go unnoticed by parents are seen in children. The cardiovascular diseases of children are commonly rheumatic or congenital; in middle age they are diabetic, syphilitic or hypertensive; in old age they are arteriosclerotic. Thromboangiitis obliterans usually occurs between the ages of 20 and 40.

Subacute combined sclerosis of the spinal cord with numbness, tingling of the hands and feet and with gradual paralysis is seen in individuals between ages 45 and 55. Multiple sclerosis is often discovered in the age group of 15 to 25.

Arteriosclerosis is generally thought to be a natural degenerative occurrence in the aged. It is described as being a degenerative fibrositis with secondary sclerotic changes in the arteries. Predisposing causes are excessive muscular activity, syphilis, alcoholism, lead poisoning, hypertension and renal disease.

Yale (3), in a radiographic study of calcification of the medial calcaneal branch of the posterior tibial artery, cited a high incidence of calcification in the age group of 20 to 40.

Mönckeberg's sclerosis occurs in the aged and in the diabetic patient. The media is degenerated, with the formation of plaques of calcium encircling the vessel. This sclerosis is believed to start at birth.

Other forms of arteriosclerosis are the senile, or atherosclerosis, and nodular sclerosis. Calcium deposition within the vessel lumen may occlude circulation with ultimate gangrene and loss of limb.

Progressive muscular atrophy may be seen during childhood and adolescence. It is hereditary and manifests itself early in the feet. The foot is in varus deformity, with shortening of the achilles tendon producing an unsteady gait that requires great muscular effort for function. The hands and feet become clawed, the arches abnormally high and the toes hyperflexed (Fig. 2.3).

Friedreich's ataxia usually occurs in adolescence up to the fifteenth year of age and may affect more than one child in a family. The gait is uncertain, limb movements are involuntary and a widespread leg posture to maintain balance is in evidence. Disturbances in speech and early loss of deep reflexes with abnormal position sense of an extremity are pathognomonic. Equinovarus of both feet occurs later in the disease.

Patients in menopause have varied complaints, some organic and others of psychosomatic origin. A common finding of unknown etiology is tenderness of the anterior lower third of the tibia in women in the climacteric who have rheumatic pains. This condition has not been found in regularly menstruating women, and it does not disappear or change in intensity during the menopausal period. It has not been observed in amenorrhea not due to menopause.

A patient in the throes of menopause may develop vague aches and pains in the hands and feet. Stiffness of the small joints of the feet is common. Dry skin with fissures about the heels has been noted.

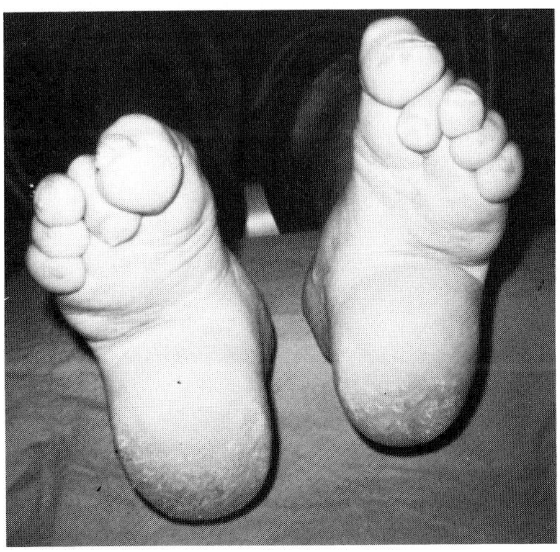

Figure 2.3. Congenital talipes equinovarus in a 40-year-old male.

Marked flexion of the toes, night cramps and alternate hot and cold lightning pains in the extremities are common. Treatment may include referral to a gynecologist if the history indicates menopausal etiology. Local symptoms of pain and stiffness may be treated symptomatically; dry, fissured and scaling skin may respond to treatment with moisturizing agents.

Sex

Sex is an important factor in diagnosis because certain conditions are more prevalent in one sex than in the other. For example, diseases of the thyroid, breasts and biliary system are more common in women. Spurs of the heels, apophysitis of the calcaneus and many other foot ailments characteristically occur in males, but may occur in females.

Arteriosclerosis obliterans and Buerger's disease are believed to be more common in males. Rheumatoid arthritis, hyperthyroidism and Raynaud's disease are predominant in the young or middle-aged female. Although gout is supposed to be more common in the male, the author feels that many cases of gout in the female are overlooked in diagnosis. Shoes worn by women aggravate foot involvements. Pregnancy and menstrual and menopausal difficulties cause varied foot disturbances. The union of epiphyses takes place about 2 years earlier in females than in males. A prostatitis must be considered in men as a possible source of infection and pain in the extremities.

A nonsuppurative acute inflammatory cutaneous and subcutaneous nodule formation occurring in females about the second to fourth decade may be erythema nodosum. It is a self-limited disorder characterized by firm, somewhat tender nodules, pink to purple in color, usually on the anterior of the legs. Temperature, sore throat and joint pains may accompany this bilateral, symmetrical lesion.

National, Ethnic and Racial Background

The patient's race, nationality and family heredity are important in making a diagnosis. Patients of Mediterranean origin may have a short, stubby and hypermobile type of foot with many minor phalangeal deformities, whereas low-arched feet are common in Semitic peoples. Blacks have a characteristic flat foot, whereas Caucasians of Nordic ancestry have abnormally high-arched, bony feet. The broad, flexible type of foot with low arch and hallux valgus deformity is typical of the Slavic peoples.

The black race shows a high incidence of untreated syphilitic infections and their complicating lesions. Ainhum, also known as dactylolysis spontanea due to its progressive gross pathology, is most commonly found in blacks. A firm constrictive band of fibrous connective tissue covered by a callus creates a cleft in the toe resulting in a swollen, bulbous end. Progressive constriction cuts off circulation, causing considerable pain, ulceration and often gangrene followed by spontaneous amputation. Pain can be relieved by early diagnosis and amputation of the toe proximal to the constricting band. The etiology is unknown. Ross (4) describes a case of ainhum and its treatment. The author has seen several cases. A smooth, shiny and elevated massive scar or keloid is also common in the black population. Occasionally helomas develop in these keloids, rendering them painful. Although bone changes rarely affect the extremities, sickle cell anemia is another condition found in blacks.

People of the Mongoloid race have tiny feet for their size. In Chinese women, especially, this condition results from the practice of binding the feet for many years. Kaposi's sarcoma commonly affects people originating from the region of the Mediterranean.

Weight

Weight is an important etiologic factor in mechanical foot imbalance. Muscular and ligamentous weakness are affected by being overweight. Improper footgear, poor posture and overwork are particularly aggravating to the feet of overweight individuals. Increased weight in pregnancy, carrying of heavy loads and the stress of lifting in certain occupations may produce mechanical foot defects. A rapid increase or decrease in weight may be due to systemic illness or metabolic or endocrine disturbances that may weaken the feet to a point of interfering with normal foot physiology.

Height

Extreme alteration in height may be of anterior pituitary origin. Height has an effect on the individual in proportion to weight and general stature. Frequently an extremely tall individual develops poor body posture that affects the feet. Short individuals may have metabolic or developmental disturbances with a faulty rate of bone growth.

Occupation

Certain muscular structures in individuals in sedentary occupations may atrophy as a result of disuse. The use of a foot pedal in certain industries results in strain or inflammation of a part because of repeated trauma to a single area. Lifting of heavy weights and changes from sedentary to active occupations produce injury to the active part. Dentists, taxi drivers, bus drivers and persons in similar occupations are subject to injury to a single extremity as a result of overuse. Men and women who walk for many hours on hard surfaces in factories, such as on concrete or metal floors, suffer fatigue readily from lack of a resilient weightbearing surface. Salespersons and counterpersons who have to stand at one counter for several hours during the day commonly develop low back pains, poor posture and aching sensations of the feet and legs from overuse or abuse of a single group of muscles.

Psychosomatic difficulties may arise from subconscious fears or dislikes concerned with one's occupation. Allergic reactions and contact dermatitis may be actively associated with occupational disorders involving the feet. Certain eczemas may be directly or indirectly associated with occupations exposing patients to irritating substances.

Working habits, vacations, use of leisure time, diet and use of drugs may influence development of a pathology (Fig. 2.4). Very often, secretaries curl their feet about the rungs of a chair while working, resulting in pressure over the extensor tendons on the dorsum of the foot. A tenosynovitis is common. If the chair presses forward at the popliteal space or if the legs are pushed back under the chair while working, a pressure neuralgia or a congestive edema of the foot and ankle may develop.

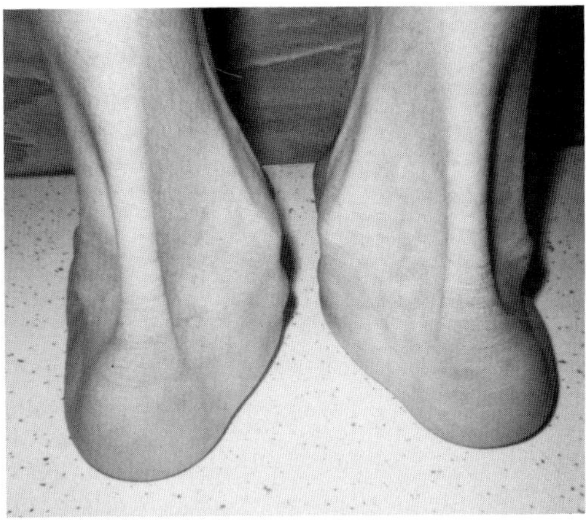

Figure 2.4. Severe calcaneal valgus secondary to generalized laxity of ligaments in a cross-country runner.

Family History and Personal Habits

The family history should contain information on the medical background of parents, siblings and other close relatives. If either of the parents is dead, the age of death and the cause should be recorded. The number of siblings and their medical backgrounds should be similarly recorded.

Does the patient smoke, drink or use narcotics and to what extent? Are these habits moderate or excessive? Smoking may affect the circulatory status of an extremity, alcohol may upset normal mental reactions and morphine or its derivatives may prove to be an excitant.

Environment

An individual accustomed to a cold or warm climate is readily affected by alterations in temperature. Symptoms of Raynaud's disease are more prevalent in the winter.

Arthritic patients are affected by alterations in atmospheric conditions, and they suffer much discomfort in a cold, humid environment. Atmospheric changes cause pain in low-grade inflammatory lesions such as helomas, tylomas and arthritis. Hyperidrosis, bromidrosis, anhidrosis and sensitivities to nylon, rubber, leather, glue, sock linings, tanning chemicals and dyes are not uncommon causes of foot trouble.

Fungi thrive in a dark, moist, warm and dirty environment. Skin, clothing and bed cloths may become infected by the mite, its eggs and wastes resulting in scabies or the itch.

Typhus fever may cause thrombosis of the blood vessels of the skin. Skin necrosis or gangrene can occur. A scratch or puncture wound on the foot makes a fine avenue of entrance of the virus from fecal deposits.

History of the Chief Complaint

This portion of the history is recorded in the patient's own words. It includes all subjective symptoms and possible etiology.

What the patient reports is of utmost importance. If the condition began suddenly, it is acute. If it developed gradually, it is chronic in nature. The subacute symptoms lie somewhere between the acute and chronic. A pathological process may develop gradually and still be acute. How long the condition had been present greatly affects the diagnosis and treatment of the trouble. The history and symptoms given by the patient may be very vague at times. It is wise to have the patient point to the area involved before weighing complaints leading toward a diagnosis. However, it must be borne in mind that the symptoms about which the patient complains may be referred pain from pathology elsewhere in the body. If these complaints have acute exacerbations with no symptoms in between, they are said to be intermittent.

A medical history, past and present and including a family history, is necessary. Many foot disabilities are the result of general illness or past involvements of a general nature. Pain in the feet as a result of psychosomatic illness may cause foot disability in some cases.

Upon noting the complaint, the patient's greatest symptoms and the patient's outward physical appearance, the podiatrist records the pertinent information as nearly as possible in the patient's own words. Considerable tact must be used to keep some patients on the subject of their complaint, whereas others require prodding in order to gather the information desired. The ideal history would be entirely in the patient's own words, although few patients stick to the point and many specific questions are necessary. The examiner may compromise by writing the history objectively in the third person while the answers to the questions are woven into the description.

Blumer (5) suggested that a better view of the duration of a chronic ailment can be gained by asking the patient, "how long is it since you felt perfectly well?" rather than "how long have you been sick?"

The initial symptoms of some of the most common chronic diseases are not known; thus the patient's sensitivity and intelligence play an important part in gathering necessary information. Neurotic patients are hypersensitive and over observant. The phlegmatic type may disregard symptoms that cause acute pain.

The podiatrist must note the location, character, intensity and extent of radiation of pain and the effects of exercise, emotion, posture and their relationship to various systems of the body.

It is necessary to know how and when the present complaint began and what the ensuing symptoms have been in order to form a diagnosis. Such information is necessary not only for medical purposes but for legal ones as well, because insurance companies request this information and expect an intelligent answer. This information may reveal the etiology of the chief complaint and may make possible removal of factors aggravating the pathology. Did the present complaint come about suddenly or slowly over a long period of time? Have the symptoms increased, decreased or changed in character? What sequence did they follow? When did the symptoms occur: during summer, winter, etc? What hour of the day did the symptoms commence? If trauma is involved, note the time and place. Careful interrogation adds to the total knowledge of the complaint.

Groups of vesicles on slightly elevated erythematous plaques distributed along one or more peripheral sensory nerves with severe pain suggest shingles or herpes zoster. This may occur in an individual who has been ill, overworked or tired.

When there has been immobilizing illness, an operation or a history of vascular disease, trauma or infection of the leg, pulmonary embolism syndrome may be suspected. A peripheral phlebitis may be a precursor to pulmonary embolism. The patient may have frequent nosebleeds that may suggest cardiac involvement. Shortness of breath and chest pains may indicate a cardiac or lung disorder. The general color and appearance of the patient are noted for corroboration. Nocturia may be due to a bladder disturbance. A great thirst, frequent urination, xanthoma, pruritus, furuncles, carbuncles, pustules or gangrene may suggest diabetes.

Constipation suggests intestinal stasis. A history of eating improperly cooked pork or bear meat may cause muscular aches and vomitus with other symptoms of trichinosis. Dizziness and frequent headaches suggest high blood pressure. Allergic reactions affecting the skin of the feet are common in individuals who suffer from hay fever and asthma. Many people are sensitive to drugs and foods. Redness and indurated swellings of the joints of the feet accompanied by exfoliation of the epidermis are not uncommon after antibiotic therapy for a systemic infection. Sharp shooting, lightning-like pains in the extremities may be a neuritis of syphilitic origin.

Hyperidrosis and late afternoon elevations in temperature with persistent cough and loss of weight suggest tuberculosis. Respiratory infections, sore throats, tooth infections, prostatitis, middle ear and gallbladder lesions may lead to painful manifestations in the extremities.

Viruses change the cells within which they grow and multiply, resulting in hyperplasia or necrosis.

The podiatrist must recognize the symptoms of the common cold, influenza, dengue, measles, herpes zoster (shingles) and acute polio as they relate to the local foot complaints. The infectious diseases produce symptoms in the extremities involving skin reactions, myalgias, thrombophlebitis, arthritis, polyneuritis and cutaneous hyperesthesia.

Medical and Surgical History

The medical history should list all pertinent information including typical childhood diseases, scarlet fever, rheumatic heart and all other diseases and infections. A record should be kept of the patient's inoculations. Listing all medications (including dosage) and allergies, especially drug allergies, is a necessity.

A past history of lung disease, asthma or emphysema should be noted. Caution should be exercised with the patient who has a history of liver disease, renal disease or alcoholism (6). The "caine" local anesthetics are detoxified in the liver. It is important to know about past history of cardiac disease. A patient with a history of cardiac arrhythmia, myocardial infarction, angina or hypertension is at greater risk during surgery. Epinephrine containing local anesthetics should not be used in patients with a history of hypertension. Patients taking antihypertensive medication are predisposed to hypertensive crisis if medication is discontinued and epinephrine containing local anesthetics are used. Patients receiving systemic corticosteroids are predisposed to adrenal crisis and severe hypotension during a foot surgical procedure.

Pregnancy

Varicose veins, phlebitis and leg, hip and low back pains together with a calcium deficiency often bring pregnant women to a podiatrist's office.

In treating a pregnant woman or a mother with other children, the number of living children and a record of previous stillbirths should be noted. Stillbirths may be indicative of syphilis or a pelvic disorder, either of which can cause a variety of foot disturbances.

The pregnant woman should do considerable walking during and after the pregnancy. The marked increase in body weight during pregnancy is a strain on the pedal extremities. However, even greater damage to physiological function is incurred by the pregnant woman who becomes sedentary or recumbent during this period.

The feet should be closely observed during pregnancy and postpartum. An examination of foot functions and posture with evaluation of their effect on body posture is necessary to appreciate some physiological changes. Many plantar warts that appear during the first trimester disappear after delivery. Complaints of foot pains, such as strained plantar fascia, cramps, fatigue and muscle soreness, are quite common. Backaches and pain in the thighs and on the medial aspect of the knees are the results of faulty foot posture, rather than simply relaxation of the pelvis joints. Swelling of the lower legs must be differentiated. Deep varicosities, lymphatic stasis, thrombophlebitis, cardiac and kidney disturbances and pressure of the fetus in the lower pelvic region may result in edema.

Wearing low-heeled shoes or flat, weightbearing inner soles and slippers causes symptoms of pulling sensations behind the knees. The heads of the gastrocnemius are pulled through the lowered position of the heel with resultant strain.

Symptoms of biomechanical dysfunction are most commonly found after the fifth month of pregnancy. Body mechanics are altered through the addition of weight and the wearing of ill-fitting footgear. Pain may be referred to the medial ligaments of the knee due to foot pronation beyond the normal range. Leg musculature may become atrophic and flabby. During the puerperium, muscular weakness becomes rapid and progressive. After parturition the patient may complain of weakness of the feet and legs. Dull aches and coldness of the feet may persist due to incomplete recuperation from physiological changes. The stretched ligaments and joint capsules, together with the elongated muscles, require several months to return to normal. In treating podiatric complaints of pregnant or postparturient women, heat and violent exercises should be avoided. Oxford shoes with freedom for toes, a firm fit in heel and arch, rigid shank, extended counter, Thomas heel or heel height of comfort, which are made of all-leather or Goodyear welt construction should be worn. Elastic stockings with open toe and closed heel and of midthigh length may alleviate symptoms. If hyperidrosis exists, a foot powder of choice should be used.

Venereal Diseases and Related Factors

When the patient's symptoms lead you to suspect a venereal infection, ask if he or she has such a disease. Never accept a denial until all suspicious diseases are investigated by a laboratory examination. If a patient is known to have syphilis, find out the date of infection. A history of inadequate treatment must be noted.

Gonorrhea is a common venereal disease. Infections of the urinary tract and prostatitis may be the result of a gonorrheal infection, with frequent involvement of the joints of the foot by a gonococcal arthritis. A chronic inflammatory dermatosis with infection of the genital tract and of the joints may be noted in patients with gonorrhea. Symmetrical eruptions of horny hyperkeratotic nodules, crusts and pustules on the palms and soles are characteristic.

If the patient is known to have syphilis or if you suspect it is present, try to elicit a history of a saucer-shaped chancre with raised, clearly demarcated, indurated margins on the genital organs. These chancres have a bloody serous discharge and usually clear up with or without treatment in 3 to 5 weeks.

Macular, papular or erythematous lesions affecting the palms and soles may occur in the secondary stages of syphilis (Fig. 2.5). Nails of the toes may lose their luster, and syphilitic onychia may be present.

The tertiary stages are characterized by gummatous lesions or general paresis, mental degeneration, delusions of grandeur, tabes dorsalis, exaggerated reflexes, loss of position sense and equilibrium with Argyll-Robertson pupil and perforating ulcers.

In a female patient it is necessary to know the number of miscarriages, if any, to establish the background for a possible diagnosis. The underlying pathology may be syphilis or Rh factor. Repeated miscarriages followed by stillbirths and finally by viable children may suggest syphilis. The child is infected in utero and may at

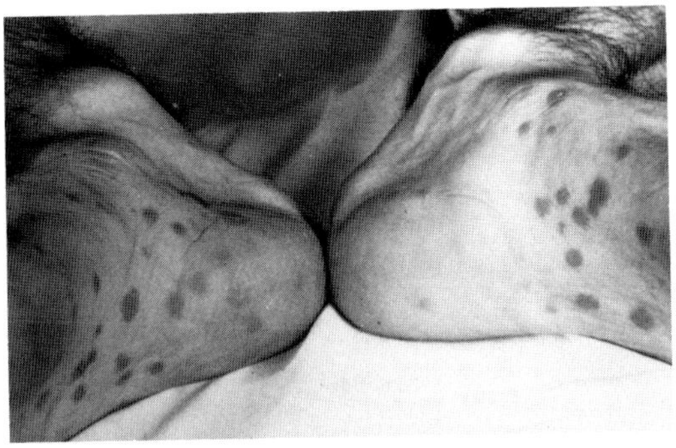

Figure 2.5. Macular lesions, bilateral and symmetrical; syphilis questionable.

birth present a saber shin and saddle nose. Notched teeth may be noted with growth and development. If the patient is a male, ask if his wife has had miscarriages. If the patient's wife has syphilis, the male patient may be infected through sexual contact. This information is of diagnostic importance.

Other related factors causing podiatric complaints should be determined. Ask a female patient if her menstrual periods are regular, if the flow is normal and what their duration is. Is the menopause causing undue difficulty?

Disturbances in the feet may be due to a pelvic disorder. One foot may get cold and clammy as a result of low pelvic tumors and edemas. Pressure on arteries, veins and nerves may cause pains to radiate down the extremity from an abdominal or pelvic mass.

Surgical History

Surgical history should include information on all operations and anesthetics administered and on accidental injuries. Hemorrhages, thrombosis or embolism point to tendencies that may be significant in subsequent illnesses. Low abdominal surgery with herniation followed by neglect results in referable damage to the pedal extremities. A history of superficial migratory phlebitis may suggest thromboangiitis obliterans.

The Patient's Record

The above outline for an adequate history does not require a thorough interrogation of the patient. It is not advisable to keep superfluous histories for minor foot involvements, and certainly a laboratory study in depth is not necessary in making a simple diagnosis. Yet it is always better to have too much information to work with than not to have enough.

The author feels strongly about the best type of history chart for establishing an accurate diagnosis, having tried many printed forms with great disappointment in recent years. The practitioner should be sufficiently well informed when taking a history to follow a pattern that allows great leeway in recording information. After recording the basic information, such as age, weight, sex and so forth, the examiner asks the necessary questions as described above to establish a complete picture of the complaint.

After noting the objective and subjective symptoms and recording them on paper, all additional information is added according to date. In this way, a running history of the patient incorporating subsequent contributory information and findings may be kept. At the initial visit, a tentative impression may be made, and at each visit additional information and complaints as of that date are also recorded. Each patient's set of history sheets is kept in a separate folder together with his or her laboratory reports, which can also be referred to according to date. Regardless of the number of visits, this file adds to the total understanding of the patient's present complaint. Consultation sheets are attached also, and the date of consultation is noted in regular order on the examination sheet.

The problem-oriented medical record developed by Dr. Lawrence Weed, University of Vermont, and the subject of a book written by Dr. H. Cross and J. Bjorn is receiving widespread acceptance. If mastered, it may well supplant the "source-oriented" medical record now in use that consists of an array of unrelated facts that are difficult to correlate from the charts.

A well-organized problem-oriented record saves the doctor time and patience in locating comprehensive material on a specific problem. Using present methods of keeping patient records, the podiatrist may be forced to wade through reams of vital data, charts, laboratory findings and unrelated radiographs and reports to find that the patient had previously complained of the symptom now at hand.

The problem-oriented record is divided into four broad categories:

1. *Establishment of a data base.* This includes the sum of the patient's complaints, a sociological and psychological history, a podiatric examination, a medical and surgical history of the patient and laboratory data.
2. *Formulation of all problems.* A list of all problems is recorded, and each is given a number. Each problem is followed by a brief comment on the subjective and objective symptoms, e.g., (1) painful swollen left hallux joint; (2) deep keratotic verrucoid lesion, plantar surface, fourth metatarsal head, right foot.

   The list of problems occurring over a period of years is numbered. Referral to these problems is made easy by using the specific number for each problem as the chart increases in size over the years.
3. *Plans for each problem.* Here the podiatrist provides further information, records anticipated treatment of each problem and numbers the treatments to correspond with the problem. The patient is advised of the significance of each problem, and this action is recorded by the problem number. Thus, each problem has its own treatment plan based on all findings.
4. *Follow-up on each problem.* This section consists of progress notes that are dated, titled and numbered by problem.

Dr. Lawrence Weed looks upon the problem-oriented record progress notes as the most important part of this structured record, for which he uses the acronym SOAP: Subjective, patient's evaluation of treatment results; Objective, results noticed by the doctor; Assessment, doctor's evaluation of the treatment and; Plans, reviewing of plans and formulating new plans to enhance treatment of each problem.

The podiatric history and physical examination should be logical and complete. It must consider the following items:

CC, chief complaint
HPI, history present illness
PMSH, past medical and surgical history
FH, family history
ROS, review of systems
HEENT, head, ears, eyes, nose, throat
CVR, cardiovascular and respiratory
GI, gastrointestinal
GYN, gynecologic
GU, genitourinary
INTEG, skin and nail
CIRC, circulation
NEUR, neurological
MUSC/SKEL/BIOMECH, musculoskeletal and biomechanical
Radiographic
Laboratory

Physical Examination

The podiatrist serving any community of patients has a responsibility extending beyond the bounds of the immediate commitment to relieve a painful foot. Be it in an office or hospital, clinic, health maintenance organization or home for the elderly or retarded, the podiatrist must consider the patient as a whole human being. Thus, a preliminary physical examination from head to toe is necessary to understand fully the physical and emotional problems that may alter the diagnosis and treatment of the foot ailment.

Examination of the patient's gait and stance will be discussed elsewhere. It is now necessary to look for physical abnormalities. The podiatrist treating an accident victim must be aware of damage to other parts of the anatomy.

HEENT (Head, Ears, Eyes, Nose and Throat)

Head Is the head markedly enlarged indicating that the patient is hydrocephalic? Is the patient a microcephalic? Is there an absence of hair as in alopecia? In a female, the presence of a beard may suggest an endocrine gland disturbance with hormonal imbalance. Dry brittle hair may be secondary to myxedema and hypothyroidism.

The forehead may be furrowed and the ears thick, suggesting lion-like features, secondary to a pituitary problem. Note the presence, absence or reduction of hearing secondary to otosclerosis or simply wax impacted in the auditory canal.

Eyes The outer eye should be observed for abnormalities before the patient has an ophthalmoscopic examination. Eyelid ptosis should be noted. Xanthomatous lesions affecting the eyelid may be secondary to hypertriglyceridemia, hypercholesterolemia, diabetes mellitus and/or primary or secondary hyperuricemia.

Opthalmoscopy has been used for medical diagnosis for over a century. The examination of the back of the human eye may be important to the podiatrist in an effort to diagnose vision disorders and upper motor neuron disturbances causing lower extremity motor and biomechanical manifestations.

The podiatrist must recognize the necessity to refer to the ophthamologist and optometrist whenever pathology is observed in a casual examination of the eye. More extensive eye examinations should be performed by the ophthamologist and optometrist, with a request for a report for your records.

Space does not permit a thorough review of the use of the opthalmoscope. It is essential that practical clinical use of this instrument be learned in the teaching laboratory, clinic and hospital. A few examination aids should help the neophyte achieve practical results with the use of the ophthalmoscope (7).

1. A semidark to dark room provides a suitable environment for examination.
2. Dilation of the pupil should be left to the eye specialist.
3. Right eye. Sit or stand at the patient's right side and place an "o" in the illuminated lens indicator. With the ophthalmoscope in a vertical position in the right hand, direct the light beam toward the patient's right eye. The right index finger is used on the lens dial to change the lenses as required. The patient is advised to fix his sight at eye level. Step back about 6 inches and shine the light into the patient's pupil. The fundus reflex, or red glow, should appear through the aperture. The red glow is kept in view as you move to within 1 or 2 inches of the patient. The lenses are rotated slowly until the optic disk is seen clearly.
4. The retina is examined methodically while avoiding the light reflected back by the patient's cornea. This is done by using the pinhole aperture or by directing the light beam toward the edge of the pupil instead of the center of the pupil. Observe vessels carefully by following them to the periphery.
5. The macula is visible when the light is moved temporally about 2 disks in diameter.
6. The extreme periphery is examined by having the patient look up for the superior retina, down for the interior retina, temporally for the temporal retina and nasally for the nasal retina.
7. A red-free filter is available to exclude the red rays from the examination field. The filter provides a better view of the eye grounds, slight alterations in the blood vessels, microscopic hemorrhages, poorly defined exudates and obscure changes of the macula. Nerve fibers that atrophy become visible. The general appearance is a yellow-green background, a white disk, intense fundus reflexes and black and sharp vessels.

(The same procedure is followed in the examination of the left eye.)

The podiatrist may find the results of an ophthalmoscopic examination enlightening in the evaluation of certain dermatologic lesions of systemic origin where capillary fragility and hemorrhage are a factor. The *diabetic* patient may demonstrate *retinopathy* when the *optic disk* outlines are clear and the smaller arteries and larger veins are irregular. The *macula* appears as spots of white exudate. The other vessels of the eye present minute, round, irregular aneurysms. The *midperiphery* shows evidence of patches of hemorrhage and exudate. Diabetics should have an eye examination every year whether insulin dependent or not.

In the *arteriosclerotic* patient, with feeble or absent pulsations in the extremity, pallor, cyanosis, coldness and intermittent claudication, ulceration, or gangrene, the eye pathology is corroborative. The optic disk is clearly outlined, and the vessels appear irregular. The *retina* is pathological with exudates and occasional hemorrhage. The *blood vessels* are thin or rarefied and irregular. Crossings are indented, and many vessels appear as fine white lines with obliteration. Streaks of light on the arteries appear widened. The *periphery* may show hemorrhages, exudates and cysts.

In the presence of a paralysis or undue weakness of the extremities with no evidence of local etiology, the patient should be evaluated for a neurological upper motor neuron lesion. Here the ophthalmoscope may show an edema of the optic papilla *(Papilledema), a choked disk* or an optic *neuritis* due to intracranial pressure without inflammation. The disk edges are blurred and elevated above the surface of the remaining retina and vessels are engorged and possibly hemorrhagic. The vessels may be tortuous, but otherwise normal. There is a generalized *retinal* edema.

A *primary optic atrophy* is demonstrated by sharp and clear margins of the dead-white-colored disk. The macula and periphery of the eye are normal, but the vessels are attenuated.

The ophthalmoscope serves as a highly desirable instrument for the podiatrist in differentiating circulatory, neurological and upper and lower motor neuron lesions from local nerve pathology and assists the podiatrist in the treatment of biomechanical foot disorders.

The eyes should move in all directions, and the pupillary reflexes should be equal and react to light and accommodation. The optic fundus is viewed for arteriolar spasm, arteriovenous nicking, hemorrhages, exudates and papilledema. The presence of a grayish-white circle around the pupil may indicate an arcus sinilis often seen in the elderly and consistent with arteriosclerosis. Using an ophthalmoscope, one may detect enlargement of the veins and occlusion of the central vein due to thrombosis secondary to atherosclerosis. The presence of a cataract may readily alter gait patterns.

Nose Does the patient have labored breathing? Are the nasal passages occluded from a cold, allergy or deviated septum, or is there a chronic lung disorder limiting proper oxygenation?

Ears Check the ears. Is the tympanic membrane (TM) intact? Is cerumen present to excess? Is the ear canal open?

Throat Note the presence of a large, hanging jaw in a tall patient, suggesting hyperpituitarism. This may be a symptom of gigantism.

A cursory look at the patient's mouth may indicate the need for extensive dental work and periodontia. This has great significance to the podiatrist concerned with nutritional and infectious disorders. Also the tonsils may be inflamed or grossly infected. In either case, the patient needs an examination by an internist, and the podiatrist should observe caution in performing foot surgery. Oral temperature should be normal. If it is a degree too high or too low, ask the patient if this is normal for him or her. Palpate for glandular enlargements, such as submaxillary and parotid glands.

The neck is examined for carotid bruits and distended veins. Enlargement of the thyroid gland is easily palpated, and if the eyes bulge slightly, hyperthyroidism is a consideration. Note whether the trachea is midline. Check for cervical adenopathy.

CVR (Cardiovascular and Respiratory)

Blood pressure should be taken while the patient is standing, sitting and lying down. Diastolic blood pressure over 90 mm Hg should be considered pathologic. A patient with a systolic pressure over 150 mm Hg may be reacting to emotional stress. The combination of an unstable systolic blood pressure and a diastolic pressure over 90 mm Hg is considered hypertension.

Essential hypertension may alter with activity, illness and emotional stress. It is fluctuating and irregular. The more difficult type of essential hypertension to treat is the stable high systolic and diastolic blood pressure that remains benign but slowly and insidiously damaging over a period of years. A malignant type of hypertension is generally acute and capable of producing serious symptoms, e.g., arterial spasms in the brain causing transient paralysis, retinopathies, occlusion of retinal veins, blurring of vision, headaches, nose bleeding, middle ear involvement and occasional paresthesis. Zier (8) reviews the pathophysiology and clinical features of the hypertensive patient in podiatric practice.

Most patients under treatment for hypertension are being medicated with depressants of the sympathetic nervous system or with a combination of depressants and diuretics.

The podiatrist must be concerned with thiazide hyperuricemias resulting in increased blood uric acids in the medicated hypertensive patient. Surgical procedures should await consultation with the internist. Sodium loss from diuresis is often accompanied by potassium depletion. The serum electrolytes are imbalanced. Diet and potassium chemicals are to be adjusted to a normal physiological balance. Periodic laboratory studies of BUN and creatinine are indicated. Renal function tests, serum cholesterol and triglyceride evaluations are mandatory. Chest radiographs, EKGs and stress tests are desirable before surgical intervention.

Chest expansion upon inspiration should be equal and symmetrical on both sides. Normal respiratory rate is 12–16 inhalations/exhalations per minute. Altered breathing patterns suggest an oxygen-carbon dioxide imbalance. Auscultation and percussion may reveal rales or rhonchi, cardiac murmurs, bruits or thrills. Bruits are the sounds heard in distant arteries as a result of cardiac murmurs as well as arterial lesions. A palpable arterial tremor or vibration may be heard on auscultation of a blood vessel as a thrill. Positive findings may indicate pleural congestion and the possibility of pneumonia (9).

Enlargement of the finger tips and ends of toes in bulbous fashion may suggest cardiopulmonary disorders. Generalized color changes of the skin and toe nails, especially cyanosis, should be investigated.

Examination of the heart for enlargement, precordial heave, atrial gallop, murmurs and arrhythmias can be diagnostically helpful.

All lower-extremity pulses should be evaluated by palpation and graded from 0 to 4 according to the strength of the pulse beat. Femoral, popliteal, posterior tibial, and dorsalis pedis pulses should be equal and symmetrical (9). Doppler, oscillometric, and/or plethysmographic studies may be helpful (10).

The podiatric surgeon, who generally performs elective surgery for the correction of disabling deformities, must evaluate his or her decisions in the light of their value to the general well-being of the patient. Complications are not uncommon in the presence of chronic pulmonary disorders.

A good history and evaluation of obvious symptoms secondary to smoking and respiratory difficulties are meaningful in the preoperative study of the patient. A chronic cough, tuberculosis, asthma, emphysema and a history of pleurisy, pneumonia, bronchiectasis, atelectasis and chest surgery should be critically reviewed. When a history of cardiac pathology is elicited or in the presence of neurological disorders, consultation is necessary to rule out altered pulmonary function. Chest radiographs are often indicated on the hospital scene with or without symptoms, and they are advisable in approaching extensive bone surgery for patients over age 30.

The examiner must have a keen sense of responsibility toward the patient. The podiatrist's ability to observe through use of all his or her senses will be reflected in the successful treatment of the patient's symptoms. A good rule to follow is to allow several minutes of examination for each minute of treatment.

In examining the patient's cardiovascular and respiratory systems, the podiatrist has the responsibility not to complicate existing problems and to refer patients to a specialist in internal medicine or family practice for treatment of systemic disorders.

GI (Gastrointestinal)

The abdomen is examined for bruits, tenderness, masses, palpable indurated liver and enlargement of the kidneys.

Assuming that the patient has or will have a careful examination of the extremities from the hips down for biomechanical, circulatory and neurological problems, the podiatrist prescribing medication or performing surgery can feel secure in knowing that his or her patient has been evaluated properly. Obviously laboratory studies are indicated before initiating treatment. Along with standard chemical and microscopic testing of the blood and urine, the podiatrist may want to order chest radiographs and an EKG to complete the examination. Whenever a systemic abnormality is noted, the podiatrist is urged to seek competent medical consultation.

Durkin (11) notes the problems attendant to patients who have been receiving steroids before surgery. He advises careful consideration of "any history of treatment with corticosteroids during the previous twelve months." If the patient receiving corticosteroids complains of fatigue, weakness and excitability, the podiatrist must assume the presence of adrenal cortex suppression. Consultation with a qualified medical specialist prior to surgery is indicated. It may be necessary to provide a corticosteroid supportive dose 24 hr before surgery and postoperatively for 48 hr with a gradual lowering of the dose to a maintenance level. Prevention of circulatory collapse is mandatory. The trauma of surgery in these patients may produce a precipitous lowering of the blood pressure, rapid pulse and a loss of consciousness resulting in death. The steroids may cause catabolic disorders involving skin, muscle and bone. Blood dyscrasias are common. Physiological dysfunctions are often masked. A variety of systemic illnesses such as atrophy, diabetes mellitus, retention of fluids and bleeding disorders in abdominal organs and the skin, are not uncommon. Symptoms of early onset of infection may also be masked. Increased difficulty in handling infections is a secondary problem requiring early consultation.

INTEG (Skin and Nail)

Abnormal changes in skin color often occur in occlusive vascular disease and must be differentiated from vitiligo and other disorders of the skin (Fig. 2.6).

Metabolic and endocrine conditions must be considered. Bilateral color differences in extremities and toes are very significant. A normal extremity demonstrates pallor on elevation with rapid return to normal on dependency.

Erlick et al. (12) describes an interesting dermatoglyphic predictive index for maturity-onset diabetes mellitus. A diagnostic test (81% specific) for diabetes based on correlation coefficients reveals that diabetics possess more large loops on their second fingertips than do nondiabetic patients.

A marked rubor on dependency with cyanosis occurring usually below the ankle and affecting an entire foot or part of the foot is indicative of chronic arterial insufficiency (Fig. 2.7). Edema, redness and heat may occur with anidrosis after a too-rapid warming of cold feet. Lividity of the toes is common in healthy persons after exposure to cold.

Neurocirculatory asthenia, which occurs after pronounced effort in work or athletic endeavors, may result in a livid, cyanotic skin surface with coldness of the extremities. This same change is noted in immersion foot, trench foot and shelter foot. Small widely spaced cyanotic patches may develop. A vivid red or yellowish-blue to black color may result.

Reddish or red-blue discoloration is a more or less normal change in the skin of

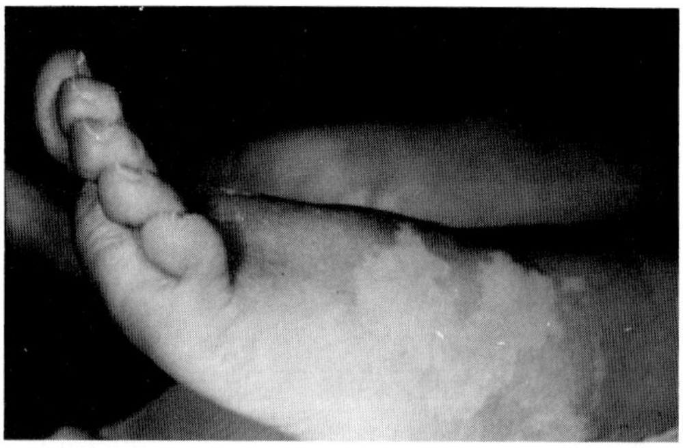

Figure 2.6. Vitiligo. Must be differentiated from circulatory disorders that produce pallor in the extremities.

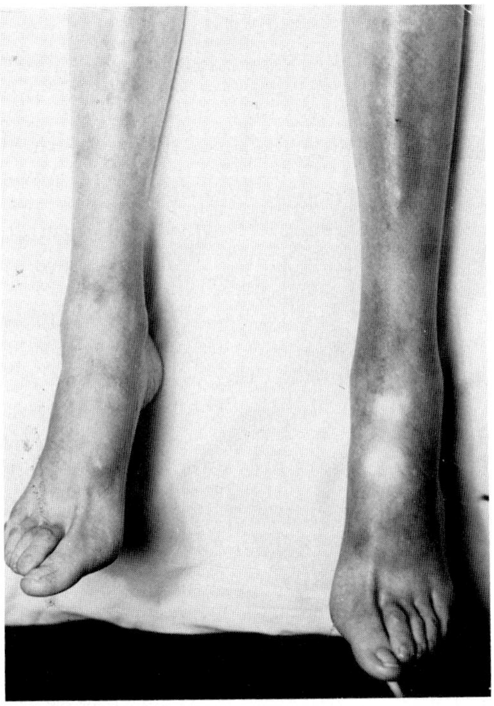

Figure 2.7. Marked rubor with blanching on digital pressure. (Courtesy of D Mowbray.)

aging persons. When it occurs in younger people it is significant of some constitutional disturbance, such as acrocyanosis, Raynaud's disease or livedo reticularis. Majocchi's disease is characterized by minute, sharply defined, rose or red to purple macules.

Slow return of blood following a blanching of the skin by pressure also suggests an imperfect blood supply requiring further study. Ischemic neuritis may produce this change. Michota developed a technique for photographing the plantar surface on weightbearing. The patient stands on a box with a heavy plate of glass or Plexiglas top. The impression created by the superimposed weight can be viewed through a large mirror tipped to 48° within the box. (Michota, personal communication, 1972).

A marble white pallor with numbness, stiffness and pain is seen early in Raynaud's disease. A local asphyxia and subsequent ulcerations and gangrene of the digits are the sequelae to this vasomotor instability. A sympathectomy or vasodilator drug may alter the pathology.

Angioneurotic edema may result in large multiple swellings of the skin varying in color from a flesh pink to dark purple. It commonly involves the tissue on the medial, dorsal and lateral aspects of the feet. Antihistamine medications by the oral route can reduce the edema. If acute, intravenous injections of minimal doses of a steroid can be lifesaving.

Redness may occur from ingestion of certain sensitizing foods or medications. Treatment consists of eliminating the sensitizing agents. The use of antihistamines may be necessary.

Elevated, itchy lesions of pink to red color may occur on the sides and dorsum of the feet and backs of the hands in granuloma annulare. The lesion measures about 5 mm and is often clear in the center. Corticosteroid topical applications should relieve symptoms of itching.

Doughy, infiltrated areas or collections of many firm bean-sized, reddish-brown or purplish nodules may be an early indication of Kaposi's sarcoma.

Erythematous lesions are seen in many eczemas and in contact dermatitis caused by shoe polish, shoe dye, sock lining dye, leather, nylon hose and leg make-up. Contact dermatitis is a reaction of the skin to chemical or vegetable irritants applied externally (Fig. 2.8). A patch test often determines the irritant. Removing the irritant and using medication to allay pruritus provide relief of symptoms.

Superficial reactions to extremes of temperature, such as a burn or frostbite, cause notable color changes. Cold and damp-

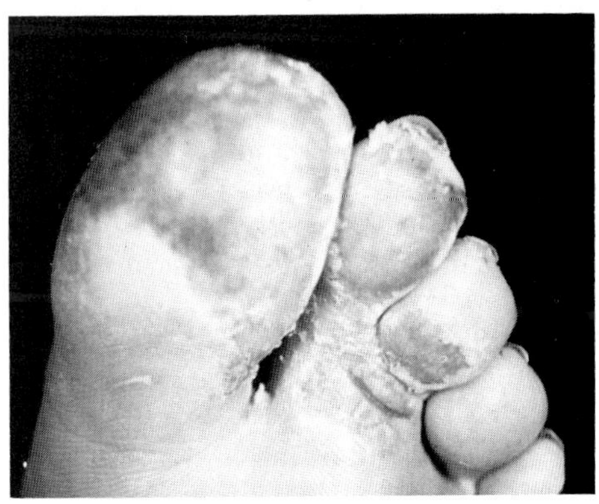

Figure 2.8. Contact dermatitis. Denuding of skin on plantar of toes is subject to secondary infection.

ness affect the local vasomotor system. A livid bluish-red color with a cushion-like swelling is the usual end result of cold and dampness; deep fissures and bullae are common associated findings. Radiant energy causes a persistent reticulated, pigmented erythema.

Colored, reddish-brown spots may be the result of the involution of indurated symmetrical cutaneous nodules in undernourished young females. They may be of tuberculous origin and the sequelae of erythema induratum. A complete physical examination by an internist is necessary. Treatment includes improved dietary habits and rest.

Ill-fitting shoes and hose may cause a redness between the fourth and fifth toes in the form of an erythema intertrigo. This condition may be alleviated by wearing correct footgear and using a mild powder to relieve chafing.

Bright red, shiny, painful nodes that are firm, elastic, oval and tense occurring in groups on the anterior aspect of the lower third of the leg may indicate erythema nodosum. They subside gradually and leave a dark red and purple discoloration followed by green or brown stains. Early use of ice bags, bedrest and elevation of the legs are indicated. Supplementary diets are necessary. The nodular lesions do not disappear readily.

Dry, scaly, imbricated, silvery scales covering red patches on the extensor surfaces of the body are indicative of psoriasis (Fig. 2.9). The thickened nails are dry, powdery, gray, yellow-brown in color, and the plate is punctate and eroded. Annointing the skin with an oil or cream, such as

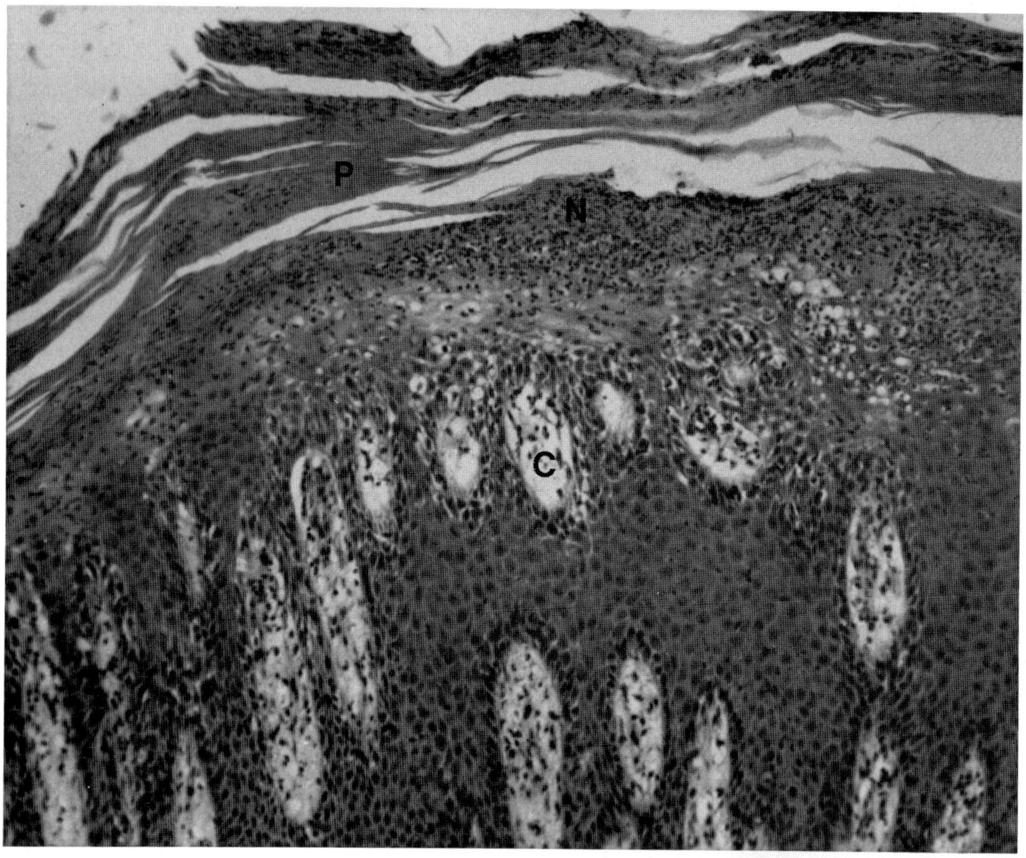

Figure 2.9. Psoriasis. Parakeratosis is noted throughout the epidermis (*P*). Collections of neutrophils are present in the lower stratum corneum (*N*). The capillaries in the dermal papillae are dilated (*C*). (100x). (Courtesy of Martin Port, MS, DPM, Veterans Administration Center, Martinsburg, W.Va.)

lanolin and cocoa butter, helps remove scales. Inflammatory changes are reduced with triamcinolone acetonide cream or hydrocortisone cream ½%. Nails are ground down, and the nail grooves are curetted out. Concomitant mycotic infections of the nails are treated by local or oral medication.

Purpuric changes brought about by escape of whole blood into the tissues producing petechiae or larger ecchymoses must be evaluated. Purpura simplex may be caused by a violent strain, such as cough or fright. Henoch's purpura may be an allergic manifestation, whereas a purpura hemorrhagica is characterized by a decrease in the number of blood platelets. Secondary purpuras may occur after acute infections and venous stasis. Careful blood studies are made to determine the cause of purpura. Purpuric lesions are best treated by good nourishment and plenty of bedrest (Fig. 2.10).

Red papules the size of a pinhead, and masses of capillary dilations covered by purplish to black hyperkeratotic caps may be an angiokeratoma resulting from trauma (Fig. 2.11). Surgical excision of the red papules is indicated.

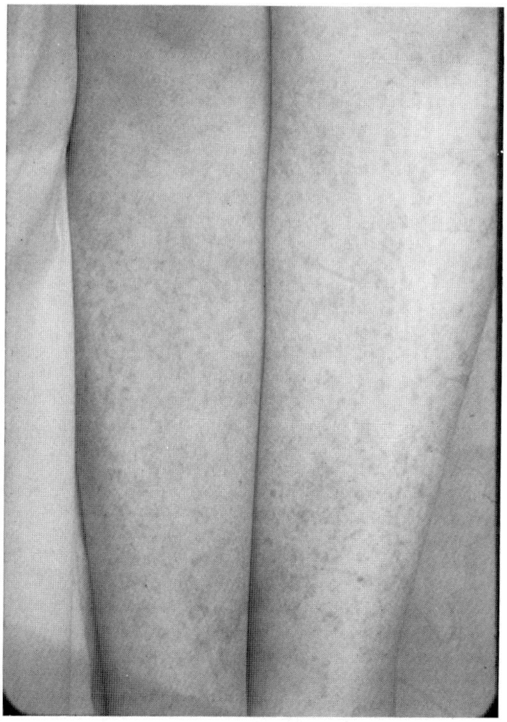

Figure 2.10. Purpura secondary to sulfanilamide.

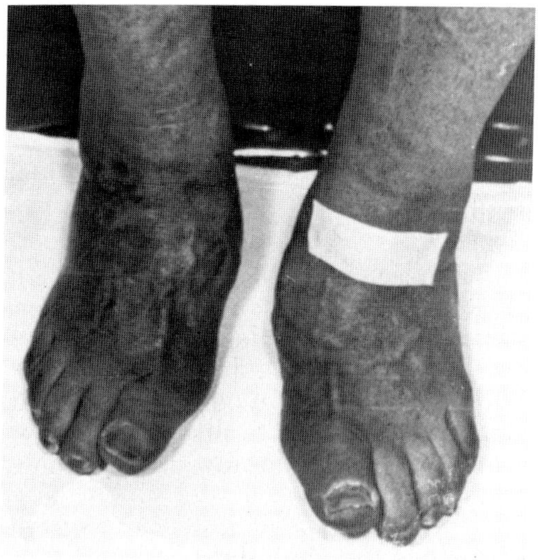

Figure 2.11. Pes planus, complicating edema, venous congestion, extensive pigmentation from fragility of capillaries—must be differentiated from angiokeratoma.

An erythema may result from occupational stress. Infection of unknown etiology may cause an erythema multiforme, which is characterized by macular, papular or vesicular lesions of bright or dark red color fading to a purplish or violaceous hue. Rest is the treatment of choice. If an infection is located, treatment depends on the location and the type of bacteria involved.

Whenever a nonspecific redness develops, the examiner must look for the possibility of a feigned irritation. Light pink, shiny plaques of angled papules with flat tops may be the result of a "stone wall worry." The papules may be caused by lichen planus, which is often seen about the ankles, soles and dorsum of the feet.

Bilateral and symmetrical plaques ranging from light to dark purple with thickening of the skin and crosspatching sometimes occur in neurodermatitis and hypopituitarism. Jaundiced individuals may present characteristic yellow color changes accompanied by severe itching.

Pallor is more significant when it only affects one foot, and when it is associated with other symptoms of vascular disease, one may look for an arterial degeneration.

Blanching can be interpreted as a diminution of blood supply to the part. Anemic individuals may have marked pallor bilaterally and symmetrically. Blood transfusions and removal of all constricting devices are helpful. Vasodilators improve peripheral circulation.

Cyanosis is due to changes in the blood of the cutaneous capillaries that are caused by an inadequately oxygenated hemoglobin. Cyanosis is very often evident in patients with impending gangrene, and a mixture of venous and arterial blood may cause it. It is usually indicative of occlusive vascular disease and is sometimes found in loss of tone in the vasomotor system. It is not only indicative of faulty blood flow but also of pathological changes in the walls of the vessels. The great toe is a common site for early cyanosis. Low-grade inflammations may produce cyanosis. Cardiac and pulmonary insufficiency may also produce cyanosis.

Constant discoloration and cyanosis distal to the ankles may indicate acrocyanosis and may occur in Raynaud's disease following color changes of that condition. A bluish-red mottling of the skin of the feet and legs known as "livedo reticularis" is present in Raynaud's disease. The mottling often extends proximally to involve the entire lower extremity and abdomen. The color changes are aggravated by cold, and ulcerations often develop at the sites of great pressure. Persistent cyanosis of an individual toe may be a manifestation of thrombosis in the distal arteries.

Vasomotor stimulators or dilators improve the functional capacity of the patient. Anticlotting medication may improve the cyanosis and prevent gangrene. Often an injection about the posterior tibial artery as it lies behind the medial malleolus provides a means of relaxing arterial spasms, as in a sympathectomy. The patient should dress warmly and avoid cold weather.

Pallor and coldness, or acroasphyxia, of the fingers and toes may occur after exposure to cold and are pathognomonic for Raynaud's disease. The color changes vary from pallor to redness and the temperature from cold to hot where acroasphyxia exists. Vasodilators are helpful in relieving discomfort and altering the spasm.

In thromboangiitis obliterans it is not the temperature but the posture of the limb that causes color changes in an entire foot. In erythromelalgia heat aggravates the degree of redness, which is relieved by cold. Pulses are generally strong and bounding. There is no tendency to gangrene as in acroasphyxia caused by Raynaud's and the obliterating diseases.

Erythema is not significant of heat or increased blood supply to the part, but results from a vasodilation from any number of causes. The minute vessels are constricted when the part is cold and dilated when hot. When it is warm and red, inflammatory changes and drug reactions are suspected.

Redness characterized by streaking or hyperemia may result from a lymphangitis. In localized severe cases, a suppurative and phlegmonous inflammation may precede gangrene. The looseness of the subcutaneous tissue on the dorsum of the foot is conducive to edema. The toes, dorsum and lateral aspect of the foot are readily affected, whereas the overhanging type of swelling on the medial aspect gives an appearance of pronation. The popliteal and inguinal glands may be tender and palpable. Lymphangitis may occur with infection, e.g., from a small puncture wound, subonychial infection, interdigital fissures, infected helomas and fungus infections of the toes.

An erythematous, butterfly-shaped area suggests systemic lupus erythematosus (Figs. 2.12 and 2.13).

Skin redness about the toes occurs when arterial circulation is slightly impaired. The discoloration may persist on elevation, although pallor is more consistent with arterial disease. An irregular reddish-brown discoloration of hemorrhagic extravasation in the skin or beneath the skin may be associated with capillary fragility. An angioneurosis, vasomotor imbalance, neurasthenia or erythromelalgia may be the cause for marked redness, for a burning throbbing engorgement of the veins and for edema in anxious and neurotic patients. Vasodilators, psycho-

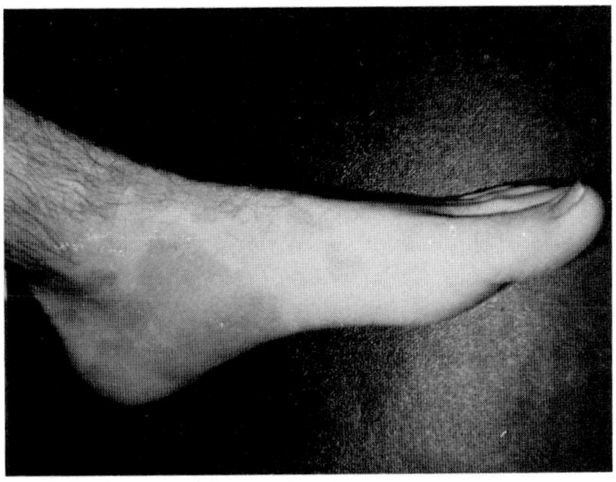

Figure 2.12. Lupus erythematosus. Note butterfly-shaped lesions. Pattern must not be confused with extensive hyperidrosis or with lack of pigment as seen in vitiligo.

therapeutic medications, sympathectomy and ingestion of vitamins C and K may be helpful. In the presence of infection, the proper antibiotics are mandatory.

Redding (13) defines erythromelalgia as a clinical entity characterized by local redness, warmth and burning pain in the distal ends of the extremities. He reports on two cases with myeloproliferative disease. Abnormally rapid platelet aggregation appears to be an etiologic factor that occludes the arteriole with thrombi. Heparin sodium and acetosalicylic acid have a pronounced effect as antiplatelet aggregating drugs. When the myeloproliferative disease is controlled, the erythromelalgia symptoms subside.

Erythema induratum is characterized by bluish-red, deep-seated nodules in the subcutaneous tissues. The nodules range in size from 1 to 6 mm and occur any place on the legs but most commonly on the posterior calf. The painful nodules ulcerate and heal slowly, leaving the surrounding tissues indurated, and a pitted, pigmented scar may remain. Corticosteroids relieve the inflammation, but the patient requires good dietary habits and plenty of rest.

Lesions of any type found on the legs or feet may help identify underlying vascular conditions. The characteristic appearances of a sinus, ulceration, dermatologic irritation, dilated veins, abnormal nails and swelling are symptomatic of various underlying conditions.

Rose spots must not be confused with dermatologic lesions of local etiology or systemic origin. Chronic venous insufficiency is seen about the ankles and is accompanied by light brown, gray to black pigmentation of the skin. Small, painless, pinkish spots on the legs or the dorsum of the foot remain for several weeks. They ultimately become dark and pigmented. Rose spots are found in diabetic patients and indicate an active process taking place in the smaller vessels. These must be differentiated from phlebitic skin lesions. Fragility of minute superficial blood vessels may result in subcutaneous hemorrhage and rose spots. Treatment of the underlying pathology is imperative. Subcutaneous hemorrhage is relieved by corticosteroids and administration of vitamins B_{12} and C.

Glossy skin produced by atrophoderma neuroticum may be secondary to neuritis, following severe trauma, disease of the spinal cord, gout or arthritis. deTakats (14) has reported several cases in which the vascular supply to the sciatic nerve was affected. Vasomotor phenomena, trophic changes and causalgia are prominent. The skin becomes bluish, glossy and eczematous, and a grayness may develop resembling an atrophic scar. Skin texture is affected by contact dermatitis.

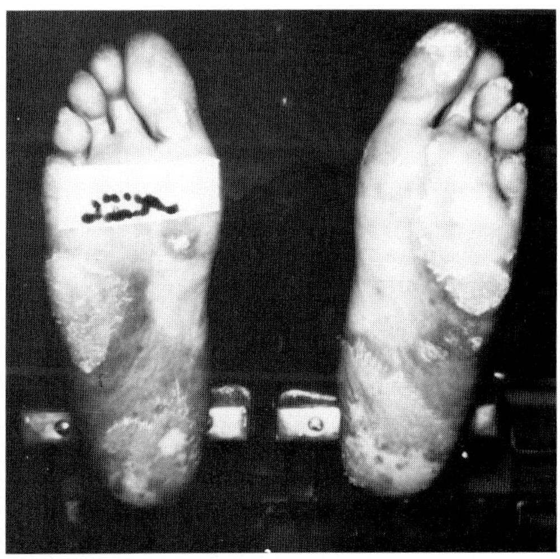

Figure 2.13. Acute discoid lupus erythematosus.

The temperature of the surface of the skin varies with environmental temperature, temperature of the body and with conditions of the skin and subcutaneous tissues. The temperature of the skin surface on the trunk varies between 92.3 and 98.4°F (33.5 and 36.9°C.). Symmetrical parts normally have identical temperature.

Temperature of the foot may be determined by placing the hand on the patient's foot or by using a thermocouple or skin thermometer for exact temperature. If both feet are above or below normal foot temperature, a systemic condition may be responsible. A difference in temperature between the left and the right foot indicates a local disturbance, although some variations may be caused by a systemic disorder. Excessive heat in one foot generally indicates inflammation. Coldness denotes improper circulation or nerve involvement affecting the vasomotor system. Excessively cold foot sweats are found in nervous people. Excessive cold or hot foot sweats are found in faulty foot mechanics.

In a case report and discussion of malignant hyperthermia, Gronen and Roda (15) emphasize the need for early diagnosis and "prompt, aggressive treatment." They conclude that therapy must consider three major objectives: "(1) Lowering of metabolism and body temperature. This can be accomplished by external cooling and by administration of cool intravenous fluids and iced gastric lavage through a stomach tube. (2) Correction of acidemia and electrolyte imbalance and, (3) Supplying 100% oxygen for hyperventilation."

It is obvious that this medical emergency requires a well-trained and skillful staff. The high incidence of fatalities suggests the need for a good case history and careful preoperative examinations. A thorough knowledge of the heat regulatory mechanism and body metabolism is essential for early recognition and treatment.

Coldness may be due to room temperature and changes in environment. The examiner's hand must be warm to determine abnormal skin temperature. Such instruments as the skin thermometer and the electric thermocouple enable the podiatrist to measure skin temperature accurately. A drop in temperature with ischemia on elevation is observed in thromboangiitis obliterans. A bilateral lowering of temperature may result from a saddle embolus.

When a single digit is cold and pale the condition may be due to a vasospasm or some organic condition of the arteries. Pressure on the vessels in the lower abdomen by tumor mass or pregnancy may produce unilateral coldness. Exposure to cold may cause a vasospastic ischemia followed by dilation and cyanosis.

Increased temperature is not always found with burning of the feet. On the contrary, if the feet are burning, the temperature of the skin is lowered. Cellulitis and phlebitis should be excluded when warmth is present along the course of an extremity. A fever of the feet associated with deep redness is suggestive of erythromelalgia. Increase in temperature is a significant finding in infectious lesions. Atmospheric warmth may increase the temperature of the feet.

An increase in temperature may occur in furunculosis when an infection of a hair follicle or a sebaceous gland causes an extensive cellulitis terminating in pus formation. This may be due to a general debility, anemia or diabetes. *Staphylococcus aureus* may be the invading organism.

A carbuncle may develop secondary to furunculosis. Carbuncles have been seen on several occasions occurring over the dorsum of the first metatarsocuneiform joint caused by irritation from prominent eyelets. Bacterial sensitivity tests are done to help determine the necessary medication. Hot packs, incision, drainage, and appropriate antibiotic usually resolve the infection.

An increased temperature accompanied by anorexia and chills may develop with erysipelas. The skin may burn and itch. The affected area is elevated, indurated, firm, erythematous and sharply marginated. Rest, elevation of the infected limb and systemic antibiotic treatment are essential.

A pustular eczema with all signs of infection may occur secondary to fungus infections, varicose eczema, contact dermatitis or dermatitis medicamentosa. Pustular eczema is best treated with the medication of choice following a sensitivity test.

Acute high fevers with a chill and steplike increases in temperature may be the result of a febrile condition in which bacteria are present in the bloodstream producing systemic symptoms of infection. This septicemia may result secondary to infectious diseases. Predisposing factors are exposure to cold and wet, fatigue, loss of sleep, chronic disease and agents that lower resistance to infection. The bacteria may enter the bloodstream through the veins and lymphatics, with the most common source of infection being infected wounds, onychocryptosis, helomas and tylomas, phlegomons, carbuncles, bedsores and blisters. Osteomyelitis may be a sequela (Fig. 2.14).

The drug of choice is based on Gram's stain and culture and sensitivity tests. The proper antibiotic must be prescribed in large enough doses orally or parenterally over long periods of time. Blood cultures may be necessary.

Local inflammation or trauma raises skin temperature. Temperature is higher over an active part or over muscles and lower over tendons or bone. Muscular exercise increases temperature response. Removal of vasoconstrictor influence by general, spinal or local anesthesia causes a higher temperature response. Acute arthritis gives a higher response to skin surface temperature. Alcohol, thyroid and amyl nitrate raise temperature response.

For a fuller discussion of skin and nail disorders, see Chapter 6, Dermatologic and Toenail Disorders.

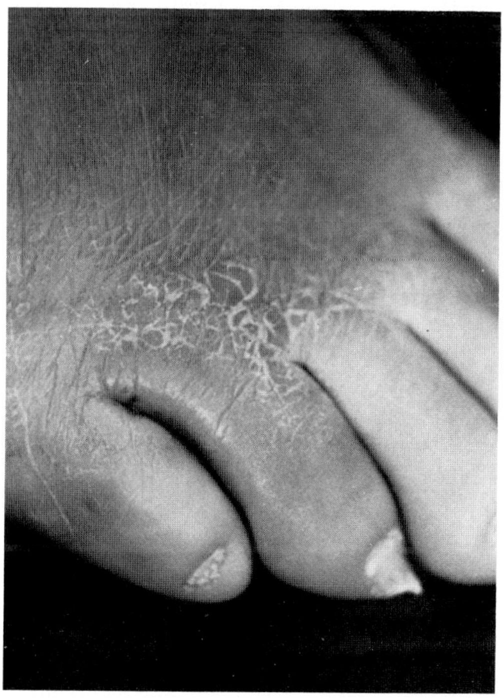

Figure 2.14. Infection of fourth and fifth toes. Note swelling, cellulitis, discoloration. Patient had inguinal lymphadenopathy.

CIRC (Circulation)

A useful practice is to grade arterial pulsations on the basis of an index of 0 to 4. *Zero* indicates complete absence of pulse; *1* indicates a marked impairment; *4* indicates normal pulsations. The examiner should not be confused by pseudopulsation in the form of pulsations from his or her own finger tip arteries.

The *pulse of the dorsalis pedis* may be felt by placing the second, third and fourth finger tips along the outer side of the extensor hallucis longus tendon behind the first metatarsal head (Fig. 2.15). Occasionally it is impalpable in normal patients, but this is often a sign of circulatory disturbances, especially if the dor-

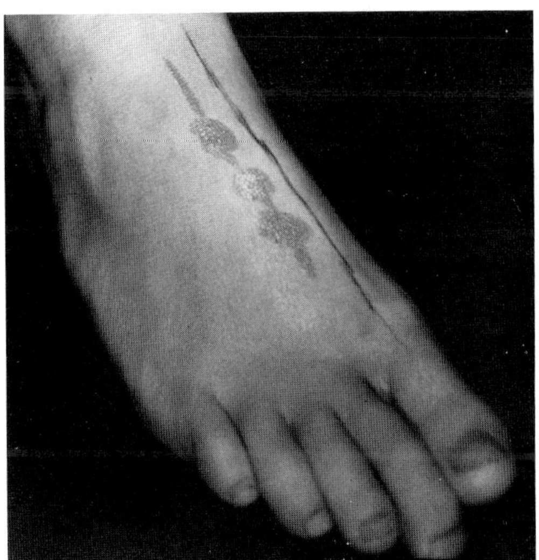

Figure 2.15. The dorsalis pedis pulse is palpated just lateral to the extensor hallucis longus tendon by placing the second, third and fourth fingers along the course of the dorsalis pedis artery.

salis pedis pulse is not present in older people.

In cases where faulty circulation is believed to be the cause of the symptoms, the patient should be referred to a specialist in circulatory diseases for consultation.

The *posterior tibial pulse* is located just distal to and slightly in back of the medial malleolus (Fig. 2.16). The patient should be seated when the podiatrist checks the posterior tibial pulse, which may be difficult to locate in obese patients.

The *popliteal pulse* is difficult to find, as it is palpated behind the knee in the popliteal space. With the patient prone, the examiner faces the patient's foot. The examiner's left hand holds the leg at the ankle in a relaxed position with slight flexion of the knee. The right hand is placed about the medial side of the extremity opposite the popliteal space, and the thumb or forefinger makes repeated pressures into the space to elicit the pulsation. This pulsation can also be palpated by the second and third fingers with the knees in slight flexion and often reveals embolic occlusion or early popliteal aneurysm.

Femoral pulse is felt below Poupart's ligament line in the groin. Normally, it is full and strong. It may be diminished in embolic or thrombotic conditions of the iliac vessels of which it is a branch. Pressure is applied with the tips of the second, third and fourth fingers in a line transverse and oblique to the axis of the limb.

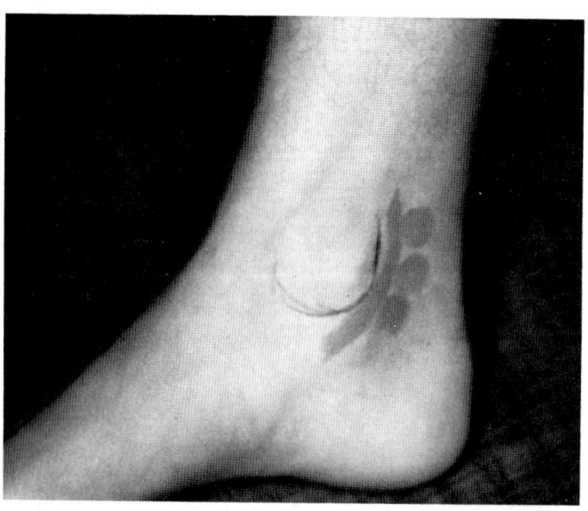

Figure 2.16. The posterior tibial pulse, which is palpated posterior to the medial malleolus.

Blood pressures in the upper and lower extremity are about equal in functional aortic insufficiency. In organic aortic insufficiency the systolic pressure in the lower extremity is from 50 to 100 mm Hg or higher than in the upper extremity. In coarctation of the aorta the blood pressure is higher in the arm than in the lower extremity. Absence of pulsations is common in thromboangiitis obliterans.

Scars that are not produced by trauma or infection may be found in individuals with impaired peripheral circulation. Small, pigmented scars that appear to be oval and punched out beneath the skin are commonly found in diabetic patients. The larger scars found usually on the crest or soft parts about the tibia, if not due to trauma, are possibly arteriosclerotic or caused by syphilis. Massive keloids may occur in blacks following surgery, lacerations or trauma. Total excision of the scar is helpful. Destruction by chemosurgical methods is desirable.

When occurring in the diabetic, blebs or bullae appear overnight without any history of injury, thermal or mechanical. Within 24 hrs the diabetic bleb becomes white and colorless. In 48 hrs the diabetic bleb fluid content becomes purple and discolored. Then, the base may become gangrenous. Most gangrene starts with bleb formation due to a change in the arteries. Blebs may occur with eczematous lesions, allergic reactions and idiosyncrasies.

Blebs must be kept clean and redressed daily. If the patient is diabetic, the lesions should be allowed to recede. Tepid soaks in 1 qt warm water and a tablespoonful of table salt are effective in providing a natural media for resolution.

The essentials of treatment are a minimum of medication, cleanliness and aseptic dressings. Bullous lesions may be caused by fungus infections, sunburn, neurodermatitis, thermal damage and separation of the dermal-epidermal juncture (Figs. 2.17–2.19). Fluid is present as a result of such skin disorders, and it accumulates by osmosis resulting from destruction of the cells.

Opening of a blister should be performed only under strict asepsis. Many podiatrists believe that the bullous lesion

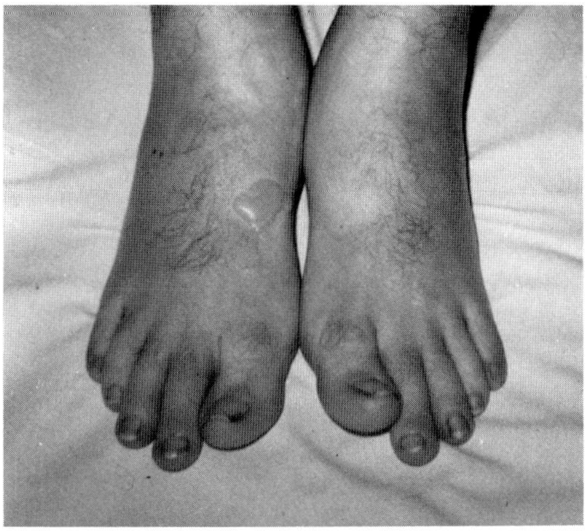

Figure 2.17. Bullous lesion. Large bulla, dorsum right foot secondary to friction.

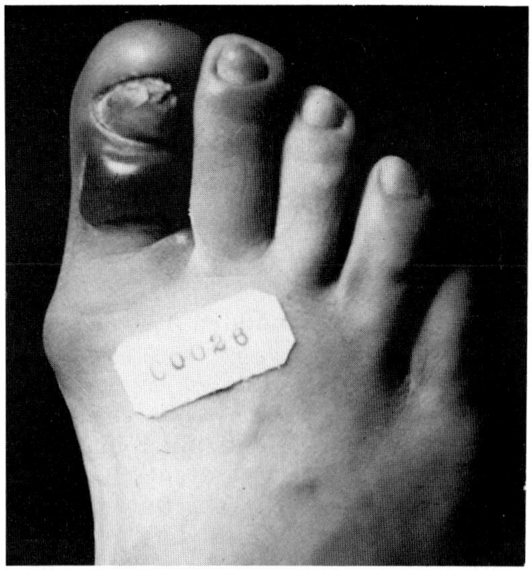

Figure 2.19. Large bulla dorsum hallux overlying eponychium.

should not be opened; however, the author prefers to remove the top of a large bleb to facilitate drainage using saline soaks to dry the base. Small blebs generally dry up with proper medication to limit inflammatory changes.

It is inadvisable to remove the top of the blister within 48 hrs of its appearance because of the marked increase in pain and susceptibility to infection. According to Cortese (16), "multiple aspiration of the blister fluid during the first 24 hrs or a single aspiration between 24 and 36 hrs is the optimal early management procedure."

Potassium permanganate soaks, aluminum subacetate and other astringent agents are helpful. In the presence of severe dermatoses, the use of oral corticosteroids in gradually decreasing dosages aids in resolution of the problem.

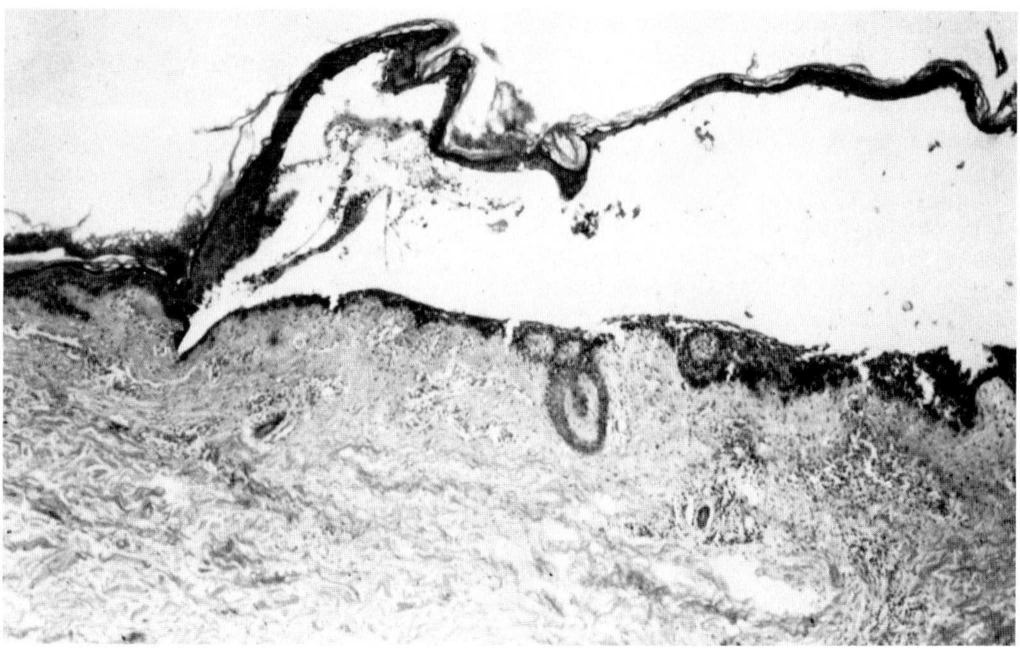

Figure 2.18. Photomicrograph of a bullous lesion. Note both acute and chronic inflammation.

Trophic changes of the skin should be noted. Palpation may detect scleroderma with taut skin and atrophy of underlying tissues. Ulceration between the toes may be an early trophic disturbance in thromboangiitis obliterans.

Nodules when palpated may be indicative of periarteritis nodosa, cysts or tumors, keratosis blennorrhagica, erythema induratum, lupus vulgaris, tertiary syphilis, acute rheumatoid arthritis, erythema nodosum or fibroma.

Pain on palpation, together with such symptoms as a fever and swelling, may establish a diagnosis of phlebitis. When the deep veins are involved one cannot palpate the vessels. However, the superficial veins can be felt as hot, indurated, cord-like structures along the normal course of the venous anatomy. Transitory phlebitis is often associated with thromboangiitis obliterans.

Impaired circulation disturbs the growth and appearance of the nails. The nails of elderly people and arteriosclerotic and diabetic patients become chalky, discolored, hypertrophied and slow growing.

The posterior tibial and dorsalis pedis arteries, when sclerosed, can sometimes be palpated. However, the fact that one vessel is hardened does not mean that all vessels are affected, that circulation is poor or that an occlusive vascular disorder is present. The necessary volume of blood may still be present to give a normal oscillometric index. A radiograph often presents many calcifications without subjective or objective symptoms.

Tenderness is present along the veins in acute or subacute phlebitis. When it is present around arteries, one must consider periarteritis nodosa as a possible diagnosis. Prominent joints may present tender bursae, and plantar fascia is often tender from inflammatory changes and strain. Frequent bathing of feet in strong antiseptic solutions causes tenderness of the skin and subcutaneous structures.

Enlarged lymph glands are due to infections in the extremities; general disease may cause swelling of all the glands. The inguinal and popliteal glands are usually inflamed and palpable when the foot is infected. A rapidly developing bright red nodule attaining full size in from 1–7 days often is noted around the nail grooves or lips. The lesion is soft and bleeds easily. It is usually caused by a staphylococcus infection of low virulence but one which is capable of causing swelling of the lymph glands in the extremities.

Lymphangitis and palpable lymph glands may be found in pustular eruptions on the feet. The sequence of infection, cellulitis, lymphangitis and lymphadenopathy is characteristic.

For a fuller description of circulatory problems, see Chapter 4, Circulatory Disorders.

NEUR (Neurological)

Deep and superficial reflexes must be evaluated. Deep patellar, Achilles, and extensor digitorum brevis (EDB) tendon reflexes are tested for reactivity and are compared bilaterally. The superficial plantar reflex is elicited. Patellar and ankle clonus are noted. Discriminative, touch, and vibratory sensation are tested (see Chapter 5, Neurological Disorders).

A generalized muscular rigidity, especially in the flexor groups, may occur in parkinsonism. This slow and progressive disease most frequently affects males over 40. The rigidity of the arms, legs, neck and back produces the characteristic stooping or hyperextended posture. The fingers and thumb pat each other in typical pill-rolling fashion. A falling forward gait and waxen masked facial expression are characteristic of this disease.

In multiple sclerosis, a disordered gait and postural instability are prominent symptoms, along with fatigue, an increase of deep reflexes, nystagmus, ataxic upper extremities, scanning speech, uncontrolled emotionalism, vague sensory disorders and remissions. Compensatory involuntary contractions of the extensor tendons may cause an abnormal high arch with pronation to maintain postural stability.

MUSC/SKEL/BIOMECH (Musculo-Skeletal and Biomechanical)

Feet should be measured for length and width because both feet are rarely alike in size and a great difference in size must be accommodated. When paralysis is present, one leg shows less circumference through the calf than the other. Shortage of one extremity may produce painful symptoms in the knee, hip or back.

A posture chart is blocked off with vertical and horizontal parallel lines. The patient stands erect and the position of shoulders, hips, knees and malleoli are noted in relation to the lines on the chart. Normally a plumb line dropped from the middle of the patella passes through the middle of the talus about 2 to 4 cm in front of the ankle and at a point midway between the base of the first and second metatarsals.

In hemiplegia alterans, the involvement of the pyramidal tract creates weakness and imbalance. The paralyzed limb may drop down, the toes may dorsiflex and the extensor tendons may contract. Tylomas usually develop under the head of the first metatarsal, and the paralyzed foot is cold to the touch.

An extremity may be longer, shorter and/or overdeveloped or atrophied as a result of disease, abnormal growth, trauma or mechanical dysfunction. When viewed from the front with the posture chart as a background, the standing patient, with limb length inequality presents one shoulder at a lower level than the other while the pelvis presents a tilt or shift. One patella may be lower than the other, and one elbow or arm may be closer to the body than the other elbow. Examination from the rear of the standing patient, with a lower extremity shortage, may reveal scoliosis. The inferior angles of the scapula are in different planes, and the gluteofemoral fold may be at a higher level on one side. The shoe on the short side shows overriding of the upper to the outside and excessive wear at the outer aspect of the heel. In the supine position measurements taken from the anterior superior iliac spine to the lower tip of the medial malleolus disclose the actual shortage of the affected limb. Note the position of the gluteal and inguinal folds for asymmetry.

1. Asymmetry of folds, gluteal and popliteal—abduction or adduction.
2. Shortened extremity on affected side—subluxation, dislocation, Legg Perthes disease, tumor, infection, muscle spasm, congenital ligamentous defect, mimickry and synovitis secondary to rheumatoid arthritis (Fig 2.20).
3. Ortolani's sign–audible and palpable click in an infant when hip is dislocated by adduction and forcibly reduced by abduction.
4. Instability of hip—check by relaxing flexor musculature and exerting thumb pressure on the hip into abduction; if the femoral head moves with pressure on the lesser trochanter the joint may be unstable.

Low back pain may be secondary to several factors. Local pathology involving the vertebral column is most prevalent. Postural instabilities secondary to stress on muscles, ligaments and intervertebral articulations resulting in structural and functional abnormalities may be aggravated by postural foot pathomechanics. Direct bone pathology and local or systemic disease are important factors to consider.

Many investigators discuss the short leg syndrome, but fail to appreciate the etiologic basis for the discomfort in the

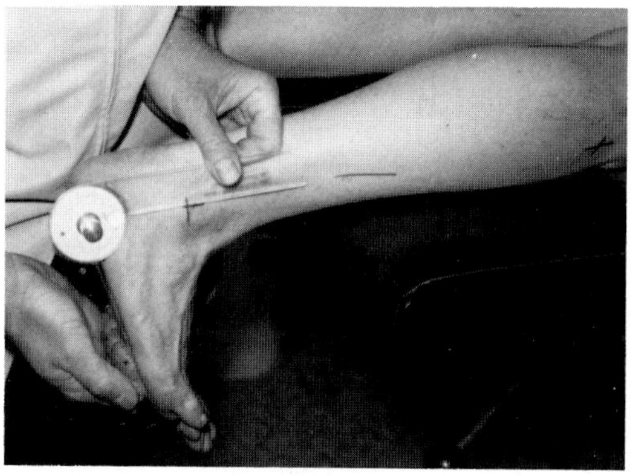

Figure 2.20. With the knee in the extended position, the tractograph is used to measure ankle joint dorsiflexion. Some practitioners become adept enough to use this instrument for most basic measurements. Marks have been made on the fibular head and fibular malleolus. The foot is dorsiflexed with the subtalar joint in a neutral position. One arm of the tractograph is held on the plantar surface and the other arm on the lateral fibular line. A 10° range of dorsiflexion is required for normal function. If 10° is not available, an equinus condition should be considered. (Courtesy of Burns Podiatric Laboratory.)

lower back. Too often the inequality of limbs is due to a lower back problem.

In the midstance phase of gait, it is imperative that the posterior musculature be of proper length. Short iliapsoas, gastrocsoleus and hamstring muscles produce knee flexion. About 10° of dorsiflexion of the foot is necessary with the knee fully extended in the gait cycle. When the knee is flexed, the amount of foot dorsiflexion is inversely proportionate to the degrees of knee flexion. Dorsiflexion of the foot generally presents an adduction, plantar flexion and forward movement of the talus in its saggital plane. The subtalar joint is in pronation, and the closed chain produces an anterior tilt of the pelvis, causing an increased lumbar lordosis. Muscle strain in the lower back is a common sequela to the pathomechanical stress in the foot. Podiatrists have been successful in relieving low back pain and knee chondromalacia in athletes by improving rearfoot structure and function.

The position of an epidermal excrescence is a good sign of the underlying bone deformity present and indicates improper footgear and poorly functioning feet. Tylomas along the inner borders of the heel and the great toe may be symptoms of an excessively pronating foot, whereas a heloma on the fifth toe denotes narrow shoes, pointed shoes or shoes with an improper last. On palpatation of the talonavicular joint, first metatarsocuneiform, cuboid and metatarsophalangeal joints, mild pressure will cause pain in pronatory foot conditions, arthritic changes and traumatic lesions. In biomechanical disorders of the joints, the foot may be painful on weightbearing and in motion. This condition should not be confused with infectious arthritis, rheumatoid arthritis or osteoarthritis.

The range of motion at ankle, midtarsal and metatarsophalangeal joints should be tested both actively and passively for any limitations present.

The examiner should test the anterior group of muscles for their ability to dorsiflex against resistance, the posterior group for plantar flexion against resistance, and the toes for both dorsiflexion and plantar flexion against resistance.

The calf muscles are shortened if the feet cannot be dorsally flexed more than at right angles to the leg. A shortened calf muscle is common to talipes plantaris. A pulling sensation is felt behind the straight knee when the foot is dorsiflexed on the ankle. An inability to dorsiflex may also result from a bony block.

Crepitation on movement of a joint may suggest an osteoarthritis with rubbing of spicules of bone at the joint margins. It may also be due to a tendon riding over bone. Destruction of cartilage in rheumatoid arthritis also causes crepitus. Crepitation is also felt in a tenosynovitis due to trauma or infection.

Palpation of the medial tubercle on the plantar surface of the calcaneus elicits pain in the presence of a calcaneal spur or bursa. A periostitis often causes tenderness on palpation at the medial and lateral aspects of the calcaneus.

Infection may cause pain on palpation of the plantar surface of the heel at the origin of the plantar fascia, on palpation of the medial and lateral aspects of the heel, and on palpation at the lower third of the tendo achilles before it inserts into the midportion of the posterior surface of the calcaneus.

Bursae found anterior to the tendo achilles between the bone and the tendon are painful and swollen when palpated during an acute inflammatory change. Bursae over the Achilles tendon between the tendon and the skin show the same signs with more edema when inflamed. Children may complain of apophyseal pain before firm union of the apophysis with the body of the calcaneus.

One of the first signs of muscle and nerve degeneration is loss of function and atrophy of the affected muscles. Atrophy, which is sometimes obscured by the subcutaneous fat, is a wasting disorder characterized by a loss of physiological function, organic substance and gross integrity. Podiatrists must utilize their powers of observation and palpation and their knowledge of abnormal muscle function and nerve reflexes to interpret atrophic changes.

Disuse of a part having a limited function results in atrophy. Limited use may be the result of a mechanical disorder that occurs from constrictive footgear, occupational stress or lack of stress, foot compensatory changes to faulty body posture, disease and paralysis.

Direct disease of the muscle itself or of the nerve tissue supplying the musculature also results in atrophy. This type of atrophy, if due to lower motor neuron disease, shows a reaction of degeneration to galvanic stimulation. Not only does atrophy affect soft tissues, but it is also seen in bone. It often indicates a lesion in the anterior horn of the spinal cord or in the central or peripheral nervous system. Peripheral nerve lesions may be a cause of atrophy.

Muscle Training Tests Joint mobility and muscle power should be tested by the use of the *goniometer.* This device, which is accurately gauged to measure angles, should be used to check the mobility of the joints of the foot and ankle in flexion, extension, inversion, eversion, adduction and abduction. The function of the joints to some extent shows the power of the foot musculature if evaluated with caution.

Toe Flexion. The patient lies on his or her back and bends the toes toward the sole of the foot. This is done both with resistance and with the foot steady and also without resistance. The examiner places a finger underneath the proximal joints and presses back.

Toe Extension. The patient lies on his or her back and bends the toes toward the dorsum of the foot with and without resistance.

Foot Dorsiflexion. The patient stands on the foot to be tested and raises the forefoot from the floor until he or she is balanced on the heel.

The patient may sit with the legs hanging free over a chair as he or she tries to flex or dorsiflex the foot. This is done with or without resistance.

The patient may lie on the affected side with the leg held firmly down on the table and with the foot in plantar flexion, attempting to bring it to dorsiflexion.

The patient lies face downward, knees flexed at right angles and the lower leg directed vertically upward, and tries to dorsiflex the foot. This is done with the examiner's hands on the dorsum of the foot resisting the movement and again with gravity assisting.

Foot Plantar Flexion. The patient stands on the affected side and is steadied by holding the examiner's hand. He or she rises on the ball of the affected foot. Note the patient walking on tiptoes.

Patient lies face down, with the knee flexed at a right angle and the lower leg directed vertically upward, and plantar flexes the foot. This is done with the examiner's hand on the plantar of the foot resisting the movement.

The patient lies on the affected side with the feet projecting over the end of the table while he or she attempts plantar flexion against the resistance of the examiner's hand.

The patient may lie on the affected side with the leg held in a tense plantar flexion at the ankle. This is done with and without resistance on the sole of the foot.

Foot Inversion. The patient lies on affected side and, while the leg is held further down on the table, tries to lift the outer border of the foot away from the table. This is accomplished with resistance on the inner border of the foot and also with the help of the examiner at the end of the movement. The patient sits on the edge of the table with the legs hanging down and the affected leg steadied by the examiner. The patient then attempts to turn the front of the foot inward and upward toward the ankle. This is done with resistance against the inner border of the foot. It is then done with resistance of gravity. For the tibialis posterior muscle the motion should be inward and downward.

The patient lies on his or her back, with the examiner holding the affected leg above the ankle to steady it, and turns the foot inward toward the other ankle. This is done without and with help.

Foot Eversion. The patient sits with the foot hanging free and the lower leg steadied by the hand as he or she everts the foot against manual resistance and with resistance of gravity alone.

The patient lies on his or her back holding the affected leg and turns the sole of the affected foot outward away from the other foot.

Gradation of Power. The relative power of muscles may be graded from one to four

1. This muscle can move without the resistance of the operator and with a lack of presence of gravity, but it cannot move against resistance.
2. Here the muscle can move against gravity, but not against both gravity and the resistance of the examiner.
3. This grade of muscle almost functions normally, but not to the extent of a normal muscle.
4. This muscle moves as all normal muscles should function. The cogwheel phenomenon is a muscle phenomenon occurring in hypertonic muscles being passively stretched. Under such conditions, the resistance of the muscle remains in irregular jerky movements.

For a fuller description of biomechanical problems, see Chapter 9, Biomechanical Disorders.

Radiographic

Standard radiographic examination of the foot and ankle includes standing angle and base of gait anterior-posterior (dorsal-plantar) and lateral views. These standard views are utilized to evaluate pathomechanical as well as pathological changes. Other views for visualization of specific areas of the foot and ankle include medial and lateral oblique foot and ankle views, anterior-posterior ankle views, axial sesamoid, posterior calcaneal, Harris-Beath and ankle stress views. Ankle arthrography and arthroscopy are becoming more helpful diagnostically as their technique is refined.

Technetium and gallium bone scans may be helpful in diagnosing stress fracture and bone infection, respectively. Computed tomography (CT) may be useful in diagnosis of tarsal synostoses, synchondroses, and syndesmoses, as well as bone and soft tissue tumors. Magnetic resonance imaging (MRI) requires no ionizing radiation, has no known biological hazards and provides high resolution and soft tissue contrast. This diagnostic tool is more sensitive than standard x-ray and CT scanning techniques. Small lesions within the foot can be detected, providing a quantum leap in rapid diagnosis.

Laboratory

Appropriate hematology, urinalysis, synovial fluid, culture and sensitivity and biopsy testing are utilized as indicated by history and physical examination. Minimal screening tests before elective podiatric surgery include a CBC, BUN, FBS, VDRL, PTT and urinalysis. Other hematology screening batteries—for example SMA-12, electrolytes etc.—may be performed according to medical indication.

Normocytic, macrocytic, microcytic and microcytic hypochromic anemias must be further evaluated. Increase or decrease in myelocytes, juvenile neutrophils, band neutrophils, segmented neutrophils, lymphocytes, eosinophils, basophils, monocytes and platelets is noted and correlated with history and physical examination. Consultation with an internist is often necessary in order to confirm a diagnosis and initiate proper treatment.

Urinalysis results are important to proper diagnosis and treatment. Findings of acetone, blood, aldosterone, amylase, calcium, casts, creatine, creatinine, cysteine, catecholamines, protein, chlorides, glucose, lactic dehydrogenase, lead, lipid or porphyrins in the urine demands further investigation and evaluation. The urine's pH and specific gravity are also of import to proper diagnosis and consultation.

See Table 2.1 for profiles or panels of screening tests that are recommended when specific pathology is suspected (17).

Normal Values Multiple normal values and ranges are included because of the variation in laboratory normals. Individual laboratory normal ranges should be used for definitive analysis of results. Medications may alter hematology, urinalysis, and blood chemistry results.

Hematology

Bleeding time	1–3 min (Duke)
	2–4 min (Ivy)
Blood volume Males	75 ml/kg of body weight
Females	67 ml/kg of body weight
Prothrombin time	70–110% of control value
Sedimentation rate	Males 0–9 mm/hr (Wintrobe)
Erythrocyte sedimentation rate (ESR)	Females 0–20 mm/hr (Wint) up to 15 mm/hr (Westergen)
Hematocrit Men	38–54%
Women	36–47%
Hemoglobin Men	14–18 gm%
Women	12–16 gm%
Children	12–14 gm%
Newborn	14.5–24.5 gm%
Red blood cell measurements	
Diameter (MCD)	5.5–5.8 microns
Mean corpuscular volume (MCV)	80–94 cu mic
Mean corpuscular hb (MCH)	27–32 micromicrograms
Mean corpuscular hb concentration (MCHC)	33–38%
Blood count	
Erythrocytes Men	5,000,000
	5×10^6/cu mm
Women	4,500,000
	4.5×10^6/cu mm
Reticulocytes	0–1%
Leukocytes, total	5,000–10,000 (100%)
Myelocytes	0 (0%)
Juvenile neutrophils	0–100 (0–1%)
Band neutrophils	0–500 (0–5%)
Segmented neutrophils	2,500–6,000 (40–60%)
Lymphocytes	1,000–4,000 (20–40%)
Eosinophils	50–300 (1–3%)
Basophils	0–100 (0–1%)
Monocytes	200–800 (4–8%)
Platelets	200,000–500,000

Table 2.2 shows the clinical significance of elevated and decreased blood count values and the differentiation of anemias by corpuscular indices is displayed in Table 2.3.

Urinalysis Urine culture and sensitivity studies are conducted on a clean-catch midstream specimen. Normally, urine does not contain protein, sugar, bile, blood or ketones. The pH is 4.6–8.0 depending on the diet, and specific gravity is 1.003–1.030.

Table 2.1.
Recommended Screening Tests[a]

Condition	Tests suggested
Injury	C-reactive protein, sedimentation rate (ESR), Bence Jones Protein, acid and alkaline phosphatase, CBC, urinalysis
Collagen disorder	ANA, latex fixation, uric acid, ASO titer, HLA-B_{27}, ESR, LE prep
Lipid disorder	Cholesterol (Chol), triglycerides, lipoprotein phenotype
Thyroid disorder	PBI, T_3, T_4, T_7, free thyroxine, chol
Cardiac disorder	CPK, SGOT, LDH
Hypertension	Urinary VMA, catecholamines, BUN, chol
Kidney disorder	BUN, Phos, LDH, creatinine, uric acid, total protein, albumin, globulin, A/G ratio, calcium, glucose, chol
Kidney function	Urinalysis, urine creatinine, uric acid, creatinine clearance
Liver disorder	Total bilirubin, alkaline phosphatase, chol, total protein, albumin, globulin, A/G ratio, SGOT, LDH, guanase, Australia antigen

[a] From Labdata Reference Manual, Labdata Service Co., Phoenix, AZ.

Table 2.2.
Clinical Significance of Abnormal Values, Complete Blood Count

Cell type	Elevated	Decreased
Red blood cells (erythrocytes) hemoglobin, hematocrit	Polycythemia, chronic oxygen deficiency, pulmonary disease, dehydration	Anemia, surgical risk, peripheral neuropathy, ulcers, cold feet, cyanosis, hemorrhage
White blood cells (leukocytes)	Acute infections, burns, leukemia, some anemias, stress, anesthesia, venoms, hemorrhage, trauma, circulatory disease, malignancy, gout, rheumatic fever, septicemia, eclampsia, uremia, meningitis, tonsillitis, abscess, menstruation, vaccination, drugs such as quinine and adrenalin	Antiobiotics, antihistamines, analgesics, antithyroid, barbiturate, griseofulvin and other drug therapy, x-ray therapy, overwhelming infection, viral infection, malaria, tuberculosis, blood dyscrasias
Neutrophils	Bacterial and parasitic infection, leukemia, acute inflammation, poisonings, acute hemorrhage, gout, burns, myocardial infarction	Drug and x-ray therapy, overwhelming infection, spleen or blood marrow damage, vitamin B_{12} and folic acid deficiency, lupus erythematosus, typhoid, malaria, paratyphoid, anaphylactic shock, viral infection, endocrine disorders
Lymphocytes	Infectious mononucleosis, leukemia, viral and febrile diseases, herpes zoster and simplex, hepatitis, gamma gobulin deficiencies, lymphatic leukemia, syphilis	Drug and x-ray therapy, lupus erythematosus, myelocytic leukemia
Monocytes	Tuberculosis, Hodgkin's disease, Gaucher's disease, monocytic leukemia, typhoid fever, malaria, undulant fever, Rocky Mountain spotted fever, collagen disorder, and viral, bacterial and parasitic infection	Not clinically significant
Eosinophils	Allergy, myalgia, skin disorders, parasites, psoriasis, neoplasias, menstruation, radiation therapy, asthma, Addison's disease, polyarteritis nodosa	Alcohol intoxication, hypersplenism, aplastic and pernicious anemia, drugs (ACTH, epinephrine, thyroxin), acute infection, infectious mononucleosis, congestive heart failure
Basophils	Polycythemia vera, myelocytic leukemia, Hodgkin's disease, myxedema, colitis, chronic inflammation	Allergies, hyperthyroidism, prolonged steroid therapy, stress reaction
Platelets	Menstruation, exercise, epinephrine injection, thrombocythemia, polycythemia vera, trauma, hemorrhage, malignancy, collagen disorders, acute infection, cirrhosis, cardiac disease	Aplastic and pernicious anemia, bone marrow depression, acute and some chronic leukemias, transfusion and transfusion reaction, infectious mononucleosis, drug therapy, radiation

Table 2.3.
Anemia Differentiation According to Corpuscular Indices[a]

Anemias	MCV[b]	MCH[c]	MCHC[d]
Normocytic	80–94	27–32	33–38
Macrocytic	94–160	32–50	32–36
Microcytic	72–80	21–24	30–37
Microcytic-hypochromic	50–80	12–29	24–30

[a] From Labdata Reference Manual, Labdata Service Co., Phoenix, AZ.
[b] Mean corpuscular volume (MCV)—red blood cell (RBC) size
males: 80–94
females: 81–99
[c] Mean corpuscular hemoglobin (MCH)—amount of hemoglobin in a single RBC
males and females: 27–32
[d] Mean corpuscular hemoglobin concentration (MCHC)—RBC proportion occupied by hemoglobin
males and females: 33–30

Table 2.4.
Clinical Significance of Presence of Substances in the Urine (18)

Substance	Indicative of
Protein	Kidney disease, polycystic disease, pyelonephritis, diabetes, lupus erythematosus, hemorrhage, tuberculosis, amyloidosis
Sugar	Diabetes, drug therapy (aspirin, morphine, phenacetin), renal glycosuria, hyperpituitarism, chronic liver disease, pregnancy, hyperthyroidism, stress
Bile	Liver disease, bile duct obstruction
Blood	Kidney or bladder disease, menstruation, glomerulonephritis, cystitis, pyelonephritis
Casts	Hyaline casts: normal; epithelial and red cell casts: renal failure; waxy, leukocyte, bacterial and fatty casts: kidney disease
Ketones	Diabetes, eclampsia, starvation, chloroform or other anesthetics, malnutrition
pH 4.6–8.0	Acid: diabetes, acidic drugs, gout, acute rheumatism, chronic nephritis, scurvy, leukemia, high-protein diet, saccharin ingestion
	Alkaline: ingestion of alkalizers, blood transfusion, cold exposure, vomiting
Specific gravity 1.003–1.030	
Increase	Low fluid intake, vomiting, sweating, diabetes mellitus, acute glomerulonephritis
Decrease	Low salt intake, high fluid intake, chronic nephritis, diabetes insipidus, primary aldosteronism

Aldosterone	6–16 mcg in 24 hrs 2–23 mcg in 24 hrs
Amylase	260–950 Somogyi units/24 hrs 2–50 Wohlgemuth units/cc 6–30 Wohlgemuth units/24 hrs Up to 5,000 Somogyi units/24 hrs
Alpha amino nitrogen	64–199 mg/24 hrs Not over 1.5% total nitrogen 100–290 mg/24 hrs
Ammonia	700 mg/24 hrs 20–70 mEq/L 10–40 gm/24 hrs
Calcium	Less than 250 mg/24 hrs on usual diet. Less than 150 mg/24 hrs low calcium diet (Bauer-Aub) Positive—1 plus (Sulkowitch)
Catecholamines	Less than 230 mcg/24 hrs
Epinephrine	Less than 10 mcg/24 hrs
Norepinephrine	Less than 100 mcg/24 hrs
Chloride	110–250 mEq/24 hrs
Creatine	Less than 100 mg/24 hrs Less than 6% of creatinine Up to 12% creatinine in pregnancy Up to 30% of creatinine in children over 1 year
Creatinine	1.0–1.6 gm/24 hrs 0.8–1.7 gm/24 hrs females 1–1.9 gms/24 hrs males
Nitrogen, total	10–16 gm/24 hrs
Phosphorus	0.9–1.3 gm/24 hrs
Magnesium	0.1–0.2 gm/24 hrs
Potassium	25–100 mEg/24 hrs
Sodium	110 mEq/24 hrs
Urea clearance	75 cc max 54 cc standard
Uric acid	0.5–1 gm/24 hrs
Urobilinogen	up to 1 Ehrlich unit/2 hrs 0–4 mg/24 hrs 2-hr specimen is collected between 1 and 3 P.M.

See Table 2.4 for the clinical significance of the presence of certain substances in the urine.

Blood Chemistry Fasting or nonfasting peripheral venous blood specimens are utilized for blood chemistry determination. The values presented below are adult values unless otherwise noted (18). Blood chemistry is altered by a variety of disease states, medication and environment. Reference is made throughout the text to abnormal blood chemistry values as they relate to lower extremity pathology.

Acetone serum	0.3–2.0 mg/100 ml 0—1 mg/100 ml
Blood	Negative
Alpha amino nitrogen, plasma	3.0–5.5 mg/100 ml
Ammonia, blood	40–70 mcg/100 ml 102 + 23 mcg/100 ml
Amylase, serum or blood	80–180 Somogyi Units (SU) 80–150 SU/100 ml 60–180 SU/100 ml
Ascorbic acid, blood	0.4–1.5 mg/100 ml 0.8–2.4 mg/100 ml
Aldolase	0.0–6.0 units 3–8 SL Units/100 ml (Sibley-Lehninger)
Bilirubin, serum, total	0.1–1.0 mg% 1.0 mg/100 ml 0.3–1.1 mg/100 ml
direct	0.1–0.4 mg/100 ml 0.2 mg/100 ml
indirect	0.2–0.7 mg/100 ml 0.1–0.6 mg/100 ml
Total minus direct = indirect	
Bromides, serum	0–toxic above 17 mEq/L
Bromsulphalein (BSP)—dye	2 mg–1% @ 30 min 5 mg–5% or less @ 45 M.
Calcium, serum	8.5–10.5 mg% 4.5–5.5 mEq/L 9.0–11.5 mg/100 ml
Calcium, ionized	4.5–5.5 mg% 2.1–2.6 mEq/L
Carbon dioxide, serum	21–30 mEq/L 26–28 mEq/L
Carbon monoxide, blood	Symptoms with 20% or over saturation. Up to 7%
Carotene, serum	20–115 mcg% 70–250 mcg/100 ml
Chloride, serum	98–106 mEq/L 355–376 mg% as Cl 585–620 mg% NaCl
Cephalin flocculation	Negative to 1+
Ceruloplasmin	15–35 units 20–35 mg%
Cholesterol, serum	150–300 mg% 150–280 mg% 220 ± 50 mg%
Cholesterol esters, serum	163 ± 36 mg% 50–70% of total
Cholinesterase	0.5–1.3 pH units (plasma) 80 to 200% (plasma) 0.5–1.0 pH units (RBCs) 80–120% (RBCs)
Copper, serum	50–250 mcg% 90–150 mcg% 65–170 mcg/100 ml
Creatine, serum	0.16–0.4 mg%
Creatine phosphokinase (CPK)	0–50 International Units 0–12 Sigma Units/ml
Creatinine, serum	0.7–1.5 mg/100 ml 1.0–2.0 mg/100 ml
Cryoglobulins, serum	0
Ethanol, blood	0.3–0.4 mg—marked intoxication 0.4–0.5 mg—alcoholic stupor 0.5 mg or above—coma

Fibrinogen, plasma	200–400 mg/100 ml
	0.2–0.4 gm%
Glucose, blood, fasting	65–110 mg%
	90–120 mg% (Folin-Wu)
	65–95 mg% (Nelson-Somogyl)
	60–105 mg% (enzymatic)
	46–94 mg% (ultramicro)
Glucose-6-phosphate dehydrogenase	100–135 units
Guanase	0.3 units/liter
17-Hydroxycorticoids, plasma	5–25 mcg/100 ml
Icterus index, serum	4–7 units
HBC, Alpha hydroxy butric acid	100–300 Rosalki Units (RU)
High-density lipoproteins (HDL)	Males, 30–60 mg/100 ml females, 35–85 mg/100 ml
Iodine, butanol extractable	3.5–6.5 mcg%
	3.2–6.4 mcg%
Iodine, protein bound (PBI)	3.5–8.8 mcg/100 ml
May be slightly higher in infants	
Iron, serum	75–175 mcg/100 ml
	60–190 mcg/100 ml
	56–183 mcg/100 ml
Iron-binding capacity,	150–300 mcg/100 ml
serum unsaturated	250–440 mcg/100 ml
transferrin	300–359 mg/100 ml
% saturation	20–55%
Isocitric dehydrogenase (ICD)	50–180 Sigma Units/ml
	50–100 S.U.
Lactic acid, serum	5–20 mg%
	6–16 mg/100 ml
arterial	3.1–7 mg/100 ml
venous	5–20 mg/100 ml
Lactic dehydrogenase (LDH)	0–250 International Units
	200–450 units/100 ml
	50–400 units/100 ml
Lead, blood	Up to 60 mcg%
	0–50 mcg/100 ml
	0–0.04 mg/100 ml
Leucine amino peptidase, serum (LAP)	75–230 GR Units (Goldbarg-Rutenburg)
Lipase, serum	0–1.0 CC Units (Cherry-Crandall)
	0–1.5 units
	Less than 1.5 units
Lipids total	450–850 mg/100 ml
	530–765 mg/100 ml
	450–1000 mg/100 ml
Lipid fractions, choles-	150–280 mg/100 ml
terol, phospholipids	150–350 mg/100 ml
	60–350 mg/100 ml
	6–12 mg/100 ml as lipid phosphorus
Total fatty acids	190–420 mg/100 ml
esterified	250–400 mg/100 ml
	8–20 mEq/L
free	0.35–1.2 mEq/L
Lithium	0.5–1.0 (Ther)
Magnesium	1.0–3.0 mg%
	1.4–2.2 mEq/L
	1.7–2.7 mg%
Mucoprotein	30–100 mg%
Nonprotein nitrogen, blood (NPN)	25–40 mg%
	15–35 mg%
Oxygen, blood capacity	
arterial	15–22 vols/100 ml
venous	11–16 vols/100 ml
Oxygen blood saturation	
arterial	98%
venous	55–71%
pH, plasma, arterial	7.35–7.45
venous	7.34–7.39
Phenylalanine, serum	Less than 3 mg/100 ml
	Less than 4 mg/100 ml
Phosphatase, acid, serum	1.0–5.0 King-Armstrong Units
	0.5–2.0 Bodansky Units (BU)
	0.5–2.0 Gutman Units
	0–1.1 Shinowara Units
	0.1–0.56 Bessey Lowry-Female
Phosphatase, alkaline, serum	1.5–4 BU
	2.0–4.5 BU
	0.8–2.3 Bessey Lowry Units
	5.0–13 King Armstrong Units
	3.0–10 Gutman Units
	2.2–8.6 Shinowara Units
	30–70 MilliUnits (mU)
	Children up to 20 BU
Phosphorus, serum	2.5–4.5 mg%
	2.6–4.8 mg%
	4.0–7.0 mg% (children)
Potassium, serum	3.8–5.1 mEq/L
Proteins, serum, total	6.0–8.0 gm%
albumin	52–68% of total
	3.5–5.5 gm%
globulin	45–55% of total
	1.5–3 gm%
paper electrophoresis	
$alpha_1$	5–8% of total
$alpha_2$	8–13% of total
beta	11–17% of total
gamma	15–25% of total
Pyruvic acid, plasma	1–2 mg/100 ml
SGOT (glutamic-oxalacetic transaminase)	0–20 International Units
	5–40 International Units
	12–36 Units
	5–40 Karmen Units%
SGPT (glutamic-pyruvic transaminase, serum)	0–20 International Units
	5–40 Karmen Units%
Sodium, serum	130–149 mEq/L
	138–146 mEq/L
Salicylate-therapeutic range	20–25 mg/100 ml
toxic range	Over 30 mg/100 ml
Sulfates, inorganic, serum	0.5–1.5 mg/100 ml
T_3 uptake (tri-iodo thyronine)	25–35%
	20–50% of dose/24 hrs
T_4 (Murphy-Pattee)	5.3–14.5 mcg%
Thymol turbidity	0–5 Todd Units
Triglycerides	20–200 mg%
	150–300 mg%
	Up to 165 mg%
Urea nitrogen, blood (BUN)	10–20 mg%
	9–17 mg%
	5–25 mg%

Uric acid, serum	
males	3.0–7.0 mg/100 ml
females	2.0–6.0 mg%
Xylose absorption	16–33%
Vitamin A, serum	30–100 units/100 ml
Zinc	50–150 mcg%

Table 2.5 displays the clinical significance of specific blood chemistry studies (15, 19).

Nutrition

The foods we eat supply us with carbohydrates, fats, proteins, vitamins and minerals (20).

Carbohydrates

Carbohydrates are mono- or polysaccharides that provide glucose to the body. Glucose is the chief sugar found in the blood.

There are two types of carbohydrates, simple and complex. Simple carbohydrates include the monosaccharides—glucose, fructose and galactose—as well as the disaccharides: sucrose = glucose + fructose, maltose = glucose + glucose and lactose = glucose + galactose.

Glucose is found in ripe fruit, roots, leaves, flowers and saps of plants. Dextrose and corn syrup are commercial glucose products that contain other carbohydrates. Fructose is found in honey, syrup, molasses and ripe fruits. Galactose is found in all foods containing lactose, as well as in grapes and legumes.

Complex carbohydrates are long-chain saccharides that are broken down in the stomach to the monosaccharide glucose. Glucose is absorbed in the small intestines. Complex carbohydrates are found in fresh fruits, vegetables, whole grains and legumes.

Carbohydrates provide the body with energy, play a role in the mobilization of fats and have a protein-sparing action.

Fats and Lipids

Fats and lipids are defined as naturally occurring substances that are insoluble in water but are soluble in organic solvents.

The important dietary lipids are triglycerides, which include esters of glycerol and fatty acids that form fats or oils; sterols, such as cholesterol and ergosterol (vitamin D_{12}); and the other fat-soluble vitamins, A, E and K.

There are two classifications of fats: saturated fats from animal sources, including palmitic acid and stearic acid, and unsaturated fats from both plant and animal sources. Sources of saturated fats include such animal products as beef, pork, cheese and milk, as well as coconut oil. Oleic acid and palmitooleic acid are found in plants, and linoleic acid and linolenic acid are found in animal sources. Unsaturated fats are found in the following animal sources—chicken, turkey, duck and fish—and the following plant sources—cotton seed, safflower, soybean, sunflower, olive and peanut oil.

The body requires three fatty acids for prostaglandin synthesis: linoleic acid, linolenic acid and arachidonic acid.

Cholesterol is the most common sterol. It plays a function in the synthesis of hormones, preservation of cell integrity and as a precursor to vitamin D. Sources of cholesterol include eggs, liver, meats, shellfish, cheese, cold cuts, sausage and frankfurters.

Protein/Amino Acids

Proteins are defined as naturally occurring, high molecular weight substances containing nitrogen, carbon, hydrogen and oxygen. They may also contain sulfur, phosphorus, zinc, iron and copper.

There are two types of proteins: complete proteins, which include all the essential amino acids, and incomplete proteins, which are missing one or more of the essential amino acids.

Protein complementation refers to the concept of combining two incomplete proteins, each of which supplies the amino acids that are missing to form a complete protein.

Protein is required for growth, tissue maintenance and repair, synthesis of enzyme proteins and nutrient transport proteins, and the proper functioning of the immune system.

Table 2.5.
Clinical Significance of Blood Chemistry Studies[a]

Substance	Increased with	Decreased with
Albumin: 3.5–5.5 gm%	Dehydration	Overdehydration Malnutrition Malabsorption Nephrosis Hepatic insufficiency and disease Burns
Alk phosphatase: 30–70 mU/ml (Bodansky/Gutman units)	Bone growth Bone diseases Osteoblastic lesions, Paget's Hepatic disease Obstructive jaundice Renal infarction Hyperparathyroidism	Hypothyroidism Hypophosphatasia Pernicious anemia Malnutrition Scurvy
Total Bilirubin: 0.1–1.0 mg%	Hemolysis Hepatic disease (metastasis) Hepatitis Cirrhosis Obstructive disease (lithiasis) Gilberts disease (Dubin-Johnson)	
BUN: 10–20 mg%	Renal disease, urinary obstruction Dehydration, hypotension Heart failure (acute MI) Diabetes Shock, infection, crush injury	Hepatic insufficiency Overhydration Malnutrition Pregnancy Liver failure
Cholesterol: 150–300 mg%	Hypothyroidism Obstructive jaundice Nephrosis Diabetes mellitus Familial/hereditary (fredrickson classification) Cardiovascular disease, atherosclerosis	Hyperthyroidism Hepatic failure Sepsis Anemia
Calcium: 8.5–10.5 mg%	Hyperparathyroidism Hyperthyroidism Excess vitamin D Bone metastases Bone lymphoma Fracture with bedrest Paget's disease Multiple myeloma Excess diuretics (thiazides) Milk-alkali syndrome Sarcoidosis Tuberculosis Acidosis	Hypoalbuminemia Hypoparathyroidism Pseudohypoparathyroidism Malabsorption Pancreatitis Renal failure Osteomalacia Rickets Medullary carcinoma of thyroid gland (excessive calcitonin levels) Alkalosis
Total Protein: 6–8 gm%	Dehydration Hyperglobulinemia Multiple myeloma Malignancy	Overhydration Hepatic insufficiency disease Malnutrition (starvation) Malabsorption

Table 2.5—*Continued*

Substance	Increased with	Decreased with
	Hepatic disease Collagen disease (RA) Infection	Burns (severe third degree) Hemorrhage (excessive) Nephrosis
Inorganic phosphate: 2.5–4.8 mg%	Renal insufficiency Hemolysis Hypoparathyroidism Pseudohypoparathyroidism Fracture healing Bone tumors Diabetes	Hyperparathyroidism (Primary, secondary and tertiary) Diabetic coma (ketosis) Vitamin D-resistant rickets Cirrhosis
LDH: 0–250 mU/ml (Wacker/Wroblewski units)	Cerebral damage/trauma Myocardial infarction Pulmonary infarction Muscle necrosis Kidney infarction Liver disease Leukemia Malignant neoplasms Hemolysis	Oxalate anticoagulant
Uric acid: 2.5–8.5 mg%	Gout Renal failure Diuretics Leukemia Lymphomas Metastatic cancer Psoriasis Nephrotic disease Alcoholism Hypothyroidism Eclampsia Ketosis	Cortisone usage Allopurinol/probenecid (uricosuric drug toxicity) Wilson's disease SIADH secretion
Glucose: 65–110 mg%	Hepatic disease (chronic) Brain damage (trauma) Hypothalmic lesions adenoma Pheochromocytoma Hyperthyroidism Cushing's disease Acute stress Pancreatitis Epinephrine Corticosteroids Thiazide diuretics	Excess insulin Insulinoma Islett cells cancer Addison's disease Malabsorption (glycogen storage disease) Neoplasms Bacterial sepsis
SGOT: 10–50 mU/ml (Sigma Frankel units)	Muscle necrosis (myositis) Muscular dystrophy Dermatomyositis Crush injuries Myocardial infarction Hepatic disease Kidney infarction Cerebral damage Pancreatitis (acute)	Pregnancy Diabetes mellitus Beri-beri

Table 2.5—*Continued*

Substance	Increased with	Decreased with
Electrolytes Sodium: 130–149 mEq/L (Na+) major cation in ECF	When H_2O is lost in excess of salt or inappropriate excessive salt replacement Profuse sweating Prolonged hyperpnea Lack of water intake Cushing's disease	Diarrhea Nephrosis Addison's disease Metabolic acidosis Diuretic therapy Polyuric states Syndrome-inappropriate ADH secretion
Potassium: 3.8–5.5 mEq/L (K+) major intracellular cation	Acute or chronic renal disease Extensive tissue injury Hemolyzed specimen Tourniquet left on too long Acidosis Burns	GI fluid losses (vomiting, diarrhea) Renal diseases (chronic) Diuretic administration Cushing's disease Alkalemia
Chloride: 98–106 mEq/L (Cl^-) major extracellular anion	Prolonged diarrhea Renal tubular diseases	Prolonged vomiting Metabolic acidosis Salt-losing renal diseases Addisonian crisis
Carbon dioxide (CO_2): arterial: 19–25 mEq/L venous: 25–30 mEq/L Acts as a buffering agent in acid-base balance of the body; can result in acidemia or alkalemia	Failure of pulmonary ventilation Metabolic alkalosis Respiratory acidosis Excess ingestion of antacids Cushing's syndrome Prolonged administration of corticosteriods	Hyperventilation Respiratory alkalosis Metabolic acidosis
Miscellaneous tests Acid phosphatase: 0–2 (Bodansky units)	Prostatic carcinoma, Gaucher's disease, osteitis	
Creatine phosphokinase (CPK): 0–50 IU	Myocardial infarction, progressive muscular dystrophy, alcoholic myopathy, delirium tremens, hypothyroidism, pulmonary edema, pulmonary infarction, exercise, carcinomas (prostate, lung, colon, esophagus), intramuscular injections, acute pyschotic reactions	
Creatinine: 0.7–1.5 mg/100ml	Young age, male gender, renal disease, skeletal muscle necrosis, atrophy, trauma, poliomyelitis, amyotrophic lateral sclerosis, amyotonia congentia, dermatomyositis, myasthenia gravis, starvation, pregnancy	

[a] From Fischback F: *A Manual of Laboratory Diagnostic Tests,* ed 2. Philadelphia, J.B. Lippincott Co., 1984 and Robbins JM (ed): *Clinical Handbook of Podiatric Medicine,* Cleveland: Ohio College of Podiatric Medicine, 1983.

Vitamins

Vitamins are nutrients required in the diet for essential metabolic function, structural integrity and physiological adaption (Table 2.6).

Water-soluble vitamins include vitamins B complex and C. Vitamin B complex plays a role as energy releasing agents, in the maturation of blood cells and hemoglobin synthesis, in the transmission of nerve impulses and in metabolism of foreign substances. Food sources for vitamin B complex include whole grains, nuts, liver, eggs, milk, potatoes, vegetables and fruits.

Vitamin C maintains structural integrity of connective tissue, acts as a reducing agent, promotes iron absorption from the intestines, and is necessary to drug metabolism. Food sources for vitamin C include citrus fruits and fruit juices, green peppers, tomatoes, cabbage, broccoli and peas.

Fat-soluble vitamins include A, D, E, and K. Vitamin A functions in the visual process, reproduction and growth and maintains structural integrity of epithelia. It is ingested in two forms—as carotene that is converted to vitamin A and as Vitamin A itself. Vitamin D is needed for calcium absorption, hemeostasis and bone growth. A sterol, vitamin D is obtained from the diet and from synthesis in the skin under ultraviolet light. Vitamin E functions as an antioxidant preventing hemolysis of red blood cells. Vitamin K functions during the blood clotting mechanism. It is supplied from the diet through animal protein and synthesis from intestinal bacteria.

Table 2.6. Vitamins[a]

Vitamin	RDA Male 23–50	RDA Female 23–50	Normal function in body	Overdosing hazards	Purported benefits from megadoses
A	1000 RE (5000 IU)	800 RE (4000 IU)	Necessary for normal vision in dim light; maintains normal structure and functions of mucous membranes; needed for growth of bones, teeth and skin	Nausea; loss of appetite; dry, cracked skin; loss of hair; joint pain; severe headache; liver damage; possible death	Cancer prevention; acne treatment; improved eyesight
B_1 (thiamine)	1.4 mg	1.0 mg	Necessary for carbohydrate metabolism; helps maintain healthy nervous system	Hypersensitivity	Increased physical performance
B_2 (riboflavin)	1.6 mg	1.2 mg	Needed for protein, fat and carbohydrate metabolism; maintains healthy skin	Unclear	—
B_3 (niacin)	18 mg	13 mg	Needed for protein, fat and carbohydrate metabolism; nervous system function; needed for oxygen use by cells	Flushing and itching of skin; irritability; tachycardia	Treatment for mental illness; improves learning disabilities; treatment for heart disease; lowers blood cholesterol

Table 2.6—*Continued*

Vitamin	RDA Male 23–50	RDA Female 23–50	Normal function in body	Overdosing hazards	Purported benefits from megadoses
B_6 (pyridoxine)	2.2 mg	2.0 mg	Needed for protein metabolism; necessary for normal growth	Neurological damage	Treatment for mental illness; treatment for menstrual edema
Folic acid	400 mcg	400 mcg	Necessary for red blood cell development; needed for tissue growth and repair	Can mask diagnosis of pernicious anemia	—
B_{12} (cyanocobalamin)	3 mcg	3 mcg	Needed for new tissue growth; red blood cells; nervous system and skin	Unclear	Improved physical performance; treatment of multiple sclerosis; slows aging
Biotin	100-200 mcg[a]	100-200 mcg[b]	Needed for normal metabolism of carbohydrates, fats and protein	None currently known	—
Pantothenic acid	4-7 mg[b]	4-7 mg[b]	Needed for normal metabolism of carbohydrates, fats and protein	None currently known	—
C	60 mg	60 mg	Needed for building the material that holds cells together; necessary for healthy gums, teeth and blood vessels	Nausea; diarrhea; kidney stones; potential mutagen	Prevention and cure of colds; immunization from diseases; cancer and heart disease treatment
D	5 mcg	5 mcg	Needed for calcium absorption; important for proper bone and teeth growth	Growth retardation; calcium deposition in soft tissue; kidney damage	Builds stronger bones
E	10 mg	10 mg	Acts as antioxidant; protects cells from damage	Fatigue; nausea; cramps; increased blood-fat levels; interferes with vitamins K and A metabolism	Prevents, cures or ameliorates aging, fertility, heart disease, balding, diabetes, cancer, arthritis; imrpoves sexual performance
K	70-140 mcg[b]	70-140 mcg[b]	Aids in blood clotting	Liver function impaired; jaundice	—

[a] From Applegate E: Vitamin overdose, *Runner's World,* 1:61, 1984.
[b] Estimated safe and adequate daily dietary intakes.

Minerals

Macronutrients, required in amounts in excess of 100 mg per day, include sodium, chloride, potassium, calcium, phosphorus, magnesium and sulfur.

Trace elements required in amounts less than 100 mg/day include iron, copper, cobalt, molybdenum, manganese, iodine, zinc, fluorine, chromium and selenium (Table 2.7).

Sodium and potassium are involved in the electrophysiology of cells, propagation of nerve impulses, and acid-base balance. Changes in extracellular sodium affect blood pressure, whereas changes in blood and tissue concentration of potassium alter cardiac function. Transport of nutrients, such as glucose, across intestinal mucosa are sodium-dependent. Protein and amino acids metabolism are also sodium and potassium-dependent. Insulin secretion is depressed by potassium depletion. High potassium foods include oranges, bananas, peas, beans and milk.

Chloride is the most important anion involved in the maintenance of fluid and electrolyte balance. It is needed to form gastric hydrochloric acid. The major source of chloride is sodium chloride.

Calcium in its soluble form is 1% of the total body calcium found outside bones and teeth. It is required for blood coagulation, skeletal muscle function, contractility of heart muscle, nerve function and enzyme system activity. Calcium is held at a constant level by vitamin D, which promotes calcium absorption; by calcitonin, which deposits excess calcium in bone; and by parathyroid hormone, which mobilizes calcium from bone when diminished states occur. High-calcium foods include milk, cheese and yogurt.

Phosphate (phosphorus) is required for formation of bone phosphate and cell synthesis. Requirements are higher during active growth. Phosphorus absorpton is dependent on vitamin D. It is found in animal foods.

Magnesium is essential during neuromuscular transmission. Magnesium sources include legumes, potatoes, dried fruits and vegetables. Magnesium deficiency is associated with an impaired utilization of thiamin and sometimes calcium and potassium depletion. Symptoms of magnesium deficiency include tremor, tetanic convulsions and coma.

Sulfate is provided in the sulfur-containing amino acids, methionine and cycteine. It is utilized in the excretion of such endogenous compounds as steroids and such foreign compounds as drugs.

Iron functions as a part of hemoglobin and other heme compounds important in oxygen transport and tissue respiration. There are two forms—heme iron from animal protein and nonheme iron from vegetable sources. Heme iron is absorbed more completely than nonheme iron. Vitamin C promotes iron absorption, whereas bran and large amounts of strong tea decrease absorption.

Iodine is required in the synthesis of iodine-containing thyroid hormones. Iodine sources include milk, iodized salt and bread containing potassium iodate.

Zinc is a constituent of enzymes concerned with metabolism of nucleic acids,

Table 2.7.
Trace Elements

Element	Function	Source
Chromium	Insulin cofactor, component of	Yeast, liver, meats
Cobalt	Vitamin B_{12} required for normal bone structure reproduction	Meats, liver, kidney, sweetbreads
Manganese	Neural function, component of	Nuts, cereals, peas
Selenium	Glutathione peroxidase	Liver, kidney, fish, cereals, legumes
Molybdenum	Protects dental enamel	Kidney, liver
Florine	Protects dental enamel	Drinking water, tea, sardines

protein, carbohydrates and alcohol. It is a structural and functional component of carboxypeptidase, a digestive enzyme present in the insulin molecule required for normal vitamin A transport and metabolism. Zinc plays an essential role in pre- and postnatal growth, wound repair, keratinization, immune function, taste acuity and visual function. Sources of zinc include meat, liver, eggs, seafood, milk and whole grains to a lesser extent.

Copper is a component of various enzymes utilized for energy generation. It is essential to connective tissue integrity and has a role in synthesis of brown pigment melanin. It is present in skin and hair. Sources of copper include shellfish, liver, kidney, nuts, cocoa, grapes and peaches.

The following dietary goals should be stressed: (20) (21) (22) (23)

1. Avoid becoming overweight; consume only as much energy in calories as is expended. If overweight, decrease energy intake and increase energy expenditure.
2. Increase consumption of complex carbohydrates and naturally occurring sugars from the current level of 28% of energy intake to about 48% of energy intake.
3. Reduce the consumption of refined and processed sugars from 24% to 10% of total energy intake.
4. Reduce overall fat consumption from 42% to about 30% of total energy intake.
5. Reduce saturated fat consumption to account for less than 10% of total energy intake and balance it with poly- and monounsaturated fats, which should account for about 10% of total energy intake each.
6. Reduce cholesterol consumption to 250–300 mg/day or less.
7. Limit the intake of sodium by reducing the intake of salt to 5 gm/day.

References

1. Kravitz H, Boehm JJ: Rhythmic habit patterns in infancy: Their sequence, age of onset, and frequency. *Child Develop* 42:399–414, 1971.
2. Gessell A, Ilg FL: *The Child from Five to Ten*. New York, Harper & Brothers, 1946.
3. Yale I: Radiographic study of calcification of the medial calcaneal branch of posterior tibial artery age group 20–40. *J Natl Assoc Chirop* 44:44–52, 1954.
4. Ross EB: Ainhum, a case report. *J Am Podiatry Assoc* 48: 255–256, 1958.
5. Blumer G: *History Taking*. New Haven, CT, Associates of the Yale Medical Library, 1949.
6. Fox HR: Podiatric management of the patient with renal disease. Medical-surgical review. *J Foot Surg* 24:148–153, 1985.
7. Welch Allyn, Inc: *Welch Allyn Ophthalmoscope Instruction Booklet*. Skaneatelas, NY, 1978.
8. Zier, G: Clinical considerations for the hypertensive patient in podiatric practice. *J Am Podiatry Assoc* 73:573–576. 1983.
9. Cangialosi, P: The podiatric history and physical examination as an effective diagnostic tool. *J Foot Surg* 21:146–152, 1982.
10. Strandness DE, McCutcheon EF, Rushmer RF: Application of a transcutaneous Doppler Flowmeter in evaluation of occlusive arterial disease. *Surg Gynecol Obstet* 122:1039, 1966.
11. Durkin, F: Patients on long-term steroid therapy. *J Am Podiatry Assoc* 66:847–849, 1976.
12. Erlick NE, et al.: A dermatoglyphic predictive index for maturity-onset diabetes mellitus. *J Am Podiatry Assoc* 73:465–474, 1983.
13. Redding KG: Thrombocythemia as a cause of erythermalgia. *Arch Dermatol* 113:468–471, 1977.
14. deTakats G: Whither vascular surgery. *Am J Surg* 134:2, 1977.
15. Gronen WW, Roda PL: Malignant hyperthemia. *J Am Podiatry Assoc* 66:31–33, 1976.
16. Cortese TA: Treatment of friction blisters. *Arch Dermatol* 97:717–721, 1968.
17. Labdata™ Reference Manual, Labdata Service Company, PO Box 26146, Phoenix, AR, 1982.
18. Fischbach F: *A Manual of Laboratory Diagnostic Tests* ed 2. Philadelphia, J. B. Lippincott Co, 1984.
19. Robbins, JM (ed): *Clinical Handbook of Podiatric Medicine*. Cleveland, Ohio College of Podiatric Medicine, 1983, pp. 120 to 123.
20. Roe, DA: *Clinical Nutrition for the Health Scientist*. CRC Press, 1979.
21. Select Committee on Nutrition and Human Needs, US Senate: *Dietary Goals for the United States*. Washington, DC, US Government Printing Office, 1977.
22. National Institutes of Health Consensus Development Conference Statement: *Lowering Blood Cholesterol to Prevent Heart Disease*, vol 5, no 7. Washington, DC, 1984.
23. Recommendations for treatment of hyperlipidemia in adults. Amer Heart Assoc, cir 69, no 5, 1984.

Suggested Readings

Arden SH: Clinical laboratory studies for the podiatric surgical patient. *J Foot Surg* 15:156–158, 1976.

Boyce-Smith G: Perioperative medical evaluation, history, and physical examination. ACFS Scientific Seminar. Las Vegas, NE. February, 1984.

Conn RF (ed): *Current Diagnosis.* Philadelphia, W.B. Saunders Co 1985.

Cortese CJ: Clinical signs in differential diagnosis of bacterial infections. *J Am Podiatry Assoc* 62:287–297, 1972.

Cross H, Bjorn J: *Problem-Oriented Private Practice of Medicine; A system for Comprehensive Care. Chicago, Modern Hospital Press, 1972.*

Delpp, MH, Manning RT: Major's Physical Diagnosis, ed 9. Philadelphia, W. B. Saunders, 1981.

Gafafer WM (ed): Occupational diseases—A guide to their recognition. Washington, DC: US Government Printing Office, Public Health Service Pub 1097:28, 1964.

Gamble FO: *Applied Foot Roentgenology.* Baltimore, Williams & Wilkins, 1957.

Gamble FO, Yale I: *Clinical Foot Roentgenology* ed 2. Huntington, NY, R. Krieger Publishing Co, 1975.

Gicker JW: Differential diagnosis of diseases of the foot. *Chirop Rec* 22:151–154, 1939.

Goss CM (ed): *Gray's Anatomy,* ed 30. Philadelphia, Lea and Febiger, 1984.

Gottlieb A: The foot during pregnancy and postpartum. *J Natl Assoc Chirop* 30:5–8, 1940.

Henry JB (ed): *Clinical Diagnosis and Management by Laboratory Methods* ed 17. Philadelphia, W.B. Saunders, 1984.

Keefer CS: Some clinical features of defciency disorders. *NY State J Med* 32:1405–1413, 1932.

Levy LA (ed): Systemic diseases affecting the foot. *Clinics in Podiatry,* 2(4), 1985.

McLaren DS, Burman D (ed): *Textbook of Paediatric Nutrition,* New York, Churchill Livingstone, 1982.

Newell RR: Roentgenology: Contrast media. In Glasser O (ed): *Medical Physics,* vol 1. Chicago, Year Book Publishers, 1944, pp. 1269-1271.

Norlander NB: Restless legs syndrome. *Br J Phys Med, New Series* 17: 160–162, 1954.

O'Brien FL, et al.: Nutrition in chiropody. *J Natl Assoc Chirop* 47:601–608, 1957.

Prior JA, Silberstein JS: *Physical Diagnosis,* ed 4. St. Louis, C.V. Mosby, 1973.

Rice JRD: Psychosomatic manifestations seen in the foot. *J Natl Assoc Chirop* 46:27, 1956.

Robertson WE, Robertson HF: *Diagnostic Signs, Reflexes and Syndromes,* ed 3. Philadelphia, F. A. Davis Co 1947.

Roetman RL: Physical examination of the podiatric patient. *J Am Podiatry Assoc* 56:271–280, 1966.

Sabiston Sr DC (ed): *Davis-Christopher Textbook of Surgery,* vols. 1 and 2, ed 12. Philadelphia, W. B. Saunders, 1981.

Seifer O, Mueller F: *Manual of Physical and Clinical Diagnosis,* ed 2. Philadelphia, J. B. Lippincott, 1934.

Strang JM: Obesity and diabetes. *Am J Med Sci* 236:405–418, 1958.

Sturm M: A theoretical explanation of the etiology of cardiovascular states. *Med Rec* 142:445–446, 1935.

Tietz, NW (ed): *Clinical Guide to Laboratory Tests.* Philadelphia, W. B. Saunders, 1983.

Wyngaarden JB, Smith LH (eds): *Cecil Textbook of Medicine,* vols I and II. Philadelphia, W. B. Saunders, 1985.

Yale I: Differential diagnosis. *Conn Chiropodist.* 11:45, 1951.

Yale I: Clinical and roentgenological interpretations in the lower extremities. *Chirop Rec* 32:186–187, 1949.

Yale I: Clinical and roentgenological interpretations in the lower extremities. *Am Podiatrist* 517, 1950.

Yale I: Clinical and roentgenological interpretations in the lower extremities. *Chirop Rec* 33:319–323, 1950.

Yale I: *Clinical and roentgenological interpretations in the lower extremities.* Ansonia, CT, Chiropody Lit, 1952.

Yale I, Yale J: *The Arthritic Foot and Related Connective Tissue Disorders.* Baltimore, Williams & Wilkins, 1984.

Yater WM: *Symptoms Diagnosis* ed 4. New York, D. Appleton-Century Co 1942.

Young JR, Humphries AW, DeWolfe VG: Restless leg syndrome. *Geriatrics* 24:167–171, 1969.

3

The Painful Foot

Subjective Symptoms

The presence of pain associated with podiatric complaint is of definite importance in making a diagnosis. If the type of pain is accurately described the podiatrist should have a reliable indicator of possible pathologies. Many general afflictions are characterized by certain sensations affecting the lower extremities. This chapter discusses the implications of the presence of different types of pain and their relationship to local and general involvements.

Pain is defined as distress or suffering; "It is a form of communication. It advises us of the presence of what purports to be a harmful situation"(1).

The cause of pain in the foot ranges from ill-fitting footgear or improper weight distribution to trauma or disease. Individuals with pernicious anemia or degeneration of the brain and spinal cord may have difficulty in interpreting painful stimuli. Circulatory diseases and peripheral nerve lesions also affect perception of stimuli, but many podiatic compliants involve characteristic pain and discomfort.

Mechanical factors, such as pressure from inflammatory exudates and swelling, result in painful irritation of local sensory nerves. A prolonged contraction of a hollow organ, such as spasm of blood vessels, results in pain of a severe nature. Pressure from a neoplasm may cause degeneration of surrounding organs or tissue, whereas hemorrhage into body tissue increases density, causing great pain. Ill-fitting clothing (shoes, hose and garters) may cause pain. Faulty foot posture may result in excessive weightbearing on a metatarsal or on the medial or lateral aspect of heels. Stress in joints as a result of poor foot function may cause degenerative lipping, spurs or osteophytes. Destruction of joint cartilage, which causes pain, may result.

Ischemia of a part as a result of emboli lodging in small arteries causes ischemic neuritis. The impoverished tissues and nerves are painful and often cause focal gangrene. Bacterial toxins result in increased temperature and infected tissue with heat, redness and pain.

Acroparesthesia may be slow or acute in onset, bilateral and characterized by "pins and needles" sensations of fingers and toes in females.

Anesthesia is a state in which there is an entire or almost complete absence of sensations. It includes hypoalgesia, tactile hypoesthesia, loss of temperature sense, loss of sense of muscular activity, absence of vibratory sensation and loss of joint sense. Loss of pain and temperature sensations are often noted in immersion foot. Anesthesia may be noted in a CNS disorder. A severed nerve, spinal cord tumor or myelitis may produce anesthesia, or it may be caused by toxic agents, such as cocaine, phenol, arsenic and belladonna, affecting the nervous system. Injection of procaine hydrochloride, lidocaine or other local anesthetics results in the loss of sensation for short periods of time. Anesthesia may occur in distal parts in the neural form of leprosy.

Analgesia is manifest when sensation of pain alone is absent. It may be present in tabes dorsalis along the distribution of the peroneal nerve. It may be brought about through the CNS and may originate from within or outside the brain. Voluntary analgesia is commonly seen in neurotic individuals who practice autosuggestion.

In functional nervous disease and especially hysteria, the patient with hysterical anesthesia of an extremity is unable to move the affected part when the eyes are closed. When eyes are open, however, and attention is directed to the involved limb, voluntary movement can be made, thus simulating a loss of muscle sense.

Classification of Pain

Subjective Pain

Subjective pain has no physical cause; it is the product of mental action arising from a disturbance in the coordinating centers of the sensory areas in the brain.

Hysterical pain is characterized by rapid changes in location, degree and severity. Pain may disappear by autosuggestion as willed by the patient. Pain appears for the same reason and is generally as severe as pain caused by a physical pathology. Emotionalism incites pain and may leave the patient exhausted. Hypnosis pain is a subjective pain. It is possible to bring forgotten pain sensations to consciousness through hypnosis and through the same mechanism to eliminate emotional or organic pain.

Objective Pain

Objective pain is excited by an agent that is foreign or abnormal to an area.

CNS objective pain may be due to a lesion in the optic thalamus, which is a relay center of the brain, or it may come from any structure within the sensory system.

Intrinsic peripheral objective pain is due to a disturbance of an axon, ganglia cells or receptors. Its cause may be organic and due to changes in structure, as in intrinsic inflammation, new growth, displacement of parts and abnormal muscular contractions.

Extrinsic peripheral objective pain may be due to displacement with pressure on adjacent organs or stretching of ligaments. Excessive use of an organ may also result in this type of pain.

Propagation of pain is the phenomenon of pain experienced in areas other than that in which the pain originated.

Referred pain is the result of irritation that occurs along the course of nerve fibers; pain is felt in the peripheral distribution of the affected nerve, e.g., imbalanced feet can cause pain in the knee; osteoma in the tibia may cause pain in the groin; pain in the ankle may be due to a tumor in Scarpa's triangle; and pain in the extremity at certain dermatomes caused by a ruptured disk suggests the level of the lesion.

Burns and decreased alkalinity of the blood cause excruciating pain. Electrical shock and other strong stimuli may result in great pain. Extremes of heat and cold with barometric variance are factors to be considered in arthritis and painful helomas. Intermittent claudication occurs in circulatory disorders and usually manifests itself as a cramp.

Roy and Tunks (2) discuss the chronic pain patient who has no presenting disease and the psychosocial aspects of the disability of chronic pain.

Perception of Pain

Pain protects from potentially harmful stimuli in environment. The loss of this protection may cause constant and repeated danger. This is especially true of the foot housed in a shoe and subject to the trauma of upright stance and gait. Pain becomes an important warning signal aided by vision, smell, touch and other senses.

The recent discovery that the body has its own pain inhibitory system, namely the *endorphins*, has created renewed interest in the body's defense mechanisms for relief of pain. Endorphin molecules are produced in the brain and by the pituitary and closely resemble morphine. Cerebrospinal fluid studies can measure the amount of endorphins being secreted and the possible extent to which endorphins are participating in the pain defense. Nerve damage caused by infection or trauma often shows a limitation of endorphin activity. However, a patient suffering a psychological or neurotic pain syndrome tends to have high endorphin levels. Patients with deficient endorphins may be treated by the transcutaneous electrical stimulation (TENS) method, an outgrowth of the old acupuncture techniques. This procedure has been shown to release endorphins and provides another approach to relief of chronic pain where certain drugs are contraindicated (3).

According to Sjölund and Eriksson (4), double-blind studies indicate that "the body possesses several mechanisms in the central nervous system to combat pain. Only some of these (i.e., acupuncture) seem to utilize endogenous morphine-like substances (endorphins)." It appears from Sjölund's studies that the narcotic antagonist Naloxane does not reverse the analgesia induced by conventional TENS, but acupuncture-like TENS analgesia was reversed in a significant number of patients.

Fink et al. (5) found that water had a local anesthetic action. They demonstrate the "existence of an osmotic block of impulse conduction that is reversible even when produced with plain water." The nerves quickly lost their ability to conduct electrical impulses, but recovered when given the chance to do so in normal saline. This approach to relief of pain awaits clinical testing before being used in practice on humans.

Ochoa of the Dartmouth-Hitchcock Medical Center, in collaboration with Professor Noordenbas (Amsterdam) and the Institute of Neurology in London (6), states that only certain types of injury lead to pain. Ochoa concludes that "(a) disruption of the nerve fibre itself results in chronic pain following local nerve injury, (b) damage to the myelin sheath alone does not cause pain, but does cause loss of sensation, (c) damage to the population of small caliber nerve fibres may either abolish pain perception or cause spontaneous pain, while the sense of touch is preserved." The studies demonstrate that injured nerves from patients with chronic pain contain excessive numbers of immature sprouts that fail to grow down the nerve and make proper reconnections with their terminals. According to Wall and Gutrick (7), in nature, these sprouts—like an epileptic focus in the brain—generate abnormal electrical impulses that might be the source of chronic pain.

The research team of Levine et al. (8) established that many patients obtain relief from pain following the use of a placebo. A series of neural events is triggered that results in the release of endorphins, the body's natural pain killer produced in the brain and the pituitary gland.

Electrostimulus acupunctural anesthesia has been created in experimental animals. Pain was relieved during and after the application of the electrostimulus by Takida et al. (9). TENS is used for relief of muscle, joint and peripheral organic pain. An advancement based on physiological concepts increased the number of electrodes from 2 or 4 to 12. With more electrodes, the optimal stimulation area could be found faster. The stimulation employs constant energy pulses, rather than constant current or voltage stimulation. The electrical nerve stimulation is therefore greater and more efficient. The new instrument in clinical studies in Israel resulted in 50% of the patients having marked relief of chronic and subacute organic pain.

In a study of peripheral nerve lesions and pain in cold injury in humans by Dash and Singh (10) reported in 1978 to the Second World Congress on Pain, the researchers found the following:

1. Cold injury affects all fibers and conduction velocity of the affected fibers is appreciably reduced.
2. Paranodal demyelination as well as degeneration and regeneration were observed.
3. Burning pain was present for about 1 year.
4. Conduction velocity of the fastest fibers in the mixed nerves (muscle afferents) recovered in 24 to 26 weeks after injury, recovery in motor fibers took about 3 years.

Tenderness is a painful condition produced by pressure; contusion may cause tenderness of connective tissue. Frequently, nails, helomas and bony prominences are irritated by ill-fitting shoes.

Hyperalgesia is an abnormal sensitivity to pain. It is commonly observed after trauma or in individuals with neurocirculatory disease. It is also common in the aged and in neurotic patients and women of menopausal age. The lightest brush of the finger over the hyperalgesic area causes extreme sensations of tenderness. Hysterical hyperalgesia is common over joints. In hysteria the sensation does not follow the distribution of peripheral nerves. Hyperalgesia is severe in gout and vasospastic disorders.

Tabes dorsalis, multiple neuritis and subacute combined degeneration of the spinal cord present early hyperalgesia. Alcoholic polyneuritis may cause pain and tenderness, increased temperature, loss of deep reflexes and paralysis. An ischemic neuritis, especially around the toe nail, may cause severe pain.

Paresthesia is a symptom that simulates pain. It is a sensation (prickling, itching, sensations of heat and cold, tingling and numbness) that is not strong enough to give the pain sensation. One may also have decreased sensation with paresthesia.

Neurasthenic patients may experience paresthesias with marked changes in type and location of the sensation. Numbness, tingling and weakness may occur in transverse myelitis. The symptoms vary with the severity of the pathology that exists. Paresthesias occur more often in females.

A feeling of walking on cotton balls with numbness of the feet is felt in peripheral neuropathy and tabes dorsalis. A traumatic neuritis often manifests itself as a pins-and-needles sensation.

Arsenical, alcoholic and diabetic neuritis and anemias cause the extremities to feel dead, with numbness, tingling and burning. Some cases of neuritis are characteristically motor or sensory.

Early symptoms of cerebral episodes are felt as paresthesia in the affected extremity. Arteriosclerosis, pernicious anemia, acroparesthesia and Raynaud's disease present symptoms of paresthesia. Paresthesias are seen in immersion foot.

Besides the primary symptoms, multiple sclerosis may present a heaviness of the limbs.

Projected pain is the sensation of pain in a part that has no feeling or in an amputated limb. Patients with projected pain may have pain sensations in amputated extremities, the so-called phantom pain. Pain may also be due to a neuroma on the amputated stump.

Description and Causes of Pain

The patient's ability to describe or to explain with similes the type of pain is important to proper diagnosis. Pain may be continuous, intermittent or remittent. Diurnal pain may be noted in involvements of the locomotor apparatus. Nocturnal pain is common in peripheral vascular problems.

Peripheral Neuropathy. Entrapment of peripheral nerves may cause a unilateral foot pain that manifests as a burning and tingling. Peripheral neuropathy must be differentiated from compressions in the lower back due to a degenerative disk, tumors or compression secondary to severe injury anywhere along a nerve trunk. When a nerve is entrapped there is generally an acute tenderness proximal to the site, with numbness distal to the compression. It is all too easy to pass off local pain or pain far removed from the site of a structural foot disturbance as being of local origin. Strain, ligamentous stress and articular pathology may be obvious, but the source of pain may be due to peripheral nerve entrapment.

Nerve entrapment may occur anywhere along its course, especially where constriction develops from anatomical distortions or trauma. Inflammation due to pressure on the nerve and its intrinsic blood supply may cause rest pain. Tenderness is noted at the site of entrapment and slightly above and below this site along the nerve trunk.

Kopell and Thompson (11) state that diagnosis can be confused by the presence of symptomatic low back derangement, diffuse nerve trunk tenderness, atypical pain distributions and secondary autonomic nervous system hyperfunction and by the presence of foot and ankle injuries causing pain and disability.

Nerve Entrapment. Johnson and Ortiz (12), in electrodiagnostic studies of the tarsal tunnel syndrome, established distal latency ranges of the medial plantar nerve. Electrodiagnostic examination usually reveals a slowed-up nerve conduction velocity and an increase in latency reaction. Because podiatrists are most commonly involved with nerves of the posterior tibial and its branches, it is clinically helpful to note that the "distal latency of the medial plantar nerve ranges from 4.5 to 6.1 msec and the lateral plantar nerve between 5 and 6.7 msec." Generally speaking, pain radiates distally, but is capable of proximal discomfort. Paresthesia, burning pain, hypoesthesia, deep or superficial sting, vague discomfort, numbness and sometimes cramps that may be acute or gradual signal the onset of entrapment neuropathies.

The podiatrist confronted with characteristic symptoms of entrapment must be aware of the anatomical origin of the nerves in the extremities and the possible sites of compression by bone, fascia, muscle or tumors, and he or she must be capable of podiatric treatment. The medical podiatrist should consult with the podiatric surgeon if medical treatment is nonproductive. Treatment varies from bed rest and/or immobilization, to injections of local anesthetics and steroids at sites of maximum discomfort, to manipulation and stretching with active and passive exercises followed by an orthotic device to hold the foot in a neutral position. Surgery includes decompression by soft tissue release, fasciotomy, neurolysis and excision of compressive masses. The podiatric consultant must determine the desirable technique after careful evaluation of the pathology. The doctor must keep in mind that the nerve and circulatory supply to the foot is not always of textbook quality and position (13, 14).

Jones (15) demonstrated a variant position of the branch of the lateral plantar nerve supplying the abductor digiti quinti muscle. In the presence of a calcaneal spur, the muscle nerve branch may be subject to continuing pressure from the exostosis, resulting in an entrapment neuropathy.

In a comprehensive study of peripheral nerve entrapment, Carrel and Davidson (16) discuss the etiology of the various nerves subject to entrapment. The validity of the electromyographic nerve conduction tests in establishing motor nerve conduction velocity and distal latency is discussed in the light of evaluating the extent of peripheral nerve entrapment. The authors describe the symptoms of compression of a peripheral nerve trunk as affecting the motor, sensory and autonomic functions of the nerve. Paralysis and/or muscle weakness, numbness, tingling and pruritus are common. Pain manifest at night as an analgesia accompanied by trophic skin changes is not uncommon. Palpation of the nerve at its site of entrapment (Valleix's phenomena) may cause pain both proximally and distally. When the pain and tingling radiate distally following percussion, a positive Tinel's sign is present.

Compression of nerves by masses, swellings and ganglia is not unusual. By far, the most common entrapment in the foot is in the tarsal tunnel. When the laciniate ligament and flexor retinaculum compress (for whatever reason) the posterior tibial nerve, its accompanying blood vessels and dynamic tibialis posterior, flexor hallucis longus and flexor digitorum longus against the medial malleolus and the calcaneus, nerve damage can be created. The groove formed by the structures above and the bones below creates the tarsal tunnel. Other entrapments common to the foot involve the deep peroneal (anterior tibial) nerve and the sural, common peroneal, superficial peroneal and common digital nerves.

Kashuk (17) discussed the nerve entrapments from the spinal nerve roots to the terminal nerve branches. His consideration of nerve entrapments include impingement of the affected nerve by anatomical alterations creating mechanical irritation. Transmission of impulses is altered, and the manifestations of the signs of clinical entrapment neuropathy prevail. Repeated irritation for long periods of time is capable of damaging the circulatory supply to the nerve, creating pathological degenerative perineural fibrosis. As long as the circulatory supply to the nerve, vaso nervorum, remains intact and unconstricted, a nerve will continue to function. Because the extrinsic and intrinsic circulation are essential to proper nerve function, compression by entrapment is capable of presenting symptoms of motor and sensory dysfunction.

Paresthesias (Tinel's sign) distal to the site of entrapment, tenderness (Valleix's phenomena) along the course of the nerve, atrophy of muscles supplied by the nerve and often a paralysis are associated with entrapment. Most hospitals and neurological centers are equipped to perform conduction velocity and nerve latency studies. Peripheral nerves have a normal conduction velocity of 43 to 58 msec.

Entrapment of the common peroneal nerve as it passes around the fibular neck may produce pain on inversion and plantar flexion of the foot and ankle. If the entrapment continues, the lateral aspect of the leg and dorsolateral aspect of the foot become painful and often numb.

The posterior tibial nerve may become entrapped, with neuropathy developing in the ankle and foot. The calcaneal branch may give symptoms of a bruised heel, and the medial and lateral plantar nerves direct symptoms to the muscles on the sole of the foot, the adjacent joints and cutaneous sensation of the sole and toes.

The digital nerves are traumatized by the transverse intermetatarsal ligament. The distal edge of the ligament often prevents the digital nerve from assuming a position of safety between the metatarsals, resulting in trauma from the metatarsal head. All intermetatarsal and digital spaces may be affected even though neuroma in the third space is the most common. Pain may be burning, lancinating, sharp and shooting or even vague.

Relief brought about by injection of a local anesthetic, corticosteroids or vitamin B_{12} is considered a confirmatory diagnosis of neuropathy. However, often the structural pathology must be corrected by manipulation, stretching exercises and mechanical devices for lasting relief. Surgical intervention may be necessary to relieve the entrapped nerve. It is essential to recognize and differentiate these problems.

Fatigue, including debility, asthenia, exhaustion, weakness, languor and lassitude, frequently arises from overstrained muscles. When foot posture is faulty and function is impaired, fatigue becomes an important symptom. Weakness may result from overstrain, disuse of certain groups of muscles, general illness, prolonged rest in bed, wearing high heels, ill-fitting shoes and hose or from occupational stress. Fatigue is an early symptom of peripheral vascular disease and usually appears months before organic occlusive vascular disease. It may also be a symptom of neurological disturbance, anemia, tuberculosis or other debilitating diseases. Emotional stress, overwork, warm and humid weather, diarrhea and abuse of alcohol, tea, coffee and tobacco may reduce the ability of the patient to withstand normal everyday muscular effort.

Dull aches may arise from muscles that are fatigued as a result of improper usage. Arthritic changes in joints and reactions to changes in climate may cause dull aches in the feet and legs. Long hours of standing and a history of injuries with resultant bone changes may cause dull aches. Vagueness of the complaint is often evident in neuroses requiring sedation for relief of the discomfort.

Sharp pains may follow the course of nerves as a result of nerve impingement, or they may occur in the joints limited in function due to degenerative joint disease. Painful joints in static foot conditions are due to the pull of ligaments on the periosteal attachments to the bone. Sudden trauma, such as a sprain, a direct blow on an exposed bony prominence or pressure on toes, may cause sharp pains. Multiple sharp, shooting pains of unknown etiology may be evidence of syphilis. Neuritis is also suggested in the presence of shooting pains. The presence of foreign bodies in the foot causes pain on weightbearing. Verrucoid tissue may cause sharp pain on weightbearing following a short period of rest.

Lancinating pain in the leg may occur in locomotor ataxia and occasionally in cerebrospinal syphilis. The examiner must ascertain whether the pain is shooting up or down the extremity in order to establish the etiology. Locomotor ataxia is usually bilateral with evidence of syphilis.

Embolism and thrombosis of the peripheral arteries can be diagnosed early on the basis of sudden intense pain in the limb. Tenderness is noted at the site of thrombus; the affected limb is cold, white and tender. Gangrene follows embolism and thrombosis of the lower extremities where there is insufficient collateral circulation.

Throbbing sensations may result from infection e.g., heloma, tyloma, furuncle or infected nail lip. Pressure on blood vessels by constricting garters or bandages may cause throbbing. The podiatrist usually finds this symptom in heloma and onychotic infections. Throbbing is common as the end result of verruca treatment when liquefaction necrosis of the growth occurs. Phlebitic changes or inflammation results in throbbing sensations. Abcess formation or acute osteomyelitis may cause throbbing.

Burning sensations, when not due to paresthesia, are attributed to abnormal pressure on blood vessels and cutaneous nerve endings that respond to mechanical treatment. These sensations are found where tylomas are present. Epidermophytosis, especially the interdigital type with its fissures, may produce burning sensations. When the skin is too dry or is hyperidrotic or when hose are too harsh on sensitive feet, burning sensations may occur. Improperly tanned leathers in footgear may also produce burning of the feet. The author has observed burning symptoms in the feet of anemic patients and occasionally in the feet of patients with hyperthyroidism. The aged often complain of burning sensations as a result of circulatory instability. Erythromelalgia and vasomotor disturbances cause burning sensations. A pressure neuritis from contraction of the fascia lata may cause pain, muscular spasm, tingling and numbness. According to Billig and Brennan (18), the peripheral nerves are involved in these symptoms. Occupations resulting in chemical contact often cause burning of the sensitized tissues.

Stiffness of muscles may be a spasticity that follows work in which the muscles have been forced to function improperly or to excess; trauma may also cause stiffness of muscles. Moderate use of muscles in an activity that is new often brings on symptoms of stiffness. It may also occur as a result of poor circulatory response to muscular effort. When a muscle is hypertonic and stretched, it may cause irregular and jerky movements. Spasms of the muscles are seen early in tuberculosis and rheumatoid arthritis.

Joint stiffness may be the result of chronic arthritis or adhesions as a consequence of static foot disability. Trauma to a joint may result in a traumatic arthritis, with possible joint mice, lipping, osteophytes and spur formation limiting normal range of motion. The metatarsophalangeal joints are usually affected. Traumatic arthritis may be caused by stubbing the great toe, a misstep, dropping an object on the metatarsophalangeal joint or from improperly fitted shoes that are either too short or too narrow. Rheumatoid arthritis, osteoarthritis, gout and many general involvements cause joint stiffness as does repair after infectious changes.

Polyarthritis. Pain in joints of the foot accompanied by urethritis, conjunctivitis and polyarthritis may be symptomatic of *Reiter's syndrome.*

Calabro (19) advises podiatrists to utilize tissue transplant compatibility tests to establish the presence or absence of histocompatibility antigen HLA B27. He states that 80 to 96% of patients with Reiter's syndrome have a positive B27. Prevention of chronic arthritis is predicated on early diagnosis of the genetic marker on the patient's lymphocytes.

The heel and great toe are often affected with indurated thickening and pain. The great toe has been described by Calabro as "sausage-like"; with swelling of the great toe and synovitis, the aspirated synovial fluid may show evidence of large macrophages and a high hemolytic complement. Reiter's syndrome can be differentiated from rheumatoid arthritis, gout and psoriatic arthritis by a careful history, examination and laboratory studies.

The judgment of the foot specialist is essential to proper utilization of medication to relieve the symptoms of pain. Systemic diseases should be properly diagnosed, and consultation with an internist is often necessary to provide continuity of comprehensive care for the sick patient. Depending on the history, the complaint and onset and duration of the symptoms, the analgesic medications discussed below are useful in relieving the painful foot. Special situations, such as treatment of infections, require specific medications that are discussed in other chapters.

Pain Relief

Drugs Used for Relief of Pain

Dibucaine hydrochloride, Nupercainal, in ointment or cream, and Quotane as a lotion may be applied to the skin to relieve painful abrasions. A 1:40 dilution of aluminum acetate and a 1:16 dilution of a Dalibour solution help reduce inflammation and swelling of trauma and superficial skin problems.

Articular, periatricular and fibrosytic inflammations are often relieved by local injections of dexamethasone (Decadron), betamethasone (Celestone) or triamcinolone acetonide (Aristocort, Kenalog). Tablets for oral use are also available for their systemic effect. These medications should be used with caution and only upon proper study of the problem to rule out contraindications and interaction with other drugs prescribed for the patient.

Short and long-acting barbiturates may be used with analgesics to control pain with neurasthenic overtones. Tranquilizers and psychotherapeutic agents are helpful in relieving anxiety associated with pain and as a preoperative and postoperative aid to recovery. Salicylates by themselves or in combination with other pain ameliorators may be the most efficacious and problem-free treatment for moderately painful symptoms. Propoxyphene hydrochloride (Darvon) in 32 mg or 65 mg capsules taken q 4 to 6 h and acetaminophen (Tylenol) in 325 mg tablets are effective pain relievers. Acetaminophen is also supplied as an elixir and in drops to accommodate the needs of the patient who is sensitive to aspirin.

Nonsteroidal anti-inflammatory drugs (NSAIDs) have been demonstrated as the medication of choice for inhibiting the action of prostaglandins. Prostaglandins are released at the site of inflammation. Other substances released at areas of inflammation, such as at the insertion of the Achilles tendon or plantar fascia, include histamine, kinins, 5-hydroxytryptamine and the toxic reactants to anaphylaxis. In addition to inhibiting protaglandins the NSAIDs limit the macrophage system, protein and calcitonin-combining reactions and have a tendency to stimulate the immunologic activity of T-lymphocytes. They do not alter the biochemistry affecting any presenting joint pathology, but do assist in providing comfort. Indomethacin (Indocin) 25–50 mg tid or 75 mg sustained release 12 hr capsules should not be used in children, in pregnant women, in the presence of gastrointestinal tract ulcer or in persons with psychiatric disturbances. Mental confusion and fatigue may occur.

Indocin may inhibit platelet formation. Prothrombin times, serum creatinine and urine protein should be monitored regularly when patients are receiving NSAIDs.

Sulindac (Clinoril) should be prescribed for a period of 1 week. It should be taken after ingestion of food, milk or a nonmagnesium-containing antacid of choice in a dose of 150 mg bid. The maximum dose is 400 mg/day. An anticoagulation effect and hypoglycemic reactions have been reported. Naproxen sodium (Anaprox), taken 550 mg to start, followed by 275 mg every 6–8 hours, should not be taken concurrently with Naprosyn. Tolmetin sodium (Tolectin) is prescribed 400 mg tid. Ibuprofen (Motrin), taken 300–800 mg qid not to exceed 3200 mg/day and ketoprofen (Orudis) taken 75 mg tid or 50 mg qid, not to exceed 300 mg/day, are also helpful.

Phenylbutasone (Butazolidin), 100 mg tid, and oxyphenylbutasone (Tandearil) are powerful anti-inflammatory drugs. These medications should be used only after other NSAIDs have proven to be ineffective. Patients should be monitored closely for blood dyscrasias and/or sodium retention. Meclofenamate sodium (Meclomen), an anthronilic acid derivative used for 1 week and taken 200–400 mg/day tid or qid, may be effective in elderly patients with reduced renal or hepatic function.

Piroxicam (Feldene), 20 mg/day, may be used as well. It may take 7–10 days for the medication to reach adequate blood levels and for therapy to be effective. Naproxen (Naprosyn) is used in varying doses of 250, 375, or 500 mg bid, depending on symptom severity and the weight of the patient. Naproxen may be used in acute gout, 750 mg initially and 250 mg every 8 hours, until relief is obtained. It is important to recognize that gastrointestinal bleeding is a possible side effect of naproxen. Platelet aggregation may be decreased and bleeding time may be increased. Acetylsalicylic acid (aspirin), 10 grains tid for 5 days after meals, milk, or the antacid of choice, should be one of the first medications prescribed for mild inflammations due to overuse syndromes in athletes. Gastric mucosa may be irritated by the ingestion of aspirin as it is absorbed in the stomach, hydrolyzed, and reacts with esters in the liver. When combined with magnesium and choline (Trilisate tablets), the salicylate is effective as a single daily dose, permitting a sustained therapeutic level (20). Two large studies undertaken by the Boston Collaborative Drug Surveillance Program reveal that NSAIDs rarely cause significant renal toxicity (21).

The following suggestions may be helpful when contemplating the use of NSAIDs for injuries or for joint inflammation of varying etiology (22).

1. If a patient has responded favorably in the past to a specific NSAID, prescribe the same medication.
2. Choose a medication that you are familiar with and have had experience prescribing.
3. Prescribe the smallest dosage to produce the desired effect; that is, a decrease in inflammatory symptoms.
4. Avoid combinations of NSAIDs.
5. Avoid changing medications without a 1–week trial.
6. If the patient's symptoms are under control with the use of one NSAID for a period of time, followed by a worsening of symptoms, do not discontinue the medication and prescribe another without first increasing the original medication dose.
7. Always be alert to side effects. Monitor the patient's prothrombin time, serum creatinine and urine protein on a regular basis when NSAIDs are being taken for extended periods of time.

Where pain is severe or intractable, such narcotic analgesics as acetylsalicylic acid with codeine (aspirin with codeine) or acetaminophen with codeine (Tylenol with codeine, 8 mg, 15 mg, 30 mg, or 60 mg) aid in proper control.

Pentazocine (Talwin) in 50 mg tablets for oral use or 1 ml ampules (30 mg), 1½ ml ampules (45 mg), 2 ml ampules (60 mg) or 10 ml multiple dose vials (30 mg/ml) is used for severe pain and has proven effective in many situations that might otherwise have required a narcotic. The oral tablet dose is one to two tablets q 4h. Its injectable form as pentazocine lactate intramuscularly is especially useful in lieu of a narcotic pain reliever. Pentazocine (25 mg) and acetaminophen (650 mg) (TALACEN) may be of benefit for severe pain control in those patients sensative to narcotic analgesics.

Other drugs used by podiatrists to relieve pain are ethoheptazine (Zactirin), 100 mg, meprobamate and ethoheptazine citrate with aspirin (Equagesic), one to two tablets q 6 h; mefenammic acid (Ponstel capsules), 250 mg for short-term analgesic activity; and chlormezanone with aspirin (Trancopal), 300 mg in tablet form. Phenaphen with codeine No. 2 (15 mg), No. 3 (30 mg), or No. 4 (60 mg) taken one capsule q 4 h prn for pain is highly effective.

Promethazine (Phenergan) in 12.5 mg, 25 mg or 50 mg strength is useful to potentiate the action of analgesics.

Promethazine (Phenergan) in 12.5 mg, 25 mg or 50 mg strength is useful to potentiate the action of analgesics.

When pain is due to muscle spasm, orphenadrine citrate (Norflex), one tablet bid, relieves rigidity and pain.

In the presence of pain, especially following foot surgery, the patient should have complete rest. Flurazepam hydrochloride (Dalmane) in a 30 mg capsule or triazolam (Halcion) in a 0.25 or 0.5 mg tablet on retiring is helpful to adults in ensuring a good night's sleep. A 15 mg Dalmane capsule or 0.125 mg Halcion tablet is more desirable for the elderly. Methyprylon (Noludar), 300 mg capsules, provides 5 to 8 hrs of sleep at night. Glutethimide (Doriden) tablets, 0.5 g, taken at night for sleep do not produce a morning hangover.

Diazepam (Valium) is useful for relief of tension, anxiety and muscle spasm associated with foot pathology. It is supplied in 2 mg, 5 mg and 10 mg tablets and may be prescribed in 2 mg and 5 mg doses tid for spasms and associated pain.

Intractable pain often requires the use of schedule II narcotics, such as meperedine hydrochloride (Demerol), 50 mg or 100 mg tablets, or parenteral administration q. 6 to 8 h prn for pain. Oxycodone hydrochloride and aspirin (Percodan) or oxycodone hydrochloride and acetaminophen (Percocet), one tablet q 4–6 h with milk, is helpful in relieving severe pain. Injection of such potent narcotics as morphine sulfate brings rapid relief of pain. As in the use of all drugs, the patient's general physical status is important when calculating dosage, and narcotics should be used in lieu of the stronger analgesics and potentiating agents only when absolutely necessary.

Allaying apprehension is perhaps the most singular factor in preparation for intravenous sedation. According to Arroyo (23) some patients need no preoperative medication. The most frequently used preoperative medication, if necessary, is 5 to 10 mg Valium (Roche), 50 to 100 mg Demerol and/or 0.4 mg atropine.

Arroyo prefers a combination of Sublimaze, thiopental and Valium. The technique depends on the skill and experience of the anesthetist in observing and regulating vital signs. Emergency resuscitation equipment and oxygen must be available at all times to maintain open airways. Following adequate sedation, the surgeon can administer a local anesthetic.

Johnson et al, (24) describe their technique for intravenous injection of Valium for preoperative sedation in outpatient surgery. In a series of over 400 cases, they found the most effective method of administration was 20 mg oral diazepam 30 min before surgery, followed by 10 mg diazepam injected slowly into the vein at the maximum rate of 5 mg (1 ml)/ min. The patient becomes drowsy and sedated. Vital signs are observed, and injections of local anesthetic are made at the operative site.

Choi and Donick (25), in their study on the changes in blood gasses, conclude that the administration of local anesthesia with intravenous sedation is a safe procedure. Patients with cardiac and/or pulmonary disorders require careful observation for hypoxia, which responds readily to the administration of oxygen. Valium appears to be the drug of choice in the older patient. It is necessary to refrain from use of pulmonary depressants for intravenous sedation in the high risk patient.

In a series of more than 3000 foot surgeries where intravenous sedation was used with local anesthesia, Donick et al, (26) note the advantages of the technique. They state that "intravenous sedation combined with local anesthesia has the advantages of both local and general anesthesia but less of the disadvantages of general anesthesia." There are some patients with systemic diseases who do not tolerate general anesthesia and would cooperate well if local anesthesia were utilized under a state of sedation administered by the intravenous route. The diabetic patients and those with renal, liver, cardiac and respiratory diseases should not receive a general anesthetic if a local or spinal anesthetic can control the surgical discomfort. The use of intravenous sedation allays the fear present with a local anesthetic, subdues neurotic behavior and limits the possibility of postoperative complications. Local anesthesia can be administered without pain when the patient is properly sedated.

The technique and choice of medication are chosen and administered by the anesthesiologist. Skilled operating room personnel should be available at all times. The patient is monitored before, during and after surgery. Valium, Pentothal sodium and Innovar provide analgesia and tranquility. During surgery, a hypnotic may be used intravenously in small doses to provide a light sleep.

Hypnosis

Block and Giorgini (27) cite the technique of hypnosis and the need for podiatrists to have a basic knowledge of hypnosis. The induction techniques are based on relaxation, which for all intents and purposes in the interpersonal practitioner-patient relationship, is most helpful. The nervous and hypersensitive patient is generally relaxed by hypnosis. The suggestion may provide a mild analgesia to a specific toe or part of a foot to allow for painless injections of an anesthetic. In minor surgery, the procedure can be performed with suggestion, rather than by the use of an anesthetic.

Block et al. (28) evaluated the effect of hypnosis on the vasodilatory and vasoconstrictive mechanism. They were able to determine by plethysmographic measurements that suggestion was capable of increasing or decreasing the dilation of the peripheral vessels depending on the depth of the hypnotic state. Increase in blood flow ranged from 21.8 to 35.6% and the decrease in flow from 29.6 to 44.0%. Using suggestion with nitrous oxide analgesia may provide greater analgesia than using the agent alone.

Hypnosis has been used by Sanders (29) for a variety of podiatric problems. He has used medical relaxation in treatment of peroneal spastic flatfoot and has found this approach more effective than the use of a local anesthetic. While the patient is under hypnotic induction, the muscle spasm is broken by gently inverting and adducting the pronated foot.

When all chemical, electrical and surgical techniques have failed in treating multiple or mosaic verruca, the author has been able to relieve and ultimately resolve the lesions by 3 to 5 min sessions of induction and suggestion on a biweekly schedule.

Vasospastic disorders are generally improved by positive suggestions.

TENS

Transcutaneous electrical nerve stimulation (TENS) complements traditional pharmacological therapy and may provide adequate analgesia by itself. Lesser amounts of postoperative medication are necessary with the concomitant use of TENS (30) (see Chapter 11, Surgery.) The Electro-Acuscope 80 (distributed by Current Medical Instruments, Point Reyes, CA) provides the conventional mode of TENS with an additional "computer-controlled circuitry with all forms of feedback."

Trigger Points

Muscle spasm is often relieved by topical ethyl chloride spray analgesia, which enables early limited motion. Harvey et al. (31) present a historical review of cryotherapy use. The effects of coldspray and stretch on hamstring and triceps surae muscle groups in 16 subjects are compared. The authors suggest that the results of mobilization may increase the functional length of muscle.

Kraus (32) described trigger points as "local tender nodules of degenerated muscle tissue." Caused by tension or muscular strain, trigger points may be found close to the origin or insertion of a muscle. Treatment for the relief of pain may consist of deep massage and/or injection of a local anesthetic combined with a nonacetylated steroid into the trigger point. MadaJet (Mada Medical Products, Inc., Carlstadt, NJ) has been used to inject small amounts of anesthetic in and around specific painful sites. The instrument is not capable of deep penetration.

Acupuncture

Pain has been successfully relieved by acupuncture and acupressure technique. Research by Laurence (33) and Lorenz et al. (34) confirms the release of enkephalins and endorphins by means of acupuncture and low-power electrical stimulation of periosteum. The release of these morphine-like substances is effective in relieving pain, reducing anxiety and lifting moods.

General Foot Discomfort

General foot discomfort can be a symptom of neurasthenia, a variety of systemic diseases, ill-fitting shoes or hose or incipient mechanical disturbances of the feet. All the arthritides, circulatory disorders and neurological disturbances may cause general foot discomfort. Occupational stress and environmental factors, such as metal floors, hot weightbearing surfaces and extreme temperature changes, often produce general foot discomfort. Atmospheric conditions and poorly constructed shoes also cause these difficulties. Leather in shoes is often tanned poorly, and shoes may be nailed or stitched irregularly. A single heloma or other excrescence on the foot may cause the patient to limp in order to favor the painful part, thus causing other foot discomfort. This general discomfort may manifest itself as cramps, paresthesias or sharp, shooting, dull aching, burning, or tingling pain.

Cramps Cramps occur in muscles as a result of unnatural anatomical positions and impaired circulation. They are involuntary muscular contractions with severe pain and partial or complete loss of function. They may occur in debilitated patients with fevers or chronic wasting diseases. Atherosclerosis, vasospasm, varicose veins and thrombophlebitis cause cramps. They are most frequent at night and are common in pregnancy, calcium-phosphorus imbalance, faulty metabolism and profound diuresis.

Deformities of the feet, nutritional deficiency—especially vitamin B and related edema—may cause cramp-like pains in the lower extremities. Heat cramps are widespread, with sudden onset affecting varying groups of muscles. They are caused by an excessive loss of sweat without sodium chloride and potassium replacement.

Unnatural anatomical positions in certain occupations result in cramps, aching pains and incoordination. Moderate shortening of the posterior calf muscle and hamstring groups often induces cramps. During tetany the toes may cramp into a flexion state, with the arch of the foot being domed by plantar contractures with inversion.

Treatment. Control foot strain and pull on the calf muscles. Triceps surae stretching exercises are often helpful. Treat underlying infection or debilitating illness. Prescribing multiple vitamins and minerals where indicated is helpful. In the presence of sodium chloride depletion, cramps are controlled by the ingestion of salt tablets. Faulty calcium metabolism is determined through blood chemistry studies. Treatment of parathyroid dysfunction and ingestion of calcium supplements are beneficial in tetany. Calcium lactate or gluconate may be given intravenously. Peripheral vascular spasms produce avascular musculature and cramps.

Quinine capsules 3 or 5 grain bid help relieve idiopathic cramping. Nylidrin hydrochloride in 6 mg tablets tid and cyclandelate (Cyclospasmol), 100 or 200 mg, help relieve cramps. If the patient smokes, limiting smoking may also effect relief. Brody and Brezak (35), after a preliminary study of the effectiveness of small doses of quinine and aminophylline in combination on nocturnal cramps, recommend the use of these drugs for effective relief to most patients. Orphenadrine hydrochloride, 25 mg bid, or if cramps occur at night, 50 mg q hs, is a most effective nontoxic muscle relaxant. Occasionally, tranquilizers, such as chlordiazepoxide hydrochloride (Librium) in 5, 10 and 25 mg capsules or tablets; meprobamate (Miltown) in 400 mg tablets up to 1600 mg daily; hydroxyzine pamoate (Vistaril) in 25, 50 and 100 mg capsules, oral suspension or by injection are useful for short-term therapy.

Lumbar sympathectomy and vasodilator relaxants are helpful. Methocarbamol, 500 mg tablets administered at bedtime or one tablet q i d or two tablets q 4 h usually relieves cramps within 72 hr. Continued relief is obtained for 3 to 4 weeks after discontinuing the drug.

Pain in the legs due to polyarteritis, which often alternately attacks each leg, that is associated with a rash and mild pyrexia is amenable to therapy. Prednisolone, 22.5 mg daily reduced subsequently to 5 mg daily, has suppressed polyarteritis. Antihistamines are often helpful for short-term therapy. The author has successfully used Benadryl in 25 and 50 mg capsules for muscle cramps. Benadryl is available also for intramuscular injection in concentrations of 10 mg or 50 mg/ml. Chlor-Trimeton in 8 and 12 mg tablets is effective, and Thephorin, 25 mg, is a helpful slow-acting antihistamine that does not cause drowsiness. Large doses of aspirin have proven helpful for relief of muscle cramps. Betamethasone, 1.5 mg daily, has given symptomatic relief according to Golding (36).

Intermittent Claudication Intermittent claudication is a cramp due to local anoxemia resulting from deficient circulation. Patients usually complain that after walking short distances or climbing a hill they become tired, their muscles get sore and their calf muscles cramp. They must stop, squeeze and rub the involved muscles and rest for a few minutes before the sensation disappears. Patients are then able to walk further, only to be afflicted again in a short time after mild exercise. Intermittent claudication is a common symptom in arteriosclerosis and thromboangiitis obliterans, varicosities, muscular fatigue, arterial spasm and anemia; it is often simulated in locomotor ataxia. Walking and standing do not cause intermittent claudication until muscular fatigue and failure of oxygenation of the muscles ensue.

This cramp-like symptom is brought on with muscular effort, such as climbing stairs and hills and by rapid or long walks; it may also be caused by severe anemia. When the cramp comes on it usually affects the calf muscles and is so severe as to cause the patient to cease walking. The cramp may vary from a severe claudication to the sensation of a tightness in the posterior group of muscles. These cramps may develop in the feet and involve the plantar muscles, interossei or the anterior tibial as well; they should be noted carefully in order to differentiate them from an imbalance of foot posture. Sometimes patients complain of experiencing cramps while at rest, especially in bed at night. Such cramps cause them to get out of bed, stamp the foot, press hard on a cold floor and to kick or massage the limb in order to bring about relief. There is no relationship between this type of cramp and intermittent claudication.

Treatment. Limit as much physical effort as possible by improving foot function. Improve circulatory status by treatment of venous insufficiency and arterial diseases. Vasodilators are prescribed, and daily use of whiskey in moderation is safe. Nylidrin, tolazoline hydrochloride (25 mg tablets) and isoxysuprine hydrochloride (10 mg tablets) as Arliden, Priscoline and Vasodilan are proven vasodilators. Pentoxifylline (Trental) 400 mg tid po, has been effective in the treatment of intermittent claudication (37). The cardiopulmonary vascular system should be examined by an internist for systemic pathology. The blood is examined for blood dyscrasias capable of causing anoxia. Corrective measures are followed if necessary.

Sympathectomy may be indicated to relieve arterial spasm. A vascular surgeon may have to perform arterial transplants, and bypass arterial prostheses may be necessary. Anticoagulants are prescribed by the internist who also treats metabolic and nutritional problems. Endocrine disorders are sought out, and if present, early treatment is given.

A cardiogram or Swan Ganz catheter study or both may be necessary in suspected myocardial infarction.

Pallor Pallor is considered a common symptom in peripheral vascular disorders, but it is not a chief complaint of a patient's condition although it is usually associated with numbness and tingling. The skin tone depends on the blood circulation. The extent of the affected area must be determined for accurate diagnosis.

Pallor may be due to an embolic occlusion in the peripheral arteries which very often occurs at the bifurcation of the popliteal artery behind the knee. Pallor after exposure to cold or due to emotional disturbances is often a symptom of Raynaud's disease.

Treatment. Removal of thrombi from an occluded artery by a vascular surgeon may be indicated. Anticoagulants may be prescribed by the internist or vascular surgeon when necessary in embolic occlusions.

Contrast foot plunges, 2 min in comfortably hot water followed by 1 min in cold water, are helpful. The process should be repeated for 20 to 30 min qid. If the patient smokes, smoking should be limited. Burger's exercises are helpful. Vasodilators such as 100 mg tablets of cyclandelate tid or nicotinic acid in 20 or 100 mg tablets, with vasospatic disorders may alleviate this type of symptom.

Nervous individuals or patients suffering from sympathetic nervous system disease may show evidence of pallor. This condition must be differentiated from thromboangiitis obliterans, which presents marked color changes on elevation. Tight garters or any constricting garment may produce pallor and should be carefully differentiated from true vasospasm. Psychotherapeutic medications may be necessary to relax hypertensive patients. Meprobamate, 200 or 400 mg tablets; chlordiazepoxide in 5, 10 and 25 mg capsules; or promethazine in 12.5, 25, or 50 mg tablets or in a syrup may be helpful.

Numbness and Tingling Numbness is a paresthesia following nerve pressure, and if the pressure is unremitting, it leads to a sensory nerve paralysis. Pressure of a tumor may cause numbness. In the feet, numbness may occur from a long-standing sciatic involvement or diabetic neuropathy. It may occur in circulatory involvements of a general nature or in a localized circulatory deficiency produced by malfunctioning feet or improperly fitted footgear. Numbness is common in Morton's neuralgia and in the feet of the elderly.

Vitamin deficiencies, pernicious anemia and dietary disturbances may cause numbness, and it may be an early symptom of tabes, arteriosclerosis obliterans, multiple neuritis, neurosis, multiple sclerosis and subacute combined degeneration of the spinal cord, Raynaud's disease and immersion foot or trench foot.

Cocaine addicts complain of paresthesias that they describe as being like "foreign bodies under the skin."

The beginnings of nerve degeneration are suggested when tingling sensations occur in the distal end of a divided nerve upon percussion over the area of division. Numbness and coldness of an extremity may be noted in rupture of the nucleus pulposus in the lumbar region. Dermatomes are carefully evaluated to ascertain the cord level of pathology.

Although characteristic mainly of a neuritis or some lesion in the posterior columns of the spinal cord, numbness and tingling are also characteristic in circulatory involvements. Usually numbness develops at night while the patient is asleep or when sitting for long periods of time, and it may be attributable to pressure on the extremity. Sometimes the numbness and tingling are symmetrical due to a vasospasm; frostbite or severe trauma may also cause these symptoms. Numbness and tingling may indicate an embolus in a large vessel of the extremity.

The sensation of numbness and tingling may suggest pernicious anemia, and it is often a symptom of causalgia. The patient suffering with a neuroma often has the neuralgic symptom early. Ill-fitting, constrictive shoes and hose may cause numbness.

Lemont (38) notes that the intermediate dorsal cutaneous nerve is very superficial and can easily be palpated when the foot is extended and inverted. Trauma is possible because of this anatomical location and can manifest as pain, numbness and tingling. If distal tingling occurs on palpation or percussion or following an injury, one must be concerned about a positive Tinel's sign. A positive sign suggests an entrapment of the nerve. Recalcitrant pain may very well be secondary to repeated lateral sprains. Injections of a local anesthetic and adhesive immobilization may be helpful.

Treatment. Correct circulatory and neurological disorders by close liaison with specialists in the respective fields. Remove tumors compressing nerve trunks, e.g., neurinomas.

Have an internist examine and prescribe for systemic diseases and blood dyscrasias and deficiencies. Examine the patient carefully and treat existing local pathology. Prescribe dietary supplements. Maintain the integrity of the musculature.

Pruritus Pruritus may be secondary to many skin diseases and may be a symptom of certain systemic diseases. It may include fungus infections, insect bites, eczema, contact dermatitis, psoriasis, lichen simplex and neurodermatitis, or it may be a result of dry skin, especially in elderly patients.

Diabetes, nephritis, diseases of the liver, malignant tumors, Hodgkin's disease, leukemia, tuberculosis, arteriosclerosis and a myriad of metabolic disorders can also cause pruritus.

Treatment is aimed at breaking up the scratch-itch syndrome. Ice packs or cold wet dressings may be helpful. Corticosteroid tablets, ointments or lotions may be prescribed to relieve symptoms. Menthol 0.1% to 0.25% or coal tar is added if necessary. Topical calamine lotion with or without 0.5% menthol or phenol 1% is helpful.

Tripelennamine (Pyribenzamine), 25 or 50 mg tablets q. 4 to 6 h for drug reaction, chlorpheniramine maleate (Chlor-Trimeton) and diphenhydramine (Benedryl) help relieve urticaria. Fifteen milligrams of phenobarbital after meals and at bedtimes may be helpful in some cases. Soothing ointments and emulsions may be the only medication necessary. Oral use of vitamin A and a topical cream are helpful. Note that the medications listed under atopic dermatitis are also suitable for pruritus. Teldrin, 8 or 12 mg spansules, may relieve symptoms.

Soreness Soreness is a symptom of overworked muscles, ligaments and joints before these structures acclimate themselves to the exercise required of them. Bruises, old scars and migrating phlebitis can cause soreness. With 12 muscles originating in the leg and inserting into the foot, a mechanically malfunctioning foot may cause soreness of one or more groups of leg muscles. Soreness develops from multiple minimal traumas to the foot. Skin lesions may be a direct cause of soreness in the foot.

Constant severe uninterrupted pain may suggest a malignancy, if no history of recent trauma is given. Neuroma and bone infection should be differentiated by careful clinical and radiographic examination. There is a strong possibility of neuritis of infectious origin.

Intermittent pain suggests a neuritis or a neuralgia caused by pressure or infection. An arteritis and arterial occlusion may cause an ischemic neuritis.

Treatment. Mild massage of overworked musculature improves muscle metabolism and relieves soreness. Contrast foot baths are helpful. Whirlpool may relieve symptoms. Low-voltage muscle stimulation relieves fatigue and sore muscles.

Eliminate traumatizing agents and locate and eliminate infection. Correct the cause of ischemic neuritis. Improve structural deformities to assist function and relieve strain.

Multiple therapeutic vitamins are helpful.

Pain On Arising Difficulty in walking after getting out of bed in the morning suggests arthritis or fibrositis. These possibilities must be investigated in all painful conditions of the feet.

Traumatic lesions are usually unilateral, whereas static foot disarrangements are commonly bilateral. However, one foot usually has been affected before the other. The podiatrist must determine whether both feet are disturbing the patient. Increased pain in one extremity often causes the patient to present only that limb for treatment. Very often, however, the foot giving the most pain is not the one presenting the greater deformity, but if so, the history should reveal that the more deformed foot was the object of severe pain at sometime in the past. If both feet are not equally affected, the treatment varies accordingly.

Pain during rest occurs before ulceration and gangrene in thromboangiitis obliterans; it consists of severe burning sensations. This is pretrophic and common with the disease.

Hereditary trophedema is a chronic edema of one or both legs, the arms or the face. It may affect a single toe or one foot and occurs most frequently in females. The nonpitting edema may cause pain if profuse; the skin is thickened with no pain or tenderness.

Causalgia due to irritation of a nerve by injury may present painful swelling, redness, sweating, trophic changes in the nails and a glossy appearance of the skin.

Treatment. Eliminate all etiologic factors. Relieve strain of poorly functioning feet and support structural defects to prevent unusual motion. Physical therapy, such as short wave, ultrasound, infrared, sinusoidal currents and contrast baths, helps relieve pain on arising after periods of rest.

The diagnosis and treatment of the arthritides are necessary for a differential diagnosis leading to adequate treatment. Immobilization by adhesive tape or construction of foot orthoses is often indicated to correct deforming states. If a localized joint is affected, injections of local anesthetics and a corticosteroid relieve acute pain.

Prescriptions of antirheumatics, analgesics, muscle relaxants and definitive medications for specific diagnoses are necessary to relieve pain on arising after periods of rest. Steroids, salicylates, NSAIDs and methocarbamol (Robaxin) can be useful. In causalgic states, Edmonson and Calandruccio (39) prescribed 15 mg of Dibenzyline qid with good results. Sympathectomy is often necessary to relieve pain. Injections of plain lidocaine for a posterior tibial block are often helpful to the patient who cannot walk. Phenoxybenzamine hydrochloride, 10 mg, and Tolazoline hydrochloride in 25 mg tablets tid serve as adrenergic blocking agents.

Sudden Severe Pain Sudden severe pain with no history of injury occurring at the site of bifurcation and along the course of an artery suggests general debility, malnutrition, endocarditis or valvular disease with embolus formation. The extremity below the embolus is cold, edematous and pulseless.

Kalish et al. (40) discussed pulmonary embolism following podiatric surgery. Massive pulmonary embolism may occur when a blood clot or a portion thereof enters a systemic vein and as an embolism lodges in the pulmonary artery or the lesser arteries in the lung. Occlusion of the pulmonary artery may develop from a venous thrombosis in the deep veins of the extremities. As single or multiple emboli of various sizes, the clot moves either slowly or rapidly to cause a pulmonary infarction and severe pressure within the chest wall. Dyspnea followed by cyanosis, shock and sudden death may occur within minutes. It is obvious that a careful preoperative examination is essential.

Prophylactic heparinization must be considered in the presence of a history of thrombophlebitis, cardiac arrhythmias, emboli and artherosclerosis. Extreme care must be exercised during surgery if preoperative heparin has been used.

Treatment. This patient may require immediate vascular surgery to remove an embolus and preserve the limb. Do not traumatize the limb with massage or manipulation. The use of extremes of cold or heat destroys the impoverished tissue leading to ulceration and gangrene.

Empirin with codeine phosphate up to 1 grain, and acetaminophen (Tylenol) potentiated by promethazine in a 12.5 to 25 mg dosage may help control this type of pain.

Neuritis Neuritis, a nerve inflammation, is characterized by various etiologic factors and symptoms that occur in all age groups. Usually it is caused by trauma, such as fracture and luxation in which there is contusion, compression and torsion of the nerve. Compression may be due to swelling of local lymph nodes or to the presence of a neoplasm, aneurism or tyloma. The extension of an inflammatory process from contiguous tissues is often the cause of neuritis. Ischemia, which leads to degeneration of the nerve, may occur in Raynaud's disease, arteriosclerosis and obliterative endarteritis causing neuritic pains. Chronic infections, such as syphilis, diphtheria, typhoid and chronic intoxications from lead or carbon dioxide, may cause a neuritic syndrome.

The primary symptom of neuritis is pain that is limited to the area of distribution of the nerve. The pains may be severe and may be brought on or intensified by local movement or pressure. The disturbance of sensation—paresthesias, hyperesthesias or complete anesthesia—is characteristic of neuritis. The impaired muscle power indicates the severity of the disease and may run from a weakness of the muscle to a paralysis. Sensation is restored before the motor function is healed. The paralyzed muscle is flaccid and flabby, and unless the conducting fibers are reestablished, it goes on to atrophy. Tendon reflexes are diminished or abolished. Flexion of the thigh on the hip followed by extension of the knee causes pain in sciatica (see Lasèque's sign). Deformities may result, such as with equinovarus. Tarsal tunnel syndrome may occur with entrapment of the posterior tibial nerve.

An altered electrical reaction occurs in neuritis. In mild cases there is only a decreased excitability of muscle, but in severe cases, partial or total degeneration is found when muscles are tested. Trophic and secretory disturbances of the skin occur in the area affected by the neuritis; the skin is smooth or glistening and red. Later it may become rough, furrowed and brittle. Hair falls out or may grow in excess, and there may be profuse sweating. A postural list to either side may be evident in sciatica, but usually it is away from the affected side. Neuritis usually lasts 10 days to 2 weeks, but it may last for months or years. The symptoms diminish with proper treatment and removal of the cause.

A thorough understanding of neuroanatomy and good judgment in the expert evaluation of electromyographic nerve conduction are necessary requisites for the diagnosis of nerve compression. Biomechanical disorders may precipitate the discomfort of a compressed or entrapped nerve.

Luke (41) describes and differentiates a neurilemoma from other nerve growths and a ganglionic cyst. The author's personal experience with the evaluation of pathology reports of nerve masses suggests that the interpretations are rather indecisive and vary, depending on the laboratory. They may vary from neurilemoma, schwannoma, neuroma, fibroma, neurofibroma or no pathology, to an inflammatory thickening of the nerve or possibly to a thickening of the nerve at its bifurcation.

Treatment. A thorough physical examination is called for to rule out or to diagnose and treat systemic disease. A neurological consultation is often necessary; a circulatory consultation may be indicated.

Localized foot problems are corrected. Faulty foot function is improved, and sites of abnormal pressure are protected. Supportive measures are used where needed if pathomechanical problems are severe. Pressure behind the knee, about the head of the fibula, over the ankle and on the dorsum of the foot and toes is relieved.

Mild galvanism is used for its sedating effect. Billig's exercises are prescribed (18). Analgesics and muscle relaxants are prescribed. The strength and frequency of medication depend on the extent of the neuritis, its acute or chronic nature, and the degree of pain.

Hypersensitivity of Superficial Nerves of the Skin Podiatrists' observations have led to the consideration of irritation of the peripheral nerve endings as a pathology in itself. It develops as a peripheral neuritis often complicated by pressure neuritis. The condition most frequently is found in high-strung, middle-aged, neurotic women. The predisposing factors are often an increase in weight, anemia, psychic phenomena, vasomotor instability and environmental anxieties.

Patients are not able to tolerate even minor pressure or friction from ill-fitting footgear; heavy shoes and improperly tanned leather cannot be tolerated; the feet burn and are hot and sensitive: they are often awakened at night with burning, hot, painful feet that are relieved only slightly by cold air and cold water foot soaks.

These patients are very nervous, and many other biomechanical disturbances develop concomitantly with minor foot disorders. Their shoes seldom fit, and color changes in the toes are observed with metatarsalgic symptoms and circulatory and neurologic manifestations. The patients are generally apprehensive.

The condition must be differentiated from Raynaud's disease, vasomotor instability, frostbite, allergic disease and metabolic disturbances.

Treatment. Place the patient at ease and concentrate on good rapport. Improve the patient's general health and refer him or her to an internist for treatment of blood dyscrasia or psychomotor instability. Larger doses of vitamin B_{12} are helpful (1000 μg. IM weekly). Warm sitz baths may also be beneficial.

Prescribe mild sedatives—sodium butabarbital (Butisol sodium), ¼ to ½ grain three to four times daily; meprobamate, 200–400 mg; or promethazine (Phenergan), 12.5–25 mg three to four times a day.

Periarticular Fibrositis This syndrome commonly affects the feet and is primarily characterized by soreness and stiffness and pain on arising after long or short periods of rest or following exercise.

On arising in the morning, the patient's first few steps are made with a limp. The limp gradually disappears only to come back after prolonged weightbearing. Objectively the joints are neither stiff nor unusually painful. In the early stages, there is no deformity of the joints or swelling or other physical findings. The fibrous connective tissues about the joints are involved. Usually a history of injury or faulty functions of the affected joints is elicited from the complaining patient.

The talocrural, first metatarsophalangeal, talonavicular, first metatarsocuneiform and second metatarsophalangeal joints are most commonly affected.

Treatment. Bedrest, shoe padding or functional adhesive immobilization is indicated. Physical therapy is helpful. Corticosteroid solutions in minimal doses of 0.3 to 0.5 ml injected into affected joints are beneficial. Analgesics, NSAIDs or muscle relaxants may be taken. Pentazocine hydrochloride (Talwin) by injection or in 50 mg tablets q 4 h prn relieves pain. Zactirin or aspirin help maintain comfort. Carisoprodol (Rela), 350 mg; methocarbamol, 500 mg, or chlorzoxazone may be used as muscle relaxants.

Restless Leg Syndrome This common complaint of an unpleasant burning or crawling sensation in the extremities may be caused by emotional strain or long periods of inactivity. It is more prevalent in women and is often experienced by persons who travel for many hours with the feet in a dependent position, as on an extended plane trip. Elevation of the lower extremities, hot and cold foot plunges and alleviation of emotional stress bring relief in most cases. The possibility of local or systemic pathology must be evaluated if symptoms persist.

Boghem (42) traced a family in which 18 relatives in five generations were affected by "restless legs." He concludes that the condition probably represents an hereditary defect.

The treatments proposed for restless legs ranges from Ayres and Mihan (43), who recommend the use of *d*-α-tocopheryl acetate or succinate in doses of 400 I.U., one to four times daily with meals, to Lutz (44) a psychiatrist, who advises limiting the use of tea and coffee for its caffeine CNS excitation. Lutz noted, "depressive manifestations, anxiety with insomnia and heightened proprioceptive awareness." He states that, "An increased striated muscle contractility interfers with the microcirculation to sensory nerve endings leading to the dysphoric sensation of restless legs." Abstinence from caffeine, a moderate use of diazepam and physical exercise generally improved the symptoms.

Increased Venous Pressure In a venographic study of 86 lower extremities, Gerlock (45) suggests that measurement of pedal venous pressure (PVP) is a useful correlation as a screening mechanism for the detection of deep vein thrombosis. The combination of venography with PVP illustrates that abnormal venographs and a PVP greater than 35 cm saline suggest a deep vein thrombosis.

Causalgia Posttraumatic reflex sympathetic dystrophy commonly occurs after severe or trivial injury. It generally follows a period of disuse secondary to the normal protective part immobility or plaster immobilization. The symptoms are characterized clinically as a swelling, rubor, painful active or passive movements, hyperidrosis or anidrosis, immobility, vasomotor instability, paresthesia, coldness of extremity and early multiple abundant spotty areas of demineralization in the bones distal to the site of trauma.

Treatment. The best treatment is early active and passive exercises. These may be assisted by injections of long-lasting anesthetics in posterior tibial and anterior tibial blocks. Occasionally a block of the peroneal at the fibular head is helpful. Sinusoidal currents producing muscle stimulation are indicated. Under all circumstances, avoid physical therapeutic hot soaks, whirlpool or heating modalities. These have a hyperemic effect, creating additional resorption of bone and painful congestion in tissues already compromised.

Gout (Figs. 3.1 and 3.2)

Gout is a systemic disorder characterized by a hyperuricemia and the body's inability to metabolize purines, resulting in acute, subacute and chronic manifestations of pain and deformity commonly affecting the feet. Gout is often accompanied by kidney stones and deposition of biurate crystals at the chondro-osseous margins of the joints. Deposits in the ear lobes are not uncommon.

Primary metabolic gout involves an overproduction of uric acid, whereas primary renal gout involves the underexcretion of uric acid. A 24 hr urinalysis—[uric acid less than 600 mg indicates an underexcretor (use uricosuric); uric acid higher than 600 mg indicates an overproducer (use allopurinol)]—helps differentiate metabolic from renal gout.

Acute gout is often precipitated by dietary and alcohol indiscretions and/or oral thiazide diuretics. Foods high in purines, such as organ parts, liver, kidneys, brains, heart and lungs, may precipitate an attack. Cytotoxic drugs in treatment of chronic leukemia and other malignant diseases or some antituberculous, antihypertensive or large amounts of nicotinic acid drugs can activiate a dormant gouty involvement. Small doses of aspirin may aggravate an acute gout, whereas large doses serve as a uricosuric agent.

Other causes of secondary gout include renal disease with renal failure, blood dys-

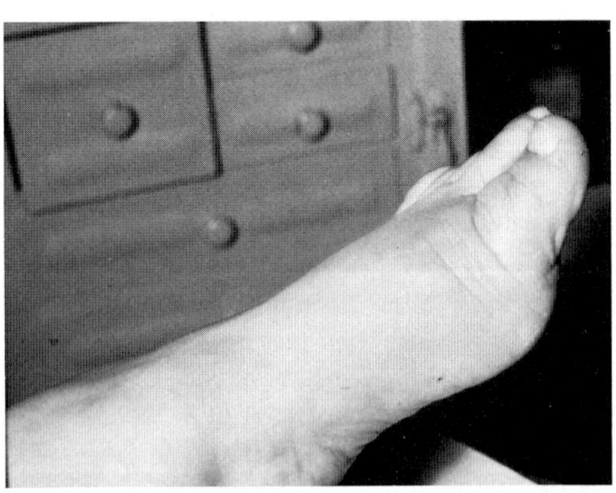

Figure 3.1. Acute gout with tenosynovitis extensor hallucis longus tendon. Area is hot, red and swollen.

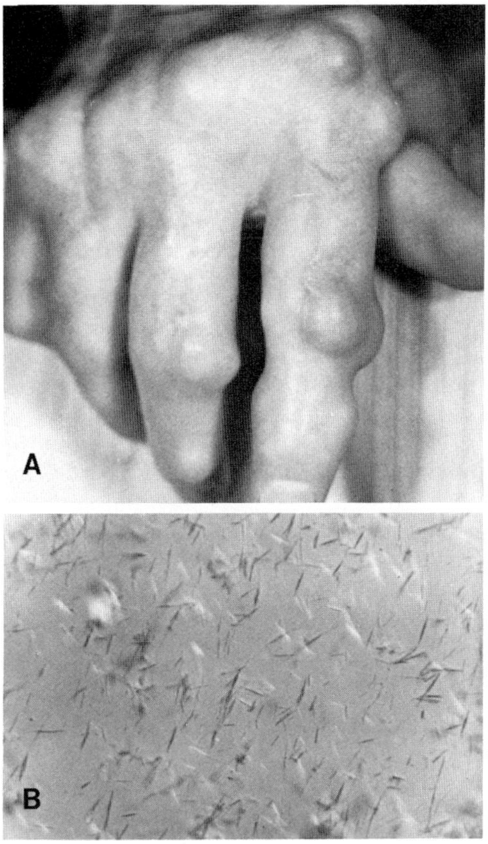

Figure 3.2. *A,* Gout, tophaceous deposits. *B,* Gout, photomicrograph of tophaceous deposit; needle-like crystals.

crasias, eclampsia, hyperlipidemia, diabetic ketoacidosis, cystinuria, glycogen storage disease, sarcoidosis, psoriasis, lead poisoning, hyperparathyroidism, pseudogout (chondrocalcinosis), dwarfism, cerebral vascular accident, mongolism and myxedema.

The attacks commonly occur in the early hours of the morning and usually affect a single joint such as the first metatarsophalangeal articulation. The ankle, knee, lesser metatarosophalangeal joints, plantar fascial or tendoachilles insertions, talonavicular joint, fingers and lesser toes may also be involved, becoming red, hot, swollen and exquisitely tender. Nerve block anesthesia followed by aspiration of the effused joint and injection of a non-acetylated steroid often results in immediate relief.

A trivial injury in the presence of hyperuricemia may produce a massive swelling and pain. Joints may appear normal between attacks. In the chronic stages, the presence of tophaceous deposits and atrophic loss of substance at the chondro-osseous margins of the affected joints create deformity.

Allopurinol is used daily to prevent the formation of increased uric acid. A 100- to 300 mg tablet of allopurinol daily provides an adequate maintenance dose.

Blood uric acid is usually greater than 6 mg/100 ml. The synovial fluid and tophi contain needle-like crystals.

Anemias and Feet

The extremities are readily affected by anemic disturbances of a systemic origin. Neurological, circulatory and gastrointestinal problems caused by anemia may produce symptoms in the feet.

Edema of the ankles is frequently seen in chronic secondary anemia that is severe. Diminution in red blood cells and hemoglobin often resulting from some chronic infection, an inability to digest and absorb food, and frequent hemorrhages are also present. The patient feels faint and complains of a "swimming head." Appetite is lost and pulse is rapid and soft. A pallor is noted, and the dyspnea produced by lack of oxygen-carrying cells is observed to be present.

In pernicious anemia, edema of the feet is common. Usually associated with it are a tingling and numbness of the feet and hands; a loss of deep sensibility and spasticity are evident, indicative of a posterior or lateral column sclerosis. The onset is insidious after 40 years of age with weakness, dyspnea, lemon-yellow pallor and gastrointestinal distrubances. The red cell count is low, color index 1+ and volume index 1+. A neuroanemic syndrome of sensory and motor disturbances exists in pernicious anemia.

Pernicious anemia when advanced may result in an awkward, jerky ataxia produced by a subacute combined degeneration of the cord. In early pernicious anemia knee jerks are increased and plantar reflexes are overactive. Later the limbs become spastic, and finally the knee jerks disappear while the plantar reflex remains.

Paresthesias are present in the early stages and are noted first by a diminished perception of vibratory sensation. Later, numbness and tingling are manifested, followed in severe cases by paresis. This involves both the legs and the feet and is a source of complaint in Addison's pernicious anemia.

The patient suffering from pernicious anemia may present chilliness, extreme fatigue and utter exhaustion and edema of the legs and ankles; the tongue is sore and atrophic. All long bones are weakened by calcium malabsorption, resulting in a broader diameter to sustain weight. The bone is tender to deep pressure.

Sickel cell anemia occurs in the black race. Sickle cells are found in many normal blacks. The bone changes rarely affect the extremities. The patient requires immediate care by an internist. Often the characteristic appearance of a foot radiograph is diagnostic.

Infectious Diseases

Viral Diseases

Although viruses are unusually small and only exist and multiply on living cells, they do not as a group cause common pathological changes. Yet, the literature groups together such viral diseases as poliomyelitis, mumps, smallpox and warts without due consideration of the diverse clinical pictures of each. Viruses exert upon the cells within which they grow and multiply a decided influence that results in hyperplasia or necrosis.

These diseases would hardly find their way into the podiatrist's office in an acute phase. It is well for the foot doctor to appreciate the sequelae of viral diseases.

Viral Hepatitis Viral hepatitis has had an increased incidence in recent years. About 10–20% of these victims have joint pain with stiffness as a prodromal sign. By the time the jaundice appears, the symptoms of bilateral and symmetrical joint pain, fatigue, and loss of appetite seem to improve. A good case history concerning drug habits and recent blood transfusions or infections helps establish the diagnosis when the symptoms are not definitive.

The Common Cold The common cold is a catarrhal inflammation of the upper respiratory tract that results from infection by a filterable virus or micro-organism. The symptoms are influenced by allergic and metabolic disorders.

The podiatrist should be interested in that part of the etiology involving environmental factors such as chilling of the body, wearing of wet footgear and body fatigue.

Frequently, the patient complains of chilly sensations with vague aching in the back and extremities. Later manifestations may result in weakness, nervousness, arthralgia, neuralgia and cutaneous hyperesthesia.

Sometimes a resistance is developed to the common cold by virtue of short doses of exposure to chilly temperatures and outdoor hardships. Experience has shown that dry, warm shoes and hose and moderate exercise are excellent prophylactic measures to be observed in susceptible individuals. Cecil's *Textbook of Medicine* (46) states, "the body, especially the feet, should be dry and warm."

When examination reveals the etiologic factors and symptoms in the extremities described above, one should suspect the common cold and refer the patient to the family physician for treatment. There is no excuse for serious errors in judgment involving the treatment of foot disturbances that manifest themselves through the inflammatory changes created by the common cold.

Influenza Influenza is a highly contagious, infectious disease occurring usually in epidemic and pandemic outbreaks. The spread of influenza is unusually rapid, and important manifestations are fever, marked prostration, respiratory inflammation, conjunctivitis and severe aches in the back and extremities. It is self-limited and of short duration.

Thrombophlebitis, arthritis, osteomyelitis and multiple neuritis affect the extremities and may occur on occasion. The severe aching pains in the back and legs are out of proportion to the catarrhal symptoms and should be recognized by the podiatrist.

Dengue This is an acute febrile disease caused by a filterable virus and transmitted by the mosquitoes of the genus *Aedes*.

During the first few hours, most of the larger joints become painful so that motion is almost impossible. The scarlatinform rash may occur about the ankles along with a periarticular swelling. Often a patchy distribution is observed on the flexor surface of the extremities. The palms and soles may be bright red and swollen while flexion is painful. A marked pruritus followed by desquamation on the soles of the feet is a common sequela to the acute phases. A neurocirculatory asthenia may occur as an aftermath of this infectious disease. A history of dengue supports the etiology of the symptoms in the extremities.

Measles This is a communicable disease characterized by epidemic occurrence usually in the winter and spring months. The lower extremities are last to be affected by skin changes. Itching and burning may occur with tiny red papules that rapidly enlarge to dusky, red macules. The macules coalesce and form blotchy areas of skin.

Encephalitis and peripheral neuritis are known sequelae to this disease. A latent branny, scaling may find its way to the podiatrist's office. A good case history identifies this sequela to the acute disease.

Rubella—German Measles Rubella is an acute, epidemic, specific disease that is highly contagious but is quite distinct from measles and scarlet fever. The rash spreads downward, but very often the legs may be affected first. It fades as rapidly as it develops and is almost clear by the time the lower extremities are involved.

Of interest to the podiatrist is the possibility of mild rheumatic pains developing in the lower extremities. On occasion, arthritis may be a sequela to this disease.

Mumps Mumps is a viral infection presenting symptoms remote from the feet. However, the author has seen arthralgic symptoms affecting the feet of an adult who was stricken at age 30. In this patient, the enlargement of the parotid glands was originally diagnosed as a bacterial infection and treated with penicillin. The patient developed a variety of symptoms that could not be differentiated as a complication of the mumps or an allergic reaction to the antibiotic. Swelling and pain in the feet were accompanied by erythema, followed by itching during the subacute phases.

Herpes Zoster—Shingles This is an acute infectious, specific disease characterized by inflammation of one or more dorsal root ganglia, accompanied by irregularly outlined groups of vesicles found along the corresponding peripheral sensory nerve.

Smallpox Smallpox is a specific infectious disease characterized by marked invasive symptoms that subside and are followed by successive stages of papule, vesicle, pustule and crust formation. When pustulation occurs the secondary temperature may return with the subjective symptoms.

Reports of osteomyelitis in the suppurative stage are not uncommon. In children edema of the feet may occur even though only few lesions are present. Itching is common about the lesions, and desquamation may be variable. Occasionally a partial cast of the foot may be removed or exfoliated.

Less common complications of interest to the podiatrist are the sequelae of hemiplegia, peripheral neuritis, gangrene and subcutaneous abscess. Arthritis may occasionally occur, and a peculiar purulant arthritis may result in infants. Necrosis of bone is possible.

Acute Anterior Poliomyelitis Acute anterior poliomyelitis is an infectious disease capable of producing widespread lesions throughout the brain and cord and also in extra neural tissues. The gray matter of the cord is especially involved. With a disease of the anterior horns, striking changes of clinical significance, such as flaccid paralysis of various groups of muscles, may result. This disease occurs most often in the summer and early autumn. It is more common in boys than girls and affects youngsters most commonly in the second year of life. Fortunately, the advent of polio vaccines has greatly reduced the numbers affected by the disease. Podiatrists may see these patients early during an acute attack accompanied by high fever, stiff neck and weakness of the extremities. The patient requires immediate hospitalization and treatment by a team of medical specialists.

Postinfectious Encephalitis Many times the only symptoms and cardinal findings of this disease are pyrexia, headache, vomiting and drowsiness. Of interest to the podiatrist for differential diagnosis is an extensive paralysis (spastic at first, followed by flaccidity or transient weakness of muscles). Incoordination and ataxia may occur. Kernig's sign may by present, and the deep and superficial reflexes are rather confused. Paralysis, anesthesia and paresthesia are common. About 50% of the patients die.

Rickettsial Disease

Typhus Fever Typhus fever is an acute infectious disease transmitted by the rat flea occasionally and, in epidemics, by the body louse. Of great interest to the podiatrist are the pathological proliferation and thrombosis of the blood vessels of skin, musculature and CNS. A scratch or puncture wound on the foot makes a fine avenue of entrance of the virus from fecal deposits. A widespread macular eruption may develop over the trunk and limbs.

Skin necrosis or gangrene is occasionally found, and there may be symmetrical gangrene of the skin covering the lower extremity. Thrombosis of large vessels often causes serious sequelae. Thrombosis of the small peripheral vessels results in necrosis and gangrene. It is suspected that predisposing exposure from pressure and cold may hasten the necrosis over bony prominences.

Rocky Mountain Spotted Fever The podiatrist must be aware of the general manifestations of this disease, especially when pain may be referred to the bones, muscles and joints, particularly the calf muscles, large joints and lower back.

The rash may appear any time from the second to the seventh day of fever; appears first on the wrists, ankles and back; then on the forehead, arms, legs and chest; and later on the hands and soles. Necrosis may occur on the toes, as well as on other peripheral organs.

Bacterial Diseases

Scarlet Fever Scarlet fever is an acute infectious disease caused by streptococcus scarlatina. It is characterized by a sore throat and a punctate rash on the skin and roof of the mouth, followed by desquamation. On the lower extremities, small areas of a punctate rash around the hair follicles on the dorsum of the foot are often the only local signs of the rash.

Desquamation is one of the most typical signs of scarlet fever. It is usually complete in about 2 or 3 weeks on the body and may continue for 4 to 7 weeks on the palms and soles of the feet. A history of this illness and its acute symptoms clearly differentiates it from other dermatologic lesions affecting the feet.

In mild forms of the disease a diagnosis can often be made by observing an indication of the disease when breaks occur in the skin below the nails of the fingers and toes. This can be seen when the ball of the toe is pulled away from the nail. Desquamation is so intense that complete casts of the hands and feet have formed in several cases.

Deficiency Involvements

One of the greatest problems the podiatrist is confronted with involving metabolism concerns the regulation of calcium and phosphorus. Although the problem is the direct responsibility of the internist, many foot diseases are indirectly related to dietary and digestive disturbances.

The physiological relation of phosphorus to calcium is maintained by the function of Vitamin D. The following discussion explains the action of vitamin D. These findings have been observed in clinical and experimental vitamin D deficiency.

There is a diminished absorption of calcium and phosphorus from the gastrointestinal tract in vitamin D deficiency. The calcium blood level remains normal whereas the phosphorus level is decreased. Phosphorus excretion in the urine is increased; the parathyroid glands enlarge and become overactive. Calcification of cartilage and bone does not take place with vitamin D deficiency.

Vitamin D directly furthers the absorption of calcium from the intestinal tract. Indirectly the parathyroids are depressed and phosphorus is reabsorbed in the kidney. Vitamin D deficiency affects metabolism by lowering calcium absorption and affects secondarily the phosphorus absorption by forming insoluble calcium phosphates. Also, vitamin D deficiency increases the activity of the parathyroid glands, and the secretion of phosphorus in the urine is increased. The body is depleted of phosphorus, resulting in a fall of the phosphorus blood level. The calcium blood level remains fairly normal in vitamin D deficiency because nearly all the calcium absorbed is not deposited in the cartilage or osteoid tissue.

The pathological changes in bone are greatest during periods of rapid growth, as in rickets in children. Osteomalacia may be seen radiographically in extensive failure of calcification due to vitamin D deficiency.

References

1. Rubin A: Periarthritis, hydrocortisone and adaptation to stress in the foot. *J Am Podiatry Assoc* 45:17–30, 1955a.
2. Roy R, Tunks E: *Chronic Pain: Psychosocial Factors in Rehabilitation.* Baltimore, Williams & Wilkins, 1982.
3. Terenius L: Endorphin mechanisms in chronic pain. Second World Congress on Pain, Montreal, Canada, August, 1978.
4. Sjolund BH, Eriksson MBE: Endorphin and analgesia produced by peripheral conditioning and stimulation. Second World Congress on Pain, Montreal, Canada, August, 1978.
5. Fink TR, Borso J, Calkins DF: Local anesthetic action of water. Second World Congress on Pain, Montreal, Canada, August, 1978.
6. Ochoa J, Noordenbas W: Pathology and disordered sensation in local nerve lesions and attempt at correlation. Second World Congress on Pain, Montreal, Canada, August, 1978.
7. Wall P, Gutrick J: Sensory physiology after various types of peripheral nerve injury. Second World Congress on Pain, Montreal, Canada, August, 1978.
8. Levine JD, Gordon NC, Fields HL: Evidence that the analgesic effect of placebos is mediated by endorphins. Second World Congress on Pain, Montreal, Canada. August, 1978.
9. Takida K, Tanigucki H, Kieriyama H, Matsuskita A: Experimental study on the mechanism of acupunctural anesthesia. Second World Congress on Pain, Montreal, Canada, August, 1978.
10. Dash MS, Singh M: Peripheral nerve lesions and pain in cold injury in man. Second World Congress on Pain, Montreal, Canada, August, 1978.
11. Kopell HP, Thompson WAL: Peripheral entrapment neuropathies of the lower extremity. *N Eng J Med* 262:56–60, 1960.
12. Johnson EW, Ortiz PR: Electrodiagnosis of tarsal tunnel syndrome. *Arch Phys Med Rehabil* 47:776, 1966.
13. Pachnik RL, Howard K: Variations of origins of the dorsalis pedis artery. *J Am Podiatry Assoc* 67:550–552, 1977.
14. Brzezinski PF, Meyn NP: The level of bifurcation of the tibial nerve into the medial and lateral plantar nerves. *J Am Podiatry Assoc* 67:553–555, 1977.
15. Jones CL: The cutaneous virulence of candida albicans of the foot. *J Foot Surg* 7:22–24, 1968.
16. Carrel JM, Davidson DM: Nerve compression syndrome of the foot and ankle: A comprehensive review of the symptoms, etiology and diagnosis utilizing nerve conduction studies. *J Am Podiatry Assoc* 65:322–341, 1975.
17. Kashuk K: Proximal peripheral nerve entrapment syndromes in the lower extremity. Northlake Surgical Seminar, December, 1975.
18. Billig HF, Brennan RL: *Foot pains. J Natl Assoc Chirop* 33:34–35, 1943.
19. Calabra JJ: A critical evaluation of the diagnostic features of the foot in rheumatoid arthritis. *Arthritis Rheum* 5:19, 1962
20. Yale I, Yale J: *The Arthritic Foot and Related Connective Tissue Disorders.* Baltimore, Williams & Wilkins, 1984.
21. Goodwin JS (ed): *Mediguide to Inflammatory Diseases,* Vol. 3, No. 3, 1984, p. 7.
22. Rosenbloom D, Craven MA: A review of nonsteroidal antiinflammatory drugs. *Can Fam Physician* 29:2121–24, 1983.
23. Arroyo J: Intravenous sedation with Sublimaze (McNeil) and Valium (Roche). *J Am Podiatry Assoc* 67:644–645, 1977.
24. Johnson JB, Cooper C, Zamy HS: Intravenous diazepam (Valium) a useful adjunct to outpatient foot procedures. *J Am Podiatry Assoc* 63:605–608, 1973.
25. Choi G, Donick I: Blood gas analysis with intravenous sedation and local anesthesia. *J Am Podiatry Assoc* 67:231–232, 1977.
26. Donick I, Choi G, Block LD, Berlin SJ, Costa A: Intravenous sedation combined with anesthesia in foot surgery. *J Am Podiatry Assoc* 67:177–185, 1977.
27. Block BH, Giorgini RJ: Medical hypnosis: Clinical application to podiatry. *J Am Podiatry Assoc* 66:23–27, 1976.
28. Block B, Levitsky DA, Teitlebaum RD, Valletta M: Hypnosis as a vasodilating and vasoconstricting agent, a plethysmographic study. *J Am Podiatry Assoc* 67:188–191, 1977.

29. Sanders SC: Acrylic nail groove protector by brush technique. *J Am Podiatry Assoc* 45:23–24, 1955.
30. Bussey JG, Jackson RN: Transcutaneous electrical nerve stimulation for relief of pain. Second General Meeting of the American Pain Society, New York, September, 1980.
31. Harvey C, et al: The use of cold spray and its effect on muscle length. *J Am Podiatry Assoc* 73:629–632, 1983.
32. Kraus H: Physical therapy to control myofascial pain. Second General Meeting of the American Pain Society, New York, 1980.
33. Laurence RM:Stimulation of the periosteum of bone for chronic pain reduction (an experimental method). Third World Congress on Pain of the International Association for the Study of Pain. Edinburgh Scotland, 1981.
34. Lorenz KY, et al: Interagency team at NJMH and NIDA studies how acupuncture works. Third World Congress on Pain, Edinburgh, Scotland, 1981.
35. Brody BJ, Brezak S: A report on the alleviation of nocturnal cramps by the combined use of quinine sulfate and aminophylline. *J Am Podiatry Assoc* 50:203–206, 1960.
36. Golding DN: Polyarteritis presenting with leg pains. *Br Med J* 1:277, 278, 1970.
37. Porter JM, et al: Pentoxifylline efficacy in the treatment of intermittent claudication: Multicenter controlled double-blind trial with objective assessment of chronic occlusive disease patients. *Am Heart Assoc* 104:66–72, 1982.
38. Lemont H: The branches of the superficial personeal nerve and their clinical significance. *J Am Podiatry Assoc* 65:310–314, 1975.
39. Edmonson AS, Calandruccio RA: Drug therapy for causalgia. *Miss Doc* 34:239–241, 1957.
40. Kalish S, et al: Pulmonary embolism after podiatric surgery. *J Am Podiatry Assoc* 64:879–889, 1974.
41. Luke RD: Neurilemoma in the foot. *J Am Podiatry Assoc* 66:547–549, 1976.
42. Boghem DR: New light on restless leg syndrome. *Medical World News*, Aug. 25, 1975.
43. Ayers S, Mihan R: Yellow nail syndrome. *Arch Dermatol* 108:267–268, 1973.
44. Lutz, personal observation.
45. Gerlock AJ, Jr: Measurement of pedal venous pressure. A screening procedure in the detection of deep-vein thrombosis and occlusion. *Radiology* 122 (Suppl):673–676, 1977.
46. Wyngaarden JB, Smith LH (eds): *Cecil Textbook of Medicine* vols. I and II. Philadelphia, W. B. Saunders, 1985.

Suggested Readings

Gilman AG, Goodman LS, Gilman A: *The Pharmacological Basis of Therapeutics*, ed 7. New York, macMillan Publishing Co, 1985.

Helfand AE, Hirt PR, Madresh AC, DeVincentis A: Triamcinolone acetonide in the treatment of bursitis and other foot disorders. *J Am Podiatry Assoc* 61:174–179, 1971.

Kollenberg LO, Hudyma EO, Robbins JM: Nonsteroidal anti-inflammatory agents. A review of the literature. *J Am Podiatry Assoc* 75-517–522, 1985.

Levine JD, Gordon MC, Fields H: Mechanism of placebo's pain-killing power. Second World Congress on Pain, Montreal, Canada, August, 1978.

Rubin A: Somatic pain. *Chirop Rec* 38:37–45, 1955.

4

Circulatory Disorders

Diagnosis of circulatory disorders is based on such subjective complaints by the patient as cramps, coldness, fatigue and numbness, as well as objective signs of rubor, cyanosis or pallor with diminished pulsations and dystrophic alterations of the skin and nails. It is not the purpose of this text to study in depth the diagnosis and treatment of peripheral vascular disease, but rather to convey the important role of podiatry in the team approach to the prevention and treatment of debilitating sequelae of circulatory disease.

The presence or absence of pulses is not in itself a good indicator of circulatory instability. Pulsations may be present in patients suffering impending gangrene, whereas, a congenital anomaly or arterial replacements may result in absence of pulsations as adequate circulation is supplied by compensating vessels.

The stethoscope, sphygmomanometer, clinical thermometer, plethysmograph and oscillometer are used to evaluate circulatory complaints. More sophisticated equipment, such as a Doppler unit, may be needed for diagnosis of borderline cases requiring surgical intervention (Fig. 4.1). Adler (1) describes the use of the Cutaneous Pressure Plethysmograph (CPP^{R}) in quantitative monitoring of blood flow to the patient's skin (Fig. 4.2).

Bartels and Rullo (2) recommend that all patients showing evidence of peripheral vascular disease should be thoroughly tested for abnormal glucose tolerance. In a study of 100 patients with symptoms of claudication, paresthesia, rest pain and gangrene, an absence of pulsations in the extremities, radiologic evidence of arterial insufficiency, rubor, slow venous filling time, blanching on elevation and ulceration, 43% showed abnormal glucose tolerance tests, indicating possible diabetes.

DeWeese (3) developed a test for arteriosclerosis in patients complaining of fatigue, aching and severe leg cramps with palpable pedal pulses at rest. He had patients run in place at the rate of 140 to 160 steps/min until claudication occurred, and he then showed that pulses disappeared with the activity. DeWeese explained the phenomenon as a "shunting of the insufficient blood supply to smaller, vasodilated arteries so that weakened pulsations are observed in the larger arteries."

The observation of color changes, temperature alterations and diminished dorsalis pedis, posterior tibial, popliteal and femoral pulsations may be followed by corroborative testing when indicated (Fig. 4.3).

If, after thorough examination and careful consideration of the symptoms, the podiatrist believes vascular disease is involved, he or she should refer the patient to a peripheral vascular consultant for further study and treatment. A cooperative attack on the problem is made by the consultant and the podiatrist.

Diagnostic Tests for Circulatory Disorders

Calorimetry

Calorimetry is the study of heat loss and skin temperatures. It has been calculated that, when the vasoconstrictor impulses

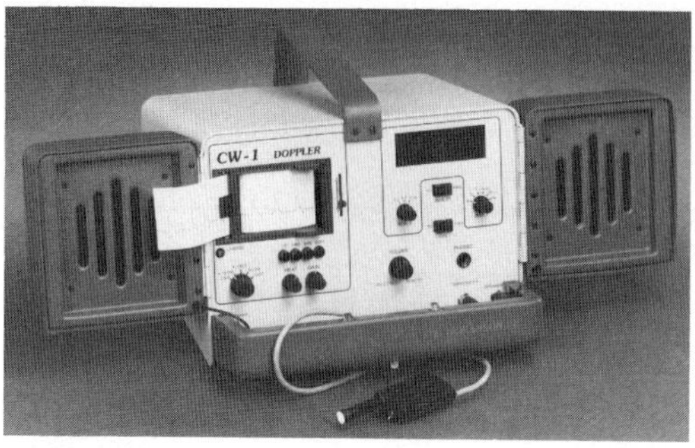

Figure 4.1. Doppler. (Courtesy of DE Hakanson, Inc.)

are blocked, there is a resulting rise in temperature that may reach 33.5 to 35°C.

Local anesthesia in the form of an infiltration of 5 to 10 ml of lidocaine in a 1% solution into or near the posterior tibial nerve as it lies below the medial malleolus serves well in evaluating the effect of the sympathetic nervous system to the toes. This local anesthetic causes a sharp rise in temperature of the toes, as well as paresthesias, numbness and motor changes. Hyperemia of the plantar surface of the foot may develop early and usually subsides readily.

Thermocouple

The thermocouple is useful in distinguishing between organic obliteration disease and spastic states because it compares the temperature of two limbs at frequent intervals. It is an important diagnostic aid in peripheral vascular diseases and also in determining progress and prognosis in therapy for peripheral vascular diseases. The thermocouple is simple to use, and any number of successive readings may be taken without any time lag or additional calculations of any kind.

Plethysmography

The podiatry digital plethysmograph provides data on the vascular system that enables the podiatrist to differentiate between vasomotor and organic arterial disease, evaluate presurgical vascular conditions, detect certain cardiac irregularities, study circulation of small arteries in the digits, locate areas of obstruction in large vessel disease, determine small artery disease, assess continuity of the sympathetic system and detail the extent of the collateral circulation. The pneumoplethysmograph was originally developed by Winsor (4).

Reflex Dilation

The findings of Landis and Gibbon have been observed by Kramer (5), who has noted excellent results with the following technique for reflex dilation. Landis and Gibbon discovered that, by immersing the forearms in warm water for 1 hr, reflex vasodilation can be produced in the lower extremities in the same manner as it is produced by local infiltration. When the temperature rises from 33.5 to 34.5°C, the condition of the circulatory disturbance is vasospastic and the spasm is overcome. When it remains unchanged after immersion, an occlusive vasular disease must be suspected.

Histamine Flare Test

Lewis (6) studied the reaction of capillaries to various stimuli and discovered

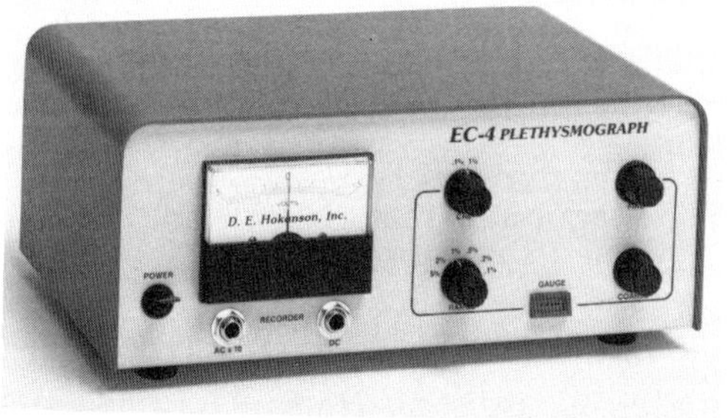

Figure 4.2. Plethysmograph. (Courtesy of DE Hakanson, Inc.)

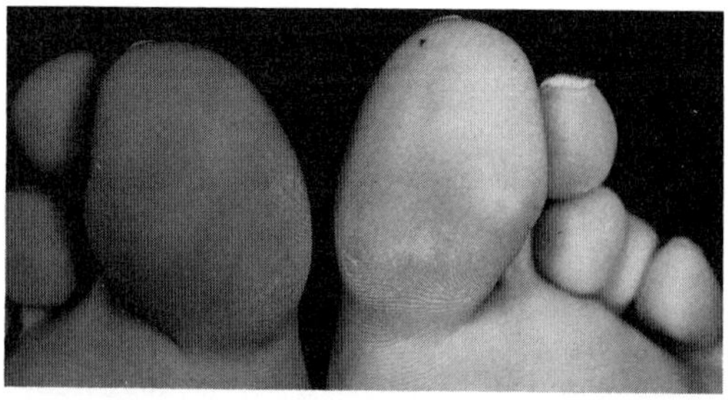

Figure 4.3. Arteriosclerosis. Note color changes in right hallux.

that, when histamine was inoculated, dilation of capillaries at the site of injection occurred, which was followed by a zone of erythema about the injection area due to relaxation of arterioles. This reaction is known as the "flare." Wheal formation from outpouring of plasma through the capillary wall usually follows.

The test is performed in the following manner. With the patient completely relaxed in a warm, well-lighted room, one drop of a 1:1000 solution of histamine acid phosphate with 0.5% Chloretone as a preservative is placed on the dorsum of the foot, above the lateral ankle and below the knee. Using a fine needle, multiple inoculations are made in these areas. Extreme care must be taken to avoid bleeding. The reaction takes place from 2 1/2–5 min after inoculation and is accompanied by itching and wheal formation. A circulatory disease may be suspected when the test fails to produce a wheal within 10 min.

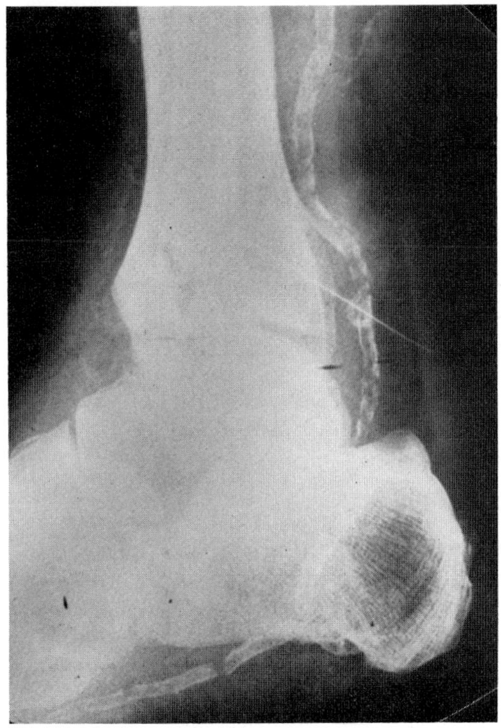

Figure 4.4. Arteriosclerosis posterior tibial artery. Calcification of posterior tibial artery represented by calcification of arterial wall. (From FO Gamble and I Yale: *Clinical Foot Roetgenology.* Baltimore, Williams & Wilkins, 1966.)

Roentgenography

A diagnosis of sclerotic vessels may be confirmed by x-rays (Fig. 4.4). Yale (7) found that many lateral roentgenograms of the foot taken to confirm a possible calcaneal spur instead disclosed a sclerosis of the medial calcaneal branch of the posterior tibial artery. The high percentage of such sclerosed vessels in patients 20 to 40 years of age who have no other evidence of circulatory changes in the feet demonstrates the need for the radiograph as a diagnostic adjunct in circulatory involvements. The presence of calcified larger vessels does not necessarily indicate the state of the arterioles. Often the nutritional state of the bones themselves indicates the presence of a circulatory fault by disclosing a general demineralization in bones of the feet. Increased circulation may cause demineralization.

Trophic osteitis or Sudeck's syndrome is a neurocirculatory disturbance. In thrombosis of the vessels, x-ray does not reveal calcifications unless arteriosclerosis exists. Phleboliths and calcified veins suggesting degenerative pathology may be visible on the radiograph. Phlebography has been useful in determining vein and vein valve status in venous insufficiency. Where infection is present, the circulatory stasis within the Volkman and Haversian canals may result in failure of resorption with subsequent condensation of the affected part.

Arteriography

This procedure is useful in observing collaterial circulation and the behavior of vessels in spasm and claudication and in determining a favorable site for amputation and arterial implants. Radio-opaque substances injected into the arterial tree allow for prompt visualization of defects and occlusions. Abnormal irritability of the injected vessel may result in spasm and local symptoms of pain, redness and increased temperature. These symptoms may persist for a few days when some of the solution is injected into the wall of the vessel or outside the vessel. The arteriogram is of great assistance in determining suspected congenital absence of an artery.

Riegelhaupt et al. (8) describe a method of evaluating lower extremity vascular status by means of the radioactive isotope technetium 99 m. This evaluation method has clinical applicability as a preoperative screening test, as a means of measuring progression of wound healing, as alternative to or in conjunction with other vascular tests and in evaluating the effects of arterial dilating medications on lower extremity circulation.

Occlusions of the vessel lumen are readily observed using arteriography. When an artery is partially occluded, a large collateral vessel arises just proximal to the occlusion. This vessel usually passes at right angles to the main artery and then turns abruptly to run a parallel course. This can be visualized in arteriography. Arteriography should be used only by highly qualified radiologists and peripheral vascular surgeons (Fig. 4.5).

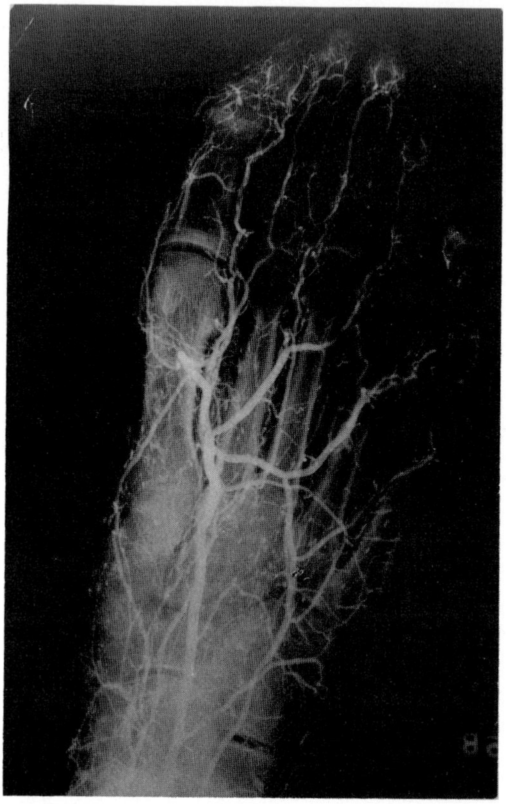

Figure 4.5. Arteriogram of the foot showing dorsalis pedis, intermetatarsal and digital vessels. (From FO Gamble and I Yale: *Clinical Foot Roentgenology.* Baltimore, Williams & Wilkins, 1966.)

Measurement of Plantar Ischemia

Samuels noted that when the patient is in a reclining position and the legs are elevated to a 90° angle and are flexed and extended 40 to 60 times, pallor occurs around the toes and soles of feet within 1 min if occlusive vascular disorders are present (9).

Claudication Time

Many times a patient cannot tell how long or how far he or she can walk before the onset of intermittent claudication. In a test devised by Baker *et al.*, the patient, after a rest, is instructed to walk 120 steps/min until claudication ensues (10).

Kisch Test

The reclining patient is asked to flex the thigh on the abdomen and the leg at the knee at the same time. The patient is then asked to extend the extremity. This action is repeated 30 times/min. Plantar ischemia and claudication time are noted.

Venous Filling Time

Collens and Wilensky (11) studied the filling time of veins in recumbent patients by having patients elevate their limbs until the veins had been drained off and then having them lower the limbs to a dependent position. Observing the medial and lateral marginal veins, they found that the filling time is normally 6 to 10 sec. A slower filling indicates an occlusive vascular disorder. Kramer (5) and his coworkers found that such other factors as venous disorders may influence the slowness of return. The slow venous filling time may affect only one toe, or it may affect the whole foot or the entire foot and leg. A patchy return of color may indicate irregular arterial occlusion or arteriolar spasm.

Homan's Sign

The symptoms of deep vein thrombophlebitis may evade the most careful examiner, but in most cases light compression of the calf muscles in the affected limb elicits pain when deep vein thrombophlebitis is the cause of symptoms. This sign must be differentiated from simple strain or myositis of the belly of the gastrocnemius or soleus. A tear or rupture of the thin string-like plantaris muscle must also be ruled out. Skin inflammation also limits the reliability of Homan's sign.

Oscillometry

The oscillometer registers the volume of pulsation in the extremity. The number of units over which the needle passes with each systole of the heart is called the index.

Since it was introduced in this country by Samuels in 1927 (12) the oscillometer has been used in an effort to be more exacting in the interpretation of a patient's circulatory status. The normal oscillometric index in the lower extremity is 8 to 15 at midthigh, 4 to 10 below the knee, 3 to 8 at midleg, 1 to 5 above the ankle and traces to 1 in the foot.

The value of oscillometry in the diagnosis of circulatory disease has been questioned. Plethysmographic and Doppler studies have proved to be more reliable. Kramer believes that the oscillometer is not the most reliable guide for determining the effect of treatment (5). In organic vascular disease, it does not readily register collateral circulation and improved nutrition after sympathectomy.

A differential diagnosis of occlusive disease from vasospastic disorders is not substantiated by oscillometry. Nor are the causes and mechanisms of circulatory disease disclosed with this technique. Clinical judgment is necessary. Goldy (13) described the value of recording oscillations of both extremities simultaneously with an oscillograph. The oscillations, recorded on graph paper, become part of the patient's permanent record.

The following factors influence the reliability of oscillometric readings. A loose-fitting cuff takes up too much buffer of the oscillometer capsule and gives a false reading. An edematous leg similarly acts as a buffer. The temperature of the room in which the extremity is exposed can also influence the reading. A cold room produces sufficient vasoconstriction to reduce the oscillometric reading. Fever, which causes diffuse vasodilation, also influences the reading in the oscillometer. Lowenberg (14) noted that patients with apparently healthy limbs who complained of pain on use of the oscillometer cuff were subsequently proven to have phlebitis.

Pratt Modification of Trendelenburg's Test

This test is used in locating incompetent communicating branches. The patient's limb is raised, and the leg and thigh are gently massaged from the distal end in order to empty all superficial veins. With the leg still in the raised position, an Ace bandage is applied from the toes to high on the thigh. The patient is instructed to stand. The bandage is now slowly unwound while the uncovered areas are carefully observed. An incompetent valve is evidenced by the sudden appearance of a saccule, or "blow out," caused by back pressure developing against the wall of the superficial vein where blood from the deep system is regurgitating into the superficial vein because of nonpatent valves in the communicating branch.

Pratt's Early Sign of Femoral Thrombosis

In over 80% of cases of pathological clotting, three dilated veins appear over the tibia. Pratt believes this to be the earliest sign of deep vein thrombosis (15). The clotting in the calf progresses to the popliteal vein, thus occluding the vessel and resulting in swelling, tenderness and cyanosis with possible extension causing a pulmonary embolism.

Perthes' Test

All cases with varicosities of the superficial veins must be tested to ascertain the competency of the communicating deep systems and valves of the veins. The deep veins must be patent before surgery is attempted on the superficial veins. Very often in a deep thrombosis the superficial veins dilate due to an inability of the deep veins to conduct blood away from the extremity.

A tourniquet is applied to the upper thigh with the patient standing to constrict the superficial veins. The patient walks around the room or flexes and extends the extremity vigorously several times. The superficial veins should collapse during the exercise and fill up from above when the tourniquet is released. When the deep veins are not patent the superficial veins remain dilated during this test and the test is negative. Injection of the superficial veins is then contraindicated.

Venous Disorders

Varicose veins are common and easily diagnosed. They are tortuous dilations of the peripheral veins with a bluish or blue-brown-red discoloration of the skin, edema and often a complicating inflammation and ulcer. Transitory phlebitis may be a feature of thromboangiitis obliterans.

Increased blood pressure, low abdominal pressure on the veins, weakened leg musculature and venous cusp degeneration may be the direct causes of varicose veins. Imbalanced feet, obesity, occupations requiring long periods of standing, trauma, constricting garters, rubber panties, and pregnancy are predisposing factors. Phlebitis may incite the formation of varicosities or be a secondary complication of varicose veins.

Varicosities usually appear between the ages of 25 and 50 and occur more often in females than in males. There are hereditary predispositions in some families. The patient complains of a heavy feeling in the extremities followed by a dull ache and often severe pain. Fatigue is common, and very often a symptom of fullness or swelling is noted. The edema that occurs after long periods of standing may be unilateral and reach its greatest severity toward the end of the day. The swelling is generally diminished in the morning or upon arising after periods of rest.

Phlebitis may occur as a complication after trauma, operative surgery or septic diseases. The vessels are cord-like and indurated, and redness, heat, swelling and severe pain are noted around the affected part. The greater saphenous vein is involved more often than the lesser saphenous vein. Phlebitis is most commonly found around the ankle and extends upward. The femoral vein is often affected, with venous thrombosis as an etiologic factor. The skin frequently becomes red or cyanotic in venous thrombosis.

A stasis dermatitis with dry scaly patches or scales and crusts with underlying oozing excoriations may complicate varicose veins. The superficial vessels break down and cause itching, burning and pain. Excoriations may result in ulcerations with secondary infections. Lymphangitis and septicemia can result from faulty care and uncleanliness; osteomyelitis is an infrequent complication (Fig. 4.6).

Phleboliths may develop in chronic venous insufficiency and are visible on radiographs. They show up as rounded calcareous bodies of increased density (Fig. 4.7). A calcified vein reveals streaks in the vein walls and must be differentiated from arteriosclerosis, in which the vein looks tube-like.

Venous thrombosis is predisposed by venous stasis, hypercoagulability and vascular endothelial damage (Virchow's triad). Thrombosis of the peripheral veins may be caused by a preexisting disease.

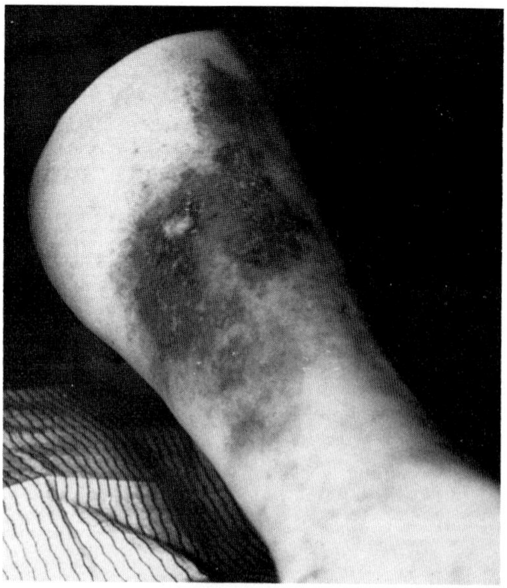

Figure 4.6. Varicose eczema secondary to ruptured and distended veins. Note extensive skin pigmentation.

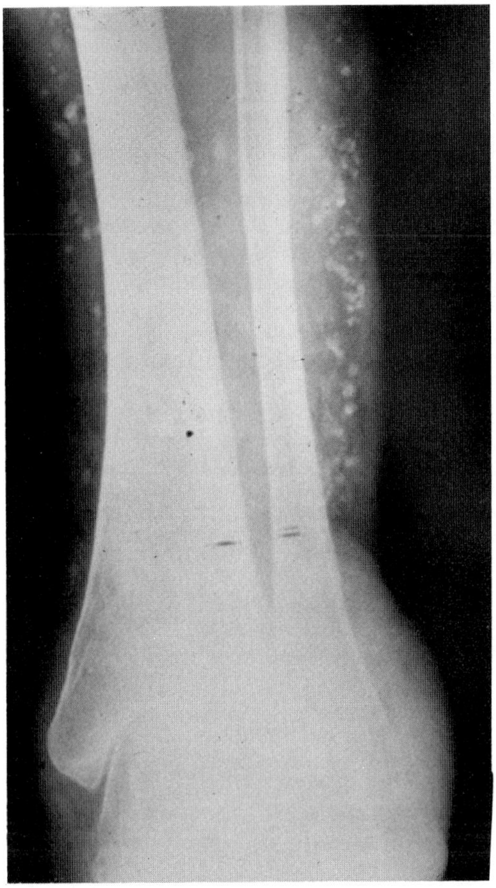

Figure 4.7. Phleboliths. Rounded calcareous deposits in superficial veins may break down and cause ulcerations. (From FO Gamble and I Yale: *Clinical Foot Roentgenology.* Baltimore, Williams & Wilkins, 1966.)

Thrombi may be septic or bland. The femoral vessels are most commonly involved, and there are irregular intervals of chills and associated moderate temperatures. In severe septic cases the temperature may rise as high as 105°F.

A deep thrombosed vein is cord-like; a dull ache, tingling, numbness and vague feeling of discomfort are noted. Edema begins in the most distal parts and extends upward; the skin becomes pale, cold and shiny.

Breneman (16) noted that on an annual basis there are at least 400,000 victims of postsurgical thromboembolic disease; of these, 18,000 patients die. Anesthesia resulting in voluntary muscle flaccidity is an important factor. The flaccidity impairs the pumping action of the leg musculature, resulting in a sluggish venous return and producing a phlebothrombotic nidus. Painter (17) notes that the more proximal the venous thrombosis, the greater the risk of pulmonary embolization. Daniels and Nash (18) present a case of venous disease and skeletal hyperostosis causing periostitis.

Thrombophlebitis and phlebothrombosis must be differentiated from varicose veins. Phlebothrombosis presents a thrombus that is loosely attached to the vein wall. It may appear after surgery, or it may occur during pregnancy or postpartum. Minimal swelling does not reflect the seriousness of the problem, which often ends in pulmonary embolism and critical illness. Chronic venous insufficiency generally follows thrombophlebitis and phlebothrombosis (Fig. 4.8).

Treatment. Compression bandages and/or elastic stockings may relieve symptoms.

Periodic elevation of the extremities decreases pressure against the expanded vein wall. In the event of an acute inflammatory episode, elevation and the use of an ice bag over the affected parts are recommended. Sometimes hot wet

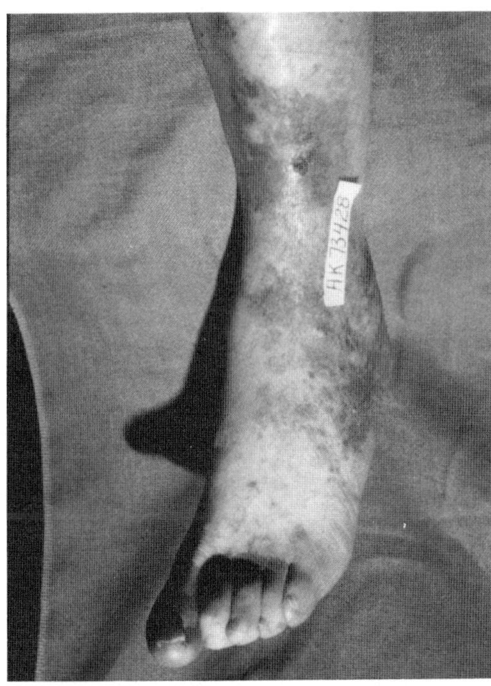

Figure 4.8. Stasis dermatitis, swelling, distention of veins; pigmentation is dark red and blue in color.

compresses are effective. The pain is relieved by systemic analgesics, and the infection is controlled by antibiotics.

Thrombosis is treated with anticoagulants under an internist's supervision. Saphenous ligation and tying off superficial veins or stripping by a vascular surgeon may be necessary. Occlusion of sacculated veins by injections of sclerosing agents may be effective in controlling further degeneration.

Elliot (19) states that injection therapy, high ligation, multiple ligation and high ligation with retrograde injection are inadequate as primary forms of treatment of varicose veins because of recurrence and such complications as deep vein thrombosis.

Ulcerations are treated by venous "heart" dressings, gelatin boots, compression bandages, bed rest and elevation, suitable antibiotic and enzymatic debriding medications, systemic antibiotics and high-protein diets to decrease capillary fragility (20).

Stasis dermatitis is treated with antipruitic anti-inflammatory corticosteroid preparations, emollients for dry, scaling skin, and mildly astringent applications where weeping exists. Occlusive gelatin compression dressings relieve the physiological dysfunction.

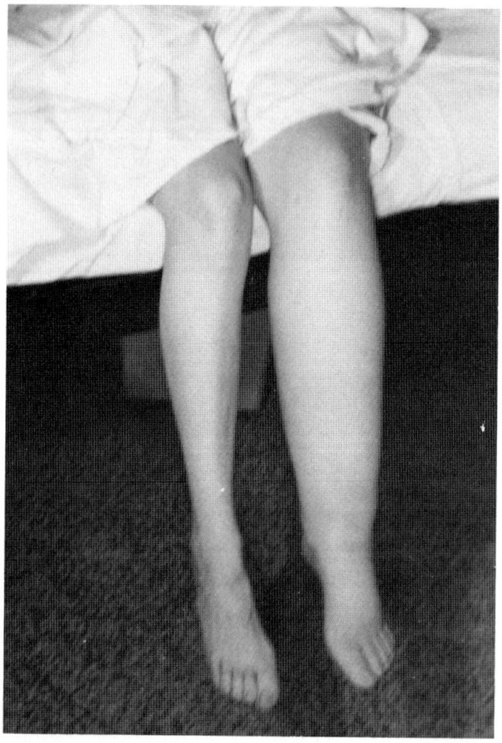

Figure 4.9. Unilateral firm, nonpitting edema commonly affecting young females in second decade. Etiology questionable.

The use of physiological saline soaks in the acute stages followed by occlusive gelatin flexible castings often relieves the dermatologic symptoms and aids in repair of ulcerations.

Gertner (21) reported the successful treatment of 20 cases of superficial thrombophlebitis by injection of a suspension of 0.5 ml. of hydrocortisone suspension and 1.0 ml. tetracaine solution directly into the painful indurated thrombotic process.

Owens (22) recommends the use of adenylic acid therapy as adnosine-5-monophosphate in the form of its sodium salt to relieve edema, inflammation, pain and pruritus resulting from thrombophlebitis. A series of intramuscular injections given daily for 3 days and then on alternate days for a total of 10 injections is suggested for mild to moderate cases. One milliliter of 20 mg/ml. is the usual daily dose followed by one or two injections weekly to maintain relief after symptoms subside.

Arteriovenous fistula occurs as a result of communication of artery and vein due to trauma and may also be of congenital etiology. The patient may be aware of a murmur in the region of a penetrating wound. The foot is a common site for such an injury. Ischemia results in atrophy and gangrene of the distal portions of the toes at an early date. Later the circulation improves to the point of increased temperatures and increased physical development of the affected side.

Varicose veins are evident in congenital arteriovenous fistula, and port wine cavernous hemangioma may be present in 50% of such cases. Increased perspiration, hair growth, enlargement of the limb, skin warmth and an oxygen saturation of venous blood are present in the affected limb. Surgical excision of the defect and very often vascular grafts are required to correct arteriovenous fistulas. Early consultation with a vascular surgeon is indicated.

Edema

Pearlman (23) offered the following definition of edema. "Edema is a condition in which the volume of extracellular water on the outside of the circulating intravascular compartment is increased. Normally there is a constant, equal, well-regulated exchange of water and electrolytes through the capillary wall from the circulation into the interstitial spaces and returning to the circulation." Generally the maintenance of fluid balance depends on the concentration of serum proteins, the amount of protein in the interstitial tissues, hydrostatic pressure in the capillaries, tissue tension and the flow of lymph.

Pitting Extracellular Edema
- Etiology
  - Increased capillary pressure
    - From venous obstruction e.g., cardiac failure (cardiac edema)
    - From arteriolar dilatation, e.g., allergic conditions (angioneurotic edema)
  - Decreased plasma protein (albumin loss)
    - From burns
    - From hepatic disease
    - From nephrosis (protein loss into the urine through the kidney)
    - From inadequate protein intake (nutritional edema)
  - Increased capillary permeability
    - From destruction of capillary endothelium, e.g., burns, allergic reactions
  - Lymphatic obstruction
    - A small amount of protein filters continually from the capillaries into the tissue spaces. It can only return to the circulatory system through the lymphatics. If the lymphatics are blocked, severe pitting edema results, e.g., filariasis or after lymphatics are removed in cancer surgery.
  - Renal Failure
    - When adequate amounts of urine are not excreted extracellular fluid increases. If it increases sufficiently, intracellular edema also occurs.

Nonpitting, Hard or Brawny Intracellular Edema
- Etiology—Local Cellular Damage
  - From trauma
  - From inflammation
    - Autolysis of cellular contents with sodium retention results in swelling. Damaged cells release toxic substances that make capillaries more permeable, resulting in pitting extracellular edema. These toxic substances also cause the protein that diffuses into the lymphatics to coagulate, which results in lymphatic obstruction and subsequent pitting extracellular edema.

Long-term inflammatory nonpitting intracellular edema caused by trauma results in extracellular pitting edema. Consequently, one cannot say that if pitting edema is present it is always related to a systemic illness.

Helfand (24) notes that an "increase in capillary blood pressure, hypoproteinemia, increased capillary permeability, venous or lymphatic obstruction, or a defect in the water balance of the body will be found in the presence of edema."

Edema may be symmetrical or asymmetrical. Swellings are classified according to etiology (Fig. 4.9 and Tables 4.1 and 4.2). Asymmetrical edema may be caused by congenital anomalies, varicosities, sprain, cellulitis (Fig. 4.10), gout, drugs, artificial ligatures, pressure from ill-fitting footgear, poor posture and pantyhose constriction.

Symmetrical types of edema are classified according to the following etiology: congestive heart failure, pernicious anemia, chronic kidney disease, hepatitis, secondary anemia, wasting diseases (carcinoma, tuberculosis), diabetes, obstruction of inferior vena cava, prolonged convalescence, Milroy's disease, myxedema and menstruation.

Sensitivity to certain foods or chemicals may cause wheals accompanied by swelling. Wheals in symmetrical edema may be uniformly rose red to purple with a white periphery. They also may be flat or elevated conical papules surrounded by vesicles. Often they are linear and several inches long.

Drug edema may occur from such drugs as aspirin, bromides, iodides, NSAIDs,

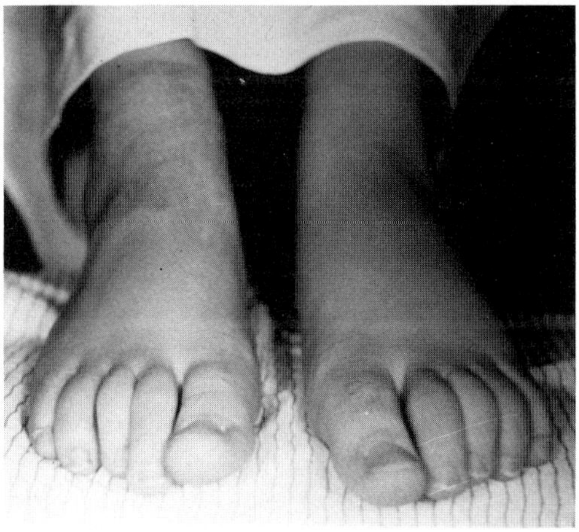

Figure 4.10. Asymmetrical cellulitis; edema with deep rubor in left foot.

Table 4.1.
Differential Diagnosis of Foot and Ankle Edema

Systemic	Regional	Miscellaneous
Congestive heart failure	Primary lymphedema	Tenosynovitis
Nephrotic syndrome	Secondary lymphedema	Neuritis
Hepatic syndrome	Chronic venous insufficiency	Drug-induced (NSAIDs, hormones, antihypertensives, antidepressants)
Acute glomerulonephritis	Trauma	Lipedema
Hypoproteinemia	Infection	Collagen vascular disease
Idiopathic cyclicedema	Chronic inflammation	Arteriosclerosis
Angioneurotic edema	Deep venous thrombosis	Livedo reticularis
	Inferior vena cava syndrome	Thromboangiitis obliterans
	After arterial surgery	Pretibial myxedema
	Compression of popliteal vein	Gravitational edema
	Tumor	

diphtheria antitoxin, mercurials, sulfa drugs, penicillin and others that cause allergic urticarial lesions accompanied by edema.

Lymphatic Obstruction

An obstruction in the removal of the lymph fluid may be caused by inflammation, the pressure of tumors, parasites and tumors of the lymphatics. Lymphangitis with occlusion of lymph vessels causes an excessive accumulation of proteins in the interstitial fluid. Growth of fibroblasts and production of scars are stimulated. Moist, warm macerated skin with fissures and vesicles between the toes may cause repeated attacks of lymphangitis and lymphatic obstruction. Dermatomycotic infections often reoccur. Young and DeWolfe (25) report on 25 consecutive cases of recurrent lymphangitis with dermatophytosis.

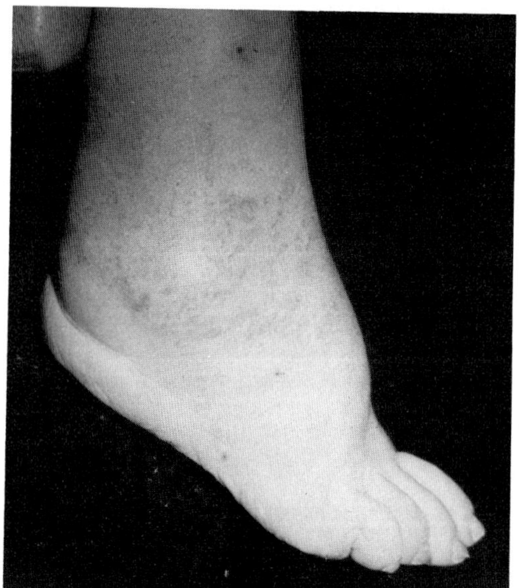

Figure 4.11. Cardiac edema showing marked swelling and distention of superficial veins.

Onset in these cases is sudden; severe symptoms of pain develop over a period of a few hours and are accompanied by chills and fever up to 106°F. The chills and fever last from a few hours to 3 days. Headache, fatigue, malaise, nausea and vomiting are common. The extremity becomes swollen and tender. Acute symptoms may persist until inflammation subsides.

Wood (26) notes the adverse effects of postoperative edema on operative results. Emphasis is placed on maintaining the integrity of the lymphatic and venous anatomy that provides for superficial drainage distally to the deeper lymphatics and more proximal on the dorsum of the foot and ankle so as to avoid lymphatic obstruction and subsequent edema. The lymphatic and venous systems work as a team in draining fluid from the interstitial spaces and into the bloodstream. Because there is no basement membrane in the lymphatics, they can fulfill an extra service that the venous capillaries are unable to perform. Fibrous protein materials are more easily absorbed where no basement membrane exists. Interstitial pressure is capable of diminished or increased function. If the force is greater than the negative pressure of −6 to 8 mm Hg present in

Table 4.2.
Differential Diagnosis of Geriatric Lower Extremity Edema[a]

Etiology of unilateral edema	Etiology of bilateral edema

Early accumulations
  Diabetes mellitus
  Congestive heart failure
  Cirrhosis
	Systemic Diseases
	  Cardiac: CHF, constrictive pericarditis
	  Renal: chronic nephrotic syndrome, insulin edema, bladder outlet obstruction
	  Hepatic: cirrhosis

Venous or lymphatic disease in presence of past injury, fracture or superficial phlebitis	Primary lymphedema
	  Simple congenital lymphedema
	  Lymphedema praecox
	  Lymphedema tarda or "idiopathic", late onset

Chronic venous insufficiency	Secondary lymphedema
	  Prostatic, GI carcinomas
	  Lymphoma
	  Filariasis
	    Lymphogranuloma venereum
	  Tuberculosis
	  Syphilis
	  Retroperitoneal fibrosis
	  Postradiation therapy

Deep vein thrombophlebitis (DVT)	Chronic venous insufficiency

Congenital amniotic bands: lymphedema	Physiological (dependent)
	  Arteriosclerosis obliterans, arterial obstruction
	  Rheumatoid arthritis and other connective tissue disorders
	  Paraplegia
	  Sudeck's atrophy
	  Causalgia, postfrostbite, postimmersion foot

Benign neoplasms: ganglionic cyst, hemangioma, fibroma, lipoma, etc Malignant neoplasms: liposarcoma, osteosarcoma, Kaposi's sarcoma, etc Other tumors: Congenital, A-V fistula, Klippel-Trenaunay-Weber syndrome, diffuse hemangio-lymphangioma, neuroepithelioma	Nutritional

Secondary venous outlet obstruction
  Inflamed Baker's cyst
  Popliteal artery aneurysm
	Drug-Induced

Physiological (dependent)
  Arteriosclerosis obliterans, arterial obstruction
  Rheumatoid arthritis and other connective tissue disorders
  Paraplegia
  Sudeck's atrophy
  Causalgia, postfrostbite, postimmersion foot
	Lipedema (painful fat syndrome)
	  Erythrocyanoid edema

Hereditary lymphedema	Nonvascular geriatric
Lymphedema praecox	Traveler's ankle

Inflammatory disorders
  Acute, chronic gout
  Tenosynovitis
  Morton's neuroma
  Bursitis
  Arterial revascularization
  Open fracture reduction
	Metabolic: pretibial myxedema

Infectious disorders
  Acute and chronic osteomyelitis
  Gas gangrene
  Deep mycoses
  Cellulitis
	Livedo reticularis

Post-traumatic
  Lower extremity surgery
  Hematoma
  Ruptured gastrocnemius
  Anterior and posterior ankle sprain
  Tibial compartment syndromes
  Shoe pressure
  Pantyhose constriction
  Artificial ligatures
	Idiopathic (cyclical)

[a] Johnson, MK, Yale, JF: The differential diagnosis of edema in the lower extremities of the elderly (Prospectives for podiatric medical care). Yale Podiatry Group, P.C. Ansonia, CT, 1984.

normal lymphatics, drainage will be adequate to reduce swelling by increasing lymphatic drainage.

An increase in the pressure outside vessel walls may present a variety of physiological problems. An increase in the protein level of interstitial tissue, along with a more positive, rather than negative, pressure in the lymphatic capillaries, may result in a limitation of drainage. However, each of these problems alone plus an increased permeability of blood capillaries is also capable of producing an edema.

Damage to the lymphatic vessels by surgical incision limits the ability of lymphatic wound drainage and disturbs normal wound healing.

The interstitial tissues become overburdened with protein, and the positive pressure in the interstitium may produce an edema. The foot surgeon should make a special effort to establish the individual patient's preoperative lymphatic drainage to ensure adequate postoperative results.

Treatment requires a thorough knowledge of the pathophysiology of the extremity, and the use of pressure bandages and the administration of proteolytic enzymes and diuretics. Early function is helpful. Care in the use of oral thiazides to minimize a hypokalemia or a thiazide-induced hyperuricemia is essential. A systemic hyperuricemia and an acute clinical gout in an already swollen local part may cause undue stress on the suture line. Sutures may have to be released, or strangulation of the tissues will ensue.

Treatment consists of bed rest and elevation of the part, local antifungal applications and systemic antibiotics for secondary infection. Inflammation is reduced with oral or parenteral anti-inflammatory or antifungal agents. The use of anticoagulants and often dissection of vascular growths or aspiration of thrombi from the lymphatics may be necessary to maintain flow of lymph in the larger vessels.

Elephantiasis

True elephantiasis, caused by *Acanthocheilonema perstans (Filaria sanguinis hominis)*, is rare in the United States. Pseudoelephantiasis is due to long-standing lymphatic obstruction of other etiologies. The skin becomes roughened, thickened and fibrous. A deep thrombosis, an operation that interferes with the lymphatics, or postfracture complications may cause pseudoelephantiasis.

Elephantiasis is an enlargement of one or both extremities or other parts where a chronic lymphatic blockage is present. The marked increase in the size of the part may be secondary to surgical injury, neoplasms, trauma or inflammation caused by a chronic filarial infection or other irritants and bacteria. The Nostras type of elephantiasis is generally due to streptococcus infections. Repeated invasion of the subcutaneous tissues results in marked increase in collagenous fibers, usually large concentrates of protein and ultimate thickening and stasis within the fibrous connective tissues.

Edema of Inflammation

Edema may be caused by increased capillary permeability resulting from inflammation that occurs when fluid accumu-

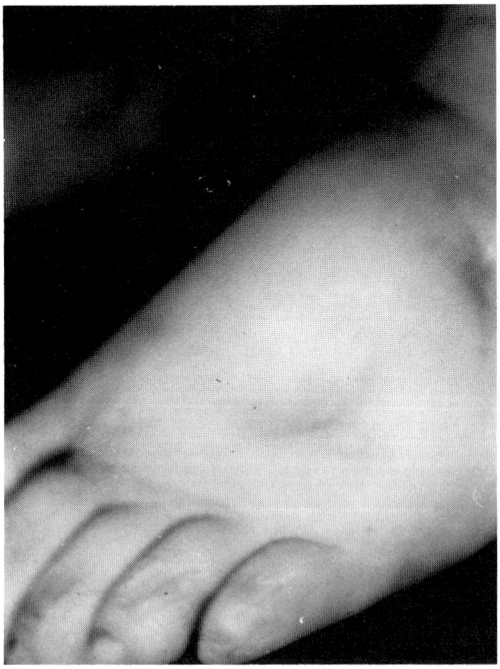

Figure 4.12. Marked pitting edema secondary to renal failure.

lates in the tissues. An infected toe, a suppurating wound, an infected mycotic lesion or collagen disorder may be present (Fig 4.12). Edema of inflammation is not influenced by gravity because of the increased fibrin in the soft tissues. The lymphatics are obstructed by clots or leukocytes and are compressed by the exudate.

Treatment. Infection must be controlled with local and oral antibiotic or antifungal agents and proteolytic enzymes when necessary to decrease capillary permeability. Resolution of thrombi and fibrin accumulations decreases the edema. Medical control of an existing collagen disorder will help decrease swelling.

Cardiac Edema

Cardiac edema is a congestive swelling caused by passive venous congestion secondary to myocardial insufficiency (Fig. 4.11). The diminished circulation causes increased venous pressure, which results in increased capillary pressure and permeability. Such myocardial insufficiency may result from long-standing valvular abnormality.

Edema is a very important sign of cardiac failure. It usually begins in the feet and legs and spreads upward at a time when the circulatory system is decompensated. As the cardiac problem worsens, the edema, which at first is slight and appears only toward the end of the day, becomes greater and more extensive. The failure of circulation in the extremities is due to insufficient cardiac strength and overly distended veins. Pulmonary engorgement produces intrathoracic pressure and impaired respiration and cardiac function. At first dyspnea subsides after rest, but later it is noted even at rest. A pitting edema is noted over the shoe tops in the early stages. The degree of cyanosis generally depends on the amount of myocardial damage. The podiatrist is often the first doctor to see and recognize this problem. Immediate referral to an internist for treatment is indicated.

Renal Edema

Because renal edema resembles cardiac edema, the swelling is difficult to differentiate (Fig. 4.12). However, the fluid is less influenced by gravity. Decreased blood protein causes decreased osmotic pressure in the blood. Osmotic pressure in the tissues remains high and edema results. The edema is present in the morning on arising. The podiatrist may note the early changes in renal edema while treating the complications of pressure produced by the swelling. Boccio et al. (27) discuss the necessity of having a high index of suspicion relative to foot swelling caused by nephrotic syndrome. Early diagnosis is emphasized in order to avoid complications.

Treatment. Maintaining a high blood protein to increase osmotic pressure in the blood may be helpful in decreasing osmotic pressure in the tissues. Consultation with a urologist or internist is indicated because local treatment is unproductive. A differential diagnosis of the etiology is essential if complications are to be avoided.

Famine Edema

In famine edema blood proteins are low because of an abnormal diet. This results in decreased osmotic pressure leading to a loss of fluids that pass to the tissues. The presence of local inflammations and infections in helomas, tylomas and nail grooves is not uncommon.

Treatment. Increase of blood protein is necessary to maintain fluids within the blood vessels. Nutritional supplements are indicated. All pressure on the toes and heels is to be avoided.

Milroy's Disease

Milroy's disease is a chronic familial and hereditary condition occurring as edema of the legs without obstruction or constitutional etiology. The swelling may be unilateral or bilateral with a solid type of edema. Milroy's disease occurs more frequently in females and is first observed early in childhood. The swollen and nonswollen parts are differentiated at joints, such as the ankle or knee. In debriding tylomas and helomas in patients with Milroy's disease, the podiatrist must exercise extreme care to avoid secondary infections and ulcers.

Treatment. Because the etiology is unknown, the best approach to treatment is even compression of the affected extremity by elastic bandages or stockings extending from behind the metatarsophalangeal joints upward to midthigh. Shoe fitting problems become critical, and allowance should be made for the edema.

Myxedema

This condition, commonly occurs in women, but it also occurs in males with hypothyroidism. The edema is bilateral with noticeably dry, thick skin. The patient is mentally dull and has precocious development of hair on the face with thinning or loss of hair elsewhere on the body. The edema is solid and of the nonpitting variety around the ankles. Skin around the heels and toes may be dry, fissured and ulcerated.

Treatment. Treatment by an internist is necessary to reverse the symptoms. There is no physiological advantage to the use of compression bandages in this condition as prescribed for Milroy's disease. The dry skin is treated with emollients and the fissures and ulcers by the use of tincture of benzoin compound and protective bandages. A plastic or rubber heel cup may protect the heel from undue stress.

Menstrual Edema

Menstrual edema is a normal finding in healthy premenopausal females. Both ankles may become swollen 1 to 3 days before menstruation, the shoes are tight and the patient has an increased body weight caused by excess water retention. The swelling may cause pressure and pain in the feet that resolve naturally as the edema subsides.

Treatment. Rest and elevation of the extremities and the use of mild diuretics beginning about 7 days prior to the onset of the menstrual flow help minimize edema. Consultation with a gynecologist should be suggested.

Pregnancy Edema

Over 50% of pregnant women show evidence of edema. In many instances the patient is toxic or presents nephritic symptoms. The edema may manifest itself as an elastic puffiness that does not pit. When the edema is generalized and is accompanied by albuminuria and hypertension, toxemia, renal or hepatic disease is possible and the patient should be referred to the obstetrician for treatment. Mechanical factors, such as tight garters, muscular weakness, obstruction of circulation by pressure from an enlarged uterus and varicose veins, may be etiologic. Abnormal foot function and faulty foot structure may contribute to edema in pregnancy and should be treated. Elastic stockings to support venous flow are beneficial.

Sprain

In sprain there is a history of trauma that results in early edema and pain. Tendon sheath inflammation may occur secondary to trauma (Fig. 4.13). Venous thrombosis caused by the trauma may cause swelling. Marked connective tissue inflammation may result in a fibrosis with development of a firm indurated edema at the site of the injury. Fracture must be ruled out to facilitate repair.

Treatment. The most common sprain affects the lateral ankle joint. Treatment of choice is adhesive tape immobilization in a neutral right-angled position. The use of an ice bag is mandatory with acute sprain. Oral enzymes aid in absorbing

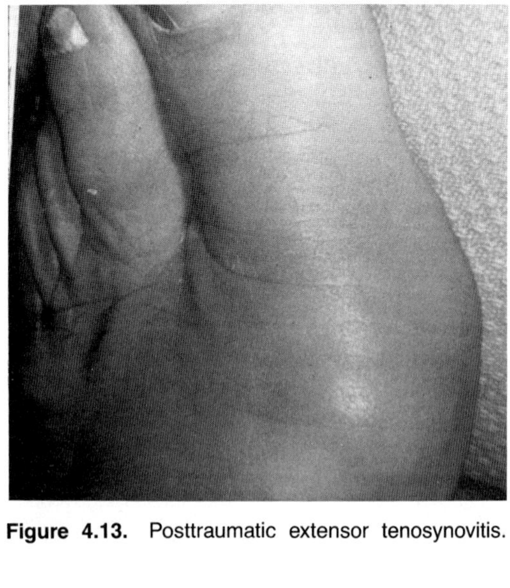

Figure 4.13. Posttraumatic extensor tenosynovitis.

and dispersing fluids. Hyaluronidase injections act as a medium for dispersion. Analgesics commensurate with the degree of pain reduce discomfort.

Cellulitis

Acute cellulitis is usually easily recognized by all the signs of infection: redness, swelling, heat and pain. However, it is often difficult to differentiate cellulitis caused by infection from cellulitis caused by primary or secondary gout (Fig. 4.14). Infections result in cellulitis around the ankle with associated edema of the affected parts. In a study by Travis and Delaney (28), 10% of the admissions to a military hospital were for foot infections. A high percentage of these admissions involved cellulitis secondary to infection by *Staphylococcus aureas*.

Treatment. Treatment of the cause of cellulitis is necessary. This may include treating severe trauma or secondary infections. There should be no pressure on the cellulitic tissue. A warm, moist dressing, elevation, incision, drainage and proper antibiotics are essential.

Phlegmasia Alba Dolens Thrombophlebitis

Thrombophlebitis of the iliac and femoral veins may be a mild or a deep phlebitis with marked swelling of the leg and ankle. The disease often complicates serious febrile disease, abortion, pelvic operation, childbirth and fracture. The patient is usually young with a history of having been confined to bed for several days.

Many cases are called to the podiatrist's attention when ill-fitting footgear, circular garters and abnormal pressure from occupational stress cause edema. Removal of local pressure relieves the stasis, which in some cases extends up to the knees. Hosiery with elastic tops pressing just below the knee that cause pressure on the saphenous veins may produce afternoon and night edema that subsides during the day. Tight shoes or straps or short-vamped pumps may cause swelling of the feet and toes from pressure on the dorsal superficial veins. One-strap shoes with an open throat cause pressure on the dorsal venous arch, producing local and generalized swelling of the limb.

Obliterative Arterial Disease (arteriosclerosis, athrosclerosis)

Calcification of the arteries in the feet may be of the tunica media type (Mönckeberg's) with few symptoms of an obliterating disease. Intermittent claudication, decreased skin temperature, absent or feeble pulsations and marked pallor, rubor and cyanosis in elderly people are the early signs of arteriosclerosis obliterans (Figs. 4.15–4.19). Gangrene is a common sequela. Jahsman (29) points out that claudication pain in hip or thigh muscles with or without leg pain arouses suspicion of segmental occlusion of the femoral or iliac arteries with or without more distal occlusive arterial disease. Important studies on arterial disease have been made by DeBakey *et al.* (30) and Pepin and Lauritzen (31).

In the presence of acute arterial thrombosis, the collateral flow is often absent or poor, not having enough time to develop. Ischemia followed by gangrene and amputation is the usual course.

The site of intermittent claudication may indicate the level of arterial occlusion. Care must be taken to differentiate a cramp in the buttocks, hips, thighs and

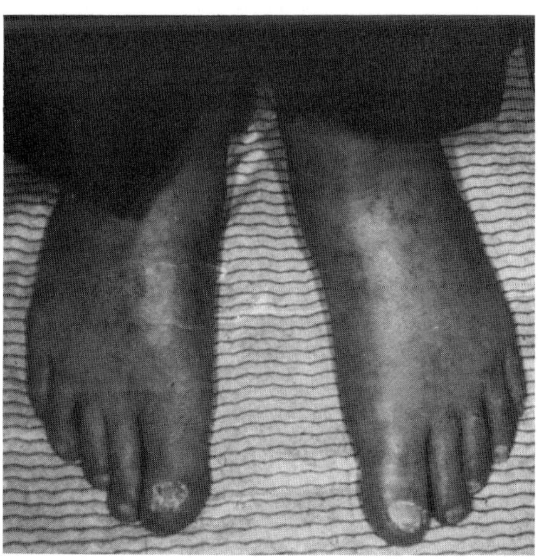

Figure 4.14. Acute attack of secondary thiazide-induced hyperuricemia.

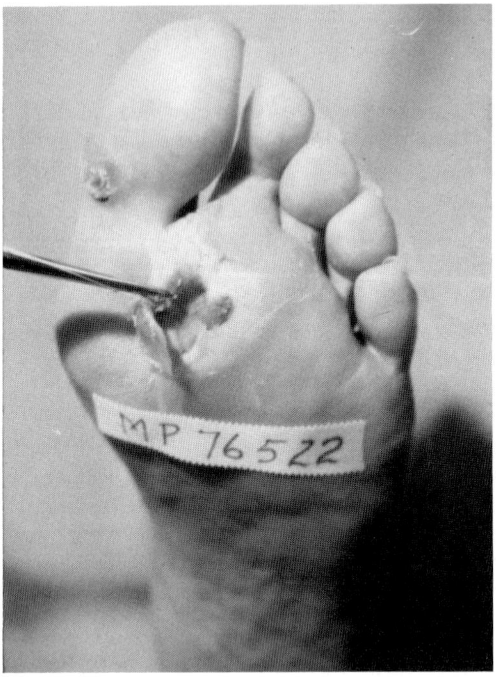

Figure 4.15. Diabetic ulcer beneath tyloma. Arteriosclerosis obliterans usually coexists with diabetes mellitus. (Courtesy of M Shapiro.)

calves due to biomechanical dysfunction from occlusion of the aorta or iliac arteries. Arteriosclerotic obliterating disease of the femoropopliteal vessels may result in claudication of the calf. With obliteration of the popliteal-posterior tibial vessels, intermittent claudication can involve the calf, leg, ankle and plantar surface of the foot.

Rest pain characteristically involves occlusion of the collateral vessels of the foot, forefoot or toes. The pain is continuous and worse when the patient is in bed, especially with legs elevated. Pain is abated when the legs are placed in a dependent position which only ultimately increases edema and extravascular pressure. Ischemia, ulceration and gangrene may develop. Pain is so severe that amputation is the usual sequela to this occlusion of the collateral vessels.

Pulses, color changes and trophic alterations of hair, skin and nails must be evaluated. The use of diagnostic instruments and techniques in an office may assist the podiatrist in corroborating the physical findings. Vascular laboratories are available to perform the more sophisticated instrumentation which may provide a numerical value of the extent of arteriosclerosis obliterans, its progress under treatment and the need for surgical intervention, as well as postsurgical results.

The brachial blood pressure is taken and noted. The systolic blood pressure is taken at the ankle by inflating the cuff above the brachial pressure and slowly allowing it to diminish while an ultrasound Doppler probe is placed over the dorsalis pedis or posterior tibial arteries. If the systolic pressure at the ankle is less than 80% and more than 50%, of the brachial pressure an early arteriosclerosis obliterans is suspected. When marked occlusions occur, the systolic pressure at the ankle may be less than 50% of the brachial pressure. The level of occlusion and extent of collateral circulation may be established by performing the blood pressure tests at the upper and lower sites of the popliteal artery and at the arteries in the foot.

Velocity wave recordings by ultrasound and pulse volume graphs using segmental plethysmography provide additional information.

When peripheral symptoms are present, consultation with an internist to review the systems for signs of atherosclerosis is often indicated.

Angiography is essential to evaluate pre- and postoperative results of anatomical studies. Modern-day instrumentation is not as important as a good history and physical examination in diagnosing ar-

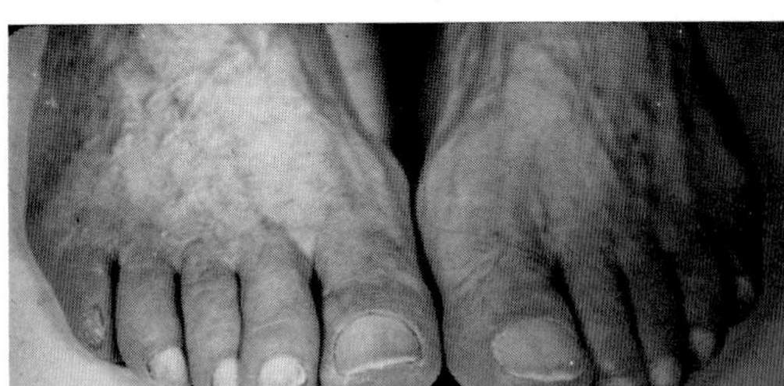

Figure 4.16. Obliterative arterial disease showing color changes ranging from rubor to cyanosis. Absence of hair on right Hallux indicates greater circulatory distress.

terial disease. deWolfe (32) tabulates angiographic patterns of arteriosclerosis obliterans and provides criteria essential for clinical diagnosis.

The angiograph demonstrates simple or multiple segmental occlusions of the aortoiliac and femoropopliteal vessels, nonsegmental occlusion of the femoropopliteal, disease from the renal area down in diffuse fashion, the site of acute thrombosis or embolism and popliteal aneurysms.

Treatment. Cranely (33) presents the following criteria for grading the severity of obliterative arterial disease of the lower extremities.

Decrease in amplitude of the dorsalis pedis and posterior tibial pulsations indicates grade one disease. Treatment consists of good foot hygiene and avoidance of extremes of heat and cold and use of tobacco (Table 4.3). Vasodilating drugs are helpful, and surgery is not usually desirable.

Absence of the dorsalis pedis and posterior tibial pulses is characteristic of grade two disease. Treatment involves lumbar sympathectomy and/or use of vasodilators, such as cyclandelate (Cyclospasmol), nylidrin hydrochloride (Arlidin) in 6 mg tablets and niacin in 25 to 100 mg tablets. Nylidrin hydrochloride in combination with vitamin E has been helpful in relieving symptoms. Quinine sulfate or Benadryl taken at bedtime can relieve cramps. Cyclospasmol is a peripheral spasmolytic and vasodilator available in 200 mg capsules and 100 mg tablets. The dosage is 400 to 800 mg/day taken in two to four doses. Porter et al. (34) report on the use of pentoxifylline (Trental) for intermittent claudication. Pentoxifylline given orally in doses up to 1200 mg/day was significantly more effective than placebo in increasing both the initial and absolute claudication distances in patients with chronic occlusive arterial disease.

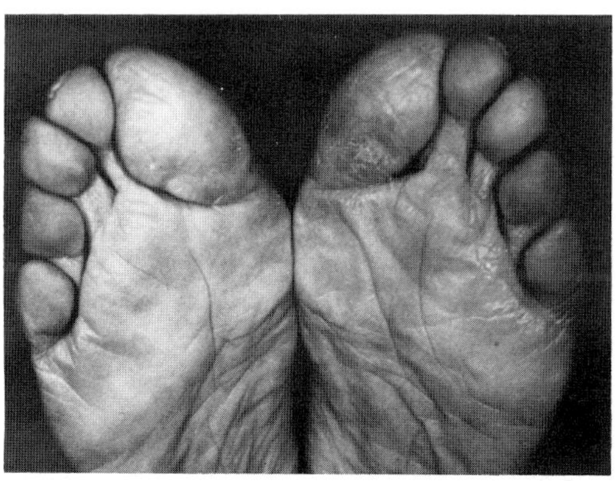

Figure 4.17. Arteriosclerosis obliterans showing cyanosis in left foot and pallor in right foot.

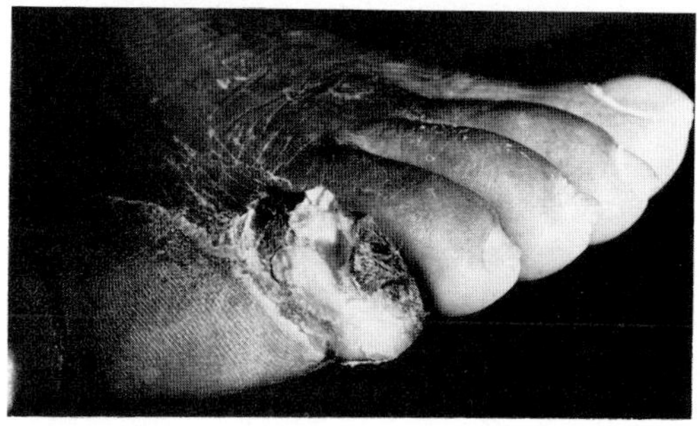

Figure 4.18. Dry gangrene in fifth toe secondary to infected heloma. Arteriosclerosis obliterans.

Definitive angiography is helpful in approaching the surgical treatment of occlusive vascular disease. Ratner et al. (35) describe percutaneous transluminal angioplasty in the treatment of ischemic disorders of the lower extremities. This nonoperative invasive procedure utilizes a Gruntzig balloon catheter for dilating stenosed or occluded large arteries in patients with occlusive arterial disease. Sengpiehl (36) aptly notes that arterial reconstruction, utilized before definitive amputation for ischemia, may permit a more distally located amputation than would have been possible without the bypass.

Absence of the dorsalis pedis, posterior tibial and popliteal pulses characterizes grade three disease. If vessels are judged suitable for bypass grafts in thigh or leg, this may be the treatment of choice. Lumbar sympathectomy and long-term use of vasodilating drugs, good foot hygiene and avoidance of infection and Buerger exercises may be indicated.

Grade four disease is indicated when there is rest pain and rubor on dependency. A femoral artery block may have to be removed. Vasodilators do not help in this stage. Quinine sulfate capsules 2 to 5 grains hs for leg cramps may be beneficial.

Grade five disease is characterized by continuous pain, petechial hemorrhages on the dorsum of the foot and gangrene. Amputation is the treatment of choice in this advanced disease.

Raynaud's Disease

Raynaud's disease, while most common in females, may occur in both males and females. The fingers and/or toes, tip of the nose, and outer ear may undergo color

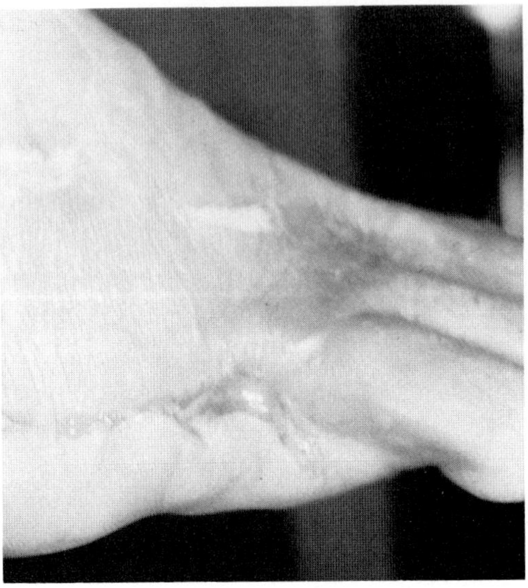

Figure 4.19. Healing by third intention following amputation. Arteriosclerosis.

changes precipitated by cold and emotional stress. These changes vary from pallor to cyanosis and a deep redness of the toes. Slight swelling, paresthesias and exessive perspiration may be seen early. The tips of the toes may undergo necrosis.

This condition is a vasospastic disorder occurring in cold-sensitive people. However, vasospastic changes on exposure to cold may also occur in arteriosclerosis and thromboangiitis obliterans. Raynaud's phenomenum may occur secondary to scleroderma and other collagen vascular diseases, arteriosclerosis obliterans, thromboangiitis obliterans, peripheral neuropathy, multiple sclerosis, syringomyelia, heavy metal poisoning, hematologic disorder, cold injury and pulmonary hypertension.

Treatment. Sympathectomy is helpful when Raynaud's is the primary disease. Treatment of local manifestations is imperative to prevent infection. Excess sweating and mycotic infections can be reduced with dilute potassium permanganate or 10% formalin in alcohol soaks. Protection of the toes and weightbearing areas from trauma prevents serious breakdown of tissue. The feet should not be exposed unnecessarily to increased temperatures or to cold. Smoking should be prohibited. Vasodilators must be used with caution because they can congest the area and create undue pressure on the embarrassed circulatory supply. Tolazoline (Priscoline) taken 23 mg four to six times daily may be beneficial.

Table 4.3.
How You Can Help Your Circulation

1. Keep your feet warm even when you are in bed. Wear warm, loose stockings, preferably made of wool, in cold weather. Cold tends to contract the blood vessels, thus slowing the circulation. However, never apply heat to the affected limb without a doctor's consent. Even moderate heat can injure the skin of a leg with poor circulation. Avoid sunburn.
2. If any redness, pain, blistering or swelling appears or if peeling and itching between your toes occurs, see your podiatrist promptly. Never apply any medication to your feet without consulting your doctor. Some medications are too strong for feet with poor circulation.
3. Wash your feet at least every other day with a mild soap and warm water. Be sure to dry thoroughly, especially between the toes, by patting, not rubbing, with a clean soft towel.
4. Apply nonmedicated talcum powder after bathing if your feet tend to be moist; if they are dry and crack easily, apply a cream, such as Nivea or other prescribed medications.
5. Cut your toe nails straight across and not too close. Do not cut into the corners.
6. Wear wide-toed shoes to avoid pressure. Be particularly careful that they are not too narrow and tight. (A low-heeled oxford shoe with laces and a round toe is the proper type.)
7. Do not wear circular garters or other tight articles of clothing on your legs or feet.
8. Do not wear stockings or socks that are too tight or short.
9. Do not sit with your legs crossed for long periods of time.
10. Do not bathe in cold water or in the ocean.
11. Do not use hot water bottles, electric pads, or any form of mechanical heating device on your feet.
12. Never use tobacco in any form. Tobacco contracts blood vessels and reduces circulation.
13. Report promptly to your podiatrist any unusual change in the condition of your feet.

Posterior tibial artery and nerve blocks often produce a helpful reflex dilation.

Livedo Reticularis

Occurring mostly in young women, Livedo Reticularis is a mottled cyanotic fishnet-appearing condition affecting the arms and legs. This vasospastic disorder may be nonpainful and idiopathic or secondary to collagen vascular disease. Exposure to cold is a predisposing factor. Peripheral pulses are normal. Treatment includes cold avoidance, use of vasodilating medications, and, in rare cases, sympathectomy.

Acrocyanosis

Acrocyanosis occurs in young women who complain that their hands and feet are cold, perspire excessively, and turn blue. This small artery and arteriolar vasospastic disorder is not associated with pain. Peripheral pulses are normal. No treatment is necessary.

Erythromelalgia

Erythromelalgia is a primary or secondary vasospastic dilative disorder of the feet and, on occasion, the hands. Primary erythromelalgia is idiopathic, affecting adult men and women equally. Secondary erythromelalgia is most often unilateral, affects the elderly, and is less painful than the primary type. It may be secondary to collagen disorder, arteriosclerosis, thromboangiitis obliterans, gout, diabetes, hypertension or polycythemia vera (37,38).

Acute attacks are initiated by exercise or heat. Arteries dilate, resulting in areas of redness, increased skin temperature and pain affecting parts of the palm, sole, or the entire foot and/or leg. The affected area is hot and is aggravated by heat or vasodilators. This condition is believed to be caused by abnormal prostaglandin synthesis in the skin; relief is attained by as little as 10 grains of aspirin or other prostaglandin-inhibiting agent. Attacks may last for a short period of time or up to 2–3 hr (38). Heat desensitization, cold application, rest, ephedrine and nitroprusside have been helpful (39).

Thromboangiitis Obliterans (TAO)

Thromboangiitis (Buerger's disease) affects men under 50 and is a generalized disease often involving the viscera, blood vessels, heart, lungs, kidneys and brain. Pain in the legs, intermittent claudication and migratory phlebitis with absent or diminished pulsations are pathognomonic. Marked rubor on dependency and pallor on elevation are noted. Ulcers followed by necrosis and gangrene of the feet are a common sequela to this systemic obliterating arterial disease (Figs. 4.20 and 4.21). Table 4.4.

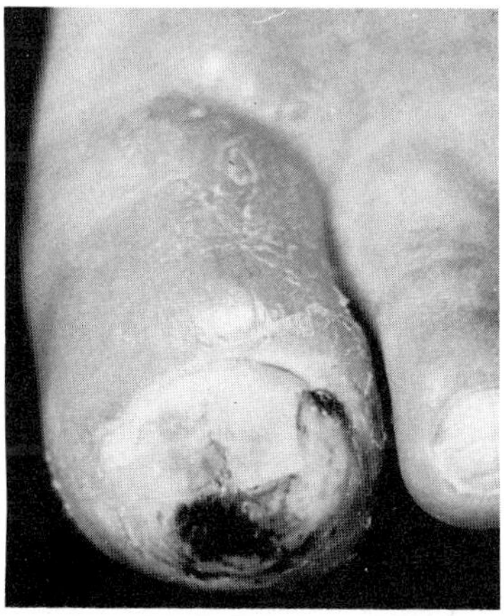

Figure 4.20. Thromboangiitis obliterans. Gangrene at distal end of hallux although part of nail is viable. Note cellulitis proximal to nail plates.

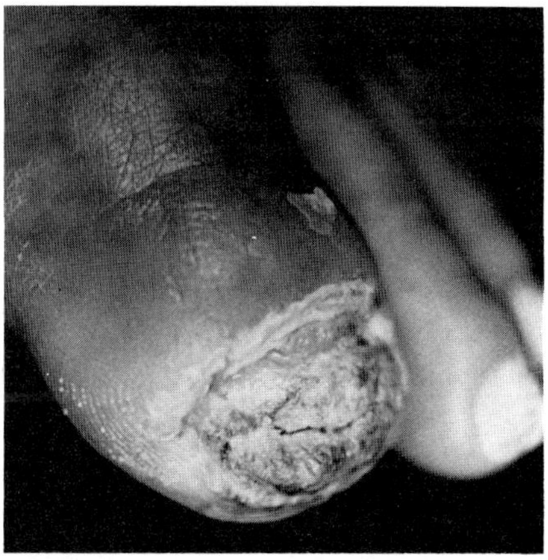

Figure 4.21. Same as Figure 4.22. Shows progressive destruction of distal phalangeal tuft.

Table 4.4.
Differential Diagnosis of Common Peripheral Vascular Disease

Feature	Arteriosclerosis obliterans (atherosclerosis)	Thromboangiitis obliterans (TAO)	Raynaud's disease
Age	Almost always over 40	20–35	Puberty to 55
Sex	75% male	Male	85% female
Involvement	Lower extremity (leg, foot, toe) common	Lower extremity, almost always (foot and toe). Upper extremity, rare	Upper and lower extremities (tips of fingers and toes)
Dorsalis pedis/ posterior tibial pulses	Absent or diminished	Absent or diminished	Present
Phlebitis	Absent	Sometimes present	Absent
Arterial calcifications	Present	Rare	Absent
Color and temperature changes	Rubor to cyanosis—cold	Rubor to cyanosis—often hot	Pallor to cyanosis to rubor—hot
Other affected areas	Heart, kidneys	Heart, lungs, kidneys	Outer ear, tip of nose
Ulcerations	Foot and toes	Ends of toes	Tips of toes
Rest pain	Present	Usually present	Absent
Predisposing factors	Diabetes mellitus, hypertension, hyperlipidemia, nephrosis, myxedema, tobacco	Tobacco	Emotional upset, temperature changes, collagen disorders in Raynaud's phenomenon
Intermittent claudication	Triceps surae—sometimes foot	Foot	Absent

Wininger (40) reviews the systemic manifestations and clinical aspects of giant cell arteritis within the lower extremities. Affecting the major arteries of the elderly, giant cell arteritis is a generalized inflammatory obliterative collagen disease.

Immersion Foot

Immersion of the feet for long periods of time in water, mud or damp shoes in temperatures above freezing may cause a variety of severe and disabling symptoms (Fig. 4.22). The colder the water, the more rapid the onset of ischemia and vasospasticity. The condition is aggravated by time, constrictive shoes and hose, dehydration and nutritional deficiencies, a decrease in systemic temperature, trauma and inactivity.

Numbness and coldness accompanied by anesthesia in localized patches, cyanosis or pallor with petechial hemorrhage are noted early. Later, the feet burn and become hot with redness. Swelling, paresthesia and intense pain followed by bullous lesions and secondary infections may occur at this time. The sequela to this pathology is a late vasospasticity. The skin temperature subsides, and vascular tone improves. The pain may persist, and the tendons contract with flexion deformities. Gangrene may occur.

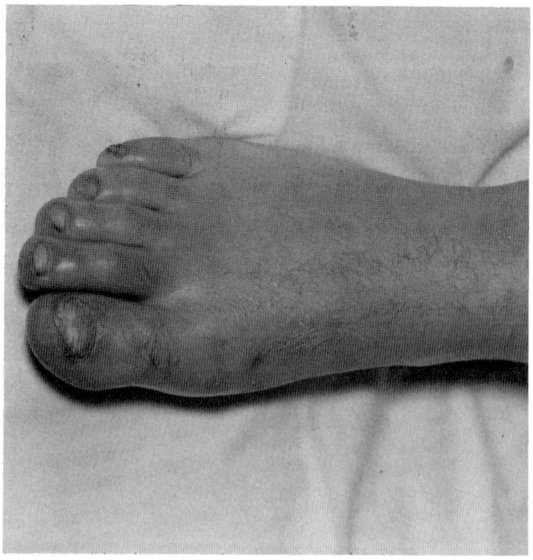

Figure 4.22. Immersion foot. Hyperemia and edema. (Courtesy of Armed Forces Institute of Pathology, #3550.)

Treatment. A comfortable body temperature should be maintained. Hose and shoes should be changed frequently. The feet should be well powdered and kept dry and warm.

If symptoms have developed, the feet should be kept dry and warm and the legs elevated. Blisters should not be broken. The feet should be exposed to room temperature and dried by cooling with a fan to reduce tissue metabolism. A hexachlorophene or dilute betadine solution is used to bathe skin lesions and maintain a diminished bacterial flora. Bacterial sensitivity tests are performed where open lesions are present. The antibiotic of choice for the bacteria present is given. The patient should not smoke. Anticoagulants should be used where thrombosis is present. Extreme cold should be avoided. A warm climate is recommended.

Ainhum

Ainhum (Fig 4.23), a condition of unknown etiology that is most frequently observed in blacks, is characterized by a firm, constrictive, fibrous band on the undersurface of the fifth toe. Eventually the entire toe is involved. The condition must be differentiated from helomas and tylomas. The end of the toe becomes bulbous and painful, and the clinically visible band may become callused and indurated. The circulation is gradually cut off, resulting in ischemia followed by dry gangrene. Repair proximal to the site of the constrictive band is usually good following removal of the distal end of the toe.

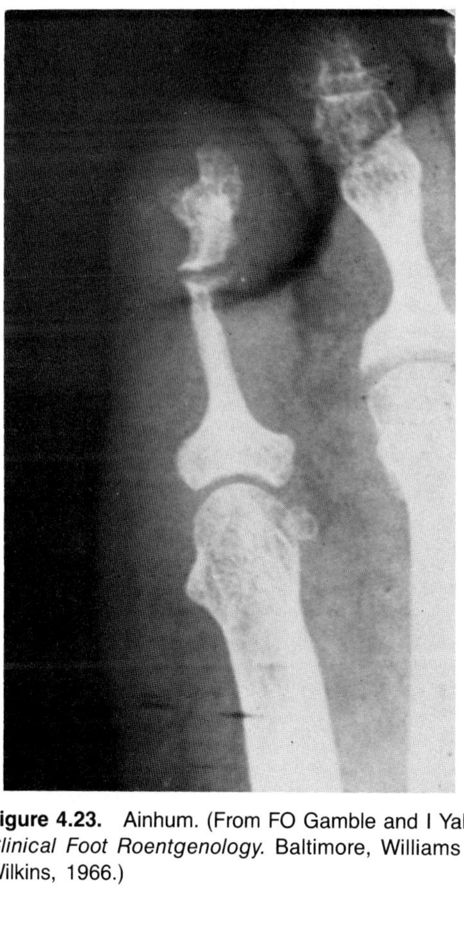

Figure 4.23. Ainhum. (From FO Gamble and I Yale: *Clinical Foot Roentgenology.* Baltimore, Williams & Wilkins, 1966.)

Constricted digits with a starfish keratosis of the dorsum of the hands and feet accompanied by hyperkeratosis of the palms and soles may be due to "keratoma hereditaria multilans" (41) and must be differentiated from ainhum if proper treatment is to be instituted.

Treatment consists of prescribing analgesics and watchful waiting for a line of demarcation. Amputation may be necessary to relieve pain.

Rossiter and Anderson (42) present a case of ainhum in which treatment with intralesional steroids provided symptomatic relief and partial resolution of the fibrotic band.

Gangrene

Gangrene is defined as the death or rotting of tissue in a part of the body resulting from insufficient blood circulation in the affected tissues. It may be caused by embolism, arterial thrombosis, diabetes (Fig. 4.24), Raynaud's disease, ergot poisoning, trauma, chemical destruction of tissue and extremes of temperature. The patient with occlusive arterial disease develops

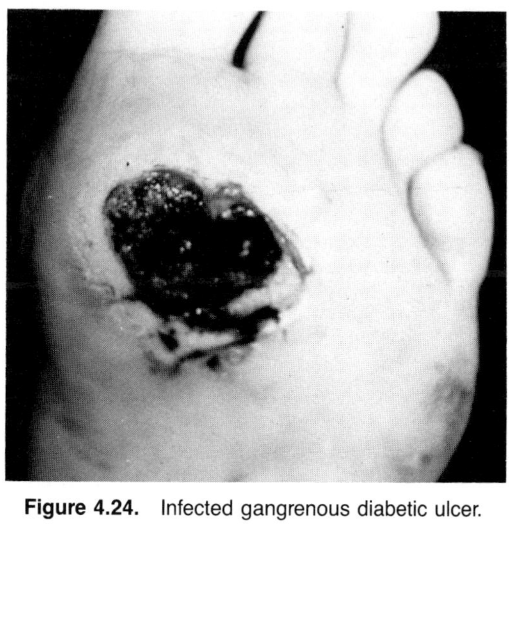

Figure 4.24. Infected gangrenous diabetic ulcer.

gangrenous areas by the occlusion of the vessels and an infarction of the tissue they fail to supply. Vasculitis may be an early sign of impending gangrene. Absence of pulsations and circulation to the part is a symptom of grangrene. The part is cool to touch; function, color and sensory perception are lost. The etiology of gangrene is based on a complete obliteration of arterial supply to the affected parts (Figs. 4.25 and 4.26). Samuels (43) recognized the presence of mycotic infection as an exciting factor in gangrene. Gangrene may be either dry or wet.

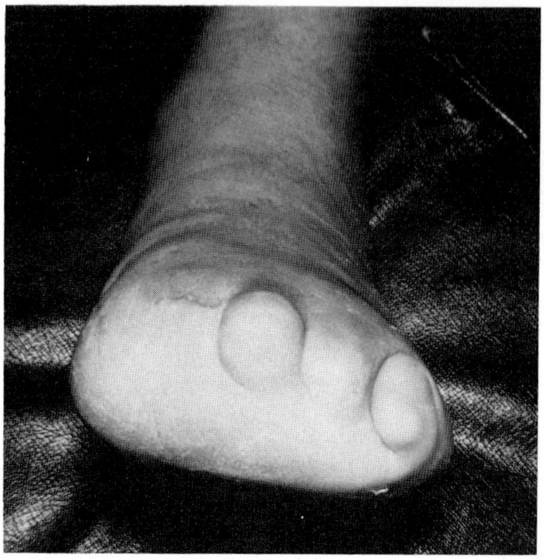

Figure 4.26. Amputation of toes—arterial embarrassment.

Dry Gangrene

This condition is caused by the loss of nourishment to a part followed by mummification (Figs. 4.27 and 4.28). The affected limb becomes dry, indurated, black, shriveled and parchment-like. Dry gangrene has little tendency to spread and is only mildly painful. Arterial occlusion results in a well-defined line of demarcation separating the healthy from the pathological tissues. The distal end of a toe in ainhum may undergo necrosis and gangrene in the advanced stages.

Treatment. Exercise is therapeutic, and vasospasm should be controlled with such drugs as sublingual nitroglycerine prescribed by the internist. A clean, dry site should be maintained to allow mummification and a line of demarcation to develop. The patient should avoid use of tobacco. Reflex vasodilation should be provided. Gravity aids blood flow.

When all soft tissues have become mummified and adjacent viable tissue appears well-vascularized, pursue the following course. Anesthesia may not be necessary if mummification is present. Nerve block anesthesia with Xylocaine 1% plain may have to be used. Care must be taken not to embarrass viable circulation. Sterile preparation includes draping of the part. With scissors, cut through necrotic tissue at the line of demarcation and remove the gangrenous part.

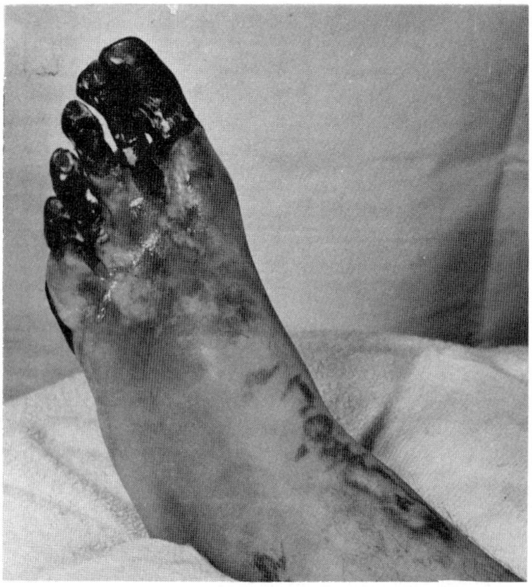

Figure 4.25. Gangrene—arterial insufficiency.

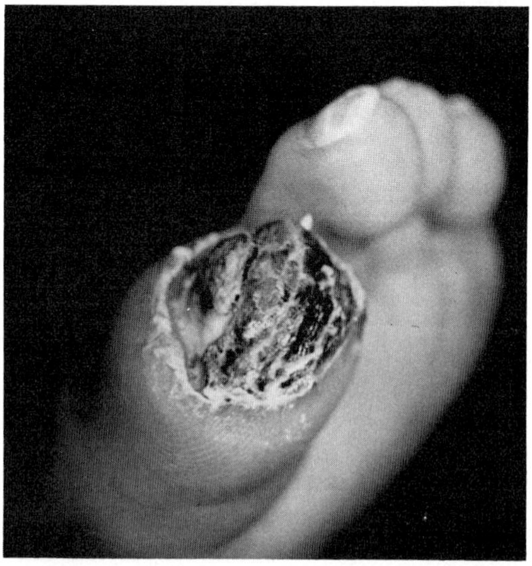

Figure 4.27. Dry gangrene distal end of hallux.

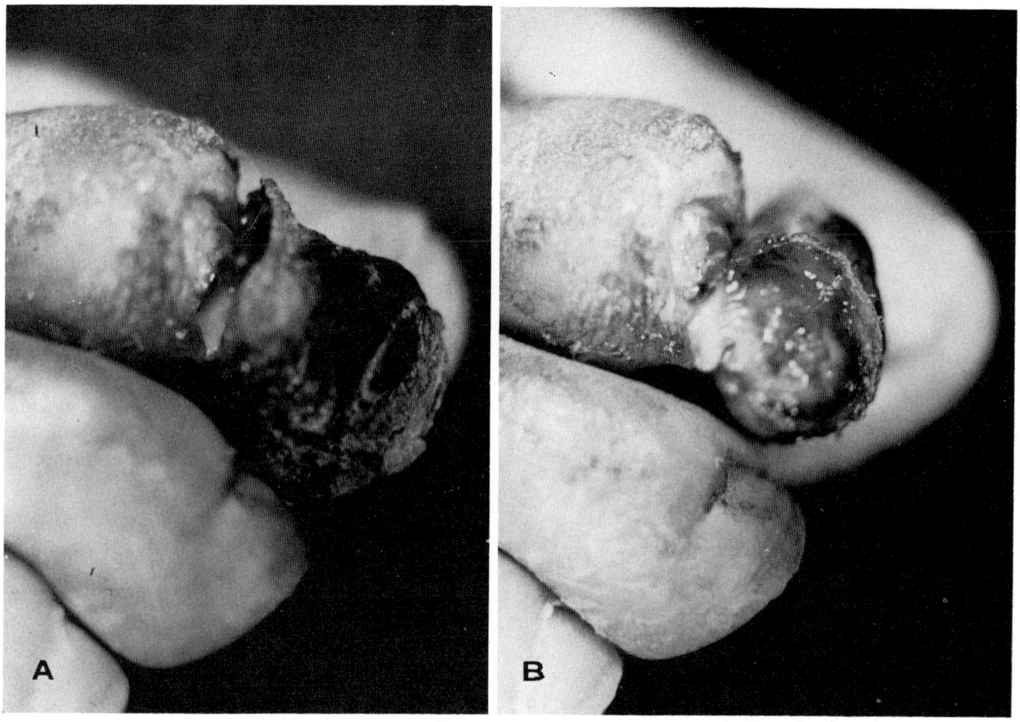

Figure 4.28. *A.* dry gangrene showing line of demarcation. *B.* distal end of toe attached only by flexor tendon.

Take care not to cut viable tissue. Dry dressing using an antibiotic powder of choice is helpful. Heat in any form should not be used.

Support of this local treatment by meticulous systemic treatment by a qualified medical doctor is mandatory. Sympathectomy is indicated. Amputation at the site of adequate circulation proximal to necrotic tissue may embarrass circulation and allow the spread of gangrene.

Foley (44) recommended walking as a treatment for gangrene of the feet and legs. He states that "one of the greatest stimuli to the development of collateral blood flow in the legs is walking."

Samuels (45) and Downie and O'Connor (46) advise the use of conservative treatment before attempting the mutilating amputation of an infected foot. Incision and drainage followed by a topical broad-spectrum antibiotic often relieve the tissue of embarrassment, allowing collateral circulation to take over. Systemic antibiotics cannot reach the infected tissue if circulation is diminished (Figs. 4.29 and 4.30).

Blau (47) describes a conservative treatment in 64 cases of vascular insufficiency and gangrenous ulceration. Treatment consists of debridement, nonirritating foot soaks, Panthoderm with 0.5% neomycin, and oral nylidrin hydrochloride, a peripheral vascular dilator. The patient was encouraged to be ambulatory to aid in vasodilation. The author has used modifications of this treatment with moderate success.

Dubois and Arterberry (48) describe five cases of gangrene due to systemic lupus erythematosus that they treated with fair success using large doses of steroids. Lassen et al. (49) cite five cases of gangrene that were improved by increasing blood pressure about 15 mm Hg. This was accomplished by using fluorocortisone or deoxycorticosterone to induce moderate hypertension.

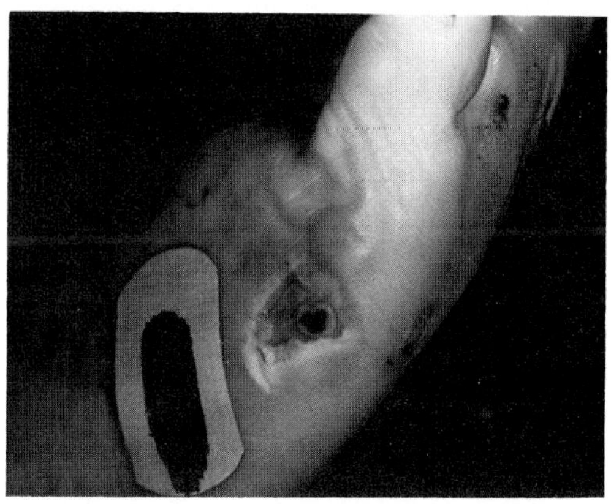

Figure 4.29. Infected gangrenous ulcer.

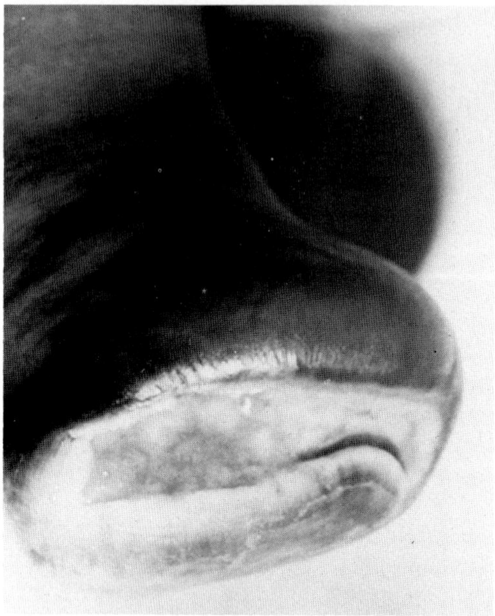

Figure 4.30. Transmetatarsal amputation with healing by third intention.

Jones et al. (51) in a review of exposure to cold, recommended rapid thawing of the frozen extremity, bed rest, nourishing diet, antibiotics and antitetanus if infection occurred. Apparent gangrene may only involve superfical layers of skin. Delays of 60 to 90 days in amputation are desirable.

Rakow (51) notes that osteopathy secondary to peripheral neuropathy must not be construed as osteomyelitis and impending gangrene. Incision and drainage may embarrass the circulation.

Wet Gangrene

This condition is a necrosis of tissue followed by destruction due to excessive moisture; decomposition occurs through the action of putrefactive bacteria. Gases accumulate in the tissues, and the line of demarcation is ill defined. The extremely painful part is purple and swollen. Wet gangrene may be due to venous thrombosis, and bullous lesions may be evident early. Diabetic patients commonly develop this type of moist gangrene when widespread infection exists.

Treatment. This type of necrosis spreads rapidly and is not easily controlled. Consultation must be sought with an internist or vascular surgeon. Bacterial sensitivity tests and early use of systemic and local antibiotics of choice may control the fulminating character of this disorder. Use of peripheral vascular dilators may be helpful. Sympathectomy is indicated.

Diabetes may cause a femoral neuropathy, autonomic nervous system symptoms, postural hypotension, diarrhea, polyneuritis (tingling, burning, restless legs and itching), atrophy and weakness.

Neuropathy is not relieved by therapy as readily as one might expect. Vit. B_{12} deficiency (Schilling test—B_{12} excretion, low percentage of oral dose)(normal is 7 to 22%), loss of vibratory sensation, unsteady gait and loss of position sense are characteristic symptoms.

Helfand (52) in an exhaustive 5-year study of a given population, demonstrated that "with appropriate foot care, patients could be kept ambulatory and free of pain in most cases, regardless of the underlying deformities and systemic diseases present." The study also points out the need for podiatric care in a comprehensive health care system.

Brenner (53) feels that diabetic patients with genetically induced biomechanical foot problems are prime candidates for neuropathic ulcerations. Circulatory problems are considered of lesser importance than the presence of multiple minimal trauma.

References

1. Adler P: Cutaneous pressure plethysmography (CPP)(R). Quantitative assessment of skin perfusion. *J Am Podiatry Assoc* 74:541–547, 1984.
2. Bartels CC, Rullo FR: Unsuspected diabetes mellitus in peripheral vascular disease. *N Engl J Med* 250:633–634, 1958.
3. DeWeese JA: Pedal pulses disappearing with exercise. A test for intermittent claudication. *N Engl J Med* 262:1214–1217, 1960.
4. Winsor T, Burch GE: An evaluation of the plethysomgraph for study of the peripheral circulation. *J Am Podiatry Assoc* 53:813–818, 1963.
5. Kramer DW: *Manual of Peripheral Vascular Disorders.* Philadelphia, Blakiston Co, 1940.
6. Lewis Sir T: *Vascular Disorders of the Limbs.* New York, Macmillan Co 1936.
7. Yale I: A statistical report on a review of 1290 foot radiographs. *J Natl Assoc Chirop* 47:61, 1957.
8. Riegelhaupt RW, et al: Lower extremity circulatory studies utilizing radioisotopes. *J of Foot Surg* 21:86–90, 1982.
9. Samuels SS: Value of oscillometry. *JAMA* 88:1780, 1927.
10. Barker WH, Barnes RW: Minor forefoot amputation in patients with low ankle pressure. *Am J Surg* 133:331–332, 1977.

11. Collens WS , Wilensky ND: *Peripheral Vascular Disease; Diagnosis and Treatment.* Springfield, IL: Charles C Thomas, 1939.
12. Samuels SS: Value of oscillometry. *J Am Podiatry Assoc* 88:1780, 1927.
13. Goldy H: Oscillographic interpretations. *J Natl Assoc Chirop* 46:826–830, 1956.
14. Lowenberg RI: Use of the cuff pain test in the early diagnosis of phlebothrombosis. *J Am Podiatry Assoc* 48:141–143, 1958.
15. Pratt, personal observation.
16. Breneman JC: Postoperative thromboembolic disease computer analysis leading to statistical prediction. *J Am Podiatry Assoc* 193:576–580, 1965.
17. Painter TD: Anticoagulation. *Postgrad Med* 74:341, 1983.
18. Daniels EG, Nash DJ: Periostitis—A manifestation of venous disease and skeletal hyperostosis. *J Am Podiatry Assoc,* 73:461–464, 1983.
19. Elliot JA: Recurrent primary varicose veins. *Can Med Assoc J* 74:388–389, 1956.
20. Block, P: Varicose ulcers—A Physiologic treatment approach. *J Am Podiatric Med Assoc* 75:166–168, 1985.
21. Gertner JJ: Treatment of superficial thrombophlebitis. *J Am Geriat Soc* 4:834, 1956.
22. Owens RE: Adenylic acid therapy for mechanical foot problems of varicose veins. *J Am Podiatry Assoc* 51:729–730, 1961.
23. Pearlman L: The importance of ankle edema in the diagnosis of cardiac and renal problems. *J Natl Assoc Chirop* 47:609–611, 1957.
24. Helfand, AE: The pathologic physiology of edema. *J Am Podiatry Assoc* 49:374–375, 1959.
25. Young JR DeWolfe VG: Recurrent lymphangitis of the leg associated with dermatophytosis: Report of 25 consecutive cases. *Cleveland Clin* 27:19–24, 1960.
26. Wood WA: Post-operative pedal edema. *J Foot Surg* 16:15–16, 1971.
27. Boccio JR, et al. Hypercoagulopathy secondary to nephrotic syndrome. *J Am Podiatry Assoc* 73:409–412, 1983.
28. Travis LO, Delaney JH: A clinical evaluation of 100 cases of infection of the lower leg and foot in military personnel. *Mil Med* 130:184–190, 1965.
29. Jahsman WE: An approach to the etiology, diagnosis and management of peripheral arteriosclerosis. *Henry Ford Hosp Med Bull* (Detroit) 4:56–61, 1956.
30. DeBakey ME, Crawford ES, Cooley DA: Chronic arterial insufficiency of the lower extremities. *DM* 1–45, 1957.
31. Pepin WA, Lauritzen WH: Can peripheral vascular disease be helped by improving foot mechanics? An early report. *J Am Podiatry Assoc* 52:202–204, 1962.
32. deWolfe VG: Assessment of the circulation in occlusive arterial disease of the lower extremities. *Mod Concepts Cardiovas Dis* 45:91–95, 1976.
33. Cranley JJ: Clinical grading of the severity of obliterative arterial disease of the lower extremities. *Geriatrics* 11:91–96, 1956.
34. Porter JM, et al. Pentoxifylline efficacy in the treatment of intermittent claudication: Multicenter controlled double blind trial with objective assessment of chronic occlusive disease patients. *Amer Heart* 104:66–72, 1982.
35. Ratner SW, Reilly CH, Gudas CJ: Percutaneous transluminal angioplasty in the treatment of ischemic disease of the lower extremity. *J Foot Surg* 22:86–91, 1983.
36. Sengpiehl KE: Improved salvage of the foot with arterial reconstruction. *J Foot Surg* 23:370–376, 1984.
37. Krupp MA, Chatton MJ (eds): *Current Medical Diagnosis and Treatment.* Los Altos, CA, Lange Medical Publications, 1983.
38. Juergen JL, Spittell JA, Fairbairn JF: *Peripheral Vascular Diseases.* Philadelphia, W B Saunders Co, 1983.
39. Dilmen U, Ceyhan M: Treatment of erythromelalgia. *Arch Dermatol* 119-793, 1983.
40. Wininger CD: The systemic manifestations of giant cell arteritis within the lower extremity. *J Foot Surg* 23:70–73, 1984.
41. Gibbs RC, Frank SE: Keratoma hereditaria mutilans. *Arch Dermatol* 94:619–625, 1966.
42. Rossiter JW, Anderson PC: Ainhum: Treatment with intralesional steroids. *Int J Dermatol* 15:379–382, 1976.
43. Samuels SS: Treatment of gangrene of the extremities. *Clin Med* 69:2635–2445, 1962.
44. Foley WT: Treatment of gangrene of the feet and legs by walking. *N Y J Podiatry* 8:10–18, 1958.
45. Samuels SS: Management of gangrene in the extremities. *Angiology* 7:532–536, 1957.
46. Downie E, O'Connor M: Infection and gangrene in the foot of diabetic patients; value of conservatism. *Aust N Z J Surg* 26:194–197, 1957.
47. Blau S: Conservative therapy in treatment of gangrenous ulcerations. *J Am Podiatry Assoc* 50:195–199, 1960.
48. Dubois EL, Arterberry JD: Gangrene as a manifestation of systemic lupus erythematosus. *J Am Podiatry Assoc* 181:366–374, 1962.
49. Lassen NA, Larson OA, Sorenson AW, Hallbrook T, Dohn I, Nilsen R, Westling H: Conservative treatment of gangrene using mineralocorticoid induced moderate hypertension. *Lancet* 1:606–609, 1968.
50. Jones RF, Watson DO, Tracy CD: "Cold injury" in a temperate climate. *Med J Aust* 1:323–327, 1970.
51. Rakow RB: Obliterative arterial disease. *J Natl Assoc Chirop* 34:17–20, 1944.
52. Helfand AE: Podiatric services for the aged. *J Am Podiatry Assoc* 63:368–373, 1973.
53. Brenner MA: An ambulatory approach to the neuropathic uleration. *J Am Podiatry Assoc* 66:862–869, 1974.

Suggested Readings

Abramson C: Normal "opportunistic" flora of the lower extremities related to post-operative surgical wound infections. *J Am Podiatry Assoc* 67:9–27, 1977.

Achauer BM, Bartlett RH, Wilson LF: Burns of the foot. *J Foot Surg* 15:43–46, 1976.

Atwell D, Pois A, Morledge J, Mahaffey H, Pawlisch DV: Severe unilateral ischemia secondary to ergot intoxication. *Wis Med J* 75:33–34, 1976.

Baden HP, Burnett JW: Injuries from sea urchins. *South Med J* 70:459–460, 1977.

Buggiani Z, Bredemeyer G: Clostridial myosities vs. clostridial cellulitis. *J Am Podiatry Assoc* 6:568–576, 1975.

Cruse, PJE, Foord R: A five year prospective study of 23,649 surgical wounds. *Arch Surg* 107:205, 1973.

Dooley DM, Kasprak M: Modification of blood flow to the extremities by electrical stimulation of the nervous system. *South Med J* 69:1309–1311, 1976.

Eaglstein WJ, Mertz P: "Inert" vehicles do affect wound healing. *J Invest Dermatol* 74:90, 1980.

Eickoff TC: Nosocomial infections. *Am J Epidemiol* 101:93–97, 1975.

Fields A: Leg cramps. *Calif Med* 92:204–206, 1960.

Fitzgerald RH, Washington JA: Contamination of the operative wound. *Ortho Clin North Am* 6:1105, 1975.

Francis D, Hubbard ER, Johnson LE: Nitroglycerine ointment as a vasodilator in the lower extremities. *J Am Podiatry Assoc* 67:874–879, 1977.

Geronemus RG, Mertz PM, Eaglstein WH: Wound healing: The effects of topical antimicrobial agents. *Arch Dermatol* 115:1311, 1979.

Hoffman AF: Noninvasive vascular evaluation. ACFS Scientific Seminar Las Vegas, NE, February 1984.

Jacobson AM, Hackett TP, Surman OS, et al.: Raynaud's phenomenon; treatment with hypnotic and operant technique. *JAMA* 225:739, 1973.

Jay, RM (ed.): *The Year Book of Podiatric Medicine and Surgery.* Chicago,Year Book Medical Publishers, Inc, 1985.

Jenkins WM: Dressings and topical agents affecting wound healing. ACFS Scientific Seminar, Las Vegas, NE, February 1984.

Jennett JH: Persistent hereditary edema of the legs—Milroy's disease. *Clin Orthop* 8:122–123, 1956.

Kozak GP: *Management of Diabetic Foot Problems.* Philadelphia, WB Saunders Publishing Co, 1984.

Meyers HL: New elastic support for stasis and stasis ulcers of the legs. *Vascular Dis* 5:188–193, 1968.

Morton JJ, Scott WJ: Methods for estimating the degree of sympathetic vasoconstriction in peripheral vascular disease. *N Eng J Med* 204:955–962, 1931.

Nomland R: Cutaneous manifestations of the circulatory disorders of the foot. A symposium, foot disorders and their treatment. *JAMA* 124:747–750, 1944.

Oshsner A, Debakey M: Thrombophlebitis, the role of vasospasm in the production of clinical manifestations. *JAMA* 114:117–124, 1940.

Perchuk E, Weinreb M, Aksu A: A new treatment for nocturnal leg cramps. *Angiology* 12:102–184, 1961.

Riccitelli ML (illustrations by Yale I): Foot problems of the aged. *J Am Geriat Soc* 14:1058–1066, 1966.

Roetman RL: Some factors in lower extremity edema. *J Am Podiatry Assoc* 58:385–387, 1968.

Rutherford RB: *Vascular Surgery,* ed 2. Philadelphia, W B Saunders Publishing Co, 1984.

Spencer AM: Report on a study of nylidrin HCl and vitamin E on the treatment of peripheral vascular disease. *J Am Podiatry Assoc* 51:341–344, 1961.

Weber DM: Occlusive arterial disease in the lower leg and foot. *J Foot Surg* 15:128–133, 1976.

Yale I: Vaso-motor imbalance. *Chirop Rec* 21:133–134, 1938.

5

Neurological Disorders

Before evaluating the lower extremities for neurological disease or disorder, it is important to determine the cerebral function of the patient. General behavior, level of consciousness, intellectual performance, emotional status and thought content should be investigated in order to obtain a general sense of the neurological cerebral functional status of the patient. Specific cerebral function tests for agnosia (cortical sensory interpretation), apraxia (cortical motor integration) and aphasia (language function) may be performed if determinations of general cerebral function dictate. Cranial nerve testing is a vital part of a thorough neurological evaluation of the patient. Olfactory, optic, oculomotor, trochlear, abducens, trigeminal, facial, acoustic, glossopharyngeal, vagus, accessory, and hypoglossal nerves are tested for their viability and possible pathology.

The neurological evaluation of the podiatric patient progresses from higher levels of integration as already noted to lower levels of integration as discussed below. The neurological examination proceeds in a step-wise fashion in order to determine the presence or absence of nervous system malfunction; the location, type and extent of nervous system lesions; and the degree to which the healthy portion of the patient's nervous system can be used for rehabilitation (1).

The neurological examination includes tests of the sensory system that measure primary forms of sensation: superficial tactile sensation, superficial pain, sensitivity to temperature, sensitivity to vibration, deep pressure pain and motion and position and cortical and discriminatory forms of sensation (two-point discrimination, point localization, texture discrimination, stereognostic function, graphesthesia and extinction phenomenon). This testing is followed by cerebellar function tests for balance and coordination and tests for the motor system, including muscle size, tone and strength and involuntary movements. The last area of neurological testing involves the reflexes (deep, superficial and pathological).

Neurological Tests

A great challenge to the skill of the podiatrist is the differentiation of the neurological syndrome from circulatory and biomechanical problems. Of great importance is the evaluation of the findings of neurological testing. The podiatrist must ascertain whether the problem is an upper or lower motor neuron lesion or a combination of each. Recognized techniques and observation are imperative for proper evaluation.

A wisp of cotton, a brush, a common pin, test tubes filled with hot and cold water, a small flashlight, galvanic or sinusoidal current, percussion hammer and a tuning fork are the necessary equipment to carry out an examination for sensory and motor involvements (Fig. 5.1).

The nervous system controls sensory discrimination, motor activity and reflex responses, and the reflex response serves as the connecting link between the sensory and motor nerves. It is possible for humans to maintain an upright posture and stance when their sensory receptors function well. This functioning is dependent on the integrity of the labyrinth of the

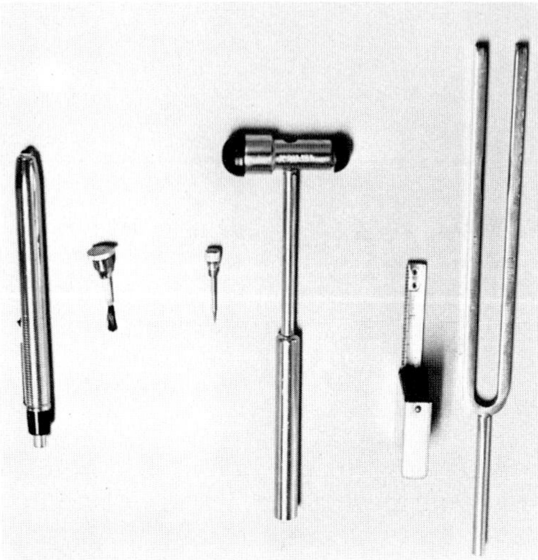

Figure 5.1. Neurological examination equipment. *Left to right:* flashlight for pupillary reflexes and examination of body orifices; brush for touch sensation; sharp, pointed object for pain perception; percussion hammer for reflexes; tape measure for mensuration; tuning fork for vibratory sensations.

ear, the retina of the eye, the proprioceptors of the neck muscles and the muscles and joints of the trunk and lower extremities.

Sensory Discrimination

This function is divided into exteroceptive impulses that give an impression of the outer world, e.g., through sight and hearing, and proprioceptive impulses associated with position and tension of muscles and tendons, and particularly with impulses from within the body. These proprioceptive impulses never reach consciousness, but receive proper reflex response. Gait and posture are dependent on their function.

Other sensory impulses are carried by mixed nerves in the form of superficial sensibility produced by impulses from the skin and as deep sensibility consisting of impulses from muscles, tendons, joints and bone. The mixed nerves carrying these impulses also supply the motor fibers to the muscles.

Superficial Sensibility. Nerves supplying the skin provide sensations of touch (pressure), pain and temperature and make possible the distinction of single or multiple stimuli. Tests for touch, pain and temperature sensitivity should be carried out with the patient's eyes closed and attention focused on what the examiner is testing. The most sensitive points of the skin seem to be at the base of hairs and on the soles and palms.

Touch. The quality of touch perception may be tested by either a wisp of cotton or a camel's hair brush used to stroke the skin. The hair follicles are receptors and therefore should be avoided. Allowances are made for the thicker skin of the palms and soles when interpreting the results.

Discriminative sensation is tested by having the patient discriminate between the pressure of one or two fingers held about ¼ inches apart. A few seconds of light pressure are put on the normal side to allow the patient to discriminate between one or two points of pressure. The abnormal side is then tested. The inability to discriminate between one or two pressure points may indicate damage to the sensory mechanism above the level of the thalamus or an absence of position sense as seen in ataxia. Dermographism or wheal formation at the site of irritation suggests a neurocirculatory lesion.

Pain. The ability to discern painful stimuli may be determined by alternately touching the skin with the pointed and dull ends of a common pin while the patient's eyes are closed. An area of sensory distribution of a nerve root is known as a dermatome. Nerve root pathology may manifest as an increased or decreased response to painful stimuli within a specific dermatome. A thorough knowledge of the sensory distribution of nerves enables the examiner to locate the level of a spinal lesion (Fig. 5.2).

In some cases, e.g., tabes dorsalis, the patient feels the touch sensation produced by the stimulus, but does not immediately perceive pain. The pain may be felt seconds after the prick of the pin because conduction of pain sense is apparently delayed in tabes. A double sensation is often experienced with the single prick of the pin.

In many disturbances of sensory perception, the border of hypoesthesia is not

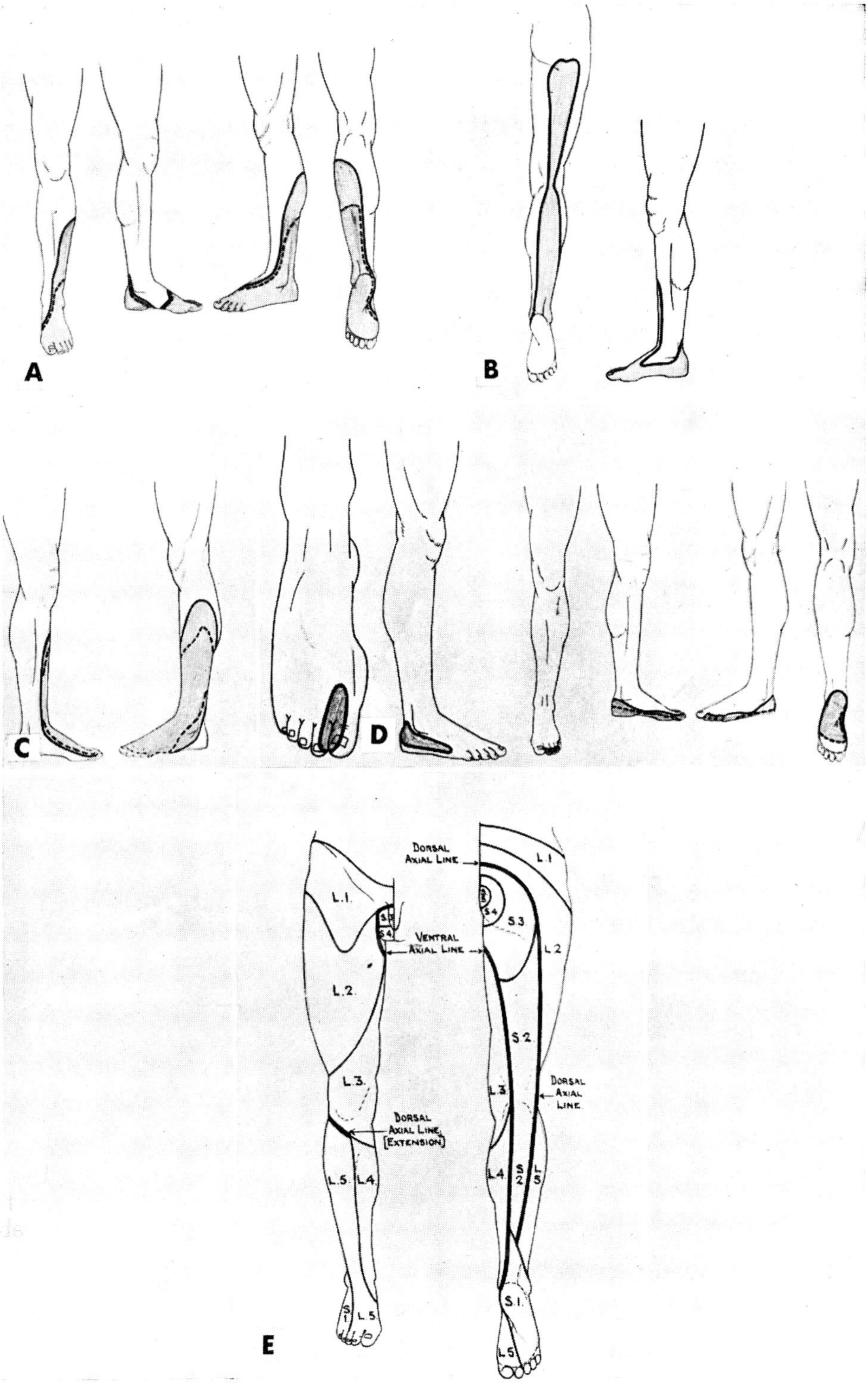

Figure 5.2. Dermatomes in extremities.

sharp, but is gradually impaired. One must note whether the loss of sensation is bilateral and symmetrical or whether mixed sensations affect the same area. Other types of sensations may be due either to a segmental loss of sensation or involvement of a particular peripheral nerve supplying the part. Perspiration, temperature and color of the skin must be noted in confirming evidence of the pathological findings. Careful examination must be made to clarify the evaluations of intensity of the pin prick and the site of irritation.

Temperature Sense. This sense is evaluated by applying test tubes filled with hot and cold water to the part being tested. This procedure tests the patient's ability to localize the site of application, as well as to distinguish between hot and cold stimuli. The area manifesting loss of heat sensation is usually larger than an area with loss of cold sensation.

Deep Sensibility. There are several methods of evaluating deep sensibility.

One test of deep sensibility is to have the patient differentiate between light touch and deep pressure on the skin. The results are obvious when squeezing the Achilles tendon. Abadie's sign is present when, in locomotor ataxia, pressure on the Achilles tendon does not produce pain. Normally the patient complains of pain and withdraws the foot.

Vibratory Sensations. The sensation from bone is limited to perception of pain and pressure and, most importantly, vibration. Vibration is tested by placing a vibrating tuning fork directly over a bony prominence. One must make sure that the patient feels the vibration or humming and not just pressure. Skeletal changes with age or the value of therapeutic approaches may be calculated by measuring the vibrating of a bone to sound.

Diminished or absent vibratory sensation is caused by injury or trophic disturbances of the peripheral nerves or the posterior columns or roots of the spinal cord. These lesions may occur in diabetes, arteriosclerosis, pernicious anemia, tabes dorsalis and multiple sclerosis.

When combined with an Argyll-Robertson pupil and a positive serology, the diagnosis is evident. Very often the bones may show evidence of syphilitic density, gummatous lesions, Charcot's joint or neurotrophic degeneration with loss of deep sensibility.

Position Sense. This is checked by passively moving the toes in a firm and definite manner, demanding that the patient describe or reproduce the motion. It is necessary to differentiate the reaction in both extremities. In severe cases of deep sensibility disturbances, patients cannot tell whether a part is flexed or extended. In spinal disease the maximum loss of position sense is in the toes and fingers. It is wise to evaluate all findings in an effort to rule out the possibility of suggestion, malingering or hysteria.

If rombergism is suspected, the patient is requested to stand with eyes closed and feet parallel and close together. Romberg's sign is present if the patient begins to sway, losing all sense of direction and balance. The sensation disappears when the eyes are opened. A positive Romberg sign is found in locomotor ataxia, cerebrospinal disease, alcoholic neuritis, pernicious anemia and diseases of the columns of Goll and Burdach.

Faulty equilibrium may result from degeneration of the dorsal roots and tracts. Afferent activity in the cerebellum may be disturbed. When loss of equilibrium is positive the examiner might suspect tertiary syphilis with neurological manifestations.

Finger-to-Nose Test. The patient stands with eyes closed, feet parallel and close together and arms outstretched. He or she brings the index finger first of one hand, then of the other to the nose. Incoordination is demonstrated by a rhythmic tremor at right angles to the line of movement in the finger-to-nose test. The heel-to-knee test may be used similarly to the finger-to-nose test to evaluate cerebellar disease. When the object is overshot and rhythmic tremors are present, a cerebellar ataxia is suspected, and if the tremors are irregular and unsteady a sensory ataxia is considered.

The André-Thomas sign, or spring-like phenomenon, is noted in the finger-to-nose test when the patient appears to touch the nose several times as if on a rebound. This same sign is observed when the patient raises his or her hand above the head. When requested to let it drop down on the head a rebound occurs in cerebellar diseases.

Another sensory symptom is seen in Lasèque's sign with the thigh flexed, when extension of the knee is accompanied by pain due to stretching of the nerve roots. Inflammation of the sciatic nerve or the perineural tissues caused either by pressure or pathology presents a positive Lasèque sign.

Motor Function

The strength of various muscles upon voluntary movement is examined by directing the patient to flex and extend a particular joint against resistance. The strength of these movements, observation of the patient's gait and familiarity with the patient's complete history contribute to an accurate diagnosis.

Early examination for motor function should include notation of posture, tremors and spasm of the extremities while at rest. This examination of the lower limbs is accomplished by asking the patient to raise first one, then the other limb from the examining table while lying in a face downward position. The patient flexes the leg at the knee to a vertical position and is instructed to maintain this posture. Failure to hold the limbs in this position is called Barre's sign. It is not, however, an indication of a specific type of motor defect.

The functions of each joint are tested for power of movement. A simple method for recording these functions is the use of a four-point scale in which 0 = no contraction; 1 = feeble contraction; 2 = ability to counteract weight of gravity; 3 = fair, but movement weaker than normal; and 4 = estimated full power of movement.

Ataxia. Due to a loss of power of coordination, the voluntary muscular movements are awkward. Swaying and irregular movements when standing or walking may be evident. Jerky and uncoordinated motions when walking and a loss of position sense of the hands and feet are all part of the ataxic syndrome. In Fournier's test for ataxic gait the patient is seated comfortably and is commanded to rise on a given signal, begin walking quickly toward the examiner and stop at a given signal. The patient then may be commanded to rise from the comfortable sitting position, walk and turn around at a given signal. During the execution of the above commands, the doctor should note any slight waverings, unsteadiness, staggering and associated abnormal movements. Owing to a loss of deep sensibility, the patient experiences difficulty in quick coordinated actions if ataxia is present. Advanced pernicious anemia is characterized by an ataxic gait.

Tremors. A tremor is a slow, rapid or moderate trembling or oscillation of parts of the body. Trembling of a part while at rest is known as passive tremor. Passive tremor may be seen in parkinsonism, or it may be a functional weakness of the musculature.

Intention tremor is trembling occurring when one is about to begin a muscular motion or is in the act of performing a voluntary function. This type of tremor often occurs in multiple sclerosis. A rapid and fine functional tremor may be seen in the fingers of an outstretched hand of one with an exophthalmic goiter.

Abuses of alcohol, tobacco, mercury, lead and other toxic substances may cause tremor. Very often in elderly persons there is a tremor of the head resembling the passive tremor.

Postural Tonus. An increase in tone causes the muscle to feel firm and thick; greatly increased tone causes the muscle to contract and shorten, resulting in deformity. The evidence of such spasticity is found in an increased activity of the tendon reflexes. Postural tone is established by noting any undue resistance of muscles to passive lengthening. In corticospinal lesions the resistance met is of the spastic type affecting the extensors of the knee and plantar flexors of the ankles; it gives way with continued passive stretch. This phenomenon remains the same from hour to hour, but varies from day to day. It is known as a hypertonicity of the muscles and should be differentiated from muscular rigidity. It has an elastic resistance to passive movement and is a result of an involvement of the pyramidal tract, whereas muscular rigidity has a lead pipe-like resistance to movement, the tendon reflexes are diminished, and the Babinski reflex and ankle clonus are absent.

Muscular rigidity may be due to widespread pyramidal and extrapyramidal involvements and may be associated with pain on manipulation. Either hysteria or a local lesion should be considered. If a passive movement is limited by firm fixation, the muscle is probably contracted permanently. Arthritic changes may limit passive motion and should be differentiated from pyramidal disease.

Hypotonicity is a decrease in muscular tone. Muscles have unusual extensibility and are abnormally flaccid. The paralyses found with hypotonia are of the flaccid variety. Here there is a loss of tendon reflexes, which is indicative either of a lower motor neuron disturbance, such as occurs in infantile paralysis, or a peripheral nerve lesion.

Atrophy. An examination to determine the normal muscle mass is very important in diagnosing nerve lesions. When muscles remain inactive for long periods of time atrophy results (Figs. 5.3 and 5.4). This may occur in severe, acquired pronatory foot conditions in which certain muscles have been inactive for years. When a joint is painful it may become fixed, resulting in inactivity and atrophy of the muscles moving the joint.

Atrophied muscles react to direct stimulation of percussion, but irritability is definitely decreased. When a motor nerve is cut or poisoned, the peripheral end degenerates in a few days and is not affected by electrical stimulation. This lack of response occurs because the striated muscles under the control of the nerve involved are removed from nervous control; with the nerves destroyed, the muscle can no longer be stimulated to perform a normal function.

Fibrillations may occur as flickering involuntary contractions of muscle fibers.

Excitability of muscles may be diminished or increased. In response to a tap on muscle substance with a percussion hammer, normal muscles present a local jerk in the fasciculi struck. Flickering may oc-

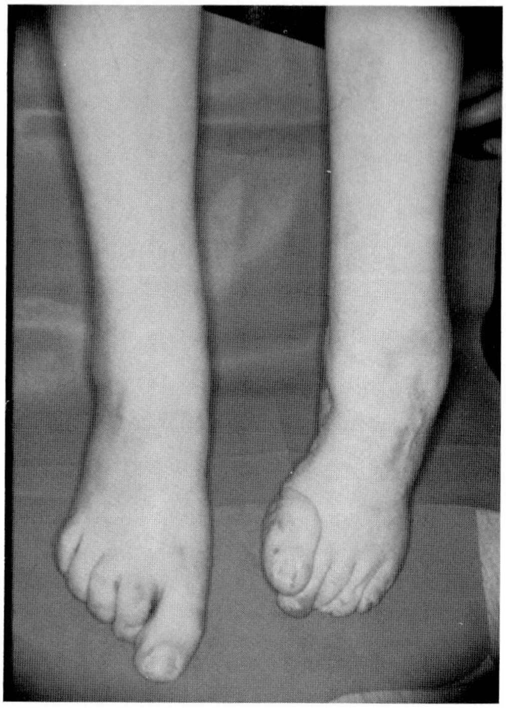

Figure 5.3. Talipes equinovarus and atrophy left limb. (Courtesy of M Shapiro.)

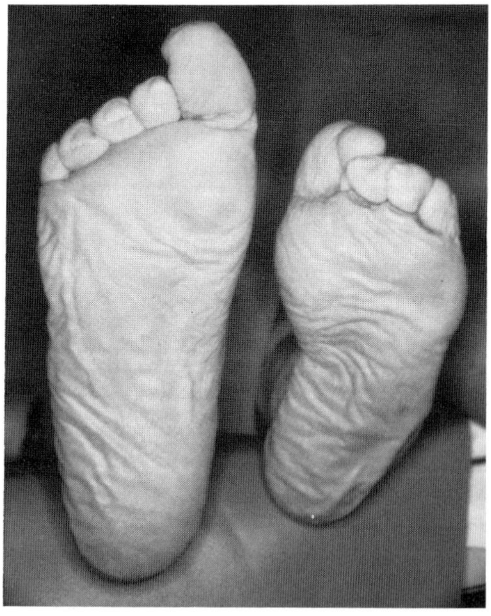

Figure 5.4. Note shortage of the left limb, atrophy, forefoot varus, flexion and adduction of toes, pes cavus and weightbearing pressure irritation at base of fifth metatarsal. (Courtesy of M Shapiro.)

cur for a few seconds in an emaciated person, but is of no value as a diagnostic sign. Atrophic muscles show slight evidence of contraction. A percussion myotonia is a sustained local contraction lasting a minute or longer in particular muscular dystrophies.

A muscle without the nerve supplying it still reacts to galvanic current, but with a slow type of contraction. This reaction is present in degeneration of the anterior horn of the cord or any lower motor neuron lesion.

Reflex Action

Reflexes give the examiner an objective group of symptoms with which to analyze the case. If the examiner is trained to understand the reflex arc and a few simple techniques, successful elicitation and interpretation of reflexes are ensured. The reflexes serve as sensitive indicators of the state of the nervous center and its pathways. The most important reflective stimulus for muscle consists of a stretching of muscle tissue upon receiving a sudden and brief concussion, resulting in a quick, longitudinal pull. This is a "muscle stretch reflex" (2) and is the so-called deep or tendon reflex. A slowly applied blow or stroke of the part is ineffective.

Reflex strength varies with the individual muscle or muscles and from one person to another. The reflex may become apparent only when there is functional or organic increase in muscle tone. Pyramidal lesions excite and increase reflexes. The presence of the "muscle stretch" must not be construed as pathological. A latent normal response may be exaggerated in the presence of pathology and may indicate pyramidal lesions.

Many methods are used to reinforce a reflex action. Among these are a cough, pulling apart clasped fingers, the patient squeezing the examiner's hand and diversion of the patient's attention to other interests in the office environment. A slight stretching of the muscle to be tapped reinforces the reflex response.

In regeneration of nerves the most distal parts are the last to regain function. Muscle tone returns first, atrophy of muscle diminishes, voluntary movements return, and, finally, the electrical reactions become normal. Unequal reflexes on the two sides between superficial and deep reflexes are more valuable in diagnosis than slight deviation from a hypothetical standard. Right and left reflexes may be evaluated using the following simple code: normal reflex = +, hyperactive reflex = + +, absent reflex = 0 and diminished reflex = dim.

Deep Muscle Reflexes. There are five deep muscle reflexes that the podiatrist should test.

Patellar Reflex. It is not possible to define a normal knee jerk as it may vary with individuals and at different times in the same individual. However, absence of the jerk or inequality of the jerk on two sides is suggestive of organic abnormality. The knee jerk may be exaggerated, diminished or lost. The presence of neurasthenia or such chronic diseases as arteriosclerosis may cause failure of pyramidal inhibition of the response to patellar tendon tapping, resulting in functional exaggeration of the reflex.

The knee jerk examination must be supplemented by examination of other reflexes. Exaggerated knee jerks that are equal on both sides and associated with a normal plantar response are not considered the result of organic loss of control of the reflex arc. However, if the plantar reflex is of the extensor type and the patellar response is exaggerated, organic changes in the motor area of the brain or in the pyramidal tracts are indicated.

When the pyramidal tract is affected equally on both sides, the patellar response in both legs is exaggerated. In hemiplegia, only the affected side is exaggerated because only one pyramidal tract is involved. The presence of a well-sustained patellar clonus indicates organic disease in the pyramidal tracts. Acute febrile and debilitating disease decreases activity of the knee jerk in children.

The knee jerk reflex is lost only in organic disease, such as involvement of the quadriceps extensor muscles or of the afferent pathway or the reflex arc. Diseases affecting the anterior horn cells, such as myelitis involving the third and fourth lumbar segments of the spinal cord, may result in loss of the knee jerk reflex. Peripheral neuritis affecting the efferent fibers may be noted when the knee jerk reflex is absent.

Complete transverse myelitis affecting the spinal cord in the dorsal region, frequently the result of severe fracture dislocation of the vertebral column, results very early in loss of the patellar reflex. However, a transverse myelitis at a level capable of deactivating the patellar reflex may not disturb the reflex arc of a deep muscle reflex below the level of damage in the cord.

When intracranial pressure is present, the knee jerk may vary with the ebb and flow of the intracranial pressure. The knee jerk may be lost in diabetes mellitus and associated peripheral neuritis.

Absence of the tendon reflex is seen in locomotor ataxia, in some spinal or cerebral diseases and in spinal cord tumors. In spinal cord tumors, absence of the tendon reflex is unilateral.

Achilles Reflex. The ball of the foot is pushed slightly against the examiner's hand while the Achilles tendon is tapped, eliciting a deep muscle reflex. The foot plantar flexes at the ankle during the "muscle stretch" with this reinforcement.

The best position for eliciting the ankle jerk is with the patient lying down, with the knee slightly flexed, the thigh rotated externally and the ankle slightly inverted. The plantar response can also be tested in this manner, but if the results are questionable the leg should be fully extended. Absence of deep tendon reflexes may be caused by myopathy, multiple sclerosis, pernicious anemia and Friedreich's ataxia.

In cases of pyramidal lesion, tapping of the patellar tendon may cause contraction in the plantar flexors of the foot and toes and sometimes of the hip extensors, in addition to contraction of the quadriceps muscle. Such a reaction to a single concussion is called a reflex of spinal automotism and is not a deep muscle reflex.

Plantar Muscle Reflex. The foot must be warm as in all other reflexes and the plantar muscles lightly stretched by exerting pressure in dorsiflexion. The stroke must be sharp and relaxed, brief and sudden with a dull, blunt or pointed object directed from the lateral plantar aspect of the heel upward to the plantar surfaces of the four lesser toes. Flexion and fanning of the lesser toes with extension of the great toe occur in pyramidal tract lesions.

The plantar muscle reflex is considered the most valuable of all physical responses in the nervous system. The normal response is a slow deliberate plantar flexion of the great toe. The stimulation is not painful except in pyramidal tract disease.

All dorsal foot reflexes act by the same mechanism as the plantar reflexes because of stretching of the plantar muscles by concussion. The plantar reflex can be produced by tapping the flexor muscles at many points of the sole.

Patellar Clonus. The leg is extended, and the patella is grasped between the thumb and the forefinger and briskly pushed down one or more times. A clonus is seen when there is a rhythmic jerking of the patella. When only a few jerks result, a clonus is said to be unsustained, and if the jerking continues as long as the patella is held it is said to be sustained. Sustained clonus is most marked in lateral cerebrospinal tract disease and disseminated sclerosis.

Ankle Clonus. The reflex center is located in the fifth lumbar and the first sacral segments of the cord. The leg is held in one hand, and the foot is grasped with the other and briskly dorsiflexed one or more times. A clonic repetition of the ankle jerk in the form of an exaggerated tremor results. Both the ankle and the patellar clonus possess the same significance.

In old spinal cord injuries, ankle clonus is present when the plantar response has again become flexor, and it appears later than other signs in progressive lesions of the cord. False ankle clonus sometimes occurs in nervous people, but in these cases the gait is not spastic.

Percussion of the tibialis anterior muscle induces dorsiflexion and supination of the foot. When the response is extremely pronounced, it indicates an organic disease of the CNS.

Leichtenstern (3) pointed out that in cerebrospinal meningitis tapping of the bones of an extremity revealed evidence of increased irritability.

Superficial Plantar Reflex. The Babinski reflex is a superficial reflex. It is negative if, when the outer sole of the foot is stroked upward and inward, there is normal plantar flexion of the toes. It is positive when this action causes fanning of all the lesser toes and dorsiflexion of the great toe.

The diagnostic significance of the Babinski reflex varies depending on age and whether temporary incapacitation or disease is present. A physiological Babinski can be elicited in infants up to 6 months and sometimes in children up to 2 to 4 years old. A temporary Babinski reflex may be found during normal sleep; during morphine, chloroform or scopolamine narcosis; or in epileptic seizures.

A pathological Babinski reflex may be the result of a pyramidal tract lesion at any part of the pyramidal tract or corticospinal pathway. A positive Babinski sign may be seen in any lesion of the pyramidal tracts either in the brain or spinal cord.

Additional Tests of Interest to the Podiatrist

Chaddok Reflex. The lateral aspect of the foot below the lateral malleolus is stroked. The pathological response is the same as for the Babinski reflex, with dorsiflexion of the hallux and fanning of the lesser toes.

Oppenheim Reflex. The anteromedial surface of the tibia is stroked. Pathological response and interpretation are the same as for the Babinski and Chaddok reflexes.

Gordon Reflex. The calf muscle is firmly squeezed. Pathological response and interpretation are the same as for the Babinski, Chaddok and Oppenheim reflex tests.

Lasèque's Sign. This is significant in diseases of the sciatic nerve. The thigh is flexed on the abdomen and the leg extended at the knee. This maneuver causes stretching of the nerve root. When there is disease of the nerve, pain and resistance on the part of the patient result.

Patrick's Test. This test indicates hip joint disease. When the patient is supine, the thigh and knee are flexed, and the external malleolus is placed on the patella of the opposite leg. On depressing the knee, pain is noted if arthritis of the hip is present.

Pupillary Reflexes. Normally a light thrown upon the retina of the eye causes the pupil of the eye being tested to contract. When the eye is shaded the pupil dilates. When looking at near objects the pupil accommodates by contracting and at a distance the pupil dilates. Abnormal pupillary reactions may be caused by luetic meningitis, tabes dorsalis, aortic or carotid aneurysm, trigeminal neuralgia, an intracranial mass, glaucoma or topical mydriatics.

Argyll-Robertson Reflex. The pupillary reflex does not react to light, but reacts to accommodation. The Argyll-Robertson reflex may be found in syphilitic patients manifesting local symptoms in the foot.

Hirschberg's Reflex. This reflex is seen in pyramidal tract disease and organic hemiplegia and is elicited by tickling the sole of the foot at the base of the great toe. It is characterized by adduction of the foot.

Many times a mild, permanent hyperextension of the great toe is noted on the affected side of a unilateral pyramidal tract disturbance. This sign may be seen before the Babinski reflex.

Tinel's Sign. Upon percussion of a nerve at the site of compression or entrapment, distal paresthesias are elicited.

Valleix Phenomenon. Sensory nerve trunk tenderness is elicited proximal and distal to the site of compression or entrapment upon percussion of the affected nerve.

Upper Motor Neuron, Lower Motor Neuron and Myopathic Disorders

There are basically two types of motor paralysis, one caused by an upper motor neuron lesion and the other caused by a lower motor neuron lesion. The upper motor neuron lesion causes a characteristic spastic paralysis, whereas the lower motor neuron lesion causes a flaccid paralysis. An evaluation of the reflexes, signs and symptoms of disease and characteristic syndromes helps differentiate neurological disorders from other diseases of the extremities.

The exact location of a lesion in the brain or spinal cord is left to the neurologist for interpretation. It will suffice for the doctor to know whether the lesion is peripheral, of lower motor neuron origin or of a cerebral spinal origin.

Peripheral paralysis may be due to nerve trauma or pressure, poliomyelitis nutritional disorders or poisoning.

Cerebral upper motor neuron lesions are caused by injuries to the motor pathways, abnormal pressures on cerebral centers by hemorrhage, tumors or emboli.

Cerebral spinal fluid (CSF) protein values are elevated in diabetes, amyloid neuropathy, Refsum's disease, and in the presence of malignancy. There is an elevation in the CSF white cell count in Guillain-Barré syndrome.

Electrodiagnostic studies confirm motor and/or sensory denervation and predict nerve regeneration (Table 5.1). Nerve conduction velocity studies are utilized diagnostically when interpreting nerve entrapment syndromes, such as, tarsal tunnel syndrome, sural nerve entrapment syndrome and medial terminal branch of the deep peroneal nerve entrapment syndrome; peripheral neuropathies, such as diabetic neuropathy (Fig. 5.5) and alcoholic neuropathy; myopathy; and anterior horn cell disease. Specific findings are noted in Guillain-Barré syndrome, genetic neuropathies, toxic and nutritional neuropathies.

Upper motor neuron, lower motor neuron (anterior horn cell, nerve), and myopathic weakness must be differentiated. In upper motor neuron disease, weakness is diffuse, there is no atrophy, muscle tone and deep tendon reflexes are increased, the plantar reflex is elicited as positive and sensory deficit is one-sided. In lower

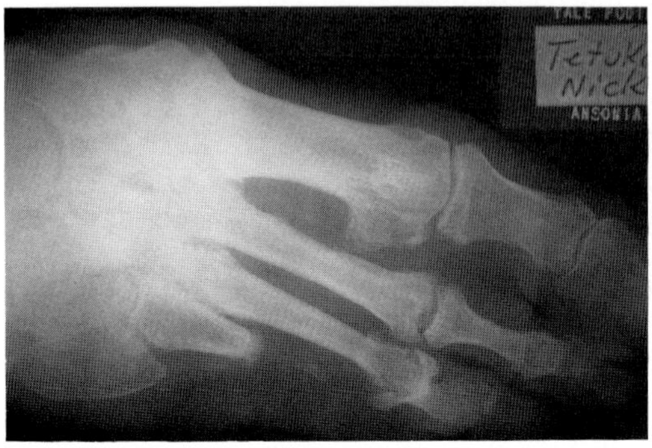

Figure 5.5. Diabetic neuropathic foot.

motor neuron disease, weakness is diffuse—(anterior horn cell) to distal (nerve)—muscle is atrophied, muscle tone is diminished, deep tendon and plantar reflexes are diminished and there is no sensory loss—(anterior horn cell) to severe sensory loss (nerve). In myopathic weakness the weakness is proximal, muscle is atrophied, muscle tone is diminished, deep tendon reflexes are normal, plantar reflex is diminished and there is no sensory loss.

Table 5.1.
Tibial Nerve: Normal Values[a]

Motor fiber conduction velocity: over 40 msec
Sensory fiber conduction velocity: over 72 ± 4 msec
Terminal latency: less than 6.7 msec
F wave (ankle to spinal cord): over 51 ± 3 msec

[a] From Levin ME, O'Neal LW (eds): *The Diabetic Foot.* St. Louis, C. V. Mosby Co, 1983.

Myopathies

Muscular dystrophy: Duchenne, fascioscapulohumeral (FSH), limb-girdle, myotonic: genetic, etiology unknown, childhood onset, progressive, contractures, equinovarus foot deformity.

Congenital: nemaline, myotubular, fingerprint body, central core disease: rare, histochemical diagnosis, cavovarus foot deformity in nemalinemyopathy.

Acquired: thyroid disease, Cushing's syndrome, hyperparathyroidism, acromegaly, diabetes, systemic lupus erythematosus, rheumatoid arthritis, periarteritis nodosa, infectious, alcoholic, carcinomatosis.

Polymyositis: muscle inflammatory disease of unknown etiology, associated with collagen vascular disease, adult onset, increased erythrocyte sedimentation rate, muscular tenderness, carcinoma associated, steroid responsive.

Myasthenia gravis: predilection for ocular and cranial muscles, episodic, myoneural junction dysfunction; diagnosis through history, examination, tensilon-chemical test, Jolly electrical test.

Poliomyelitis

The onset of the general disease is usually in childhood, but it may affect adults. There is a marked atrophy of muscles, and symptoms of a lower motor neuron lesion rapidly develop. Sometimes the muscle or group of muscles affected is flaccid for only a few months and then returns to normal. When the attack is in childhood, there is usually a shortness in the limb due to a lagging of bony growth caused by faulty nutrition. A foot drop generally develops, resulting in faulty weight distribution. Tylomas may develop under the first or fifth metatarsal heads, and helomas are common on the dorsum of the toes and along the lateral border of the fifth toe nail. Toes are dorsiflexed and extensor tendons contracted (Fig. 5.6).

Polyneuritis

Synonyms: acute febrile neuritis, alcoholic neuritis, diphtheritic neuritis, diabetic neuritis, infective neuritis, plumbic or lead neuritis and arsenical neuritis.

This disease demonstrates a bilateral foot drop due to a weakness of the dorsiflexors. In walking the toes catch on the ground, giving the characteristic steppage gait. A wrist drop may also be present. Symmetrical pains in the extremities, numbness and tingling are also characteristic. The degree of weakness of the muscle is out of proportion to the minimal atrophy.

Polyneuritis may be secondary to vitamin B_1, pyridoxine, nicotinamide, pantothenic acid or vitamin B_{12} deficiency (4). Localized etiology for a plantar burning sensation includes trauma, tylomas, burns, neuroma, contact dermatitis, herpes zoster, dermatomycosis, erysipelas, sciatica, arterial or venous insufficiency, phlebitis, causalgia, and Sudeck's atrophy.

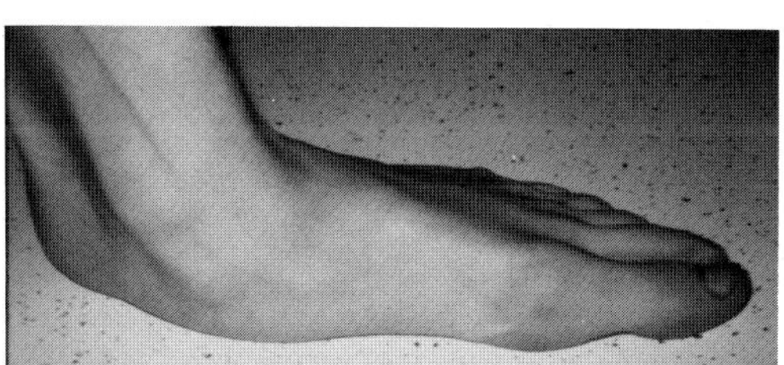

Figure 5.6. Severe calcaneal valgus scondary to poliomyelitis with atrophy and pes planovalgus. Head of talus palpable medially. Limp.

Diabetic polyneuritis affects the distal leg and foot. There is sensory loss and often motor weakness. (See Chapter 6 for a more detailed discussion of pedal manifestations and treatment of diabetes.) Mild adult onset diabetic patients sometimes suffer a mononeuritis involving the femoral or tibial nerve. Control of the diabetic process is essential to the treatment of diabetic polyneuritis and mononeuritis. The prognosis is not favorable for diabetic polyneuritis, whereas diabetic mononeuritis often disappears in several months.

Idiopathic polyneuritis may occur subsequent to viral or bacterial infection. There may be motor weakness, numbness and tingling paresthesias in the fingers and/or toes. Sensory symptoms are minimal. Deep tendon reflexes are often lost. The neurological deficit progresses for 2–3 weeks and then slowly resolves over the next several weeks. The clinician must be alert to concurrent respiratory depression.

Other causes of peripheral neuropathy with subsequent burning sensation in the feet include Raynaud's phenomenon or disease, cold injury, chronic venous insufficiency, acrocyanosis, heat injury, erythromelalgia, pheochromocytoma, Déjérine-Sottas disease, hypothyroidism, hemophilia, hyperthyroidism, polycythemia vera, pernicious anemia, alcoholism, collagen disorder, sarcoidosis, temporal arteritis and psychogenic factors (5).

Genetic disorders may result in hypertrophic neuropathies, such as peroneal muscular atrophy, Charcot-Marie-Tooth, interstitial neuritis and Refsum's disease; acute porphric polyneuritis; and amyloid neuropathy.

Peripheral neuritis may be a sequela to chemical or heavy metal poisoning (arsenic, lead, mercury, benzene, CO_2, etc), medication use (isoniazid, Apresoline, nitrofuran, Antabuse and the chemotherapeutic agents used in malignancy treatment), and toxin ingestion (solvents, fumigants, acrylamide and carbon disulfide). Renal impairment may result in a peripheral uremic neuropathy, and carcinoma in situ may result in a carcinomatous neuropathy.

Common Peroneal Nerve Injuries

Trauma involving the head of the fibula may lead to the development of talipes equinovarus with a flexor contraction of the toes. A history of an operation in that area with prolonged use of bandages or splints is common. Anesthesia of the outer side and dorsum of the foot is present. Sensory perception is diminished, and a numb, dead feeling is noted. When present for a long time, abnormal pressure of weightbearing results in development of a tyloma under the fifth metatarsal head. A digiti quinti varus is common, and digiti flexus of the lesser toes is usual.

Paralysis often occurs in elderly individuals who habitually cross one leg over the opposite knee. Wedged between the ipsilateral fibula and the external condyle of the heterolateral femur and heterolateral patella, the common peroneal nerve is traumatized by repeated pressure.

Patients convalescing from a severe illness, hyperthyroidism and mental depression are particularly susceptible to this lesion. Minor operations on the foot and postinjection therapy for varicosities have been reported as etiologic.

Complete Transverse Myelitis

Bilateral foot drop occurs in complete transverse myelitis. There is a loss of deep reflexes and very often a history of syphilis or trauma to vertebrae. This disorder also presents an anesthesia or impairment of sensation at definite levels below the paralysis. The extensor muscles are affected, resulting in a flaccid paralysis and bilateral drop foot.

Peroneal Muscle Atrophy

Onset of drop foot caused by peroneal muscle atrophy occurs before the age of 25. The condition tends to be familial and pursues a slow progressive course with an atrophy of the small muscles of the feet. Similar atrophy occurs in the hands. Peroneal muscular atrophy may result from trauma, alienation of the muscle in polio, disuse, alcoholism, neuritis and acute febrile disease.

Peroneal Spastic Flatfoot

Johnson (6), in an interesting review of peroneal spastic flatfoot syndrome, concludes that "tarsal coalitions are not the sole cause of peroneal spastic flatfoot, and any irritative lesion in the peritalar area can induce protective contraction of any or all of the muscles bridging the peritalar joints. True muscular peroneal spasm has been shown to be present on a clinical basis in this entity. Where tarsal coalitions are not present, neoplasm should be included in the differential diagnosis of the rigid flatfoot deformity."

Charcot-Marie-Tooth Disease

This condition, also known as progressive peroneal muscular atrophy, is a posterior column disease characterized by fatigue, insidious clubfoot or peroneal drop foot with stork-like lower legs, atrophy of the peroneals, tibials or muscles of the hands, impairment of position sense and vibratory sensation (Fig. 5.7). Deep tendon reflexes are diminished or gone. The disease is slow and progressive.

Treatment. Treatment instituted must depend on whether experience indicates that corrective forces can be exerted with some reasonable assurance of positive results. In a flaccid paralysis such as may develop with a polio or peripheral nerve injury, it is essential to try to coordinate the mind and body in bringing about active motion in the affected part during the early stages. At all

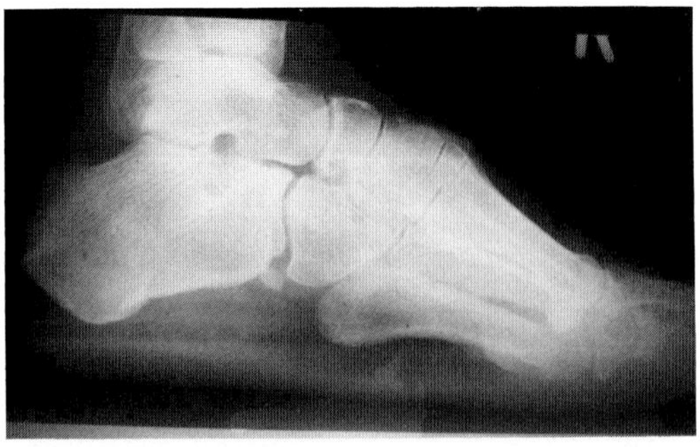

Figure 5.7. Cavovarus foot type associated with Charcot-Marie-Tooth disease.

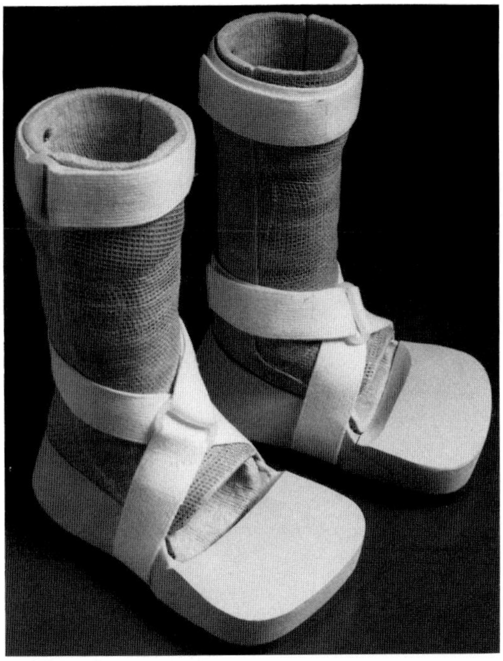

Figure 5.8. Tone Reducing Ankle-Foot Orthosis (TRAFO)®. Helps reduce spasticity and improve limb stability in victims of stroke or cerebral palsy.

times a firm shoe should be fitted to the affected part. It is essential that a knee-length brace be utilized on the affected extremity either by a double bar or a posterior bar inserted into the shoe to maintain the foot in a functional position without dropping. In a peripheral neuritis, proper medical treatment should be instituted to offset the damaging effect of pathology on the peripheral nerve. This treatment must be aided by the utilization of a foot drop orthosis in gait. While at rest, maintenance of the foot at right angles to the leg is essential. An early attempt should be made to maintain the length of the Achilles tendon. If this tendon is allowed to shorten, it may be lengthened by surgical intervention.

Patients with ataxic gait must be referred to the neurologist who can establish the etiology and provide systemic care. Podiatrists can maintain the foot at right angles to the leg by utilizing knee-length braces (Fig. 5.8). In gaits of various types, the prime approach to the treatment is an attempt to maintain the foot at right angles to the leg and to add sufficient support through use of proper orthoses to maintain confidence and improve gait.

Cooperative treatment by the internist, neurologist, orthopaedic surgeon, psychiatrist, physiatrist and podiatrist usually relieves pain and restores some function.

Gait

According to Durcoquet et al. (7), when discussing the work of their father, Charles Durcoquet, equilibrium on two feet in the standing position is best served when the heels are separated about 12 cm, creating a quadrilateral above which the center of gravity can be shifted. Equilibrium becomes altered during the gait cycle when standing on one foot, taking the step in the swing phase, heel strike and with toe off. When bearing weight on one foot, the maintenance of equilibrium is assisted by the arms, which extend away from the body. Painful feet and certain deformities result in shortened periods of single-foot support during gait. The affected part increases the duration of the stance phase held by the opposing pain-free limb, causing a limp.

Forward and backward movements above the equilibrium of the limbs through the line of gravity extending from the thoracic region in the saggital plane downward occur as a measure of compensatory motion secondary to functional disabilities. Lateral oscillations result in transfer of weight from one foot to the other, which results in reactive functions of the muscles around the subtalar joint, the pelvis and the vertebral column (tibialis posterior, peronei, gluteus medius and minimus, adductors at the hip and abdominal muscles).

The nerve centers initiate gait and maintain equilibrium by balancing opposing forces. The backward limb thrusts the body into disequilibrium. The forward limb serves as a brake to compensate for the loss of static equilibrium beyond the base of support. The proprioceptive mechanism attempts to maintain the body in the upright posture.

Examination of the functional capacity of a part or of the total body is essential before embarking on a treatment regime. The patient should be examined in stance from the front, back and in profile, both left and right. Also, examination of the subject on one foot may uncover instabilities. The total posture is considered relative to the influence of age, weight, height, limb lengths, joint deformities, atrophy, hypertrophy, paralysis, etc. The length, width and angle of gait are documented.

According to the Gait Analysis Laboratory (9), the average percentage of the walk cycle events are as follows: heel strike 0 to 7%, flatfoot 7 to 12%, opposite toe off to heel off 12 to 34%, until opposite heel strike at 50 to 62% with toe off, followed by heel strike once again at 100% of the cycle. From heel strike to toe off is known as the stance phase, and from toe off to heel strike, the swing phase.

In patients with a normal gait, the weight of the body is supported by one foot while the other is advanced. The heel of the weightbearing foot touches the ground first; the toes touch last as the heel raises. Repeated alternations of this pattern result in a smooth and rhythmic locomotive process.

Variations in gait may have a hereditary basis involving skeletal, muscular or nervous system peculiarities, or they may simply be acquired through imitation of a parent. Abnormal gaits are the result of wearing improper footgear, trauma, arthritis, motor neuron lesions, congenital or hereditary disorders, muscular dystrophies, atrophy and faulty adipose distribution (Fig. 5.9).

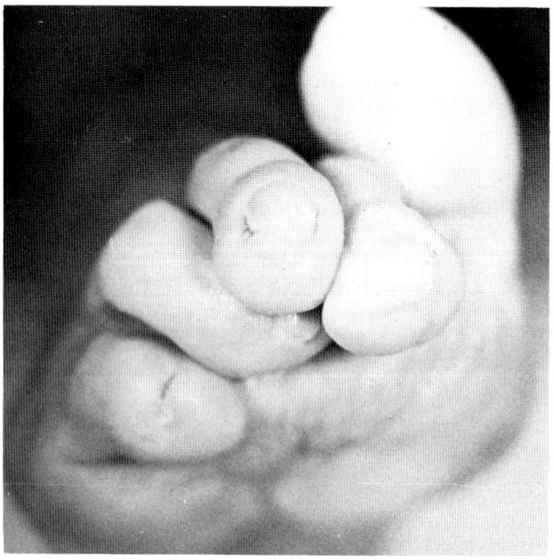

Figure 5.9. Underlapping, overlapping toes secondary to contractures caused by upper motor neuron lesion.

Dyskinesias are movement disorders. **Hyperkinesia** is an acceleration of movement whereas **bradykinesia** is a reduction of movement. Several types of dyskinesias are listed below.

1. Chorea: variable, sudden, quick, jerky movements, e.g., Huntington's chorea
2. Asterixis: flopping hand movement when wrist is extended, e.g., liver cirrhosis
3. Athetosis: slow, writhing movements, e.g., cerebral palsy
4. Dystonia: fixed postural distortions
5. Tic: brief, recurrent, compulsive spasms, e.g., psychogenic
6. Hemiballismus: rare violent jerking movement of one-half of the body
7. Myoclonus: brief isolated muscle jerks, e.g., during nerve regeneration, post-CVA, fatigue, normal movement
8. Fasciculation: fine twitching movement
9. Tremor: slow, rapid or moderate trembling
   - Resting: parkinsonism, "pill rolling", basal ganglia
   - Intentional: occurs at termination of movement, cerebellar disease
   - Statokinetic: occurs from anxiety, hyperthyroidism, alcohol toxicity

Cavus feet and subsequent hallux hammertoe development are associated with muscular dystrophy, peripheral nerve lesions, anterior horn cell lesions and spinocerebellar lesions (see Chapter 9, Biomechanical Disorders).

A slow exaggerated gait with staggering toward support may be evidence of loss of confidence in the patient's legs. A long-term illness, cerebral pathology or peripheral neuropathy may cause this gait.

A spraddle-legged gait in children is actually compensatory to give the child a broader base for balance in the early days of progression. Infants learning to walk usually spread their legs apart, lift their elbows up in wing-like fashion and adopt a spraddle-legged gait.

The **hemiplegic** patient has a short phase of support on the paralyzed side with a slow, spastic propulsion, resulting in a long progression on the same side. The patient holds the leg stiff, and the progressive phase of walking is in circumduction; the arms also move more than normally. Sometimes the affected limb is dragged because of the secondary muscular involvement in the paretic, the knee is stiffer and the foot scrapes the ground.

In **tabes dorsalis** the progressive phase is long because of the time element required in observation by the patients of how high they are raising their feet and how hard they place them down. Tabetic patients must watch their step to see where they are going due to loss of proprioception.

In **steppage gait** the toes strike the ground first, followed by a slapping down of the heel. This type of gait is very common and is usually the result of a flaccid paralysis. Infantile paralysis, peripheral neuritis, Charcot-Marie-Tooth disease, trauma to the external popliteal and muscular dystrophy may result in a foot drop; an alcoholic neuritis predisposes to drop foot. The Achilles tendon may be shortened; the patient is unable to stand on his or her heels. Flexion of the leg on the thigh is increased while the foot is raised high when walking.

An **ataxic gait** is a jerky, unsteady support and progression in which the patient may reel and lose his or her balance. A test for ataxia is to have the patient walk sideways with eyes closed and then, with open eyes, walk forward, backward and sideways. The ataxia will manifest itself at all times. If it disappears with the eyes closed, the ataxia may be hysterical in etiology.

Spastic gait is a slow, stiff-legged gait with legs extended and feet shuffling. It is due to an upper motor neuron lesion and it may be noted in hemiplegics.

Scissors gait is characterized by crossed leg progression with spastic shuffling; the hips and knees are flexed, and the legs have a tendency to cross in gait. This gait is seen in patients suffering chronic muscular disease or cerebral palsy.

Waskin et al. (8), in a review of the podiatric concerns in the cerebral palsy patient, note that the most frequently seen foot deformities are equinus, equinovalgus, and equinovarus (Fig. 5.10). The purpose of treatment is to stabilize the lower extremity and allow the patient to ambulate as independently as possible. Although the basic approach to treatment is conservative, both osseous and soft tissue surgical procedures may be indicated to increase the efficiency of ambulation.

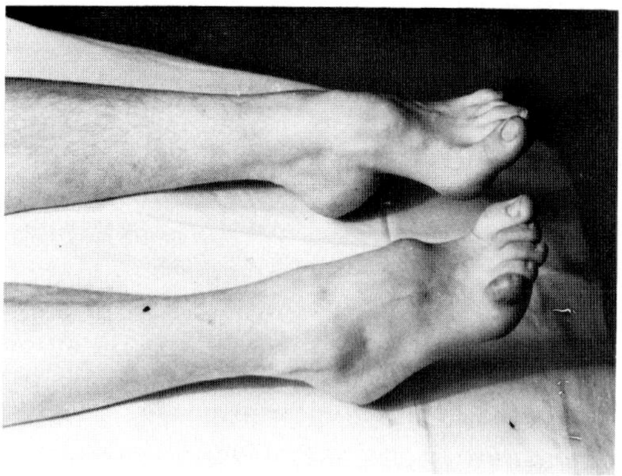

Figure 5.10. Talipes equinovarus.

Short steps may be seen in cerebral arteriosclerosis. The patient appears to hesitate with each step before shifting to the opposite foot.

Waddling gaits give the impression of being very top heavy, with a resultant sway above the hips. This gait occurs in patients with muscular dystrophy, spinal muscular atrophy or bilateral dislocation of the hips and in the very tall and obese patient.

Festinating gait is seen in parkinsonism. It is characterized by a falling forward of the body resulting in the center of gravity being forward of the midline. In an effort to maintain balance the patient progresses faster and faster, resulting in either a fall or bump into an object. This represents basal ganglia disease.

Apraxic gait is seen in cerebral hemisphere disease. It is a gait of small steps associated with impairment of walking ability in the face of intact motor, sensory and coordination testing.

Hysterical gait may be suspected when the gait is marked by hesitating foot movements followed by sudden shuffling and grotesque balancing movements. It is a bizarre, atypical gait.

In the absence of rigidity and spasticity, lack of swinging of an arm while walking—**cerebellar gait**—may be seen in cerebellar disease of the same side. The patient with a disorder of the cerebellum may present with an unsteady gait, loss of balance with the eyes closed, an unsteady route when bringing the finger to the nose and a positive Romberg sign. Spinocerebellar disease includes Friedreich's ataxia and Roussy-Levy syndrome. Cavovarus foot deformity and hallux hammer toe are associated.

Antalgic gait or painful gait is seen with hyperesthetic painful foot conditions. It is a short-stepped, halting, limping gait. The feet compensate during gait in order to avoid weightbearing on the soles. Antalgic gait is seen following trauma, in biomechanically induced pain syndromes, alcoholic peripheral neuropathy, polyneuropathy and Sudeck's atrophy.

References

1. Vazuka A: Essentials of the Neurological Examination. Philadelphia, Smith, Kline, and French Laboratories, 1968.
2. Wartenberg R: *The Examination of Reflexes*, Chicago, Year Book Publishers, 1945.
3. Leichtenstern: *Diagnostic Signs of Reflexes and Syndromes* (standardized by HF Robertson), ed 3. Philadelphia, F A Davis Co, 1947.
4. D'Orazio L, D'Orazio P: Nutritional polyneuropathy and its manifestations in the lower extremity. *J Am Podiatric Med Assoc* 75:28–30, 1985.
5. Pack LG: Burning feet: A partial guide to diagnosis. *Arch Podiatric Med Foot Surg* 2:78–79, 1974.
6. Johnson JC: Peroneal spastic flatfoot syndrome. *South Med J* 69:807–809, 1976.
7. Durcoquet R, Durcoquet J, Durcoquet P: *Walking and Limping*. Philadelphia, Lippincott, 1968.
8. Waskin MR, Frost JP, Hatalowich GS: Cerebral palsy: A podiatric overview. *J Foot Surg* 22:362–365, 1983.
9. Mann R, Inman VT: Phasic activity of intrinsic muscles of the foot. *J Bone Joint Surg* 46A:469–481, 1964.

Suggested Readings

Brachman PR: *Podiatric Orthopedics—Principles and Practices*. Park Ridge IL, Podiatry Book Co, 1984.

Chasen JL: *Nervous System and Skeletal muscle*. In Anderson WAD (ed): *Pathology*, ed 6. St. Louis, C V Mosby Co 1971.

Degomin, Degomin: *Bedside Diagnostic Examination*. New York, MacMillan, 1976.

DeJong RM: *The Neurologic Examination*, ed. 2. New York, 1958.

Denny-Brown D: *Handbook of Neurological Examination and Case Recording*. Cambridge, MA., Harvard University Press, 1957.

Kozak GP, et al.: *Management of Diabetic Foot Problems*. Philadelphia, W B Saunders. Co, 1984.

Levin ME, O'Neal LW: *The Diabetic Foot*, ed 3. St. Louis, C V Mosby Co, 1983.

McNamara G, Shor RI: Diabetic neuropathic osteoarthropathy. *J Am Podiatry Assoc* 73:485–489, 1983.

Mooney V, Wagner FW, Jr: Neurocirculatory disorders of the foot. *Clin Orthop* 122:53–61, 1977.

Reeves A: *Disorders of the Nervous System*. Chicago, Yearbook Medical Publishers 1981.

Simpson J, Magee K: *Clinical Evaluation of the Nervous System*. Boston, Little, Brown and Co, 1973.

Steinberg MD, Pack LG: Burning feet—A partial guide to diagnosis. Symposium on Neurological Diseases as They Relate to the Foot. San Francisco, March, 1974.

Tax H: *Podopediatrics*. Baltimore, Williams & Wilkins, 1980.

Tuccio AT, Wertheimer SJ: Noninfectious osseous alterations in the diabetic foot. *J Foot Surg* 24:154–157, 1985.

White H: Some aspects of the neural integration involved in gait and posture. *J Am Podiatry Assoc* 57:157–163, 1967.

Wolf J: *Segmented Neurology*. Baltimore, University Park Press, 1981.

6

Dermatologic and Toenail Disorders

Many years of podiatric practice have shown the importance of alterations in color, texture and physiology of the skin in evaluating foot health. When the foot is examined with the patient in a recumbent position, the general color and texture of the skin are observed. The significance of marked specific color changes and texture of the skin is described in earlier chapters. These changes, especially those of rubor, cyanosis and pallor, in addition to the presence or absence of hair and the evaluation of texture and deformity of the foot and toenails, are vital clues to a patient's foot pathology.

Skin Structure and Composition

The skin is made up of the epidermis and dermis. The outermost layer of the skin is the stratum corneum, developed from a cornification process of the viable epidermal cells. The deeper layer of the stratum corneum is highly specialized and is capable of serving as a barrier to absorption of substances through the skin. This layer is called the **barrier area**.

The granular layer beneath the stratum corneum is a cellular layer containing basophilic granules. Below the granular layer is the cellular epidermis consisting of the stratum Malpighian and the palisading layer stratum germinativum.

The dermoepidermal juncture is where the epidermal cells meet the connective tissue beneath. The dermis (corium) is that section of the skin lying between the subcutaneous fat and the epidermis. This layer of the skin contains blood vessels, nerves and such specialized epithelial tissues as sweat glands and ducts and hair follicles and their sebaceous glands.

The surface film on the epidermis is the product of the metabolic functions of the skin; it interferes with absorption of noxious agents, serves as an antiseptic, lubricates the corneous layer while it maintains adequate moisture and buffers acid and alkali.

Stoughton (1) notes that the chemical content of the surface film differs on different parts of the body. Some of the contents of the surface film have been analyzed as being derived from the following: sweat glands, lactic acid, amino acids, urea, uric acid, ammonia, sebaceous glands (not found on the soles of feet), triglycerides, free fatty acids and wax alcohols, cornification processes, sterols, pentoses, phospholipids and complex polypeptides.

Sano et al (2) in a study of pathological keratinization, evaluated glycogen, pentose, hexosamine and β-glucuronidase in normal and pathological keratinization. In noninflammatory keratoses these substances were present in normal amounts, but in the scales of psoriasis, erythrodermia and eczemas, abnormally high amounts were present. Sano et al. concluded that abnormal products of metabolism may be excreted from the epidermis as a scale.

Keratin is a fibrous protein in the horny layer of the skin and is probably derived from cytoplasmic filaments in the granular layer. Although fungus infections commonly occur on the soles of the feet, free fatty acids—which are highly fungistatic—are not normally found on the soles.

The horny layer of skin on the soles of the feet is thickest where external trauma is greatest. The stratum corneum increases in thickness with trauma. The outer layers peel off as new cells are formed continuously to maintain the thickness. It is not clearly understood what binds these loose, non-nucleated cells together. This binding process may very well contribute to the development of helomas and tylomas.

The nerve supply of the skin serves both sensory and motor functions. The sensory nerves provide for perception of touch, temperature and pain. The involuntary sympathetic motor nerves control the sweat glands, arterioles and smooth muscle of the skin.

McCarthy and Habowsky (3) evaluated the dermoepidermal interface in human skin from the feet of male and female specimens aged 44 to 80 years. Skin samples from 10 regions of the foot that perform different functions were reviewed. Light microscope measurements and dermoepidermal interface studies add to the current knowledge about the skin of the foot.

The investigators hypothesize that "the function which skin serves, in part, directs or determines its structural characteristics." The data compiled suggest that "epidermal thickness and length of the rete Malpighii are directly proportioned to the work load placed upon the particular skin part." The epidermis of the heel was the thickest of all sites studied. Here the stratum corneum makes up 90% of the skin's total thickness. Of special interest was the average length of the Malpighian rete, "0.23 mm, the greatest of all sites studied." The epidermis on the plantar surface of the first metatarsal heads is "about two-thirds the thickness of the heel." In other areas of the foot the average length of the rete ridges as evaluated by McCarthy and Habowsky are as follows: "measured on the plantar toe fold, 0.10 mm; midplantar arch, 0.09 mm; Achilles tendon, 0.07 mm; dorsum of the toe, 0.06 mm; inferior to the malleolus, 0.05 mm; dorsum of arch, 0.04 mm; midanterior ankle, 0.04 mm; and malleolar prominence, 0.03 mm. The researchers dramatically illustrate the dermoepidermal interface in each area examined.

Skin Cultures

Interpretation of clinical findings obtained through the use of skin tests and sophisticated diagnostic equipment is essential to early diagnosis and treatment. The lesions seen on the extremities can be magnified by a high-power magnifying lens or by smears, sections and cultures of lesions examined grossly and under the microscope. The presence of a specific type of bacteria can be ascertained by careful macro- and microscopic examinations of cultures and smears.

One of the common uses of the microscope in podiatry is to examine in a few minutes a scale, skin scraping, or fluid from a suspicious vesicle, in looking for the presence of mycelia in mycotic skin disorders. In this examination the skin is first cleansed with 70% alcohol. The infected material is obtained from the spreading margins of the skin lesion or from the roofs of vesicles and placed on a clean slide. Potassium hydroxide in a 10% strength is applied by dropper to dissolve the specimen. The use of ink in combination with potassium hydroxide may allow for better visualization of the mounted specimen. After several minutes, microscopic examination reveals hyphae as networks of threads and filaments in chains and interspersed spores or clumps of spores if the smear is positive. One must be trained in differentiating mycelial threads from cotton fibers, wool fibers, hair or feathers. Mycelial threads are usually thin, light green and refractile.

In *Epidermophyton* invasions, the mycelia may be numerous. In *Trichophyton rubrum* infections there are few threads. In *Candida (Monilia) albicans* infections, one may see budding cells in the specimen.

Test tube cultures are made by implanting the tissue or scraping into a medium previously selected for growth of the suspected organism. The medium must be free of impurities and incubated at 37°C. for 2 days before using to rule out contamination. Beef extract broth is a frequently used liquid medium. Beef extract, agar and gelatin are used in the solid medium. Sabouraud's slants and Dermatophyte Testing Media (DTM) are widely used in raising colonies of fungi. Conrad (4), in a series of experiments to produce a more luxuriant growth, found that potato broth and carrot broth in combination with vitamin B complex gave best results.

Growth Reactions in Culture Media

The following changes are seen and may be interpreted in the colony growth of fungi.

Trichophyton gypseum. On culture media, the surface of the colony is white to cream colored and may have a powdery or fluffy surface. The substrate pigment changes from red to brown in old colonies. In new colonies there is very little pigment.

Trichophyton rubrum. On culture media, the fluffy surface of the colony may be white to rose or purple. The substrate pigment is red or purple.

Epidermophyton floccosum. On culture, the colony is green to buff colored. The surface is velvety or felt-like. There are usually many irregular folds in the surface; at times there are small, white fluffy areas present on the colony.

Candida (Monilia) albicans. On culture media the colony appears as a cream-colored, moist, yeast-like growth.

Methods for diagnosis of fungus disease include direct examination, where pus, exudate, scrapings, scales and hair may be examined microscopically after careful but simple preparation of a slide.

The magnifying glass is an aid in differentiating gross lesions that are small in size and difficult to see with the naked eye. Very often petechial hemorrhages, uncommonly shaped skin lesions and other characteristic skin changes may be noted on examination by magnification under good light, preferably daylight.

The culture method discussed above shows characteristic colonies and thereby identifies the species.

Filtered ultraviolet radiation creates a fluorescence of the fungi in the infected tissues. Wood's black light is used for this purpose. Normal skin appears as a weak blue color under Wood's light. The presence of fungus shows up as a greenish yellow, and in erythrasma a pink fluorescence is noted.

Tests for Hypersensitivity

Patch Test

The patch test is used primarily to demonstrate the etiologic basis for contact dermatitis or allergies. A **primary cutaneous irritant** is an agent that causes dermatitis by direct action on the normal skin at the site of contact, if it is permitted to act in sufficient intensity or quantity for a sufficient length of time. A **cutaneous sensitizer** is an agent that does not necessarily cause demonstrable cutaneous changes on first contact, but may effect such specific changes in the skin after 5 to 7 days or more; further contact on the skin of other parts of the body will cause dermatitis.

A small portion of the suspected sensitizer material is applied to normal skin, covered with impermeable material, such as plastic wrap, and sealed to the skin by nonallergenic tape. The test varies in accordance with the materials being tested. When a liquid sensitizer is being used for the test, a piece of ¼-inch square gauze is saturated with the solution and covered by cellophane. One must make sure that the adhesive binding on the patch is not setting up a reaction that may interfere with the real test.

Powders are placed on a small gauze patch that has previously been dampened to hold the powder better. Solids are dissolved in a suitable solvent, and the remaining saturated solution is used for the patch. Ointments are tested in the same manner as liquids. In all tests the examiner must determine the extent of the sensitivity, and a careful evaluation is made of the skin changes that result.

The reaction to the patch tests is graded as 1+, erythema under the patch; 2+, erythema and edema; 3+, erythema, edema, papules and a few vesicles; 4+, erythema, edema, many vesicles and sometimes ulcerations. The same individual may have different reactions to different concentrations of the same material. Reactions should be checked after 48 hrs and for delayed action at least 5 to 7 days after the patch has been removed.

Contact dermatitis is rarely seen on the soles of the feet. Allergic dermatitis occurs where the keratin is thinnest.

In a shoe, the backing, tongue, inner sole and lining may be the cause for sensitivity, but rarely is the outer leather the cause. Often the tanning chemicals, shoe dyes and adhesive materials are at fault. Patch tests of sock and sock lining are indicated in suspicious foot dermatitis.

Tuberculin patch tests can be used by the podiatrist in a commercially prepared form when a foot lesion suggests tuberculous infection.

Scratch Test

After selecting a suitable place that is free of hair, such as the forearm, upper arm or back, it is cleansed with alcohol and dried. Two or three series of very superficial scratches about ⅛ inch in length and 1 inch apart are made with no bleeding. One drop of 0.1% sodium hydroxide is placed beside each scratch. The proteins of suspected materials in powder form are carefully combined with the sodium hydroxide and rubbed into the scratch using plain sodium hydroxide as a control. A positive reaction shows up in about 30 min if the protein used is the offender. The reaction is shown by a wheal and surrounding erythema larger than that in the control.

Intradermal Test

In this procedure, about 0.05 ml of an extract diluted 0.001 mg of protein to 1 ml is injected intradermally. Care must be taken to inject the protein into the dermis and not under the skin.

Trichophyton Test

An antigen prepared commercially from fungi grown from mycotic skin infections is injected intradermally. About 0.05 ml of the standard preparation is used either by injection or by a patch test. The positive intradermal test presents an erythematous area from 1 to 3.5 cm in diameter within 45 hr. The patch test results in a papulovesicular dermatitis in from 4 days to 2 weeks. The value of this test is questionable.

Culture and Sensitivity Tests

Podiatrists must at all times have sterile swabs and transport media available. When an ulceration or infection does not respond readily to conventional treatment it is necessary to ascertain quickly the type of antibiotic that is most suitable in combatting the offending organism. Under proper incubation in the laboratory and with aerobic and anaerobic testing of the colony growth for sensitivity to different antibiotic agents, the podiatrist prescribes the medication that serves best as a bacteriostatic or bacteriocidal agent.

Biopsy

Wherever pathological tissues present a problem in interpretation, it is best to do a biopsy. This procedure can be readily performed in a pathology laboratory. A small portion of the diseased tissue is removed, stained and examined. At the hospital operating table a frozen section sent for evaluation helps determine the presence of malignancy.

Using sterile technique and a suitable skin punch, the podiatrist can remove a small section of marginal skin along with lesional tissue. The punch-biopsied tissue is placed in an alcohol or other suitable preservative and submitted for pathological study (Figs. 6.1 and 6.2). Specialized podiatric pathology laboratories are available for this purpose.

Heloma Durum

The uncomplicated heloma durum or hard corn can be described as a thickness of the skin composed of desquamated, impacted, crenated, distorted and keratinized dead cells of the epidermis localized at a site of great pressure and friction (Fig. 6.3). The lesion is found most commonly about the toes and can occur wherever great pressure and friction are present. The color may vary from a white to gray-yellow, brown or red. The texture may vary from a dry, horny mass to a waxy, hyaline appearance.

Helomas may be caused by a variety of extrinsic factors. The more common etiologic factors are shoe pressure from ill-fitting footgear and irritations from irregularities in the shoes or hose. Intrinsic problems, such as bony prominences, enlarged bursae or faulty foot function and structure, may cause helomas. Altered foot physiology due to occupational stress, deformity and pathology of the skin and underlying structures creates friction and pressure, producing helomas.

Gamble and Yale (5) noted several types of bone involvements as being etiologic. They described irregularly shaped toe bones, roughened bone margins, exostoses and malalignments. Toes are often entirely in varus, or parts assume a varus position.

Bonavilla (6) supported the concept that heloma dura occur where there is inflammation rather than degeneration of cells. He demonstrated by histologic study the presence of a thickened layer of cornified epithelium. Polymorphonuclear leukocytes invade the thickened epithelium. The dermis demonstrates an increase in capillary vessels, arterioles and collagen fibers. Bonavilla also concluded that the pain and chronicity of a heloma durum is probably due to perineural scarring of the nerve filaments in the skin.

The author has recognized a rotation of the proximal phalanx on its long axis with a prominent condyle serving as the source of intrinsic irritation and heloma formation on the fifth toe. Helomas and tylomas may be the result of multiple minimal trauma sufficiently severe to disturb the mechanism that releases the horny layer cells from each other. Thus, instead of desquamation, there is an over activity of the binding process, resulting in a laying

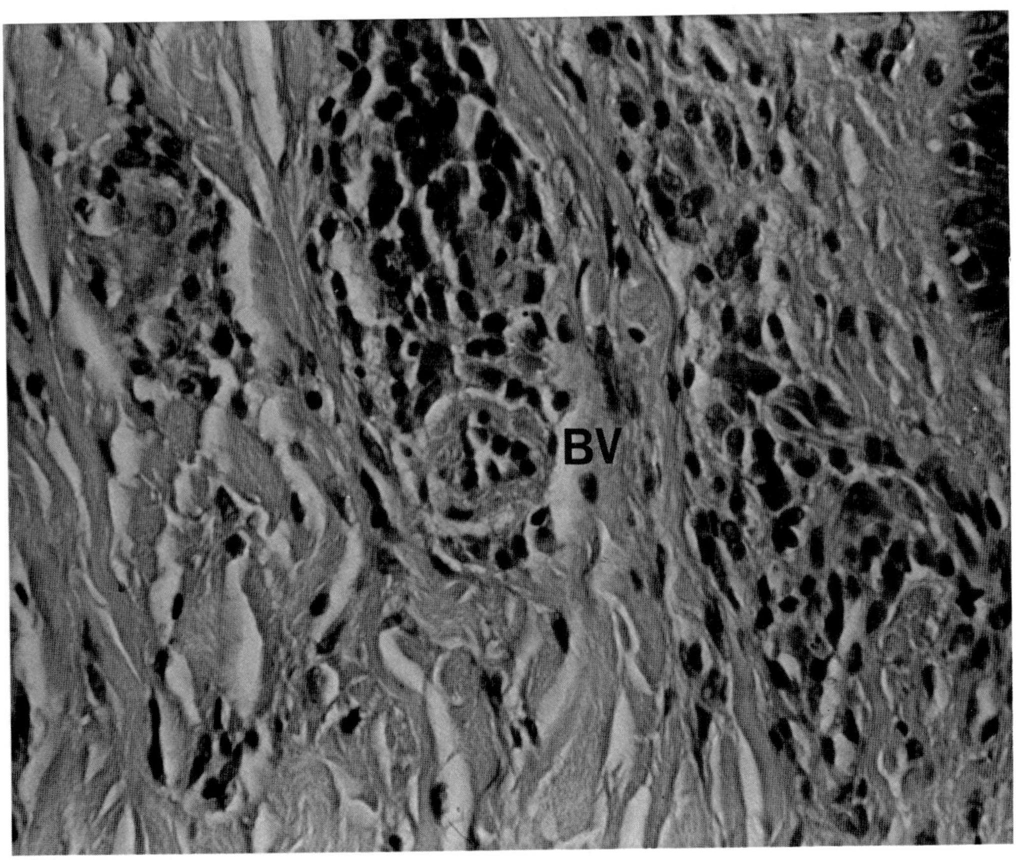

Figure 6.1. Necrobiosis lipoidica diabeticorum. A blood vessel showing thickening of the wall with proliferation of the endothelial cells resulting in a narrowed lumen (*BV*) Vascular changes of this type are conspicuous in the lower legs. (400×) (Courtesty of Martin Port, MS, DPM Veterans Administration Center, Martinsburg, WV.)

down of one cell upon the other that causes the development of a hard, horny mass.

Penneys et al. (7) noted that cell proliferation is not limited to the basal layers, but also occurs in the more superficial

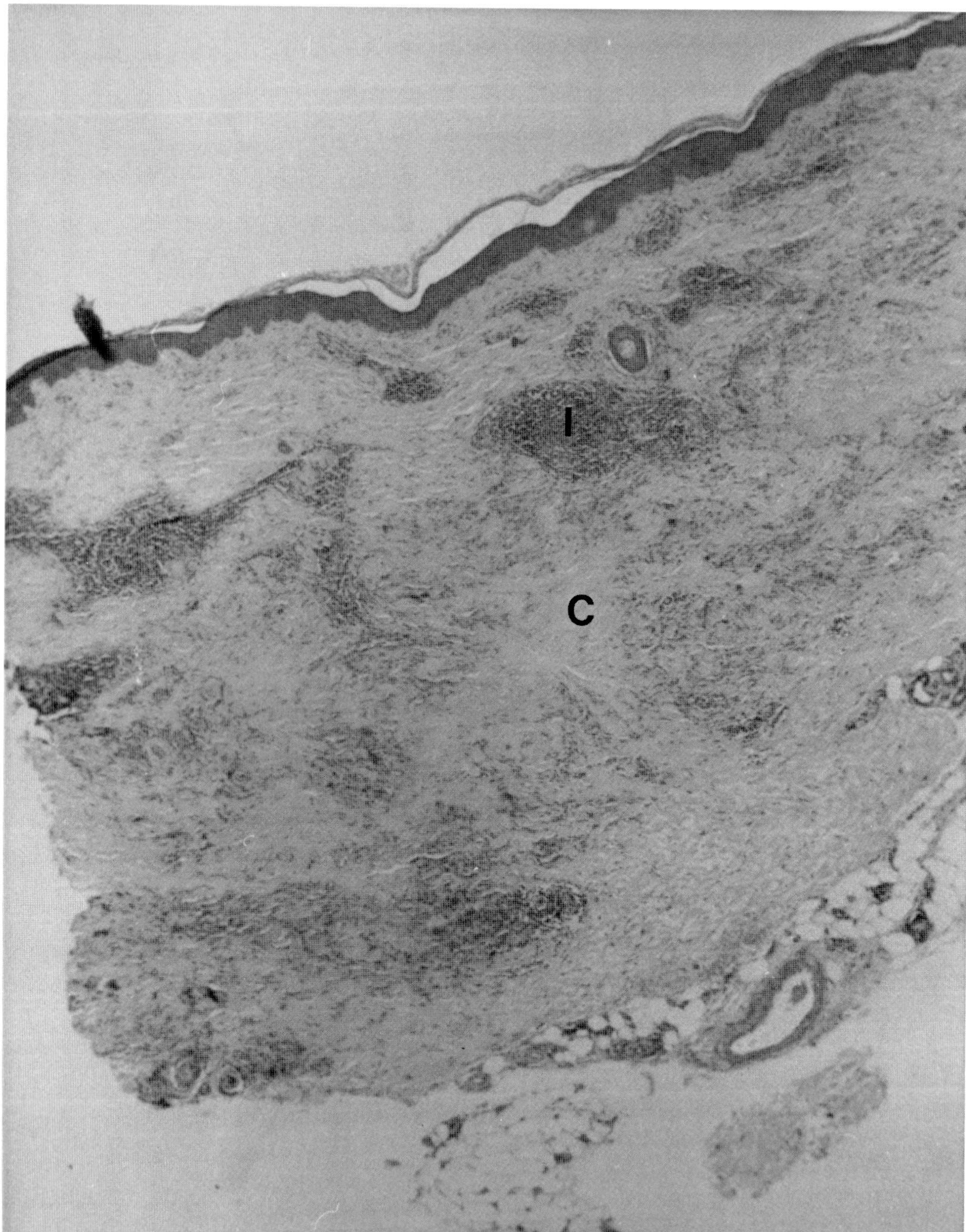

Figure 6.2. Necrobiosis lipoidica diabeticorum. The right one-third of the dermis has a relatively normal appearance. On the left mid and lower dermis can be seen irregular patches of homogenized degenerated collagen (*C*) with a reduced number of fibrocytes. Note nonspecific focal areas of infiltration of chronic inflammatory cells (*I*). (40×) (Courtesy of Martin Port, MS, DPM, Veterans Administration Center, Martinsburg, WV.)

cells. Mitotic division in the stratum germinativum is stimulated by removing a few of the many layers of the stratum corneum (8). McCarthy and Habowsky (9) studied the structure of the heloma durum and presented electromicroscopic evidence of their findings (Figs. 6.3–6.7).

Pathogenesis

Repeated trauma may result in dilation of capillaries and redness of the skin. If the trauma occurs over a long period of time, the subcutaneous tissue reacts to create an adventitious bursa to cushion the underlying bone. The irritation may go on to develop into a bullous lesion. In most instances, the trauma is so subtle that the superficial epidermal cells pack down as a thickened mass. Repeated trauma disturbs the binding functions of the exfoliating stratum corneum, which results in a localized thickening of the skin painful to digital pressure. The surrounding skin shows evidence of inflammation, and the subcutaneous tissue is edematous. Complicating bursitis, traumatic arthritis, lipping, osteophytes, exotosis, sinus tract formation and ulcerations may require treatment for relief and cure of the heloma. On microscopic examination of 76 toes from cadavers, Freed (10) noted the following sequence of events: (1) inflammation of soft tissues about the bone, (2) enlargement of cortical bone by homoplastic bone formation and (3) swelling of the skin and corn formation.

A broad conical hard hornified mass of thickened stratum corneum is noted. It may be white, yellow, red or brown in color. A heloma may be dry or waxy in appearance. It appears over a bony prominence or at a site of pressure from ill-fitting footgear or malaligned toes (Fig. 6.8). The lesion may be compressed so that its superficial surface is even with the skin surface, or it may be elevated with a broad base and peaked top. Digital pressure from side to side is not as painful as direct compression into the underlying inflamed skin, bursa and bone. Helomas may occur

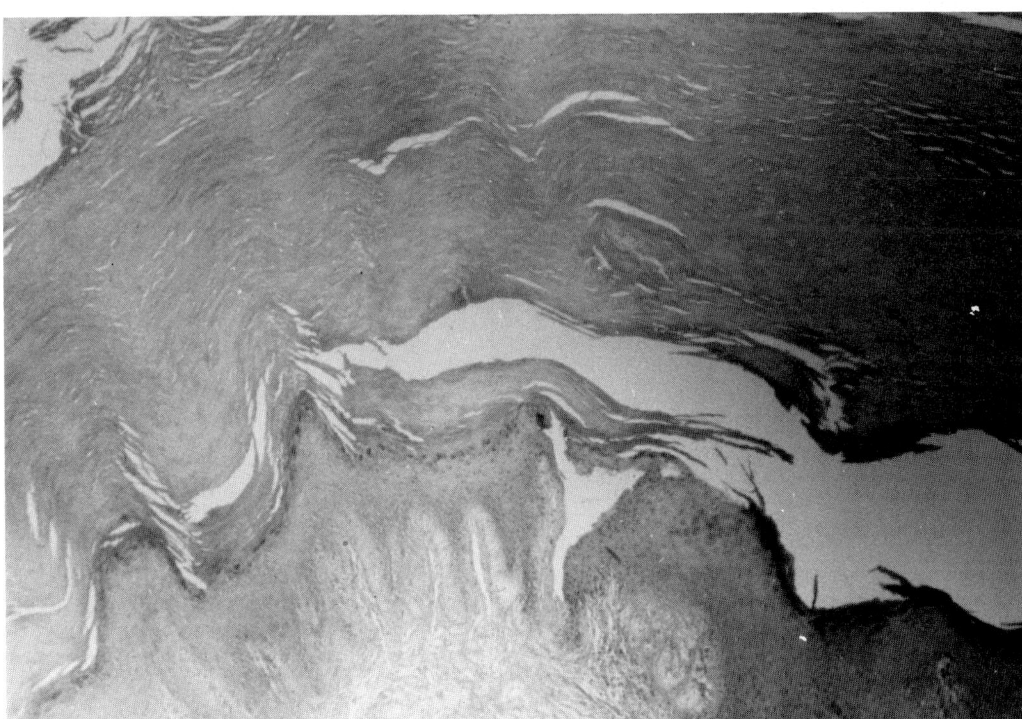

Figure 6.3. Low-power magnification of heloma durum. Note the typical thickening of the epidermis consistent with hyperkeratosis.

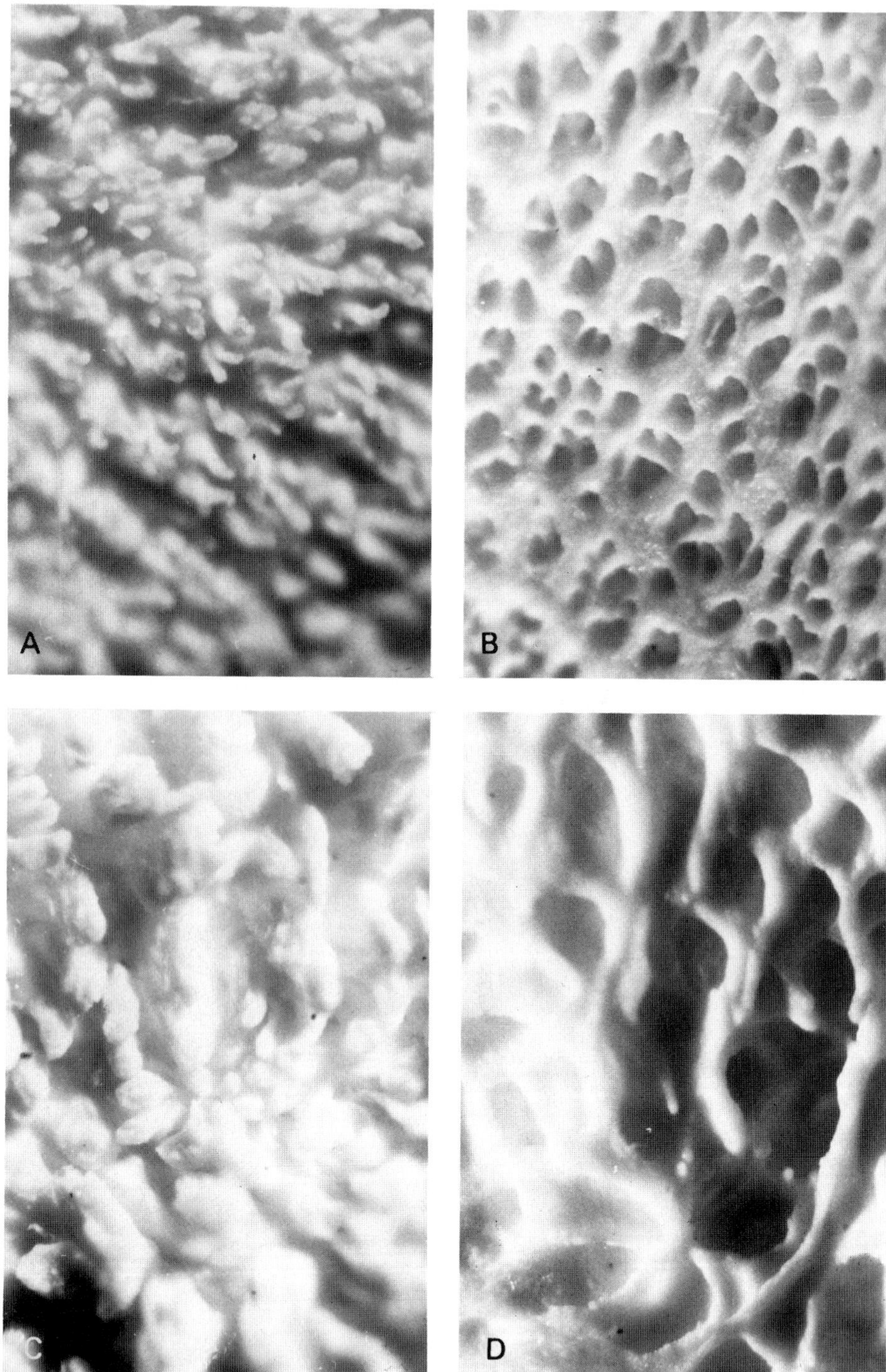

Figure 6.4. Incident light photomicrographs ×35 of normal skin and heloma durum. *A,* dermal portion of dermoepidermal interface of skin excised from the interphalangeal region of a normal fifth digit. Dermal papillae show a uniformity of height and are spaced with regularity. *B,* epidermal portion of dermoepidermal interface of skin excised from the interphalangeal region of a normal fifth digit. Rete ridges are interconnected in an orderly fashion and are structurally discrete. *C,* dermal portion of dermoepidermal interface of surgically excised heloma durum of the fifth digit. The dermal papillae are hypertrophied with foot-like projections on the superior aspect seemingly from a coalescence of several papillae. Papillae orient in several directions. *D,* epidermal portion of dermoepidermal interface of surgically excised heloma durum of the fifth digit. Rete ridges are considerably wider and irregular making a bizarre pattern for receiving the grossly altered dermal papillae. (From DJ McCarthy, JE Habowsky: Alterations in skin morphology in heloma dura utilizing maceration technique for examination of epidermal-dermal interface. *J Am Podiatry Assoc* 62:305, 1972.

beneath a toenail (Fig. 6.9), at the distal ends of the toes—usually the second, third and fourth toes—and on the dorsum of all the lesser toes and over their proximal and distal interphalangeal joints. Misuse of commercial corn remedies may produce a heloma overlaid with white, macerated and necrotic tissue (Fig. 6.10).

Heloma dura located at the distal ends of the second, third and fourth toes often pose a major problem. This type of lesion is commonly found in elderly patients with degenerative disease involving the interphalangeal joints. The flexion deformity is generally accompanied by a dorsal prominence, contraction of both the skin and flexor musculature on their plantar surface and a broadened distal end of the toe. Intermittent trauma to the distal end of the digit creates a painful heloma or tyloma. The toenail is often hypertrophied by trauma, and the toe takes on the typical appearance of a modified or well-advanced hammertoe. The lesion at this site may break down with multiple minimal irritation and eventually ulcerate. This occurs especially frequently in patients with diabetes or peripheral vascular problems because fragility of the capillaries predisposes to ulceration.

The patient may become a "heel walker" in an attempt to relieve pressure. Adaptation becomes a subconscious command. With continuing pain, the stress and irritation must be removed early to avoid complications. This removal is accomplished palliatively or surgically, depending on the patient and the attendant risk. Treatment must embody an active or passive adaptation for the pathology.

Gibbs (11) briefly defines confusing terminology when the podiatrist, dermatologist or orthopaedist discusses hyperkeratosis. Gibbs used hyperkeratosis to

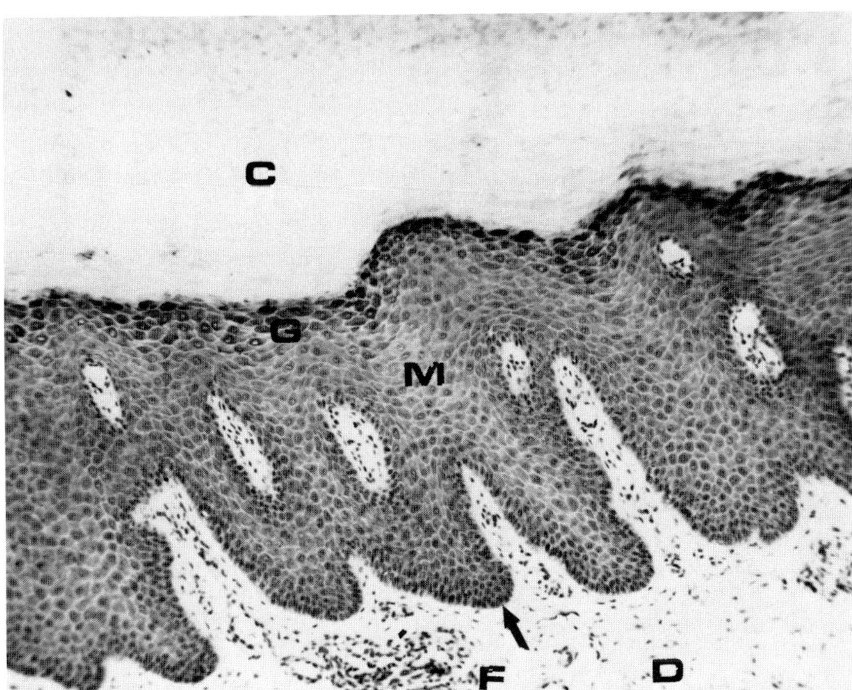

Figure 6.5. Human heloma durum stained by hematoxylin and eosin stratum corneum (*C*) is hypertrophied over an acanthotic stratum Malpighi (*M*) in which all cells are well formed. Stratum granulosum (*G*) is deeply basophilic and regular throughout the lesion. Rete ridges (*arrow*) are elongated and orient essentially perpendicular to the free surface of the skin. Dermis (*D*) is rich with fibrocytes (*F*). Islands of dermis in the epidermis are more apparent than real because they are dermal papillae oriented on a plane somewhat parallel or tangential to the free surface of the skin and cross-sectioned in the preparation. Light microscopy ×100. (Courtesy of Luther Gilliam and Daniel J McCarthy, DPM PhD Veterans Administration Medical Center, Perry Point, MD.)

include traumatically induced thickening of the skin, e.g., helomas and tylomas. However, he differentiates keratoses, or keratodermas, as the nontraumatically induced thickening of the skin either of infectious origin, hereditary or possibly of systemic etiology.

Treatment. Treatment of these painful helomas depends on their etiology, size, consistency, number and location and on the patient's age and health.

The heloma durum, wherever its location and regardless of other circumstances, must be treated judiciously by a podiatrist. A hyperkeratotic skin mass by its very pathological state is capable of causing further difficulty. Treatment is simple and is accomplished by softening the hyperkeratosis with a keratolytic, analgesic, antiseptic solution before debridement.

The heloma may be excised by sharp dissection using a sharp scalpel, a small sharp chisel or sharp skin forceps. A line of demarcation is noted between the dead horny mass and the healthy pink underlying skin. Removal of the keratotic mass is often accomplished by use of sandpaper disks or diamond or steel burrs. In the more painful lesions a complete toe block or field block anesthesia is used to relieve pain. The author uses lidocaine or carbocaine, 1% solution plain. A 1:200,000 epinephrine solution can be used in combination with the anesthetic where the circulation is good; however, the constriction causes slower absorption and often increases postoperative pain.

Once this treatment has been accomplished, the site of debridement is properly shielded, and a cream or ointment dressing is applied. A crest pad may be used for lesions on the ends of the toes. (Fig. 6.11). Sansone (12) described the very successful shielding of excrescences of all types and on all locations by parallel strips of adhesive felt (Fig. 6.12). These are placed behind and in front of the lesion or in parallel fashion to each side.

After debridement of the heloma, it is the responsibility of the operator to evaluate the etiology, the degree of damage to the skin, the extent of inflammation of a bursa that commonly forms beneath the

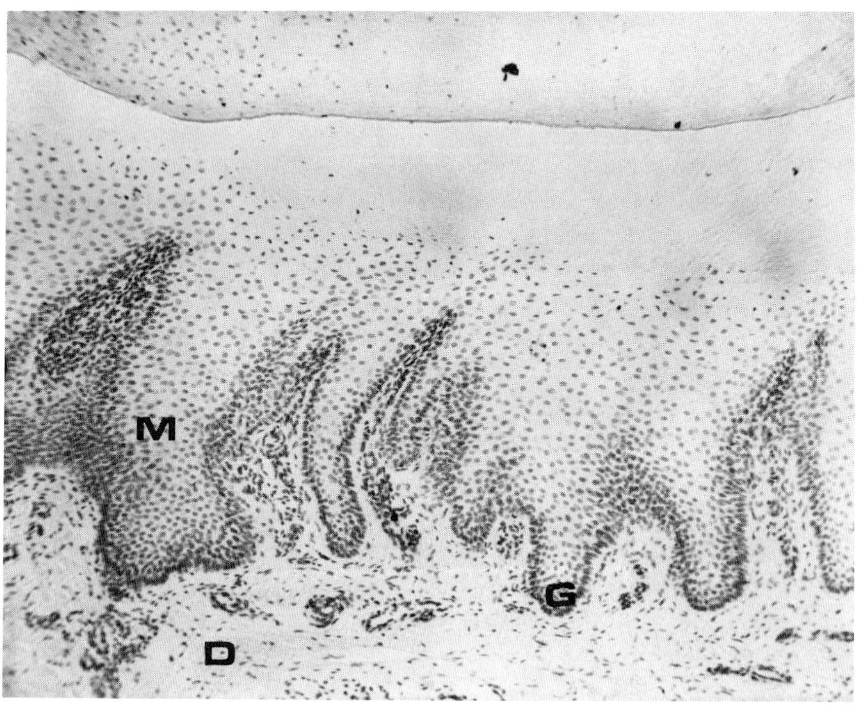

Figure 6.6. Human heloma durum stained by the Feulgen reaction for DNA. The stratum Malpighi (*M*) is acanthotic, and DNA cannot be seen superficial to the stratum granulosum. The stratum germinativum (*G*) demonstrates heavy concentrations of DNA/RNA. The dermis (*D*) is rich in fibroblasts that also are rich in DNA/RNA. Light microscopy ×100. (Courtesy of Luther Gilliam and Daniel J McCarthy, DPM, PhD, Veterans Administration Medical Center, Perry Point, MD.)

heloma, the presence of a toe deformity and the size of bone enlargements on the underlying phalanges. Very often the phalanges are rotated on their longitudinal axis. Radiographs are taken to ascertain the extent of the underlying pathology.

Deffinger (13) describes neuromas occurring on the digital nerves to the toes as being the primary cause of severe pain in a heloma.

At this point in treatment, the podiatrist plans the desirable treatment for the par-

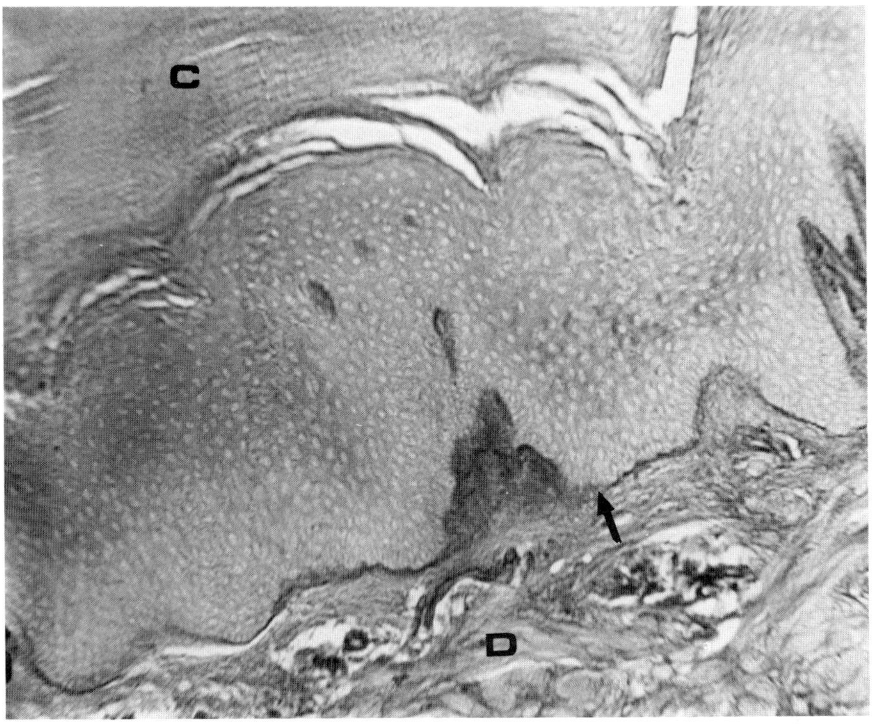

Figure 6.7. Human heloma durum stained by Periodic Acid-Schiff (PAS) reaction for mucopolysaccharides. The dermis (*D*) is rich in mucopolysaccharides, and the basement membrane (*arrow*) is deeply stained. The dermal-influencing factor stimulating epidermal cell mitosis is know to be a mucopolysaccharide. Cells of the acanthotic stratum Malpighi are well stained by PAS reaction at the intercellular boundaries, whereas the ergastoplasm does not stain. Stratum corneum (*C*) is not reactive to PAS stain. Light microscopy ×100. (Courtesy of Luther Gilliam and Daniel J McCarthy, DPM, PhD, Veterans Administration Medical Center, Perry Point, MD.)

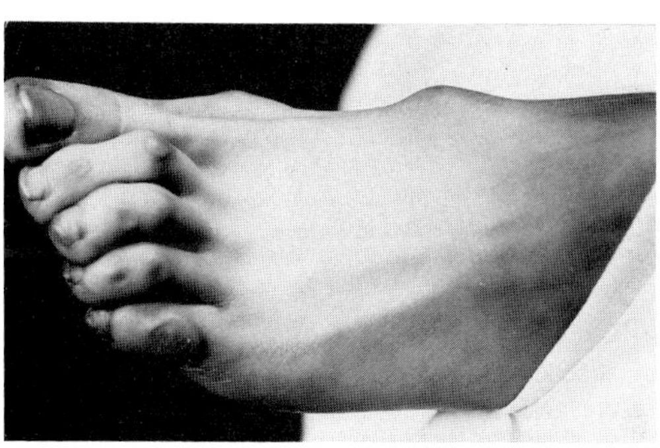

Figure 6.8. Hypertrophied first metatarsocuneiform joint with keratotic mass overlying prominence.

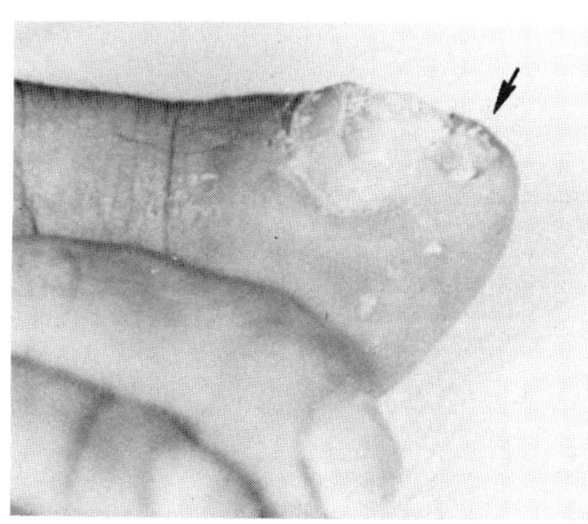

Figure 6.9. Subungual heloma uncovered following removal of hypertropied plate and debridement of nail bed.

ticular pathology. The patient is usually relieved by the skillful excision, debridement and shielding of the lesion, but complete eradication of the heloma must be sought. Treatment may require consideration of the degree of faulty functioning of the foot, which must be corrected. Ill-fitting footgear must also be replaced according to the podiatrist's instructions or prescription. If a complicating circulatory or diabetic problem exists, further treatment is conservative. It may include periodic examination and reduction of the excrescence and instruction of the patient in

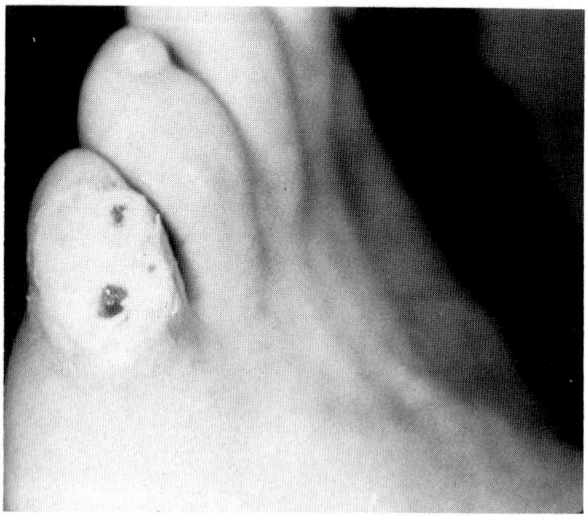

Figure 6.10. Salicylic acid burn due to commercial "corn cure."

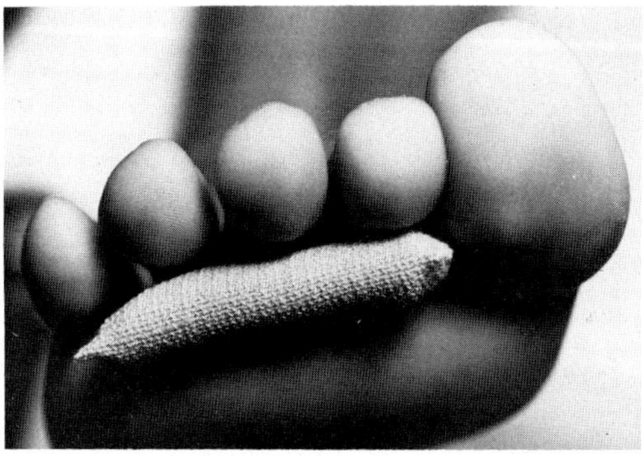

Figure 6.11. Crest pad. This pad can be dipped in latex after it has been worn and shaped for 5 days. It may also be covered with silicone paste, closed in plastic to keep from adhering to hose and completed with subsequent coatings of silicone.

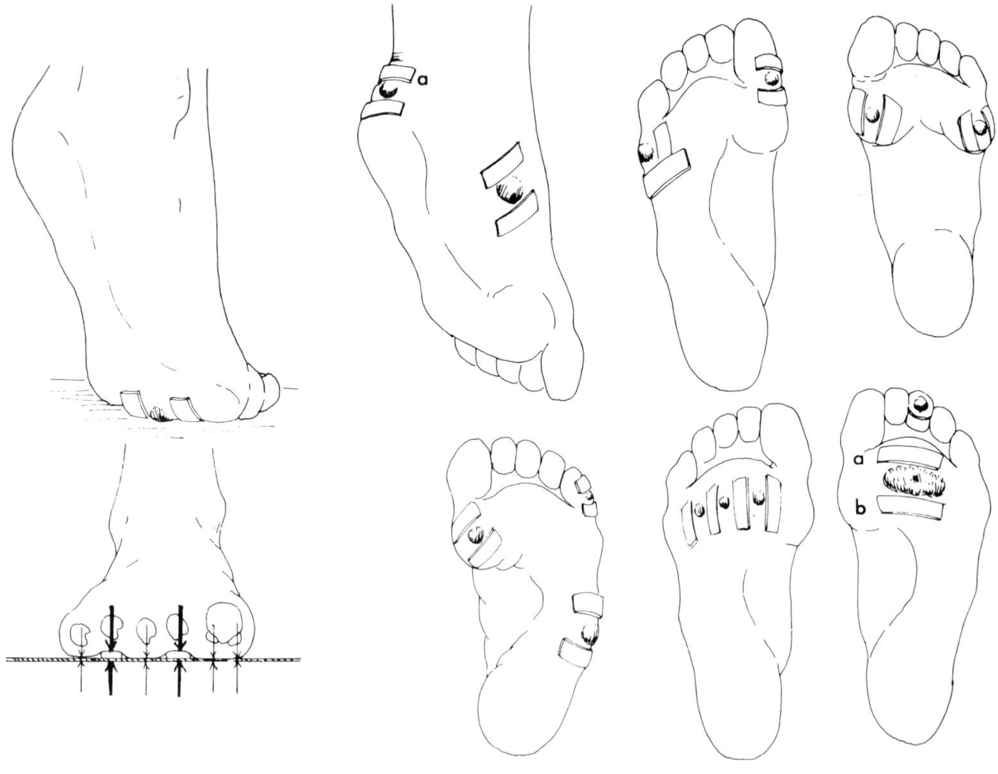

Figure 6.12. Parallel pads and strip pontoons as described by Sansone. (Courtesy of R Sansone.)

basic rules for foot care. The patient and family are taught to recognize incipient problems and are advised to refrain from use of home remedies and "bathroom surgery." The uncomplicated heloma in a patient with arteriosclerosis, diabetes or other peripheral vascular disorder may be protected by permanent removable shields and pads that are constructed to plaster impressions or made over the affected toe. These are made of liquid latex, liquid plastic, silicone, foam, sponge rubber, felt, self-adherent bandages and a variety of other materials.

Construction of Permanent Shields

Sivitz (14) describes the construction of crests and shields from acrylic plastic resin (Figs. 6.13–6.15)

Polokoff (15) describes a latex shield made with tubular gauze directly on the affected toe. Many variants can be constructed based on Polokoff's original techniques.

The following method is a typical approach to permanent shielding of the painful excresense that is not amenable to surgery.

A 4 inch length of no. 1 tube gauze is slit around 2 inches at one end. The toe is coated with rubber cement, and the tube end of the gauze is slipped over the toe and cemented down. An aperture pad or a suitable shield shape designed by the podiatrist is placed around the excrescence for protection. The shield and tube gauze on the toe are covered with rubber ce-

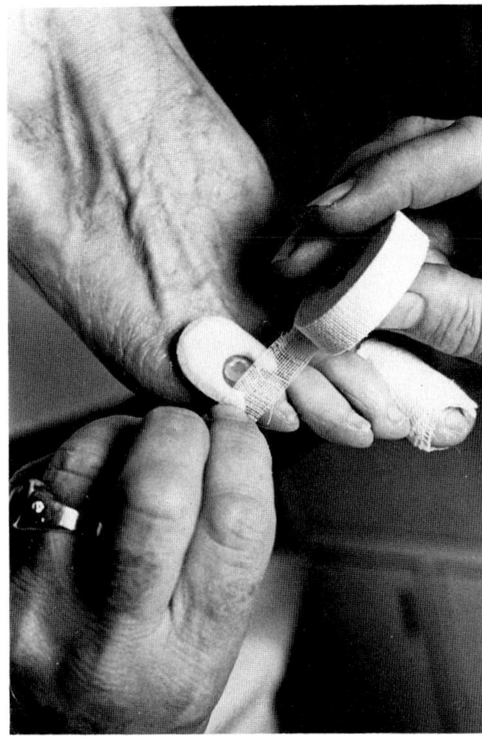

Figure 6.14. Heloma shield.

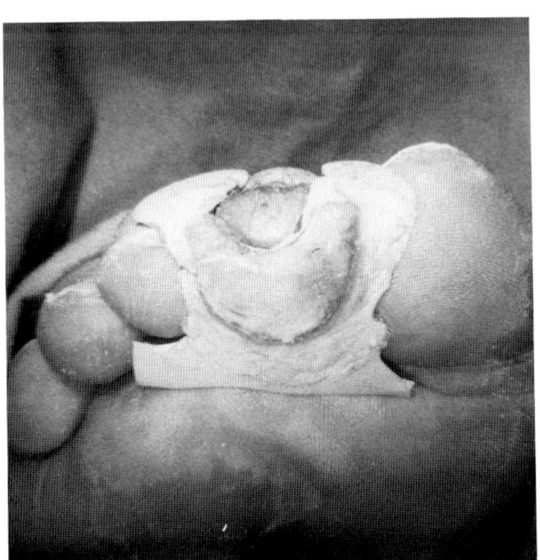

Figure 6.13. Moldable podiatric compound with 1/16-inch felt pad covered with bathtub caulk—distal heloma durum accommodation.

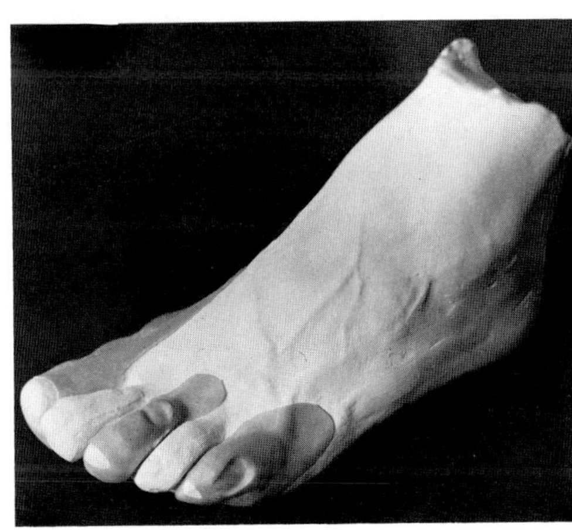

Figure 6.15. Latex prosthesis. In diabetic or arteriosclerotic patients or in those unable to tolerate surgical correction, the use of latex prostheses constructed to plaster casts is advisable. Impressions are taken of individual toes and sent to the laboratory for construction of prosthesis. (Courtesy of Liquid Rubber Appliance Laboratory.)

ment. The split end is given a half-twist, worked back over the pad-covered toe and adhered on the dorsum of the foot behind the toe.

The entire shield is then coated with liquid latex and covered with thin plastic sheeting to protect the hose. The shield is kept on the toe for about 4 days. When the patient returns, the shield is trimmed, coated once again and dried with a hot air blower or a spray of equal parts acetic acid and alcohol to speed up curing of the latex. The podiatrist may wish to use silicone gel or other plastic substances in lieu of liquid latex (see Chapter 13, Podiatric Treatment).

Ulcer and Sinus Tract Formation. If the subhelomal tissue presents an ulceration or sinus tract, it is imperative that the operator stimulate repair with suitable medication and physical measures. The sinus tract may be cauterized with silver nitrate from 5 to 50% to stimulate or destroy the fibrous tract. If an infection is present, incision and drainage may be necessary. Total excision of the sinus tract may be the desirable approach if the tract is calcified and intractable. Wet dressings of aluminum subacetate, physiological saline or dilute boric acid solutions may be necessary to facilitate drainage. Hexylresorcinol as a wet dressing is best used for only short periods of time. If an ulceration exists, follow the principles outlined for ulcerations. If an infection is present, bacterial sensitivity tests are performed to ascertain the antibiotic of choice.

Sinus Tract (Figs. 6.16–6.19). Stratified squamous epithelium grows down the tract from the skin and may line the marrow cavity in the presence of chronic osteomyelitis. A squamous cell epithelioma can develop in a chronic sinus. An early sinus tract may be excised because a chronic sinus can be premalignant.

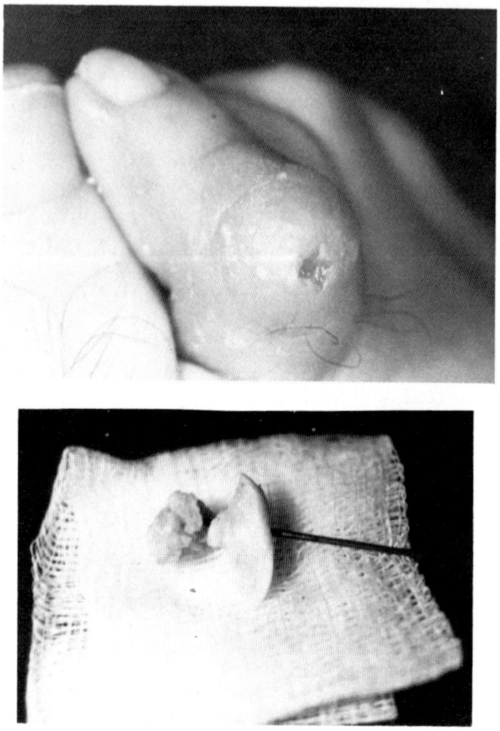

Figure 6.17. *A,* hammertoe. Sinus tract beneath heloma durum. *B,* gross specimen, sinus tract, osteomyelitis.

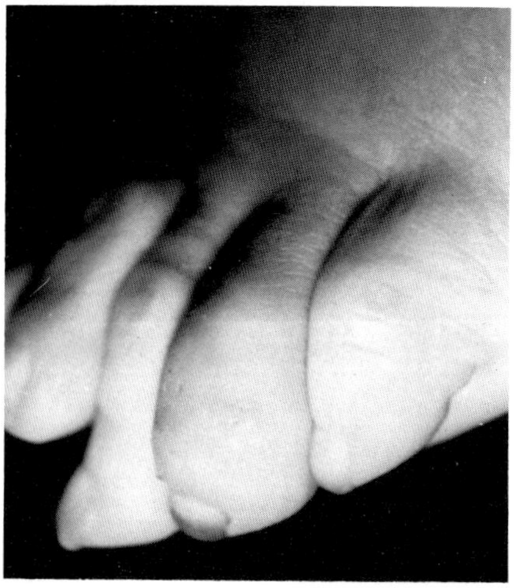

Figure 6.16. Swollen fourth toe, osteomyelitis, sinus tract.

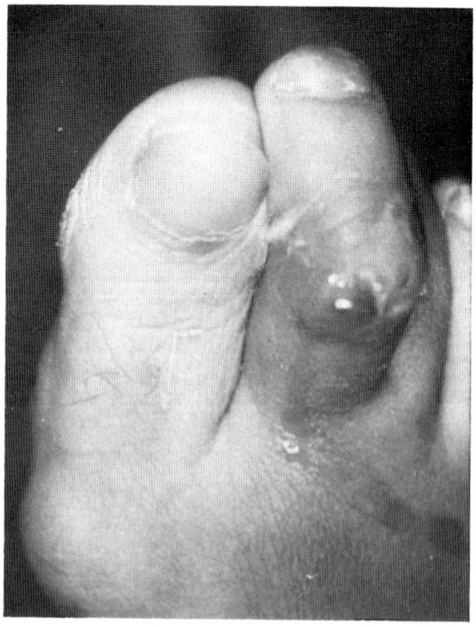

Figure 6.18. Infection, cellulitis, swelling, discoloration, draining sinus tract, second toe. Pain with impending gangrene.

Subheloma Bursitis

Very often an adventitious bursa develops in the subcutaneous tissue beneath the heloma (Figs. 6.20–6.23). If acutely inflamed, the toe is swollen in circumscribed fashion around the perimeter of the keratotic mass. It may be red, indurated or fluctuant and exquisitely painful to touch. If the lesion is chronic, a radiograph may disclose a calcareous degeneration of the bursa, osteochondroma and often a secondary osteomyelitis (Figs. 6.24–6.26).

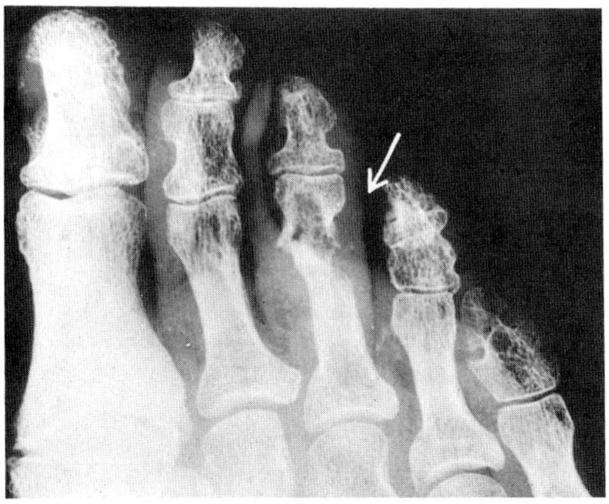

Figure 6.19. Heloma durum, proximal interphalangeal joint. Osteomyelitis secondary to infected sinus tract. (From FO Gamble and I Yale: *Clinical Foot Roentgenology.* Baltimore, Williams & Wilkins, 1966.

Treatment of the bursitis may be necessary to relieve pain. This is accomplished by meticulously aseptic use of field block anesthesia and infiltration of lidocaine 1% plain into the bursal tissue. If calcific deposits are present, they must be broken up by needling multiple subcutaneous punctures of the calcified bursa following the initial injection. Needling is followed by aspiration of the intrabursal fluid using an 18 to 20 gauge 1 inch needle.

With the aspirating needle within the bursa, the barrel of the syringe is replaced by one containing 0.3 to 0.5 ml of a corticosteroid antiinflammatory solution, which is injected into and around the bursal sac. Results have been gratifying where betamethosone (Celestone), triamcinolone (Aristocort, Kenalog) and methylprednisolone (Medrol) have been used. Chymotrypsin, 0.2–0.6 ml, may be used instead of a cor-

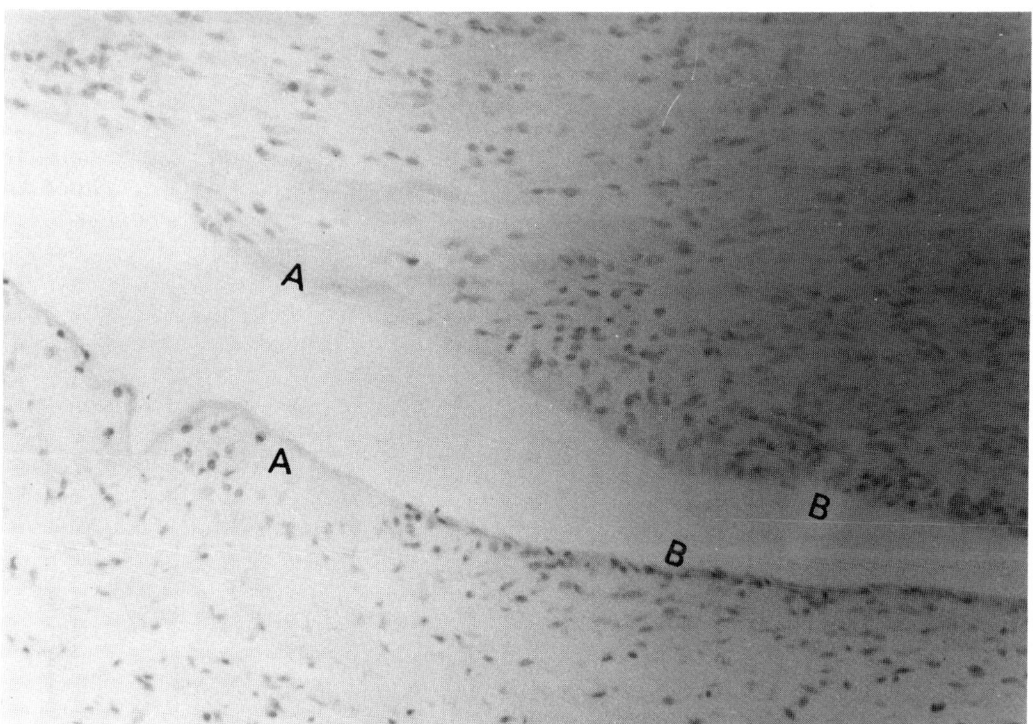

Figure 6.20. Bursal lining. *A,* Epithelium has degenerated consistent with late change; *B,* note the epithelial cells lining bursa.

ticosteroid. Streiker (16) was impressed by the results of chymotrypsin injections in treating helomas and related disorders. A suitable protective dressing is applied to relieve pressure. Physical therapeutic measures consisting of saline soaks—hot or cold—infrared rays, short wave and ultrasound may be used for fast relief of pain. Oral analgesics or combinations of analgesics and narcotics, such as aspirin with codeine or Tylenol with codeine potentiated by promethazine, are indicated where the pain is severe.

On occasion, the treatment of choice is surgical excision of the chronic bursa or calcific deposits. This may be accomplished by semielliptical incisions around the heloma to remove an elliptical section of tissue and expose the bursa. The bursa is grasped by Allis forceps and sharply and bluntly dissected out by Sistrunk scissors. If a prominence of bone, either thickened cortex, and exostosis, or osteochondroma, is present, the overgrowth is removed by bone forceps and rasping. Closure is completed by suturing with 5-0 nylon.

Palliative treatment for heloma dura on the dorsum of the interphalangeal joints of the lesser toes includes debridement of the excrescence and adequate protection and use of a corrective

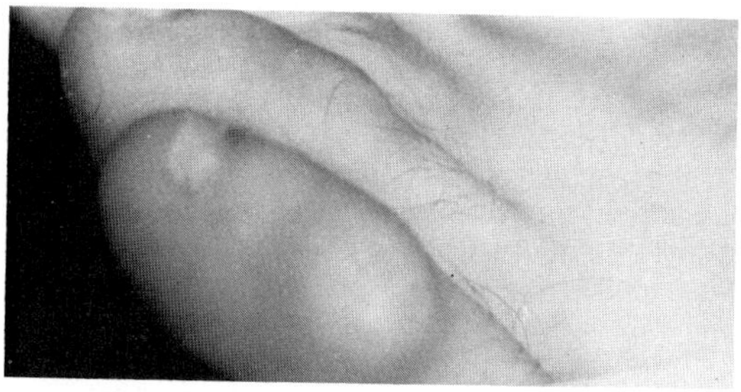

Figure 6.21. Distended bursa beneath heloma.

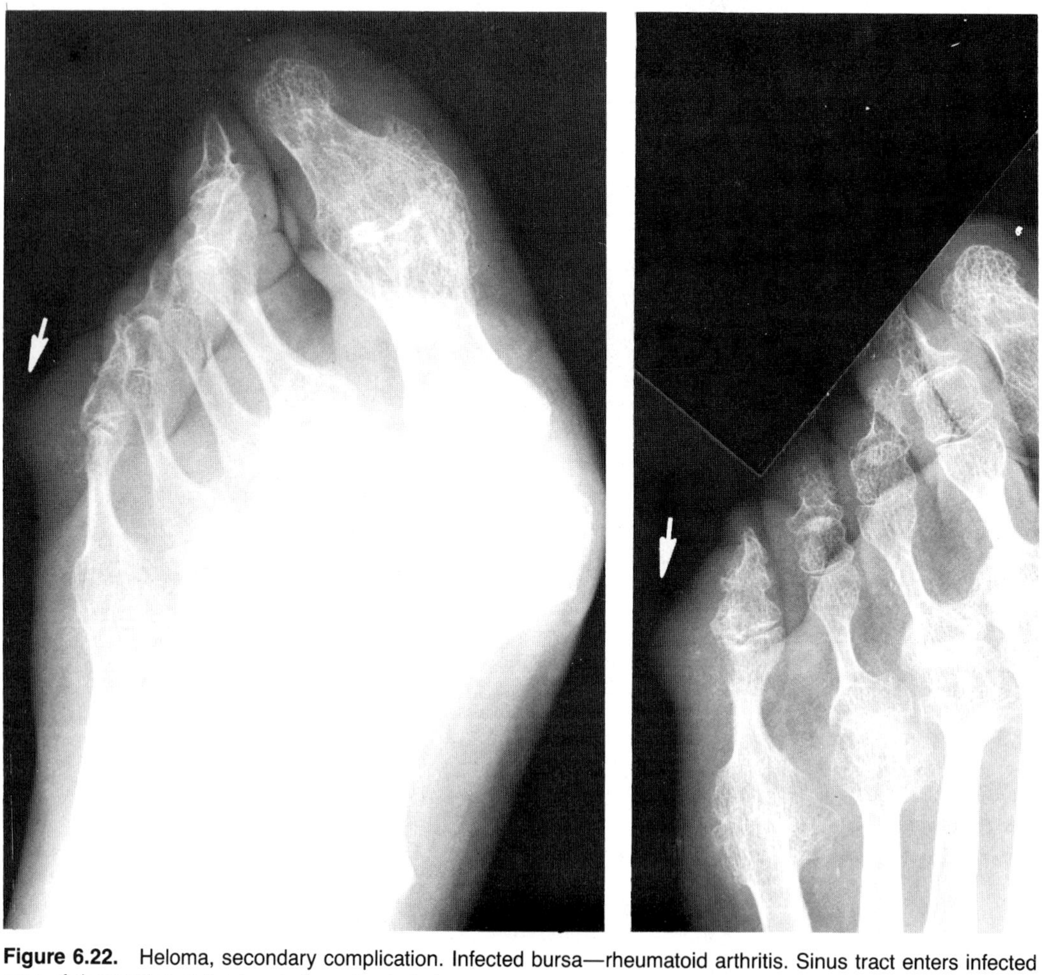

Figure 6.22. Heloma, secondary complication. Infected bursa—rheumatoid arthritis. Sinus tract enters infected area of destruction at the head of proximal phalanx.

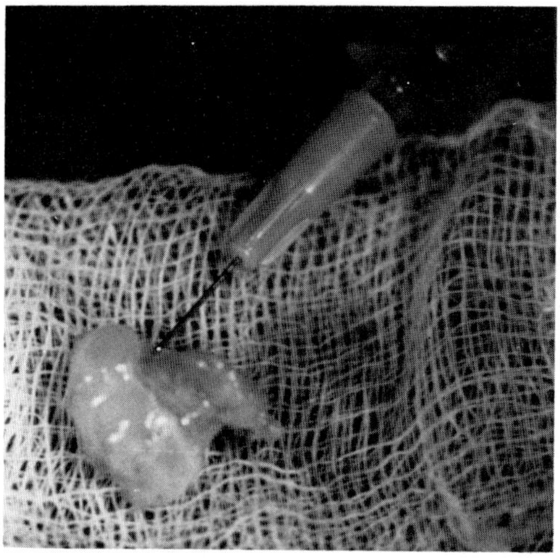

Figure 6.23. Distended bursa beneath heloma durum. Gross specimen.

force to realign the deformity. Debridement is accomplished in the usual manner. Pain is relieved by injections of local anesthesia and corticosteroids. Shields of a variety of materials, including felt, moleskin, foam, adhesive and latex are used.

Splinting the toe or using adhesive strapping to bring a flexed toe into better forefoot relationship is often necessary to facilitate relief. Construction of a crest pad to realign the toes is

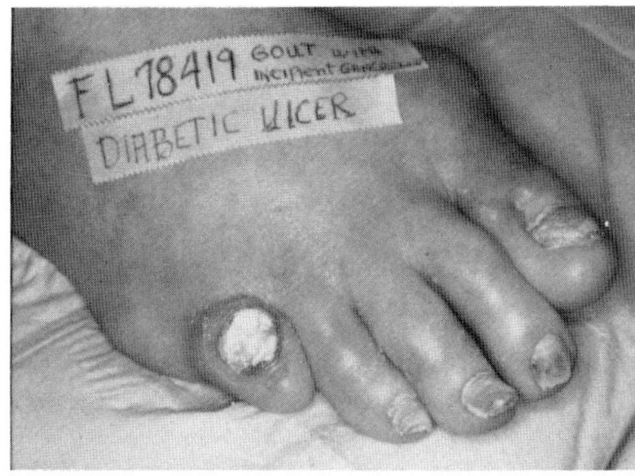

Figure 6.25. Heloma dura—incipient gangrene; tophaceous deposits fifth toe—gout. (Courtesy of M Shapiro.)

helpful. Shoes with extra depth relieve pressure from dorsiflexed toes by providing an additional ¼ inch in the toe region when properly corrected. The ¼-inch insole is removed and the forepart removed or ground to a feather edge. Acker (17) did some early research on subcutaneous implantation of silicon for the relief of helomas. To date, the treatment has not been approved. However, subdermal collagen injections have been approved for the symptomatic treatment of helomas (see Chapter 13, Podiatric Treatment).

There are many treatment approaches for helomas including surgical correction of defor-

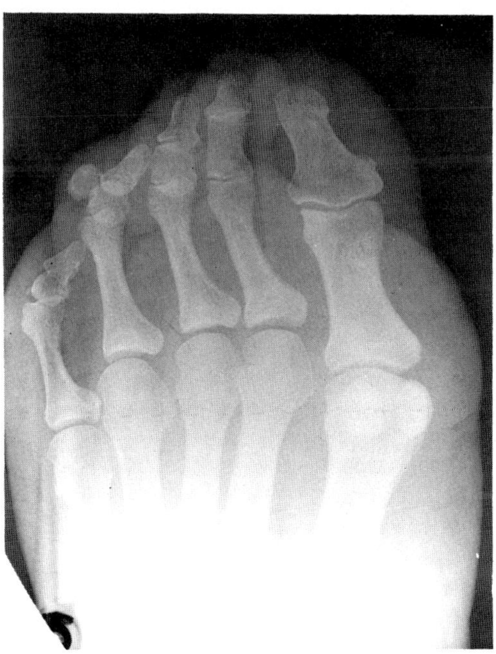

Figure 6.24. Osteochondroma fourth toe. Heloma durum occurs over deformity.

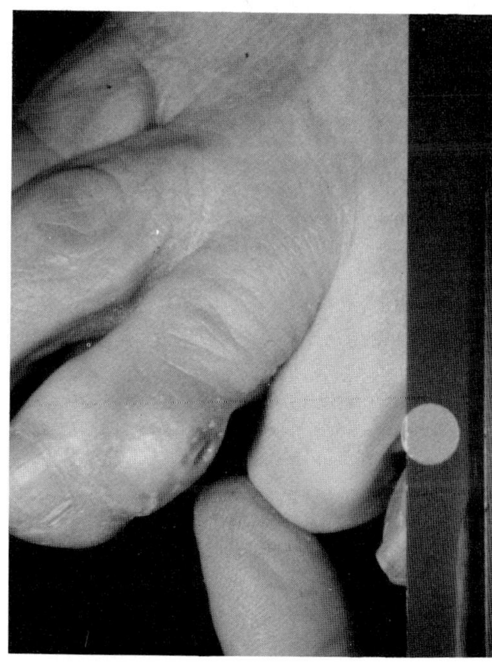

Figure 6.26. Calcified bursa markedly distended and acutely inflamed with underlying osteomyelitis.

mities and the injection of local anesthesia, sclerosing agents, dispersion media, corticosteroids and vitamin A for the relief of pain or alteration of the subhelomal pathology. The techniques are described below.

In a painful heloma with an underlying bursitis or capsulitis without bone pathology or infection, the use of a local anesthetic by infiltration or field block is often helpful (Fig. 6.27). The hyperemia created by the local inflammatory reaction to stress is often relieved by alterations in the local tissue chemistry following use of local anesthesia. Injection is best made by using a tuberculin syringe and 25 to 26 gauge 1 inch needle. The author prefers the solution of lidocaine 1% with 1:100,000 epinephrine. Epinephrine must be used with care, especially when circulatory inadequacies are present. However, the use of epinephrine to constrict the markedly distended capillaries is essential to the relief of symptoms. The amount of anesthesia is kept at a minimum. About 0.5 ml of anesthetic per lesion is adequate.

Kaplan and Kashuk (18) report no serious complications either systemically or locally in over 65,000 digital surgical procedures where epinephrine in proper concentration was used with the anesthetic for vasoconstriction. Steinberg and Block (19) report the successful use of lidocaine with epinephrine in over 200,000 injections with proper selection of the patient and good injection technique.

The injection is directed from the proximal side of the lesion, infiltrating behind, beneath and to the outer sides of the heloma and its underlying bursitis. The injection has the immediate effect of relieving pain. Gross appearance is blanching of

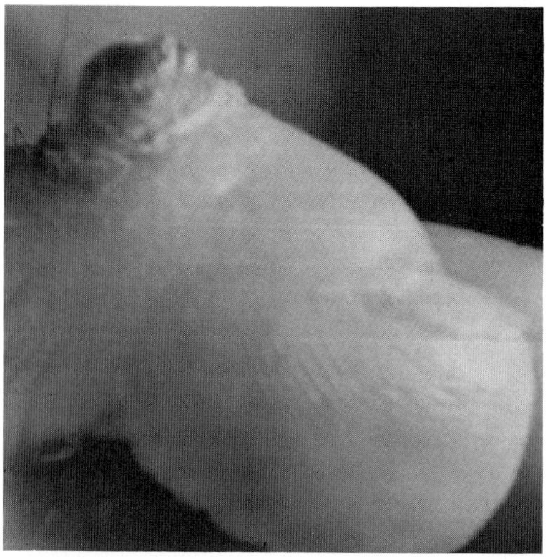

Figure 6.27. Heloma durum, cutaneous horn with underlying bursitis.

the area injected as the distended capillaries constrict. Subsequent observation reveals a decrease in swelling and inflammation. Bursae are usually reduced in size.

Austin (20) demonstrated fibrous adhesions between the chronic heloma and the underlying fascial or capsular tissue. He recommended the infiltration of local anesthesia by pooling beneath the heloma. This, in effect, results in a mechanical stretching and tearing of the fibrous adhesions beneath the excrescence. Austin also suggested incising the fibrous adhesions. To obtain the same effect, Jacobs (21) treated 107 cases by suction, using specially prepared applicators attached to a ⅙-horsepower aspirator-suction machine. He notes that "severing adhesions will very likely go on to result in more adhesions. Repeated administration of negative pressure at regular intervals should mobilize the adhesion so that the surface tissue will not be bound down, but will be freely movable." The reflex hyperemia produces an alteration in tissue fluid chemistry and relief from pain.

Sclerosing agents must be used with great care. The author finds little use for this technique in the treatment of helomas. Hyaluronidase (Alidase) in 250-unit vials acts as a dispersing media when used with other drugs. When injected under a heloma in combination with a local anesthetic, one can expect better and more complete infiltration of the degenerated subhelomal tissue. Corticosteroids in intradermal, intrabursal and intracapillary injections, as recommended by Locke (22, 23) and by Ashur and Farrar (24), have been found useful as an anti-inflammatory agent in acutely sensitive noninfected helomas. Locke (23) notes that the "newest water soluble corticosteroids have proven of special value in soft tissue injections." Cameron (25) reported the use of an aqueous suspension of betamethasone disodium phosphate by injection, claiming a 10 to 15 times greater anti-inflammatory effect than prednisolone produced. The average dose is 0.2 to 0.4 ml. If the excrescence is complicated by a calcareous deposit beneath the heloma, it is often possible to break up the calcium deposit through needling, multiple injections of a local anesthetic under the excrescence into the calcareous deposit. The deposit is broken up, and aspiration may be productive.

Multiple punctures without withdrawing the needle from its original site of insertion are made into the calcium deposit to break up the mass into small fragments. A wide-bore 18 gauge needle is used for this purpose, and an attempt is made alternately to inject and aspirate the anesthetic, with the purpose of trying to remove some of the flaky or paste-like calcareous deposit. When the deposit is in an early paste-like state, this treatment is adequate for relief of pain and removal of the deposit. When the calcareous deposit is extensive or old, it is advisable to resect the mass in toto.

Levy (26) studied the efficacy and safety of the corticosteroids injected in the treatment of clavi and callosities. He compared a group treated with injectable steroids with a control group. Levy states that "in the control group, 58.6% of the sites were successes. This is compared to 42% of the sites which were successes in the steroid treated group. Forty-two percent of the sites treated with corticosteroid solutions developed the following side effects: ulcers 12%, severe pain 16%, subdermal atrophy 14%. There were no side effects in the control group injected with the vehicle alone."

The oral use of vitamin A, 50,000 to 100,000 units daily, has been prescribed by many as an antihyperkeratotic agent, and it has been effective in decreasing the extensive hyperkeratosis in many helomas. The injection of Steinberg's solution, Keramin, has been used successfully in decreasing the keratinization in inflamed helomas (Fig. 6.28).

Silverman et al. (27) cites patients who were successfully treated with injections of a high-potency, aqueous solution of synthetic vitamin A palmitate containing 50,000 U.S.P. units/ml. The heloma is anesthetized by infiltration with an anesthetic of choice. Keramin solution is then injected intradermally under the heloma. The direction of the 25 gauge needle is practically on a horizontal plane. The author prefers a field block or complete toe block prior to injections of vitamin A. This block is followed by infiltration of the vitamin solution from the periphery of the lesion intradermally using from 0.1 to 0.3 ml according to the size of the heloma. The needle is held in its puncture for 2 min before removing it quickly to avoid loss of the injected fluid. Injections are repeated if necessary for 2 to 6 successive weeks.

Surgical treatment (see Chapter 11, Podiatric Surgery) depends to a great degree upon the presence or absence of pathology as visualized on the radiograph. If the distal interphalangeal joint is involved, removal of the middle phalanx is in order (Fig. 6.29). Middle phalangectomy has been used with success by many podiatrists. In this technique, the resection of the middle phalanx enables the podiatrist to bring about a normal alignment when the middle phalanx is disarticulated and removed. The flexion deformity and pressure on the distal end of the toe are corrected.

Another surgical technique, the condylectomy or arthroplasty, is performed by removing the head of the proximal phalanx. A longitudinal or tranverse semielliptical incision is the usual surgical approach to the bone. When the heloma

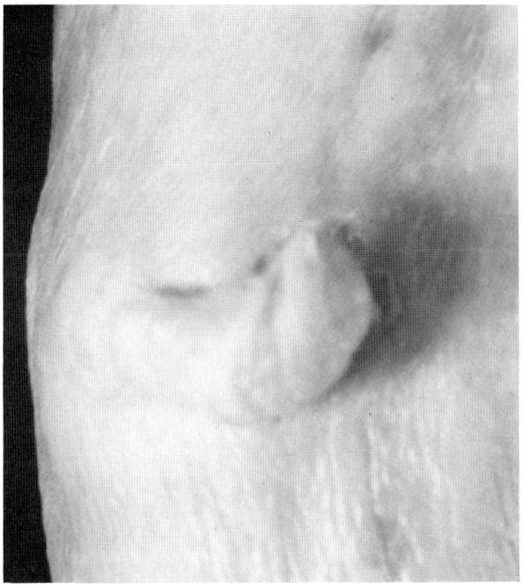

Figure 6.28. Cutaneous horn dorsum first metatarsal head.

occurs on the plantar surface, it may be excised in a similar fashion.

McCain (28) illustrates a technique where the flexor digitorum brevis is severed at its attachments and split; following removal of the proximal phalangeal head, the tendon is carried upward, overlapping and attaching to the neck of the proximal phalanx. As a result the proximal phalanx is brought down to a more horizontal plane.

Polokoff (29) describes his technique of "raspostectomy" in removing exostoses that develop beneath excrescences. Following toe block anesthesia, he makes a small incision in the skin adjacent to the lesion and passes a narrow chisel through the skin opening to the pathology. The exostosis is chiseled down, a file of the necessary size is inserted through the same wound and the exostosis is rasped smooth. The grit and coarseness of the files and rasp depend on the size of the bony prominence. Polokoff states that results have been favorable in 600 "raspostectomies" of lesser toes and 20 subungual exostoses. Osteotripsy is the term for this technique (Fig. 6.30). This minimal incision surgery has been popularized by Probber and Perrone (30) and a growing group of their disciples. Hymes has also demonstrated the value of rasp techniques in podiatry. Power equipment has been developed for definitive minimal incision surgery.

Selecting the proper treatment for the individual pathology is mandatory. There is no special technique or best procedure

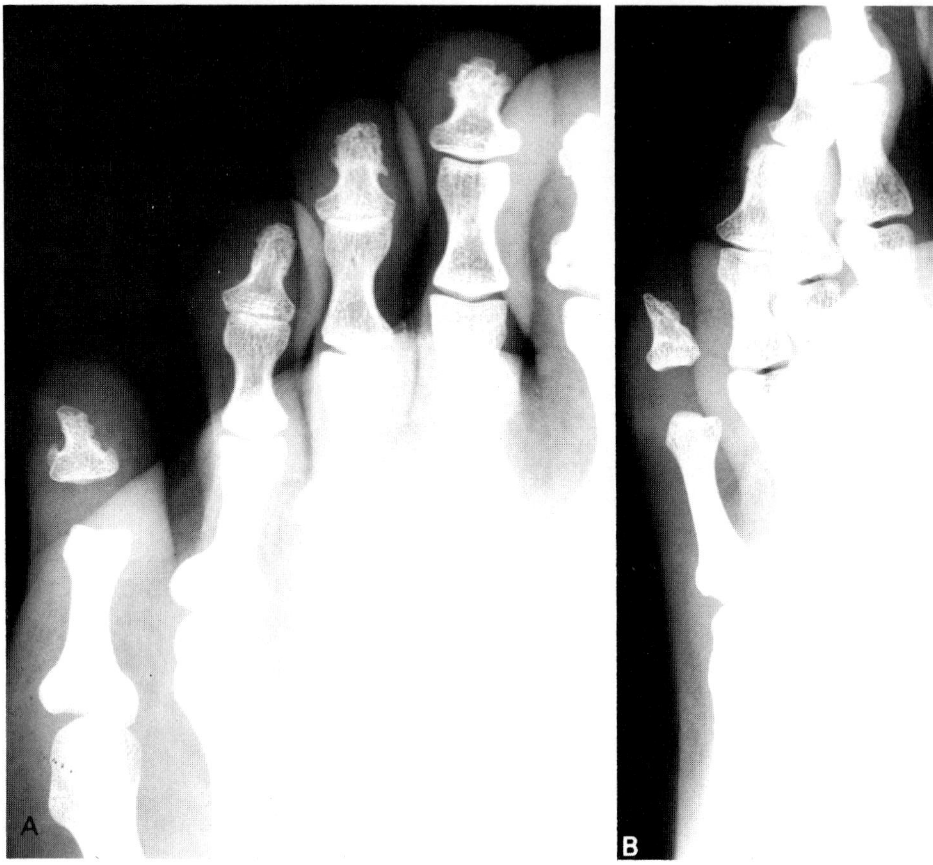

Figure 6.29. Correction of chronic heloma durum, middle phalangectomy fifth toe. *A,* dorsoplantar view; *B,* lateral view.

for eradicating helomas. Levin (31) briefly lists acceptable procedures as follows: condylectomy, midphalangectomy, partial midphalangectomy, complete removal head of proximal phalanx, smoothing of the base of the middle phalanx, and a variety of combinations of the above (Fig. 6.31).

Treatment of helomas on the dorsum of the toes depends on the location, pathology and operative technique. Austin (32) suggested placing a scalpel under the heloma in such a manner as to cut the subheloma fibrous strands. This is done under local anesthesia using a puncture wound at the periphery of the lesion and then inserting the blade.

In the event of contraction of the extensor tendons creating stress on the dorsum of the toe or toes, it is practical to do a tenectomy or tenotomy to bring the toe down to a proper relationship. Very often this procedure is accompanied by a

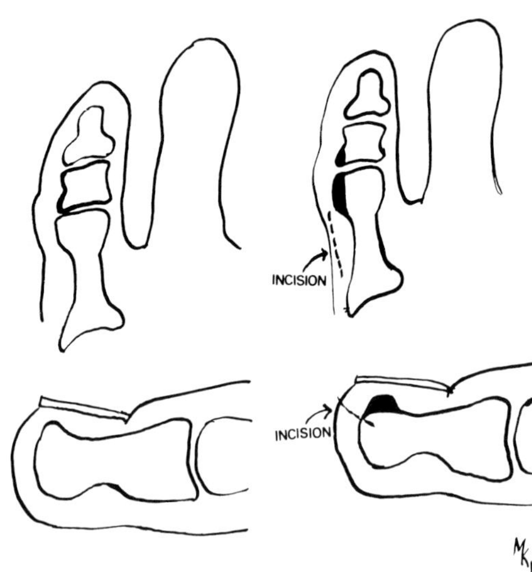

Figure 6.30. Osteotripsy for removal of enlarged condyles at the articular margins of phalanges has proven successful. Note the entrance site for the condyles and also a subungual exostosis. Technique after Polokoff.

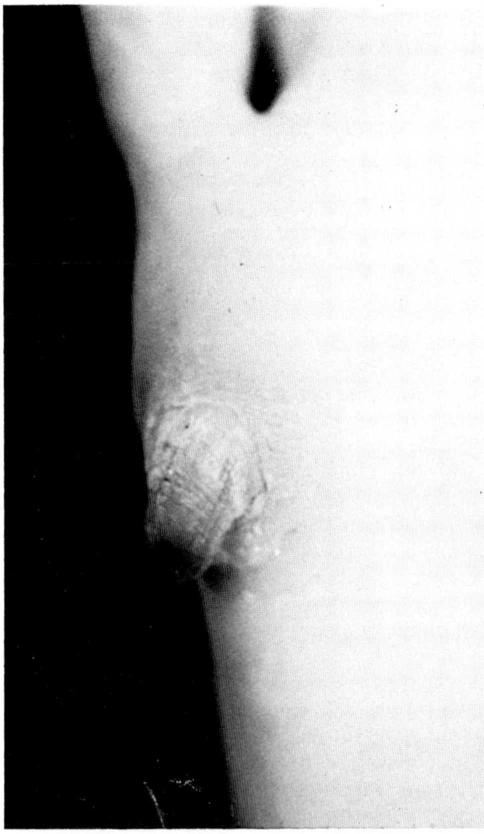

Figure 6.31. Intractable plantar keratosis (heloma) on the head of fifth metatarsal. Treatment is radical excision and suturing. Plantar condylectomy based on x-ray findings. Construction of balanced accommodative orthosis. Skin graft may be indicated.

"Z" plasty of the skin in order to correct the contraction of the skin. Infiltration of anesthesia is effected with a 1% solution of lidocaine. The site selected is about 1⁄16 inch to one side of the extensor tendon over the metatarsophalangeal joint. The incision is only long enough through the skin and superficial fascia to expose the extensor tendon. A 1⁄4-inch incision using a no. 15 blade is usually adequate and least traumatizing. The exposed tendon is grasped by Allis forceps and pulled up into the surgical wound. An incision is made at the distal margin of the forceps through the tendon. The toe is thus released. A second incision on the proximal side of the Allis forceps allows for removal of about 0.5 cm of the extensor tendon.

The author does not believe that the so-called punch tenotomy is a good or adequate technique in most cases. The blind plunge of a narrow scalpel blade through the skin and tendon can prove to be dangerous.

In the punch tenotomy, the skin incision is to one side of the tendon, thereby diminishing the possibility of scar tissue developing over the incised tendon. The incision is small enough to close by sterile Steri-Strips, butterfly suture or a single interrupted subdermal 4-0 dexon suture.

It may be necessary to do a "Z" skin plasty with the tenectomy for best results. Through infiltration, field block or nerve block anesthesia, a longitudinal incision about 1 inch long is made to one side of the tendon and is deepened to include the superficial fascia exposing the tendon; the tendon is grasped by Allis forceps and is incised. A small section is removed as stated above. The dorsal capsule is incised. Subcutaneous closure is accomplished by interrupted 4–0 dexon sutures. The skin is closed with 5–0 nylon. However, the ends of the longitudinal incision are allowed to remain open. The toe is flexed to a maximum, indicating the extent of the tendon correction. The amount of skin contraction is noted, and skin plasty is accomplished to allow further release. A transverse incision about 1⁄4–1⁄2 inch is made through the skin only at right angles and laterally from the distal incision. A second transverse incision as above is made medially to join the proximal end of the long incision. Now when the toe is flexed, the transverse skin incisions open wide, removing the previous restriction. No sutures are used; repair is by second intention while the toe is kept flexed or splinted in a correct position until complete repair takes place. The completed incision looks like a "Z" with the center sutured and the ends healing by second and third intention.

Another approach to the surgical cure of helomas is the removal of the subheloma bursa. The technique is used in the uncomplicated heloma without bone pathology. It is an operative procedure that can be instituted together with the tenectomy. The heloma is excised by the elliptical incision around the excrescence and deeply around the underlying bursa. The skin margins are sutured using 5–0 nylon. Repair is rapid and results are good.

Still another technique is the use of a semielliptical incision around the heloma. The underlying bursa is exposed and dissected out. Any underlying exostosis is removed by rongeur and/or bone rasp. The incision is closed, a dry adaptic dressing is applied and the usual postoperative care is followed. More radical procedures for correction of dorsal heloma are the same ones used for the correction of hammertoes.

The incisional approach for condylectomy may be either longitudinal, elliptical, semielliptical or transverse. These may be a single incision or may take in an elliptical section overlying the affected tissue. The longitudinal incision over a hypertrophied, markedly flexed joint is made on the dorsum of the toe medially or laterally to the hyperplasia. It extends ¼ to ½ inch behind or in front of the joint and exposes the extensor tendons over the neck and head of the proximal phalanx and the base and shaft of the middle phalanx.

The transverse elliptical incisions are made directly in front of the highest point in the hypertrophied joint and in front of and behind the heloma. The incision is confined to the dorsum of the toe, and care is taken not to incise the digital vessels on either side of the toe.

If a chronic heloma and/or bursa is to be resected, an elliptical incision is made around the lesion as previously described and a section of tissue is removed. This incision may be either longitudinal or transverse. The dorsal aponeurosis is thus exposed. Here a transverse incision is made through the flat fibrotendinous tissue and the joint capsule. It is wise to make this incision anterior to the prominence of the joint because experience has shown that the lipping at the joint margin obscures the joint space. Such an incision facilitates easy division of the articular ligaments. Also, one must keep the scalpel close to the bone to avoid damage to the circulatory supply. Transverse incisions are then made through the lateral collateral ligaments on either side of the joint resulting in an immediate release of the articulations. The head of the proximal phalanx is delivered up through the surgical wound. The capsule is retracted and the neck exposed. The head and neck are excised by bone rongeur, forceps or saw. The margins are rasped smooth and corners are rounded. Care must be taken to remove all bone fragments and debris from the wound. Flushing with physiological saline is advisable. A trial coaptation is made, and if there is a restriction to correction or to motion, more bone should be removed. Locke and Strauss (33) recommend local instillation of corticosteroids in minimal dosage for reduction of postoperative pain and edema.

The author uses interrupted sutures exclusively in uncomplicated digital surgery. A single, deep vertical mattress suture may be used for closure of the joint. If the incisions have been transverse, the capsule may be picked up with a vertical mattress or interrupted deep suture. Further closure is based on one's appreciation of the need. Sutures are actual splints for the toe, and skillful closure facilitates maintenance of position and early uneventful repair.

A middle phalangectomy is accomplished as above. incisions are the same. However, the dissection of the middle phalanx must be close to the bone to avoid the digital vessels. A good technique makes for minimal trauma and rapid repair. The author's experiences has shown that a middle phalangectomy is less traumatizing than resection of the head of the proximal phalanx (Fig. 6.32). Thus, when faced with a choice of surgical technique for correction of hammertoe, removal of the middle phalanx is advised. This is especially desirable if the middle phalanx is short.

Kaplan (34) corrected overlapping toes by detaching the extensor digitorum tendon from its attachment to the proximal and middle phalanx. The head of the proximal phalanx is resected, a capsulotomy at the metatarsophalangeal joint is performed and the extensor tendon is sutured to the proximal third of the proximal phalanx. The skin is closed, and an elliptical section of tissue is removed on the plantar surface of the toe at the crease in the web. The toe is then sutured down into position.

Proximal phalangectomy can be used to correct a hammertoe with a dislocation dorsally at the metatarsophalangeal joint. The author does not believe this surgery should be used—except on special occasions—in hammertoes involving the interphalangeal joint. The approach to proximal phalangectomy may be a dorsal, medial or lateral plantar longitudinal incision. The dorsal approach is as described for hammertoe except that the incision is extended back over the metatarsophalangeal joint. The proximal phalanx is sharply dissected out, and if damaged, the tendon tissue is repaired with 4–0 dexon. The skin is closed in the usual manner. This results in an unstable toe unless surgical syndactyly to an adjoining toe is accomplished.

The lateral or medial plantar approach is made by an incision along the side of the shaft of the proximal phalanx. The phalanx is disected out, and the toe is surgically syndactylised to the adjacent toe.

Whatever the approach or technique, the foot surgeon must evaluate the need for either severing or lengthening the flexor digitorum longus tendon. A "Z" plasty on the plantar skin may also be necessary to obtain correction.

Fusion or arthrodesis is accomplished by removing the head of the proximal phalanx and the base of the middle. Thus, the two opposing bleeding surfaces are free of cartilage and are opposed. According to the author's experience, the use of a Kirschner wire is unnecessary for these small joints. Splinting of the part following suturing usually suffices to bring about arthrodesis. The use of bone cement may also serve to obtain fusion.

Subotnick (35) in a well-illustrated but brief dissertation on the etiology and treatment of digital deformities, describes a variety of bone and soft tissue deformities of both young and elderly patients that are amenable to surgical correction. Subotnick concludes that "resection arthroplasties" are suitable for younger patients, and

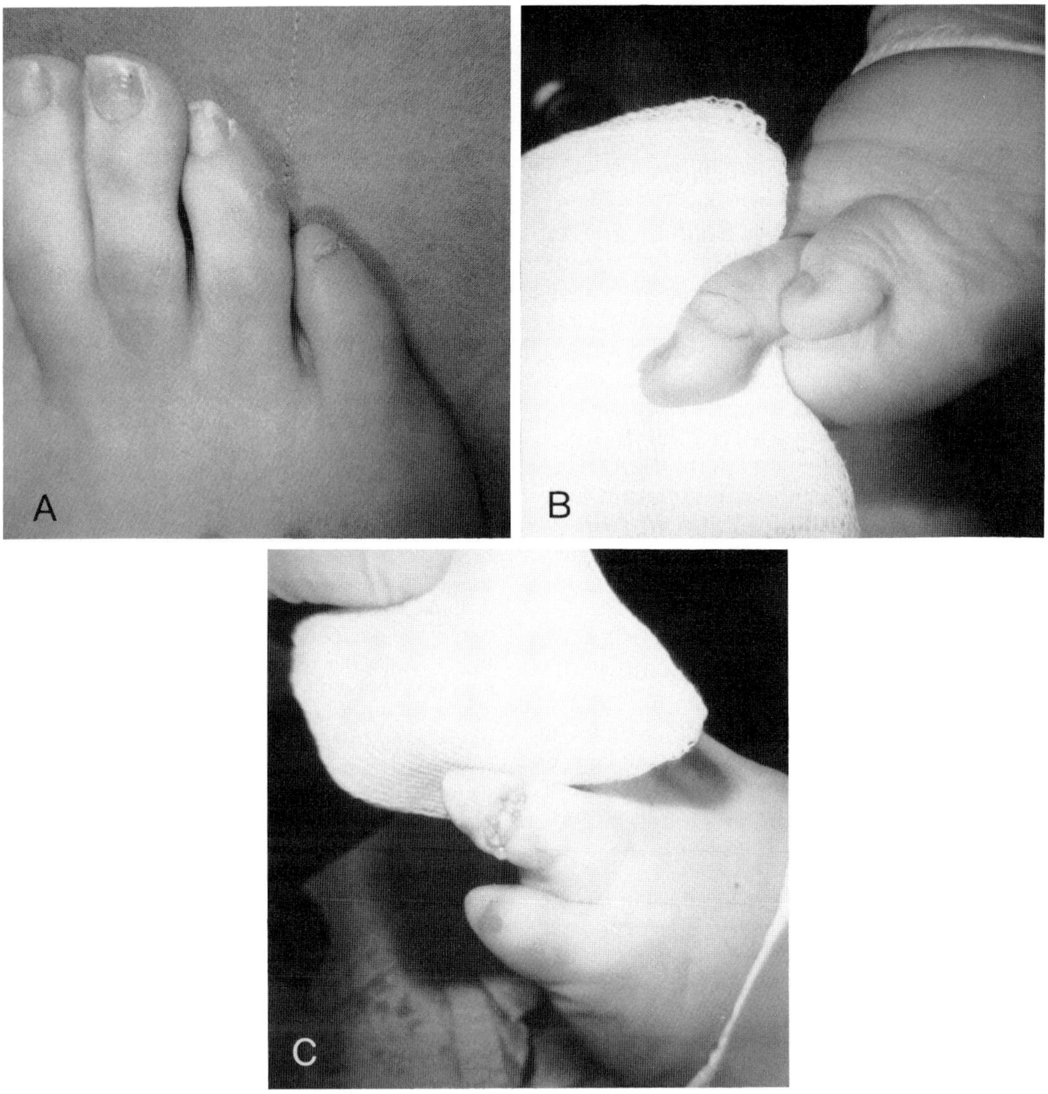

Figure 6.32. *A,* Heloma durum overlying middle phalanx on varus fourth toe. *B* and *C,* Skin plasty with excision of middle phalanx for correction.

soft tissue "palliative surgery" is recommended for the geriatric patient. This article is an historical approach to an ever-improving surgical technology.

Medication. Preoperative medication must provide mild sedation and rest for the anxious patient. Diazapem (Valium), 5 mg, the night before surgery and 5 mg 1 hr before anesthesia may help relieve a patient's anxiety. Short-acting barbiturates are helpful preoperatively. Pentobarbital (Nembutal), in 30, 50 and 100 mg capsules or by injection and secobarbital (Seconal), 50 and 100 mg capsules, provide the desired effects.

In foot surgery that is traumatizing, administration of anti-inflammatory enzymes 24 hr before surgery and after surgery helps reduce pain and swelling. Chymoral tablets, 100 mg bid, Papase, Orenzyme and other natural enzymes are absorbed readily when taken 1 hr before mealtime.

Postoperative daytime sedation may be provided by Valium, 2½ to 5 mg, tid after meals. Other nonbarbiturates for postoperative rest are ethinomate (Valmid), 0.5 mg, and ethchloroynol (Placidyl) in 100, 200 and 500 mg capsules.

Analgesics and sedatives essential for relief of pain are described in detail elsewhere in this text.

Keratotic Implants

Often after surgery on the foot or the nails, fine, deep-seated, horny plugs of cornified tissue develop at the site of suture markings. Faulty technique in suturing skin may result in a few dermal cells being carried deeply into the subcutaneous tissue where they begin to grow. A dull hypodermic or suture needle or poor apposition of the skin may create this problem. Radical nail surgery with removal of the nail lip may result in subsequent epithelial implants when technique is faulty. In the subcutaneous tissue the displaced cells grow and proliferate, producing an irritating sharp implant. The presence of a low-grade inflammation that is aggravated by pressure and friction is noted early at the previous site of surgery or at the suture markings. Dry skin is an etiologic factor.

These implants differ from the ordinary heloma in that they grow from within outward to the external surface. When removed they usually measure 0.75 to 1 cm in length and rarely exceed 2 mm in diameter. Usually, they are straight and long, but often curve with the outline of subcutaneous structures such as bone.

The author has found that frictionizing the affected skin area with a sanding burr separates the implant from the surrounding tissue and allows for easy removal by scalpel or tissue forceps.

Field block or infiltrating anesthesia followed by sharp curettage or sharp excision is often a successful procedure. Local intradermal injections of aqueous solutions of vitamin A, 50,000 USP units, have proven helpful. Subcutaneous injections of a nonacetylated corticosteroid may relieve discomfort.

Electrodessication, fulgeration or coagulation followed by sharp curettage of the necrotic tissue may destroy the lesion. Good judgment must be exercised when a lesion is over a bony prominence or prominent weightbearing area.

Shielding and padding the painful lesion are indicated. The use of foot orthoses to accommodate the pathology is necessary where there is a loss of adipose tissue.

Treatment of keratotic implants may include treatment for extremely dry skin (Fig. 6.33). A vitamin deficiency should be corrected by prescribing emollients, such as oils, 20% urea cream, lanolin and Acid Mantle-based vitamin A creams. These emollients are fortified by daily oral use of 50,000 units of high-potency vitamin A capsules. Foot baths in moisturizing agent-reinforced solutions are generally helpful. A variety of bath oils and over-the-counter or prescribed products for dry skin may be used.

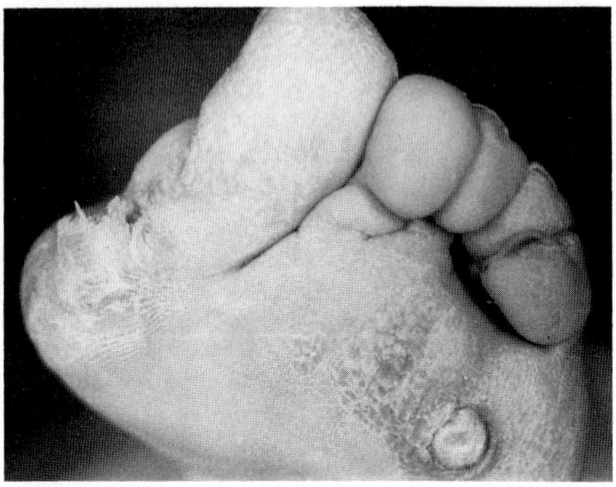

Figure 6.33. Keratotic implant—tyloma, dry skin at base of rotated hallux. Deep keratoma of the fourth metatarsal. Anidrosis—arteriosclerosis.

If it is necessary to remove chronic keratotic plugs, they may be burned out with strong keratolytics and acids capable of creating a liquefaction necrosis. Monochloroacetic acid, bichloracetic acid, fuming nitric acid, salicylic acid in highly concentrated 20 to 70% strengths and compounds of vesicants such as cantharides may be used.

It is occasionally necessary to apply 20 to 40% salicylic acid to the lesion in a plaster. The patient returns in 5 days, the foot is soaked in warm water and the implant may lift out with the plaster. Several treatments may be indicated, and sharp section or curettage may be necessary to complete the treatment. Occasionally the keratotic implant has a large inclusion cyst attached to its base. Metatarsal osteotomy is often indicated.

Heloma Milliare

Miliary helomas consist of multiple localized spotty areas of hyperkeratosis measuring about 1 to 3 mm in diameter (Fig. 6.34). They are found alone or in tylomas, helomas or tissues that are markedly anhydrotic. They occur on the plantar surface of the balls and heels of the feet, but are capable of developing on any site. Occasionally miliary helomas are located over a hallux joint, in a heloma or tyloma on the dorsum and distal ends of the toes.

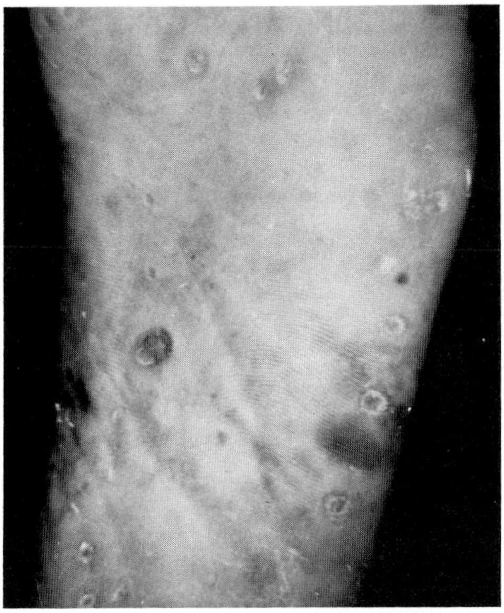

Figure 6.34. Diffuse heloma milliare.

Pathogenesis

Either single or multiple lesions are noted over weightbearing areas with tylomas and helomas. The skin is dry and presents a marked scaling and hyperkeratosis over areas that are not necessarily subjected to trauma. Miliary helomas are pearly-white to yellow, pinpoint to pinhead in size. They are multiple, deeply imbedded hyperkeratotic lesions in the feet and often on the palms at sites of friction and pressure. Mibelli lesions, according to Wheeless (36), become hyperkeratotic and slowly enlarge to a diameter of 1 to 2 cm. coalescing to form larger plaques. They may become verruca-like and itch and break down at the heel, causing deep fissures. Mullens (37) noted resolution of this lesion following 3 to 5 injections of vitamin A (Steinberg's solution) beneath the lesion. Hall (38) anesthetized and injected the solution from the dorsum to the plantar, depositing the medication subjacent to the lesion. Locke (22) advised the injection of corticosteroids beneath this recalcitrant lesion. Results appeared promising at that time. To date, corticosteroids have proven helpful in eradicating the lesion or relieving pain for longer periods of time following treatment. The author prefers to anesthetize the lesion by field block and inject a corticosteroid sublesionally. About 0.2 to 0.3 ml of a dexamethasone solution is the average dosage required for relief of pain.

Injection techniques are of no value in the presence of an inclusion cyst.

Etiology

It is believed that loose threads in hose or irregularity in insoles may contribute to this lesion. Evidence of this type of keratosis has been observed in patients suffering from avitaminosis A.

Trice (39) noted complete resolution of miliary helomas in patients undergoing treatment for fungus infections. In further studies, he cited cures of this condition in 25 cases using undecylenic acid compounds and other forms of antimycotic treatment. Of those 25 cases 23 exhibited microscopic evidence of fungus conditions, and 21 had clinical evidence of the disease.

Treatment. To treat miliary helomas, the tissue is softened with a keratolytic solution. Each lesion is enucleated by scalpel or sharp tissue forceps using sharp section, sharp curettage or sharply pointed tissue forceps. Antimycotic treatment as prescribed by Trice (39) may be used. Kleiman (40) applied a 10% silver nitrate ointment with good results. Sharp curettage under local anesthesia may cure the lesions.

Heloma Neurofibrosum

Heloma neurofibrosum is the common name of lesions that pathologically resemble verrucas, but in clinical appearance look like helomas with ill-defined hyperkeratotic margins and a central core of fibrous, verrucoid tissue. It is an excruciatingly painful lesion with a throbbing, burning and stabbing pain found in the area of extreme friction and pressure or at a site of direct trauma. The underlying heloma takes on a yellowish-gray to white appearance with vascular elements that appear to be a superficial plexus of nerves following along the course of the capillary plexus in the skin.

Pathogenesis

The heloma neurofibrosum has a rather irregular outline and an appearance of hyperkeratosis that differs from the usual heloma. It is both superficial and deep, with hypertrophy of the capillary layer and extreme fibrosis of the deeper layers of the skin. This neurofibrous lesion may be related to warty masses, and it may also be secondary to tylomas that have hemorrhaged or been irritated from injudicious cutting or extremes of trauma. The lesion is very often seen in a patient with endocrine disorders and is often characterized by its mosaic appearance and fibrous characteristics. It may occur at points of great friction and pressure, such as the dorsum of the fifth toe, medial aspect of the hallux joint, lateral aspect of the fifth metatarsophalangeal joint and the plantar of the first and fifth metatarsal head. On surgical resection of these lesions where the heloma was localized, compact and conical, the author has noted that an underlying bursa and frequently an inclusion cyst were present in the deeper layers of the skin. Resection of these tissues cures the condition.

Treatment. There are several approaches to removal of a heloma neurofibrosum. One method involves debridement of the overlying callus to expose the painful lesion. This is followed by the application of concentrated silver nitrate and 40% salicylic acid plaster slightly larger than the mass. The patient returns in 3 to 5 days, and the necrotic tissue is removed by sharp section. Treatment is repeated until the entire verrucoid lesion is cleared of pathological tissue. However, other escharotics may also be used to destroy the pathological tissue. Sixty percent salicylic acid in a suitable base, pyrogallic acid and many vesicants, such as cantharides, dry ice and monochloroacetic acid, have been used. Liquefaction necrosis often occurs.

It has been the author's experience that, if the lesion is excruciatingly painful under careful treatment, a subcutaneous inclusion cyst may be found in the center of the lesion. Its superficial, sharply demarcated, white fibrous elements is deceiving. A local anesthetic and deep probing often uncover an inclusion cyst beneath the corium.

Another approach to treating heloma neurofibrosum consists of local anesthesia by nerve block or field block followed by excision by sharp section or curettage of the pathological tissue. The wound is cauterized by electrodesiccation and a dry dressing is applied.

The author has excised these lesions by removing an elliptical section of tissue including an underlying inclusion cyst, chronic bursa or fibrolipomatous mass. The wound requires suturing in most cases, but sometimes may be allowed to granulate in by third intention. Gelfoam controls bleeding.

Permanent results may require supportive therapy, such as foot orthoses, for relieving pressure on the affected part.

Heloma Vascularis

Heloma vascularis is similar to heloma durum, but the hyperkeratotic tissue becomes hemorrhagic. The extravasations, which stand out as orange, red to yellow linear discolorations, are separated by a callus and covered with dry or moist hyperkeratotic tissue.

The pathogenesis of heloma vascularis is similar to that of heloma durum with this exception: The presence of vascular elements within the heloma may be secondary to severe pressure and friction or injudicious cutting of the heloma. On occasion, the splitting of the superficial capillaries beneath the heloma may be secondary to systemic disorders that create fragility of the capillaries. These disorders may be classified as metabolic, endocrine or circulatory disturbances of the extremities. The presence of vascular elements may also be the result of previous infection with resultant hypertrophy of the papillary layer of the skin.

The pain in this lesion is more severe than that of a typical heloma durum. The pain may be excruciating and sometimes throbbing and burning in nature. The usual site for the development of these lesions is at points of great pressure, such as the dorsum of the fifth toe, the plantar surface of the first and fifth metatarsal heads, the distal ends of the lesser toes or the plantar surface of the interphalangeal joint of the hallux. These lesions may be compact, conical, vascular, hyperkeratotic masses. They are characterized by the presence of capillary loops and a coagulum beneath and within the hyperkeratotic mass. The surrounding tissues may be mildly red due to inflammatory changes. A sinus tract may be found along the course of one of the capillary loops.

Pathogenesis

The presence of a heloma durum with underlying capillary loops that appear thickened, together with a hemorrhagic coagulum within the hyperkeratotic mass, is typical of heloma vascularis.

Treatment. Debriding the hyperkeratotic tissue without creating hemorrhage often relieves pain in these lesions. The metabolism of the localized tissue must be decreased, the hypertrophied capillaries should be destroyed or decreased in size and the underlying systemic problems must be treated to alleviate capillary fragility. Subhelomal ulceration may be present. Shielding and padding of the part are used to relieve continuing trauma. The construction of orthoses designed to remove pressure from the part is also indicated. Large doses of vitamin C and systemic medications for reducing capillary fragility are helpful. In the acute phases of this lesion, adequate protection and use of 25 to 50% silver nitrate stick or solution decrease the size of the hypertrophied capillary layer of the skin. If the patient is a good surgical risk, it is often advisable to perform corrective surgery as in a heloma durum. Surgery must include complete dissection of the pathological tissue.

Occasionally, painful helomas or tylomas become infected, and the patient develops cellulitis, lymphadenopathy, lymphangitis, ulceration or even gangrene. Antibiotic therapy is given when infection is present. Treatment of local infections may be by warm saline soaks or with betadine soaks as a wet dressing. Enzymatic debridement using an antibiotic-enzyme combination is useful.

Systemic antibiotics are prescribed as dictated by bacterial sensitivity and extension of the infection, cellulitis and evidence of systemic symptoms. Penicillinase resistant penicillin, tetracycline, erythromycin and cephalexin monohydrate (Keflex) are often useful systemically where needed to combat sensitive bacteria.

Topical antibiotics, such as Bacitracin, neomycin, gentamicin sulfate (Garamycin) and corticosteroids, may be necessary. Nitrofurazone as Furacin may be used as a pad, powder, solution, cream, soluble dressing or stretch gauze roll. Nitrofurazone is available with hydrocortisone or as a cream.

Locke (41) recommended shoe sponging as an aid in removing pressure from plantar lesions. The technique consists of applying an indelible marking on the sole of the foot at the site of the painful lesion and having the patient step into the shoe to locate the site on the insole that falls beneath the lesion. When this area is located, the site of weight transfer is ground out of the insole into the shoe filler by a drill. A piece of sponge is cemented into the ground-out section of the insole, enabling the patient to walk in comfort. The ground-out insole area should be larger than the lesion to provide for movement during gait.

Heloma Molle

A heloma molle or soft corn is essentially a heloma that has absorbed a considerable amount of skin moisture, which produces a slight edema and increased dermal pressure (Figs. 6.35 and 6.36). The skin may have a dull redness that progresses to acute irritation and a bullous lesion that may eventually dry, become atrophied and develop into a mild hyperkeratosis. Continued pressure results in an additional moist, hyperkeratotic mass developing over the primary site of irritation. In the presence of moisture, pressure may create a heloma molle, usually on the interdigital abutting surfaces of the toes. The lesion may be white, gray or yellow and spongy in texture. It may be localized and circumscribed over a bony enlargement, usually the head of the proximal phalanx of the fifth toe or at the base and the head of the proximal phalanx of the fourth toe. On occasion, a diffuse type of excrescence may develop within the web itself secondary to friction in that area. Secondary infections are common with cellulitis and the development of ulcerations and sinus

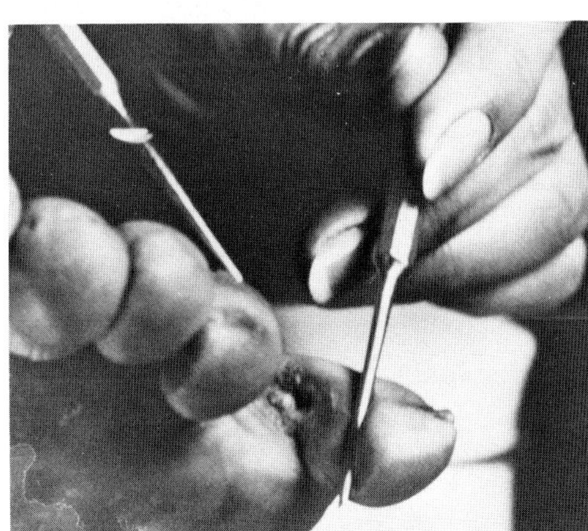

Figure 6.35. Ulcerated heloma molle.

tracts. A heloma molle may develop between any of the toes, especially where excessive perspiration has been permitted. Cellulitis, lymphangitis, inguinal lymphadenopathy and osteomyelitis are not uncommon with infection of the soft tissues.

Palliative Treatment. The affected tissue may be resected by the judicious use of a scalpel and a tissue forceps. Many podiatrists use a special instrument called a soft corn spoon that is quite effective in the resection of this spongy hyperkeratosis. Following debridement of the hyperkeratotic tissue, the hyperidrotic underlying skin may be dried thoroughly by the use of a 5 to 10% silver nitrate solution. This solution also decreases the metabolism of the skin. Protecting the opposing toe surfaces by inserting lamb's wool, foam rubber, moldable podiatric compound or a similar substance may be quite effective in relieving irritation. When an ulceration or sinus infection exists beneath the excrescence, it is wise to use an antibiotic to control infection. Wet dressings of an astringent, such as potassium permanganate or aluminum subacetate solution, should also be used in such cases.

The physical treatment of a heloma molle may necessitate the shielding and padding of the excrescence and the underlying enlargement of bone. It may also require the use of an anti-inflammant to decrease the inflammatory changes within a bursa common over the bony enlargement under the heloma itself (Figs. 6.37 and 6.38). Very often the elevation of the fourth metatarsal has a tendency to alter the relationship of the fourth and fifth toes, eliminating some of the abnormal pressure that exists. Certainly the removal of such irritating forces as ill-fitting footgear, including stretch hose, is indicated.

Surgical Treatment. Many of the surgical techniques used for removing a heloma durum are indicated in the treatment of a complicated heloma molle. However, where an exostosis exists, an incision should be made over an area that is not easily irritated or aggravated by friction or pressure from adjacent toes. Occasionally, resection of the base of the proximal phalanx of the fourth toe is indicated. Resection of the head of the proximal phalanx of the fourth toe is often necessary where there is hypertrophy of the head or an exostosis. Resection of the proximal interphalangeal joint of the fifth toe for the permanent removal of a heloma durum is equally effective for removal of some soft corns. A surgical syndactyly of the abutting toes is useful in some intractable cases (42).

Surgical excision by "raspostectomy" or osteotripsy has proven successful in some cases.

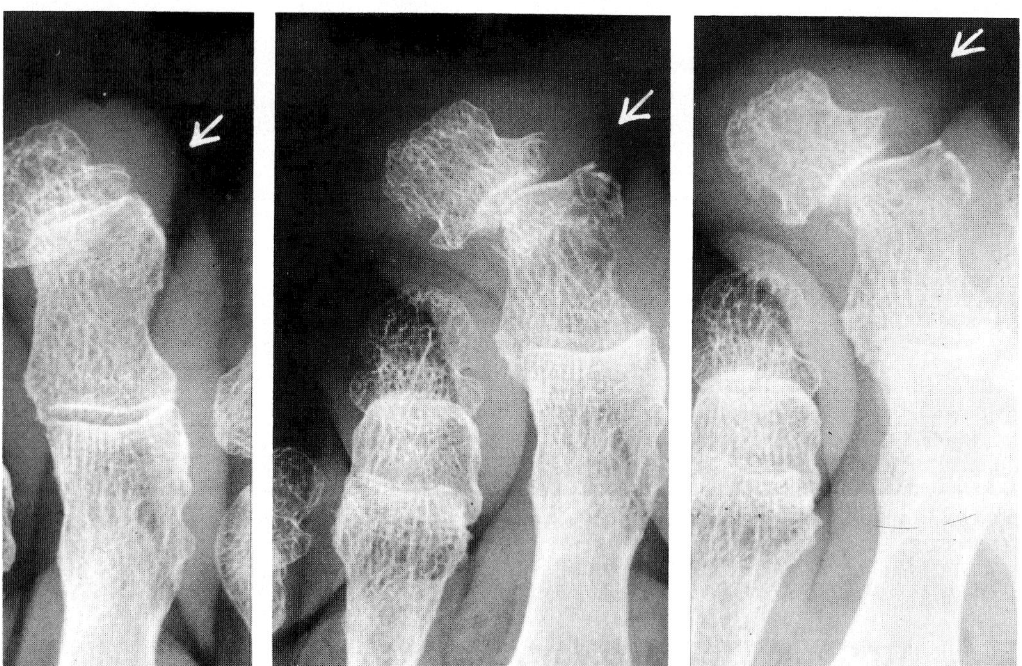

Figure 6.36. Infected heloma molle, sinus tract, and osteomyelitis distal interphalangeal joint. As destruction increases, the joint becomes dislocated. (From FO Gamble and I Yale: *Clinical Foot Roentgenology.* Baltimore, Williams & Wilkins, 1966.)

Tyloma

A tyloma or callus is a broad-based hyperkeratotic mass commonly found at the ball of the foot at a site of friction, irritation or pressure (Fig. 6.39). It occurs often over a bony enlargement or at a site of abnormal weight distribution. Symptoms include burning, tenderness or a throbbing ache.

Common sites for a tyloma may be at the perimeter of the heel, at the medial aspect of the heel, at the talar head or a prominent tuberosity of the navicular, the dorsal surface of the first metatarsocuneiform joint, the medial aspect of the hallux joint, the plantar medial aspect of the first metatarsophalangeal joint, the medial and plantar aspect of the great toe, the plantar surfaces of each of the metatarsal heads, especially under the first, second and fifth heads, the lateral aspect of the fifth metatarsal head and occasionally at a prominent base of the fifth metatarsal. The yellowish-gray lesion is flat, often raised and spread over a wide area (Figs. 6.40 and 6.41).

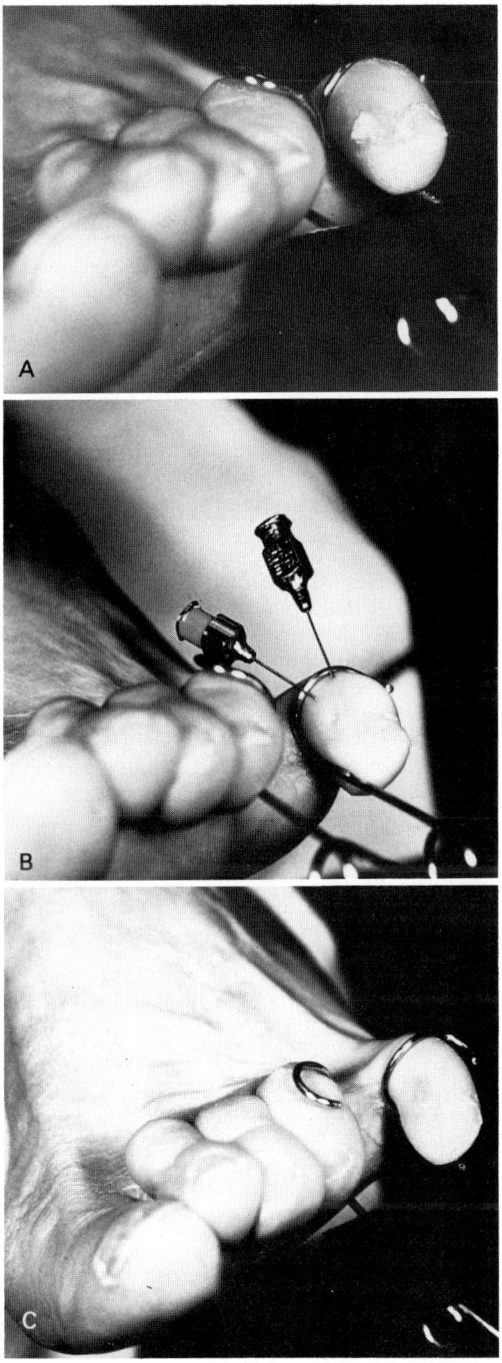

Figure 6.37. Treatment of heloma molle. *A*, lesion; *B*, anesthesia and injection of corticosteroid; *C*, regression of lesion. (Courtesy of RK Locke.)

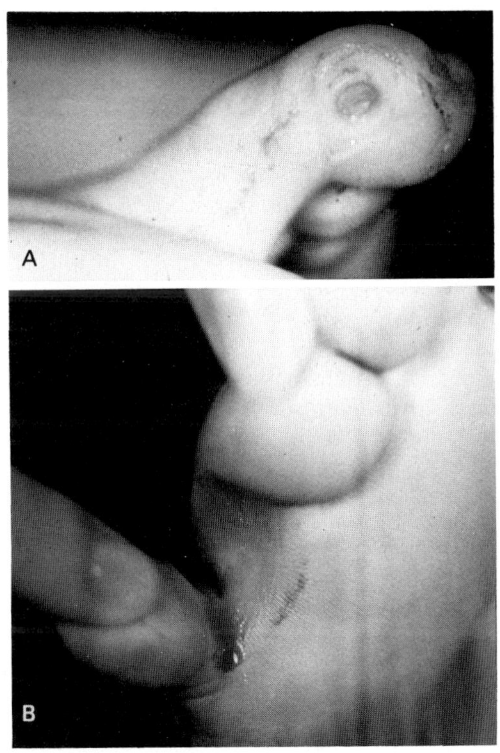

Figure 6.38. *A*, Ulceration secondary to multiple minimal trauma in diabetic patient with heloma molles. *B*, Infected fourth interdigital space. Staphylococcus cellulitis secondary to infected heloma molle.

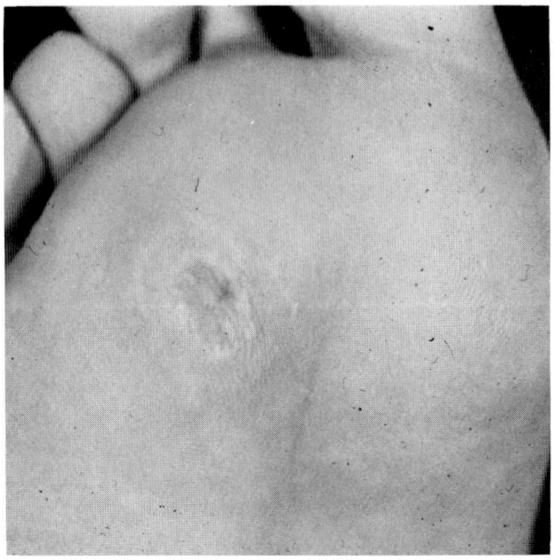

Figure 6.39. Typical tyloma.

Pathogenesis

At first a hyperemia is present, followed by a thickening of the skin. Later a packing down of the superficial layers of the skin is noted as desquamation takes place, creating a broad hyperkeratotic mass. Unlike the discrete margins of helomas, the margins of tylomas are not clearly defined. Surgical reduction may reveal an adventitious bursa; sometimes a sinus or suppurating ulceration is found beneath the thickened callus tissue. An intractable plantar keratosis is often a complication of a simple tyloma.

Microscopic examination shows hyperemia with increased epithelial cell formation, cornification with dehydration of the localized tissue and atrophy of the sudoriferous glands (Fig. 6.42).

X-ray examination of the foot may disclose a biomechanical problem resulting in abnormal stress on the affected parts. There may also be an exostosis present or calcareous deposit on the bone or within the soft tissues beneath the affected part.

Palliative treatment of painful tylomas is generally used concomitantly with measures to correct the etiologic basis for the development of the lesion because the callus is the objective reaction to the stress of friction, pressure and irritation caused by faulty weight distribution and deforming pathology.

The following procedures are used in palliative treatment of tylomas. Absorbent cotton is placed over the thickened excresence, and a suitable liquid antiseptic keratolytic agent is applied to the cotton and allowed to remain for at least 3 min. The agent used may be an aqueous solution of 2 to 5% phenol, a solution of tincture of green soap in warm water, a softening and wetting agent, moisturizing solutions, hydrogen peroxide, or one of the numerous commercial products compounded for this purpose. The ideal solution is one that has the properties of being keratolytic, antiseptic, germicidal, analgesic and relatively nonsensitizing.

After the initial contact with the softened callused tissue, the moist cotton is removed, and a suitable instrument is used to debride and excise the tyloma. Some podiatrists use chisel blades; others prefer a scalpel. Electrically powered burrs and disks may also be used (Fig. 6.43).

Surgical Treatment. Two surgical techniques are commonly used to reduce tylomas. Total excision of the tyloma in one section requires an initial incision at a line of demarcation at the periphery. This initial incision loosens and separates the pathological mass from the underlying healthy skin. The loosened margin is grasped with forceps, hemostat or thumb forceps held with the left hand and gently retracted. As the tyloma is retracted, the blade of the scalpel or chisel in the right hand follows the line of cleavage between the pathological hyperkeratosis and the pink, healthy underlying skin. As the scalpel advances, the tyloma is gently pulled up and away until the entire mass is removed (Fig. 6.44). This technique is only suitable for thick tylomas and deep-seated nuclei.

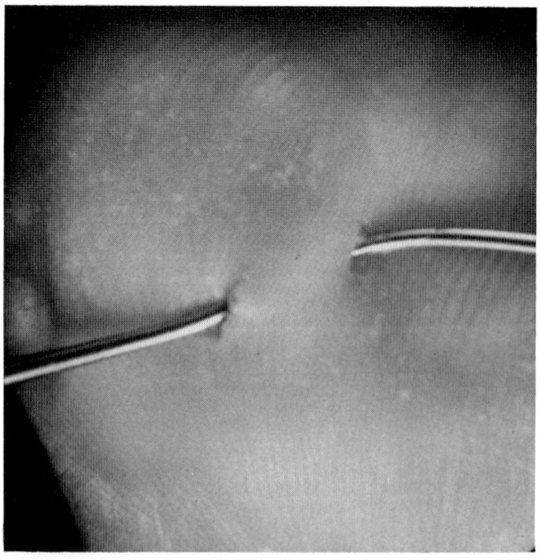

Figure 6.40. Spontaneous rupture of epidermoid cyst through sinus tract in tyloma.

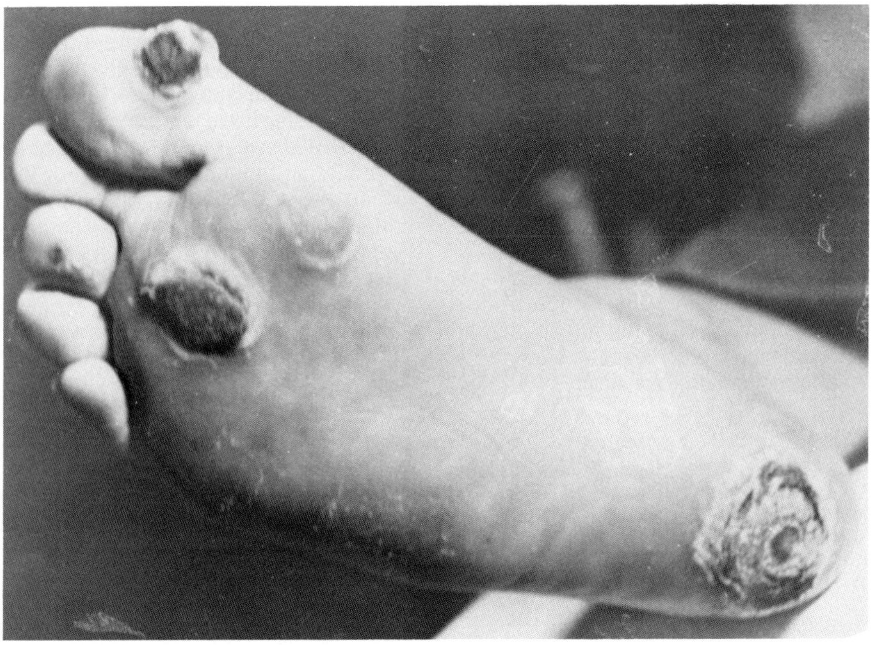

Figure 6.41. Large hyperkeratotic lesions overlying verrucoid masses.

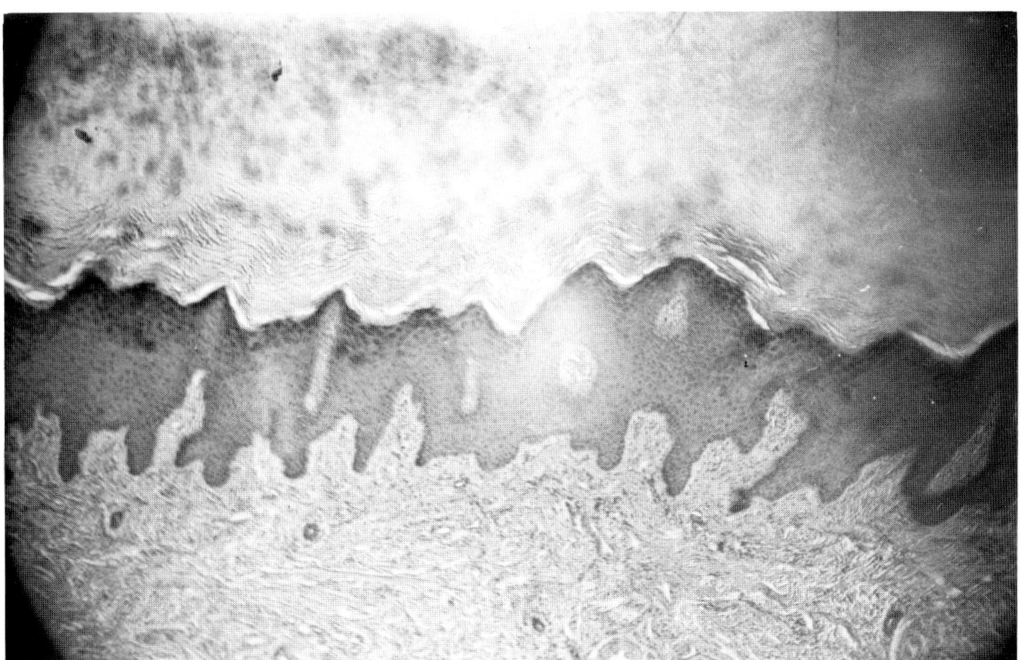

Figure 6.42. Low-power cross-section, plantar tyloma. Note thickened corneum (hyperplasia); exaggerated and hyperchromatic stratum granulosum (dysplasia); engorgement, edema, cloudy swelling of dermis. (Courtesy AT Sharpe, Department of Pathology, Pennsylvania College of Podiatric Medicine.)

Woolf (43) reports favorable results with the use of Ureacin-20 cream. Sixty patients were treated with Ureacin-20 cream after enucleation of a plantar keratoma over a prescribed period of time. In 40 patients the plantar keratoma was resolved. Eight lesions were greatly improved. The remaining cases were lost to follow-up.

The second method of surgical treatment is universally used by podiatrists and consists of removing the softened tyloma by scalpel or chisel in small slices. The skill of the Podiatrist is demonstrated by his or her knowledge of how deep to cut and how close to debride the hyperkeratosis in order to obtain relief of symptoms. The technique requires the sensitivity of a violinist to feel the different textures of the underlying tissues through the operative instrument. Proper wrist motion, finger dexterity and sensory perception are developed only after years of practice. The palliative surgical debridement of inflamed tylomas may be necessary as often as monthly or as infrequently as four times a year when the patient has diabetes, collagen disorder, arterial insufficiency, vascular compromise, severe foot deformity, morbid obesity, endocrine disorder, plantar forefoot fatty pad deficit, or any condition that prevents deeper surgical intervention.

Other methods for debriding heavy keratoses are the use of such keratolytic agents as salicylic

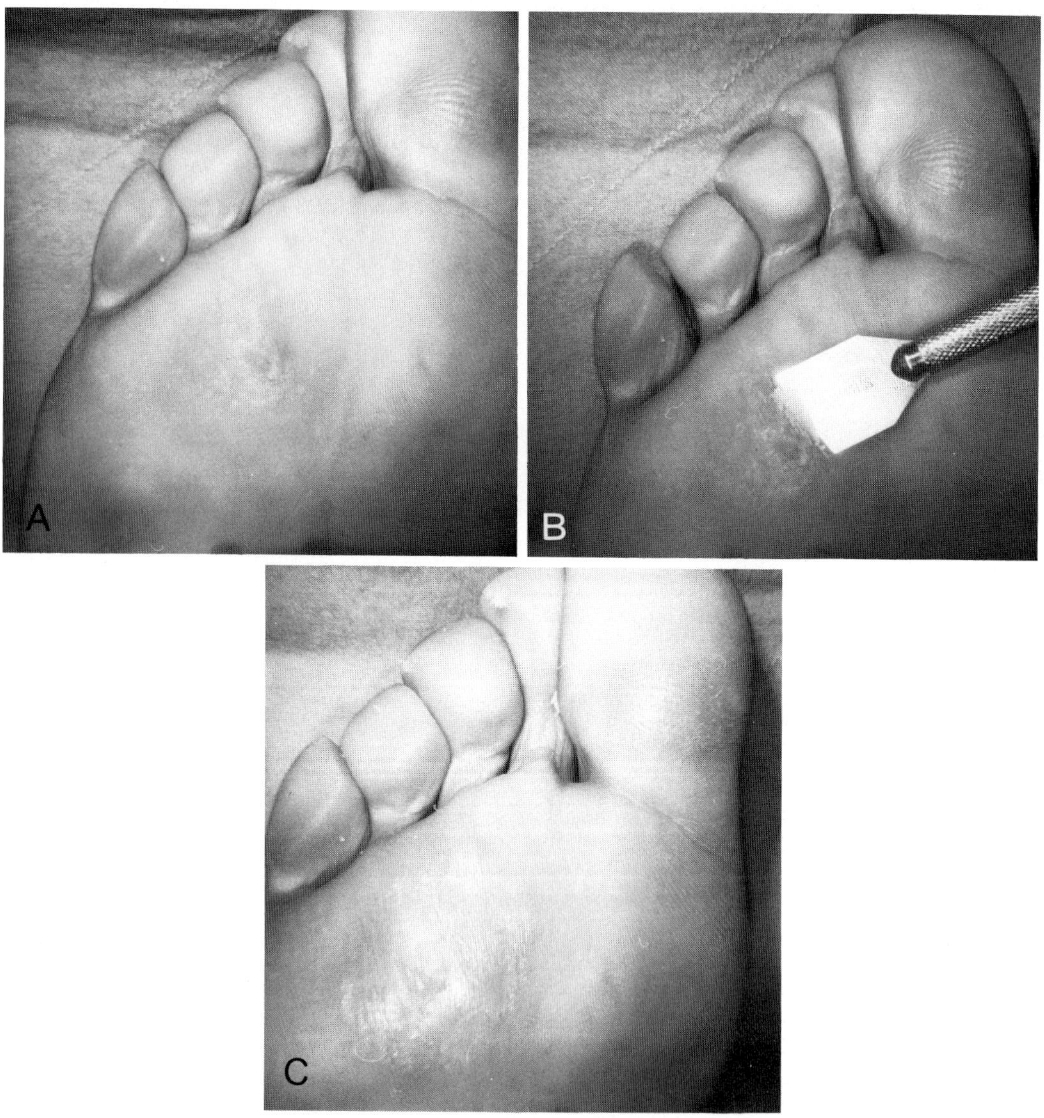

Figure 6.43. *A,* Plantar tyloma. *B,* Aseptic debridement with no. 312 chisel blade. *C,* Postdebridement.

acid in 10 to 30% solutions or ointments. Twenty to 40% salicylic acid plaster is often applied to a tyloma for 3 to 5 days, followed by hot soaks and removal of the white necrotic tissue by sharp scalpel.

Some foot specialists use a podiatric drill with a diamond or steel burr and a variety of fine and coarse sandpaper disks to debride the painful lesion dependent on skin texture.

Balkin (44), in a preliminary report, discussed the use of liquid silicone injections beneath the plantar keratosis. Local anesthesia is induced by field block or posterior tibial nerve block. An 18 gauge needle is used to remove the liquid silicone from its vial. Using a 25 gauge 1 inch needle, 0.5 to 1.0 ml of the silicone preparation is deposited beneath the lesion from a proximal insertion of the needle. Doing so minimizes migration of the solution because the tendency in walking is to force the fluid forward. This treatment with refinements may prove to be most effective in the resolution of plantar keratosis. A new subdermal collagen (keragen) injected between the skin and boney prominence shows promise for the temporary and sometimes permanent relief from painful plantar tylomas (see Chapter 13, Podiatric Treatment).

Regardless of the treatment used to remove the tyloma for palliative relief, the etiology must be understood. The etiologic basis for tyloma development is stress over the affected part beyond physiological limits. This stress is primarily initiated by disease, deformity, injury or biomechanical dysfunction.

It is not the purpose of this text to delve deeply into the realm of foot biomechanics; yet it is imperative that broad factors leading to production of the tyloma be discussed. Faulty weight distribution acts as a *stressor* and, therefore, must be corrected. Obviously, this stressor creates other problems in the tissues immediately subjacent to the tyloma. For example, one must be concerned with inflammation of the true skin, verrucoid lesions in the dermis not of viral origin but related to pressure, subcutaneous bursae, calcifications, tenosynovitis, fasciitis, neuromas, inclusion cysts, ganglia, giant cell tumors, capsulitis, fibrositis, degenerative changes in the affected joint secondary to trauma, spurs, exostoses, osteophytes and lippings. These lesions often occur beneath tylomas and must be relieved and corrected.

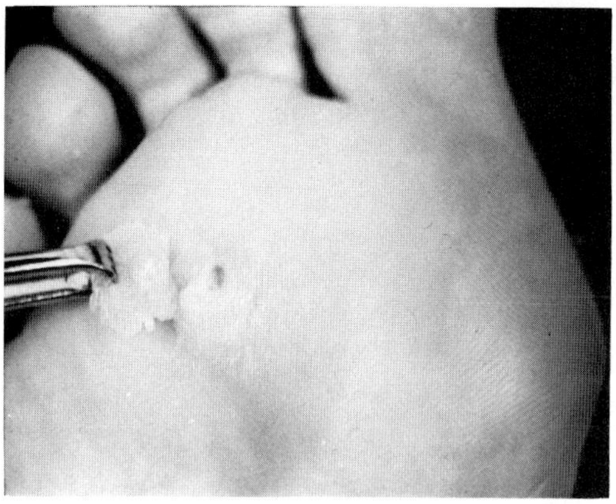

Figure 6.44. Intractable plantar keratosis—total excision of hyperkeratoses. Must be differentiated from verruca.

The stressors are reviewed below in broad fashion. Ill-fitting footgear may force the toes back or limit function at the metatarsophalangeal joints, creating faulty function of the forefoot. High-heeled shoes often throw undue stress on one or more metatarsal heads or on the bases of the phalanges and cause tylomas to develop. Soft, flexible soles fail to protect the malfunctioning foot and allow for abnormal stress. Elasticized stockings may force toes back, causing friction at the ball of the foot. Narrow shoes often cause the medial and lateral borders of the foot to bear weight on seams where the upper and the insole of the shoe come together. It is necessary to recognize here that imbalanced feet, foot deformities, toe deformities, paralysis, shortages, traumatic disturbances, functional and structural weaknesses and developmental and acquired disorders may also act as stressors. The reaction to this stress may manifest itself in the objective finding of tylomas and their sequelae. Adaptation to the stressor may be demonstrated by a conscious or subconscious effort to offset the pathology. Alterations in gait to remove pressure and friction from the tyloma, using foot and leg musculature incorrectly, and acquiring sedentary habits are but a few of the adaptations to the reaction of stress. Tylomas may also be idiopathic and chronic (Fig. 6.45).

Treatment of the Marginal Heel Tyloma. Shoes with a well-constructed heel seat, a firm

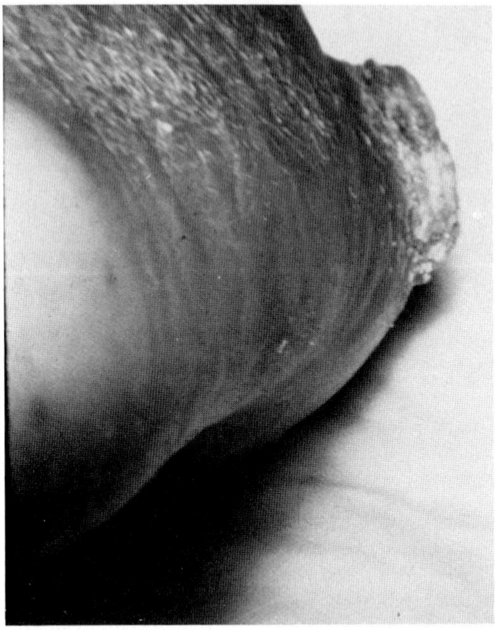

Figure 6.45. Cutaneous horn secondary to marked idiopathic hyperkeratosis. Chronic.

rubber heel and a fit that allows for a broad distribution of body weight often relieve pressure from the marginal heel tyloma. A plastic heel cup may be necessary to reinforce the lateral spreading of the soft tissue in the heel. The wearing of open back shoes should be discontinued. A pendulous abdomen and lordosis of the spine in obese individuals throws the center of gravity backward on the heels, and this must be corrected. Loss of weight is indicated. A full-foot orthosis worn in the shoe, constructed for the foot to a cast or by a variety of molding methods, may be necessary to control weight distribution.

Tylomas at the medial plantar aspect of the heel are generally the result of rotation of the calcaneus in foot disorders involving pronation with a positive Helbing's sign. Correction of the foot disorder to restore physiological functions is necessary to keep an excised tyloma from recurring. Thomas heels and extended counters are helpful in controlling subtalar pronation.

Tylomas overlying prominent talar heads require maintenance of the integrity of the midtarsal and subtalar joints through adequate footgear, corrective orthotic thrusts, and, in old, uncorrectable subluxations, accommodative foot orthoses to remove pressure.

Spence and Shields (45) describe a closed cellular Neoprene insole that absorbs 1 cm of fore, aft and lateral shear with 25° of rotary shear. The insoles and material from which they are made are commercially available for professional use. An inlay depth shoe with a ¼-inch Neoprene insole covering the metatarsal heads is helpful.

Felt pads may be designed to relieve weight-bearing stress on painful tylomas. Sansone (46) presented a system of parallel strip padding with adhesive felt of various widths, lengths and thicknesses—3/16 inch, 1/16 inch, ⅛ inch. This technique is used following the debridement of tylomas to protect the area from friction, irritation and pressure. With time and persistent effort, the excrescence should undergo resolution. According to Sansone, these pads act as pontoon stabilizers, disbursing and diffusing the weight stresses. They induce flowing action over tissues of various densities. The pontoon strip pads act as a buttress and encourage the flow of weight to follow the line of least resistance.

The parallel pads assist weight distribution and exert little pressure upon the structures of the foot (Fig. 6.46). Because of their minimal bulk, accommodation is relatively simple. They detour weight from the areas of pain to the pontoons. They are intended to accept the additional stress and remove it from the area of insult (see Fig. 6.12)

Tyloma formation on the dorsum of the foot over the first metatarsocuneiform joint may be due to an accessory ossicle, exostosis or simple hypertrophy of bone. Wearing low-cut shoes may help. However, these problems usu-

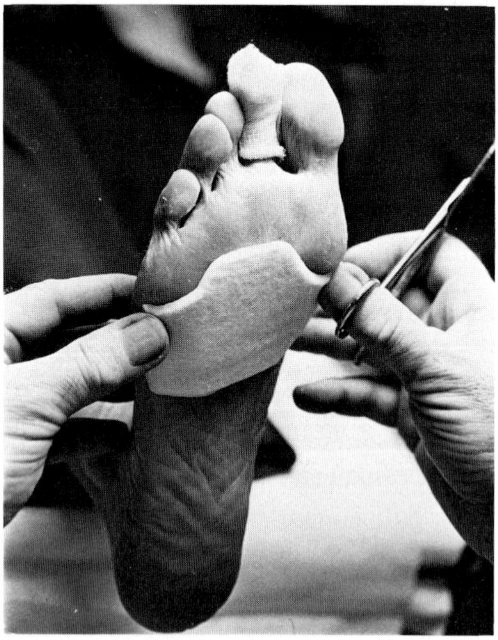

Figure 6.46. Typical pad for relief of tylomas under first, second and fifth metatarsals. May also be useful for sesamoiditis.

ally occur in a structurally disabled foot that requires a firm, highly laced 5 to 6 eyelet tie. It may be necessary either to remove the metal eyelets overlying the bony prominence or to lace the shoe in a manner to avoid the callused area.

Correction can be provided by surgically excising the extra ossicle or bony prominence and correcting the faulty foot function. This procedure may also be necessary at a prominent tuberosity of the navicular or where an os tibiale externum is present at the medial aspect of the foot (Fig. 6.47). Full-foot radiographs are essential for study. Occasionally accessory ossicles create pressure and hyperkeratosis formation.

Where tylomas develop over a bunion joint, accommodation by bunion-last shoes may eliminate the lesion. A bunion shield is helpful in relieving pressure from the part. Surgical correction is necessary if the joint is markedly enlarged and deformed as in hallux abductovalgus.

Tyloma at the medial plantar aspect of the first metatarsophalangeal joint is generally secondary to excessive subtalar pronation, which must be controlled.

Tylomas at the plantar and plantar medial aspect of the hallux at the interphalangeal joint result from the part acting as a fulcrum due to a limitation of motion of the hallux at the metatarsophalangeal joint or an equinus deformity of the first metatarsal. A plantar interphalangeal joint sesamoid may be etiologic. A hallux limitus or rigidus does not allow dorsiflexion of the metatarsophalangeal joint and results in the hallux taking the brunt of the stress in the "take-off phase" of walking (Fig. 6.48).

Cavus or cavovarus feet usually cause the weight of the body to be borne on the heel and ball of the foot in stance. This often results in **tyloma formation around the rim of the heel and under the first and fifth metatarsal heads,** especially beneath the sesamoids. An intractable keratosis may be formed.

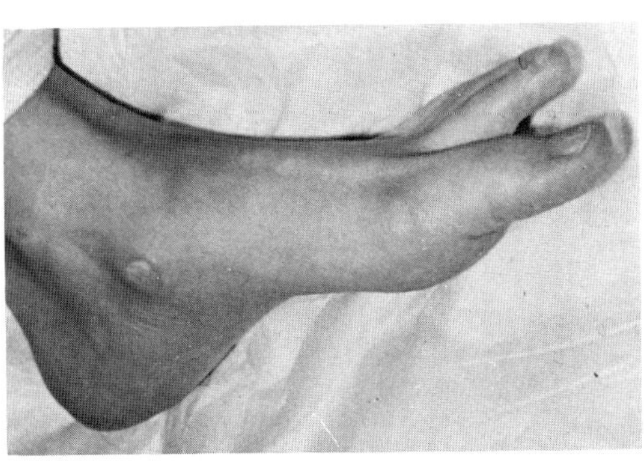

Figure 6.47. Os tibiale externum. Note tyloma on prominence.

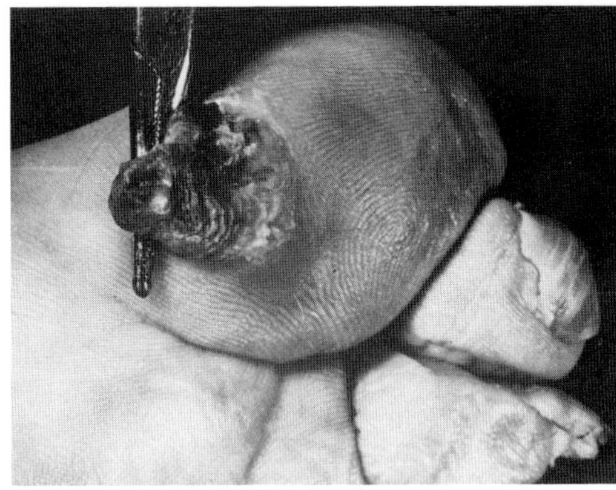

Figure 6.48. Keratoma—cutaneous horn.

After palliative debridement, the tyloma is relieved by constructing a foot orthosis to allow distribution of the weight broadly across the foot. Often the orthosis provides for cutouts under the first and fifth metatarsal heads to take pressure off the callused parts. A rigid orthotic device may be used to control the usual forefoot varus.

Polokoff (47) described a removable shield for lesions around the fifth metatarsal. He refers to it as "MH5" and again in a simple approach he fashions a suitable pad from ⅛-inch Polokoff felt measuring 2 × 3 inches. An off-center oval is cut out of the pad so the base of the fifth toe is encircled by a soft felt and the tyloma on the plantar surface of the metatarsal head is suitably protected. The pad is trimmed and beveled to conform to the shape of the metatarsal head. A ½-inch elastic adhesive is placed around the base of the toe and encircles the foot with the adhesive side up. Rubber cement is placed on the skin and the pad. The pad is then slipped over the fifth toe and adhered. A second strip of elastic tape covers the first, enveloping the pad. Excess material is trimmed, and the entire pad and encircling strap is coated with latex. The pad may be built up and covered with plastic solutions to complete the protection.

When the normal metatarsal parabola is disturbed and in the presence of erratic metatarsal length patterns, tylomas develop below those metatarsal heads receiving the greatest stress. Where hypermobility of the first and fifth metatarsal segments exists tylomas form below the central metatarsophalangeal joints. Thus, wherever possible, foot deformities and abnormal structural and functional states must be corrected or accommodated to remove pressure and stress that cause the painful tyloma. Improved foot mechanics may be augmented by shoe therapy, shielding, padding, wedging and metatarsal build-ups.

Mixtures of rubber butter (liquid latex and cork or wood dust) spatulated into a shoe or on a Celastic insole are often used to create dynamic molds. Dynamic molds can be constructed for plantar tylomas and placed in shoes much like an insole. They are usually a rubberized or vinyl material capable of being compressed and shaped by the weightbearing foot. (See Chapter 13, Podiatric Treatment) (Fig. 6.49).

Roven (48) describes a latex forefoot device made to a plaster impression cast in dental stone. The particular orthosis was constructed to remove pressure from a painful bursa overlying the hallux, dissipated pressure from a painful plantar heloma neurofibrosum and compensated by biplane pads for the imbalance of the forefoot.

Surgical Resection of the Metatarsal Head. Surgical correction techniques consisting of resection of the metatarsal head for intractable plantar tyloma or keratosis have had excellent results in many cases (Figs. 6.50 and 6.51). Amberry (49) described a technique used in 1,200 resections with fine results. French surgeons have been using variations of this technique for many years. Plantar condylectomy described by DuVries (50) has met with varied success. Hennefeld and Walkes (51) described a modification of DuVries' plantar condylectomy that involves removal of the base of the proximal phalanx as well as the plantar condyle. Proximal or distal metatarsal extension osteotomies have been helpful in eradicating painful plantar tylomas.

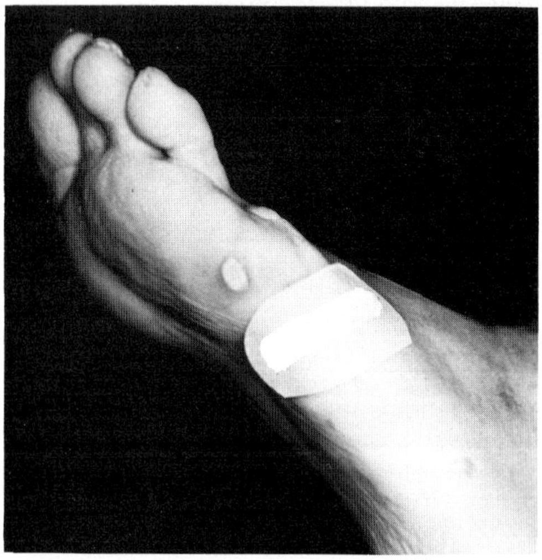

Figure 6.49. Reactive chronic keratosis—amputated fifth toe followed by localized reactive keratosis head of fifth metatarsal that acts as a fulcrum in gait. Note grayish-white scar tissue in base with irregular border. Gunshot wound and keloid resulting in deformity requiring accommodation.

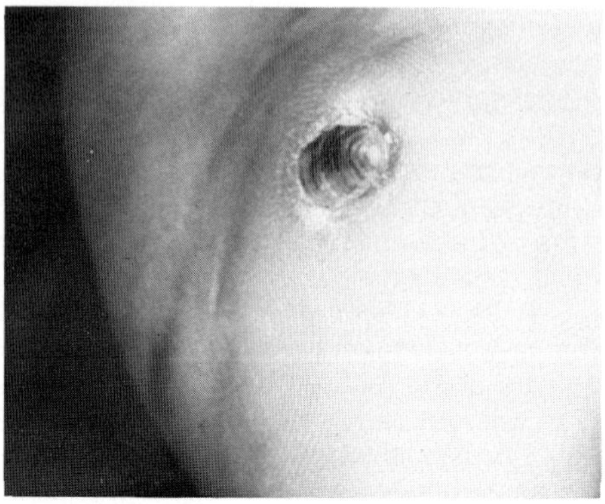

Figure 6.50. Intractable plantar keratosis.

The author has noted the presence of an adventitious bursa under chronic, deep-seated tylomas. The excrescence is resected by semi-elliptical incisions around the mass to include the subcutaneous tissue. Invariably a bursa is found beneath the excrescence. The entire mass is excised by sharp and blunt dissection and sutured.

Excision of Plantar Tylomas. Although surgery on the plantar surface has generally been discouraged, the author feels that excision of plantar lesions can be a useful procedure when it is attempted after careful evaluation of previous treatment results and in those cases where pain remains acute and that have proven resistant to palliative treatment.

Hennefeld and Walkes (52) recommended excision of the proximal phalanx where subluxations of the metatarsophalangeal joints exist. They note marked improvement in the pathology on the plantar surface of a metatarsal head where a callus exists, correction of a hammertoe and elimination of a dorsal excrescence, as well as reduction of the subluxation. The author has

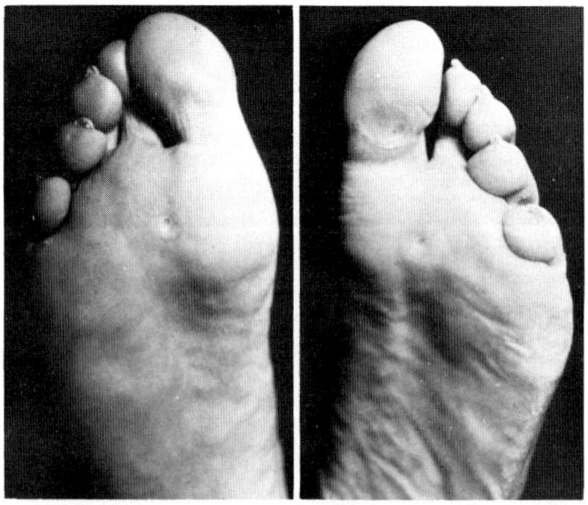

Figure 6.51. Intractable plantar keratosis.

used this technique successfully to relieve forefoot keratosis.

In nucleated plantar tylomas (Fig. 6.52), Bronston (53) recommended a soft tissue approach in selected cases. Using a 2% lidocaine solution mixed with Decadron in a 10:1 ratio, he induced anesthesia from the dorsum over the involved metatarsophalangeal joint and continued to infiltrate the plantar site of the nucleated tyloma. A snap tenotomy is accomplished on the extensor tendon dorsally through a ¼-inch linear incision. A second incision on the plantar surface distal to the lesion is used as an approach for adhesiotomy between the tyloma and its underlying attachments. The incisions are closed with a single suture, and a length of tube gauze is applied to the toe and bound down. The end of the tube gauze is carried under the foot and adhered to the ball of the foot with the toe in flexion.

Promising results may be obtained in intractable plantar keratoses by inducing a surgical fracture (osteoclasis) of the affected metatarsal at the surgical neck. Repair generally results in a slight elevation of the head of the metatarsal following immobilization. Osteotomy performed at the base of a metatarsal is also effective if proper postoperative care is given.

Balkin (54, 55) discusses 11 years of observation of treatment of plantar tylomas by injection of fluid silicone. One hundred and two cases were treated, and five patients have been followed since 1964. Though this research is still under surveillance by the Food and Drug Administration, this technique seems promising as an alternative to surgical intervention and as a means of relief in a high percentage of cases. According to Balkin, there has not been a single rejection or serious problem. A cushioning remains beneath the tyloma with minimal drift of the silicone following repeated interval injections of a minimum of solution.

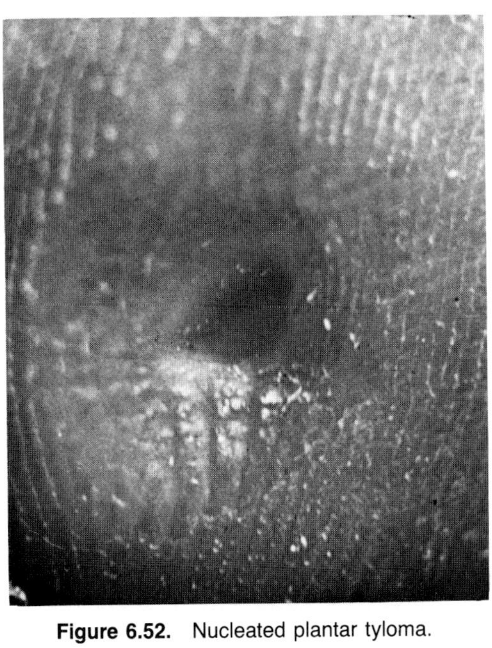

Figure 6.52. Nucleated plantar tyloma.

Levine (56) includes in the treatment of 50 cases of plantar keratoses (tylomas) soft tissue excision, DuVries' plantar condylectomy, metatarsal head resection, osteotomy, osteoclasis and collectomy.

Weinstock (57), in a brief report, cites the necessity for the surgeon to assume responsibility for the osteotomy site for elimination of intractable plantar keratoses. In order to prevent the development of transfer lesion, he urges pre- and postoperative biomechanical evaluation and proper orthoses. Above all, Weinstock's contribution to the foot surgeons armamentarium is "good surgical judgment." He states, "There is no one acceptable procedure which may be used routinely."

Porokeratosis Plantaris Discreta

Steinberg and Taub (58) described porokeratosis plantaris discreta (Fig. 6.53) as an obstruction by pressure of the terminal portion of the plantar sweat pore with the formation of a lamellated horny plug com-

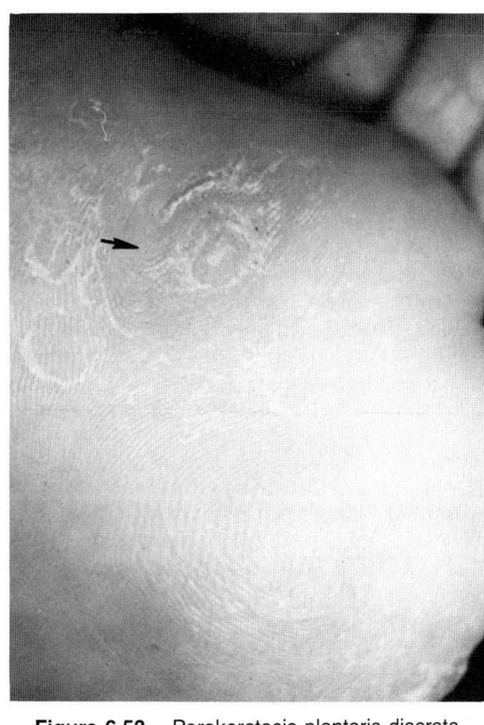

Figure 6.53. Porokeratosis plantaris discreta.

monly occurring in the age group 22 to 55. Their exhaustive studies of 649 consecutive biopsies indicate that the lesion penetrates about 1.5 cm in depth. Pressure so great as to obstruct a sweat gland is thought to be the exciting etiologic factor. The investigators concluded that this pathological entity was characterized by a "hyperkeratosis of the epidermal sweat duct with the formation of a cornoid lamella, absence of stratum granulosum and acanthosis of the epidermis and dilitation of the sweat apparatus in the corresponding deep dermis."

In a study of 60 cases diagnosed as porokeratosis plantaris discreta, Michota et al (59) consider the history as the "most striking aspect" of this condition. They state that pain is excruciating, sharp and quite constant. A history of several years duration is common.

In gross anatomical terms, they describe the porokeratosis as a central plug of hyperkeratosis that is definitely demarcated from the surrounding tissue. The pain is more severe on palpation from side to side. The plug appears white, gray or yellowish-white and presents little or no central vascularization such as seen in verrucas.

Treatment consists of field block local anesthesia, a Betadine scrub and a circumscribed incision about the lesion, followed by a wide sharp excision of the mass sufficient to include the secretory gland and excretory duct. All white-gray fibrous connective attachments are dissected out. Some surgeons prefer to desicate the base to control bleeding. The author has used this technique for many years. The remaining cavity may be packed with Gelfoam. The Gelfoam is left intact under a compression bandage for about 5 days. Removal of the dressing entails debridement of the soft coagulum without inducing hemmorrhage. Enzymatic debridement and proper felt shielding allow for healing.

Cryosurgery utilizing dry ice or liquid nitrogen has also proved to be effective in eradicating porokeratotic lesions. Drawbacks include the formation of a superficial bulla, with the lesion still intact beneath it, and postapplication pain (60).

Eccrine Poroma

Eccrine poromas appear as painless, nonpigmented, superficial, partially flattened lesions with intertwined bundles of small cells with dark-staining nuclei from the epidermis down into the corium. No keratinization or melanin has been seen in the reported cases. Only two of the ten cases reported occurred in males. Kipping (61) reported a case of eccrine poroma in which the lesion occurred on the sole of the foot and was believed to have originated from the "intraepidermal sweat duct unit."

Okun and Ansell (62) note that eccrine poroma is a benign slow-growing tumor composed of poral-epithelium that occurs generally in patients over the age of 40. It resembles a granuloma pyogenicum, amelanotic melanoma, scar tissue with telangiectasia and dermatofibroma. The lesions are solitary with a sessile or pedunculated base.

Tanenbaum (63) reported the first five cases of poroma on the glabrous surfaces of the foot and toes. They may appear on the soles, palms and digits. They enlarge slowly, are soft, gray or red, and by their appearance and location suggest a benign neoplasm. Gibbs (64) describes the lesion as being a smooth-surfaced and pedunculated mass that is usually located interdigitally.

Treatment. Treatment of choice is complete surgical extirpation by wide excision with field block anesthesia or infiltration of 1% lidocaine hydrochloride, 1:100,000 epinephrine solution.

A curette is placed at the line of cleavage and pressed deeply into the lesion with a sweeping type of motion. The hard mass with its characteristic pearly base is removed en masse. Steinberg and Taub (58) recommend that extirpation extend subcutaneously to include 1/16-inch of normal tissue. A dry compression bandage is applied and repair is usually uneventful. If bleeding persists, the cavity is packed with surgical sterile coagulating gelatin foams, powders or cellular coagulants. Gelfoam, an absorbable gelatin, and Surgicel, an oxidized cellulose, have proven useful in podiatric procedures.

Verruca

Verrucas (warts) are benign, highly vascular epithelial neoplasms occurring singly or multiply; they are characterized by excruciating pain on weightbearing, especially when arising after a period of rest. They may be classified according to anatomical location, such as verruca digiti, metatarsi, plantaris, calcanei, etc, or according to their characteristic texture, as moist (humida) or dry (verruca arida). When warty lesions are moistened with alcohol or glycerine, their topography is sufficient to differentiate them from helomas or tylomas.

The etiology of these lesions is obscure, with many theories having been proposed as possible etiologic factors. Recent study has shown the cause to be a filterable virus. Irritation by stone bruises, shell cuts, improper weight distribution and ill-fitting shoes are believed to be contributing causes. Psychologists point to the possibility of a psychosomatic factor being etiologic, as these growths are often cured by psychotherapy. Other investigators feel that the endocrine and metabolic disorders in children of adolescent age are etiologic.

McConaly (65) states that "the papovavirus is present in the nuclei and neucleoli of the stratum granulosum in spontaneously regressing warts only." It is not present in nonregressing warts. The papovavirus is not capable of producing its own antigen antibody response. The epidermis shields it from the human immune system. McConaly feels that the destruction of warts by chemotherapy is capable of inducing a resolution of untreated warts at a distance (Fig. 6.54).

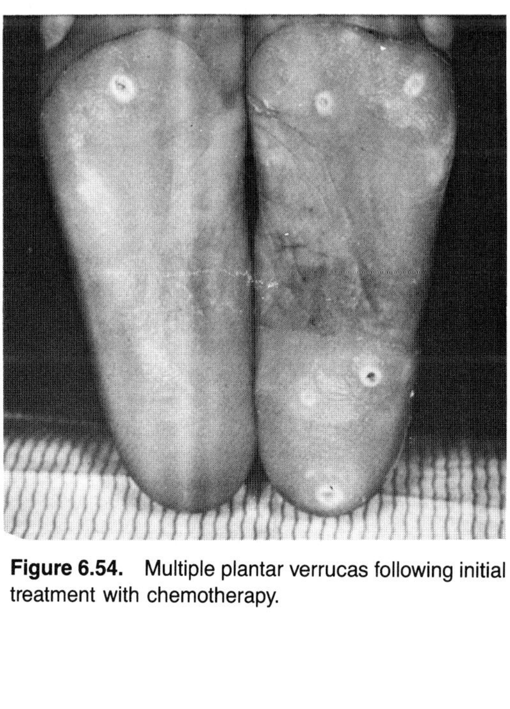

Figure 6.54. Multiple plantar verrucas following initial treatment with chemotherapy.

Carrel and Davidson (66) report a high success rate and shortened treatment time for treatment of recalcitrant verruca using topical immunotherapy. However, this technique has not been used sufficiently to make a scholarly or clinical judgment of its value. However, when faced with a challenging lesion, the immunotherapy approach should be considered.

McCarthy (67) in referring to the studies of Goodheart (68) and others, such as Almeida et al. (69), states that "the verruca virus belongs to the polyoma-papilloma group, is large, filterable and characterized by a typical 72 unit capsomere."

Using a special preparation technique for electron microscopic examination of verrucous tissue, McCarthy observed and studied the dermoepidermal interfaces. He had difficulty in studying plantar specimens due to the "marked compression changes." Ontogenetic studies were possible on verrucas on semipressure sites of the foot, such a the dorsolateral aspect of the fifth metatarsal.

Significant findings by McCarthy (67) are briefly discussed here. The student and researcher should review the complete text of the research effort by McCarthy to fully appreciate this scholarly effort. Table 6.1 explains briefly a few of the differences noted in the study between verrucas and heloma dura.

These warts are most commonly found in adolescents, in young married woman and in extremely anxious individuals. Several cases in pregnant women disappeared without treatment after delivery. Conversely, in many other cases, growths have appeared after delivery of a baby. Generally, the patient comes into the podiatrist's office after many weeks or months of neglect with a history of having had a single small growth the size of a pinhead that has since enlarged. Often the enlargement proves to be a coalescing of two or more growths with many satellite tumors about the periphery. These growths may vary from size of 1 mm to as much as 1.5 cm.

Under electron microscopic study, plantar warts present unusual cytologic variations, such as virus-like particles, intranuclear inclusion bodies and growth characteristics (Fig. 6.55). Clinical ap-

Table 6.1.
Scanning Electron Microscopy[a]

	Heloma Dura	Verruca
1. Acanthosis suprapapillary stratum Malpighi	×	×
2. Hypertrophy rete pegs	×	×
3. Broad rete pegs and right angles to free surface of skin	×	0
4. Rete ridges elongate and converge in certripetal fashion	0	×
5. Unusual arborizations small blood vessels epidermal portion—alters epidermal-dermal interface	0	×
6. Coalescing long and thin rete pegs converge and leave a structureless cap of inverted dome epidermal portion of interface	0	×

[a] After McCarthy DJ: Alterations in the morphology of dermo-epidermal interface of pedal verrucae as revealed by scanning electron microscopy. *J Am Podiatry Assoc* 66:505–514, 1976.

pearance and reactions to treatment may vary with cellular characteristics. It is conceivable that antibodies may develop in the presence of infectious agents. Verrucas in other parts of the body are known to stimulate antiviral or other immunologic reactions.

Warts are believed to be ectotropic, affecting only skin and mucous membranes, and they invade only cells of epithelial origin. Papillary acanthosis and hyperkeratosis (Fig. 6.56) are characteristic with elongated rete ridges and papillary processes that appear to come together at the base in cone-like fashion. Microscopic examination also reveals a thick stratum corneum, enlarged cells and many mitotic figures. There is much controversy about the appearance of the nucleus, cytoplasmic and intranuclear processes (Fig. 6.57). Lyell and Miles (70) noted that the whole verruca was not uniformly affected. The central part appears to be more involved with less pathology at the periphery. Mendelson and Klingman (71) demonstrated the isolation of wart virus in tissue culture. When the ultrafiltrate of the infected tissue culture was injected with human skin, wart developed.

Where virus-like particles are found, it is also noted that the lower layers of the stratum corneum are nucleated directly above the verruca. The parakeratosis is characteristic of only those warts that present cytologic changes (viral-particles and intranuclear inclusion bodies). Apparently the viral particles interfere with the normal development of epidermal cells from the basal cells to keratinization. Fluorescent microscopy studies have been conducted confirming the presence of wart virus antigenic material in the nuclei of the upper prickle layer, the granular layer and the nuclear residues of the keratin layer (Figs. 6.58–6.60).

The individual lesions are usually clearly circumscribed papillary masses, characterized by a corrugated and somewhat spongy surface of fibrous tissue intermingled with hypertrophic papillae. The lesions may be clear, wax-like or translucent in character. Plantar verrucas are surrounded and covered by a keratotic tissue. Verrucas involving the periungual and subungual tissues require special treatment to avoid permanent damage to the nail.

The mosaic verruca is a patchy lesion with an irregular border and dry, granular, friable, horny top (Figs. 6.61–6.65). The surface appears rough and hemorrhages readily on reduction.

Treatment. Verrucas are treated successfully by many techniques. Specific treatment for the etiologic viral infection has not yet been developed. Removal of warts may be achieved through excision or destruction or a combination of both methods.

Treatment depends on the patient's general health and the number of warts and their location, type and size. Treatment may range from chemotherapeutic techniques (a variety of acids and strong salts) to treatment with carbon dioxide snow, surgical excision, sharp curettage, electrodesiccation, fulgeration, coagulation, electrosection, negative galvanism (electrolysis), injection techniques, oral vitamin A therapy, psychotherapy and ultrasound therapy.

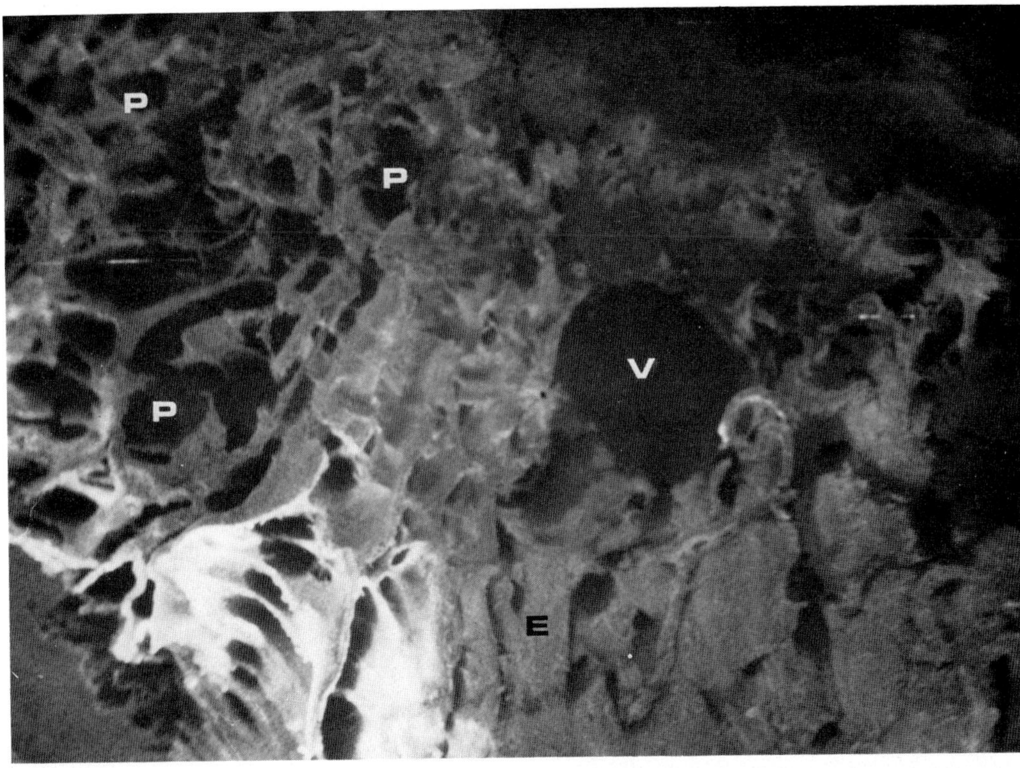

Figure 6.55. Epidermal interface in human verruca plantaris. The epidermis (*E*) has formed an inverted dome as the rete pegs converge in centripetal fashion and coalesce. Peripheral areas are more normal as the epidermis demonstrates crater-like depressions for the reception of dermal papillae (*P*). The large central aperture is for the reception of principal vascular elements (*V*) that typically seem to invade the epidermis. Scanning electron micrograph × 50. (Courtesy of Luther Gillam and Daniel J McCarthy, DPM, PhD, Veterans Administration Medical Center, Perry Point, MD.)

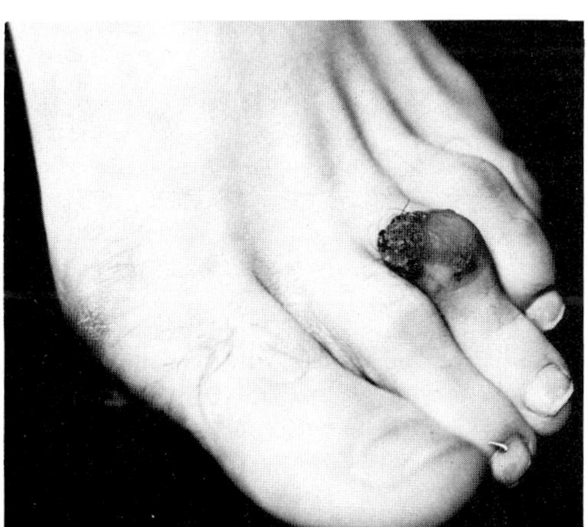

Figure 6.56. Verruca dorsum third toe—digiti flexus.

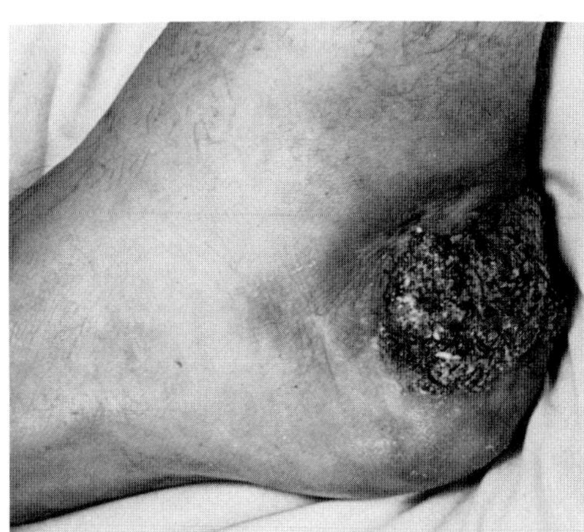

Figure 6.57. Tuberculosis verrucosa cutis.

The most popular treatment and one that has proven effective in the majority of cases is chemotherapy. Many chemicals, including monochloroacetic, bichloroacetic, fuming nitric, pyrogallic and salicylic acids; cantharidin, vitamin A, and silver nitrate and a variety of sclerosing agents, are used alone or in combination.

Surgical excision of verrucas is practical when a single lesion exists or if multiple lesions are widely separated. Excision of lesions over bony prominences or on weightbearing areas of the foot must be properly evaluated to eliminate scar formation. The author has found excision (excochleation) superficial to the superficial fascia, by means of a small sharp bone curette with mild electrodesiccation of the surgical site, to be most effective. In cases of mosaic verruca, a "planing" procedure, utilizing a no. 312 chisel blade and remaining superficial to the superficial fascia, is most effective. Mild electrodesiccation of the large remaining concavity is performed. Care should be taken not to pierce the superficial fascia so as to minimize scar formation and to protect adequately the surgical sites as they heal by third intention. (Fig. 6.66).

Liquid nitrogen or liquid oxygen applied to a plantar verruca causes instantaneous freezing (73). This application is painless, but pain commences with thawing and is increased for several hours. A bullous lesion develops, and the patient returns in 1 week for excision of necrotic tissue. The wound is dressed daily and may take 3 to 4 weeks to heal. This treatment is especially effective for mosaic warts (Fig. 6.67).

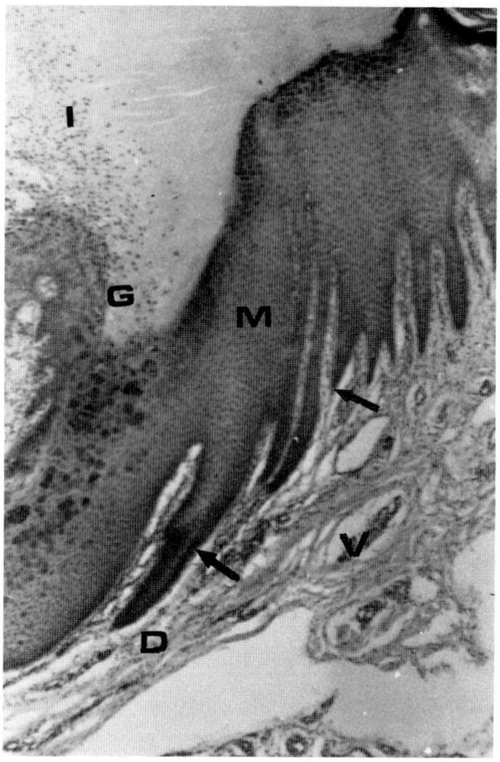

Figure 6.58. Human verruca plantaris stained by hematoxylin and eosin for general morphology. Rete ridges (*black arrow*) assume a distinctly centripetal orientation. Suprapapillary stratum Malpighi (*M*) is acanthotic and demonstrates vesicular cells in the central portion of the lesion. DNA inclusion bodies (*I*) are deeply basophilic and stream toward the free surface of the skin. The stratum granulosum (*G*) is ill defined centrally, but well organized at the periphery. Venous sinusoids (*V*) are abundant in the dermis (*D*) and may occasionally appear in parts of the epidermis as well as in verruca. (Courtesy of Luther Gilliam and Daniel J McCarthy, DPM, PhD, Veterans Administration Medical Center, Perry Point, MD.)

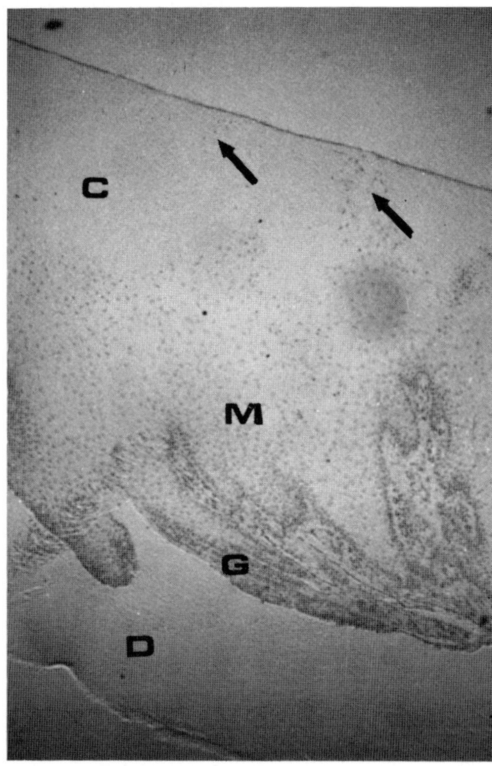

Figure 6.59. Human verruca plantaris stained by the Feulgen method for DNA. Cells of the stratum germinativum (*G*) are actively synthetic and replicative. As cells proliferate through the Malipighian layer (*M*), these activities are reduced. DNA bodies (*arrows*), the products of viral activities, can be seen streaming through the stratum corneum (*C*). The dermis (*D*) is relatively free of Feulgen positive material. Light microscopy × 100. (Courtesy of Luther Gilliam and Daniel J McCarthy, DPM, PhD, Veterans Administration Medical Center, Perry Point, MD.)

The presence of scar tissue following surgery may well plague the patient throughout his or her life. However, when handled judiciously, chemosurgical approaches rarely cause scar formation.

Chemosurgical Technique (Fig. 6.68). A circular adhesive cutout, slightly larger than the wart, is placed over the lesion to cover the healthy tissue and expose the wart. An applicator

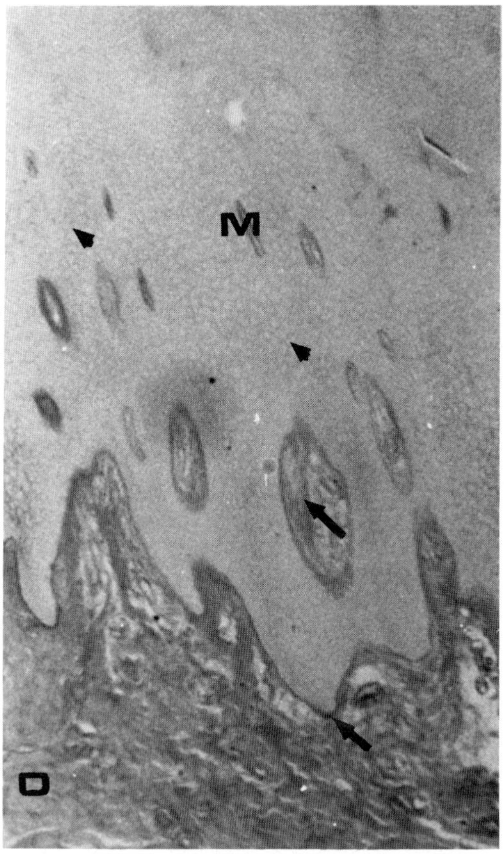

Figure 6.60. Human verruca plantaris stained for mucopolysaccharides and related substances by the Periodic Acid Schiff (PAS) reaction. The dermis (*D*) is deeply reactive. "Islands" of dermal elements (*arrows*) appear to be in the stratum Malpighi (*M*). These are the result of cross-sectioning papillae that are centripetally inclined with reference to the free surface of the skin. The basement membrane (*arrows*) is deeply PAS positive, most probably due to high concentrations of the "Dermal Influencing Factor" that stimulates mitotic activity in the germinativum. Intercellular boundaries (*arrow heads*) of the Malpighian layer are also deeply PAS positive, indicating a high degree of adherence of the cells, one to another. Light microscopy × 100. (Courtesy of Luther Gilliam and Daniel J McCarthy, DPM, PhD, Veterans Administration Medical Center, Perry Point, MD.)

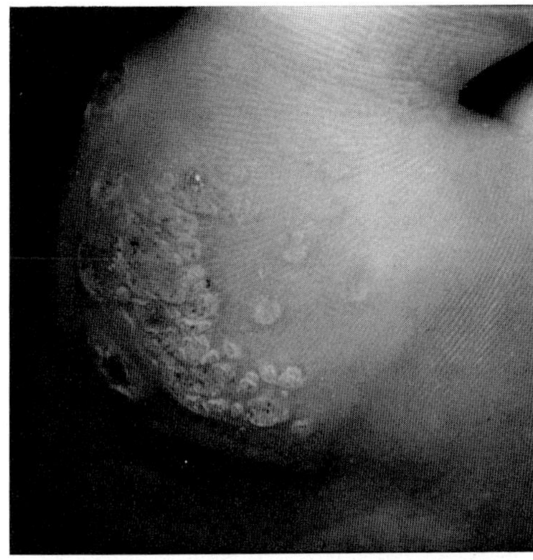

Figure 6.61. Mosaic verruca.

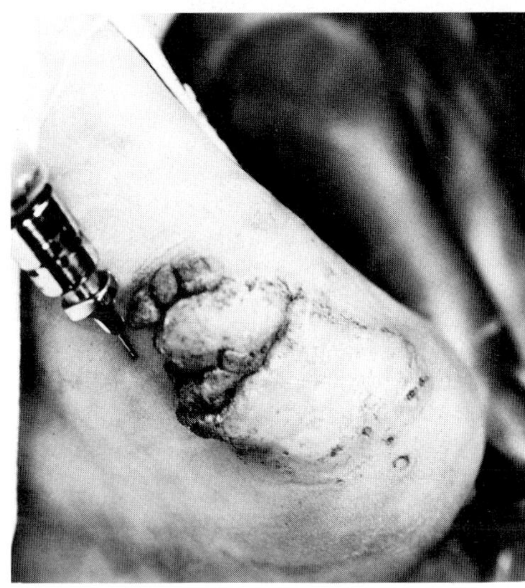

Figure 6.62. Verruca vulgaris and keloid posterior heel. (Courtesy of D Mowbray.)

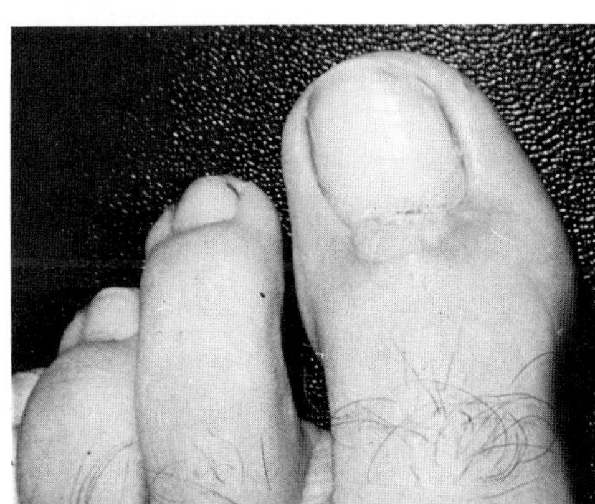

Figure 6.63. Verruca, posterior nail fold.

or capillary tube (74) is dipped into the agent of choice and applied to the wart. The hole in the adhesive is filled with 60 to 70% salicylic acid ointment or suitable commercial compounds, and a protective ⅛- or ¼-inch U-shaped felt pad is applied to the part to relieve weightbearing. The entire dressing is covered, and the patient is cautioned to keep the part dry.

After 3 to 5 days, the wart appears slightly raised, white, soft and spongy and often has undergone a partial necrosis. A liquefaction necrosis may not occur until several applications of the above treatment have been completed. Debridement usually discloses an ulceration.

Repair of the ulceration caused by the acid is usually rapid, and if a severe destructive reaction takes place with cellulitis and severe pain, it can be relieved by warm saline soaks.

Churney (75) advised against destruction of plantar warts and recommended shielding in "anticipation of spontaneous remission."

In 180 cases of mosaic verruca, Lieberman (76) reported good results in 165 cases with a half-cup of sea salt to a quart of warm water as a foot soak daily for 15 min and vitamin A, 50,000 units bid. The average cure took place in 2 to 10 weeks. The lesions were seen weekly and cauterized with silver nitrate.

Levy (77) recommended the use of topical applications of 3% formaldehyde with oral vitamin A capsules as a regimen for selected cases of plantar warts.

Lerner (78) claimed a 91% rate of success using a method of excision and curettage and believed that recurrences are the result of faulty technique. The technique consists of a posterior tibial nerve block or direct infiltration of a local anesthetic of choice. A no. 11 or 15 scalpel blade is used to incise around the perimeter of the wart. This incision is deepened to include the entire mass. An iris scissors is used to excise the mass and trim the wound. A mastoid curette of desired size is used to remove verrucous elements. A compression (Gelfoam) dressing is applied (Fig. 6.69).

Bornstein (79) in describing the procedure by Lerner, noted that he had a 43% decrease in healing time when oral chymotrypsin was prescribed, e.g., 2 tablets Chymoral qid 2 days preoperatively and 4 to 6 days postoperatively.

Antahades (80) used refrigeration anesthesia in the surgical excision of plantar verruca of nonmosaic type. He applied dry ice to organize, solidify and anesthetize the wart and ensure hemostasis. With a sharp curette, the lesion was immediately excised while hard and anesthetized. Three or four sterile gauze pads were applied with pressure for hemostasis. Postoperative pain is negligible and repair is rapid with this procedure.

Suppan and Besterman (81) described a similar approach to the treatment of verrucas using curettage and chemocautery. This procedure essentially consists of field block or infiltration anesthesia, followed by sharp curettage of the wart. The base is then cauterized for from 3 to 5 min with a cotton swab and 88% phenol solution.

Buske (82) cited bismuth cevitamate as his method of choice for injection into the verrucous mass. He cautions the operator to use no more than 0.5 to 1.0 minim on the toes, but he demonstrates the effective use of 1.0 to 3.0 minims on other parts of the foot. The 27 gauge needle is injected from the periphery directly into the base of the lesion. Resistance is felt if the medication is being properly placed. Smernoff (83) used successfully a combination of bismuth cevitamate and 1% Sotradecol mixed with an anesthetic and administered by Panjet. This application is followed by a 60% salicylic acid ointment

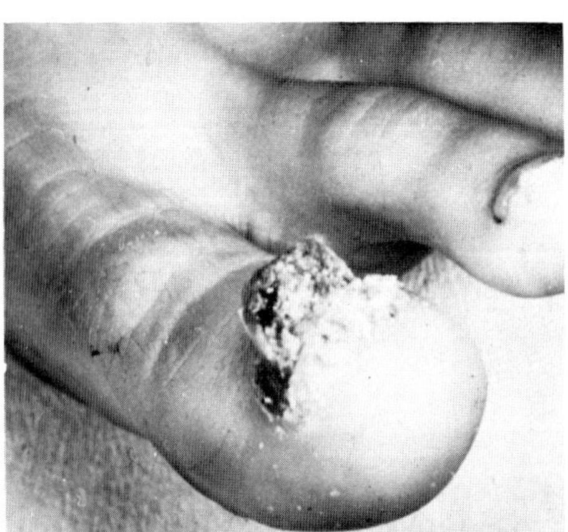

Figure 6.64. Verruca in nail bed.

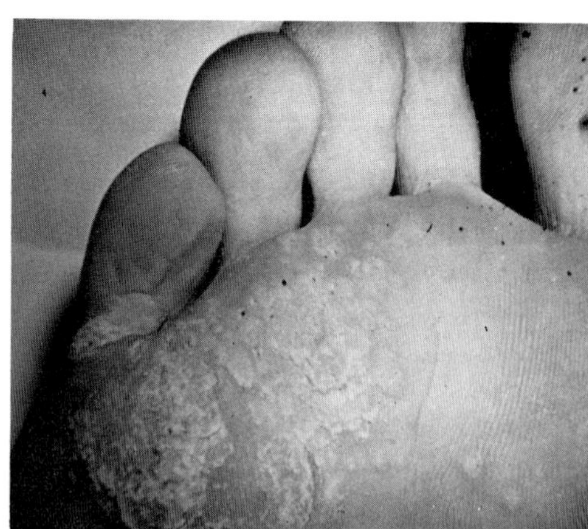

Figure 6.65. Mosaic verruca, ball of foot.

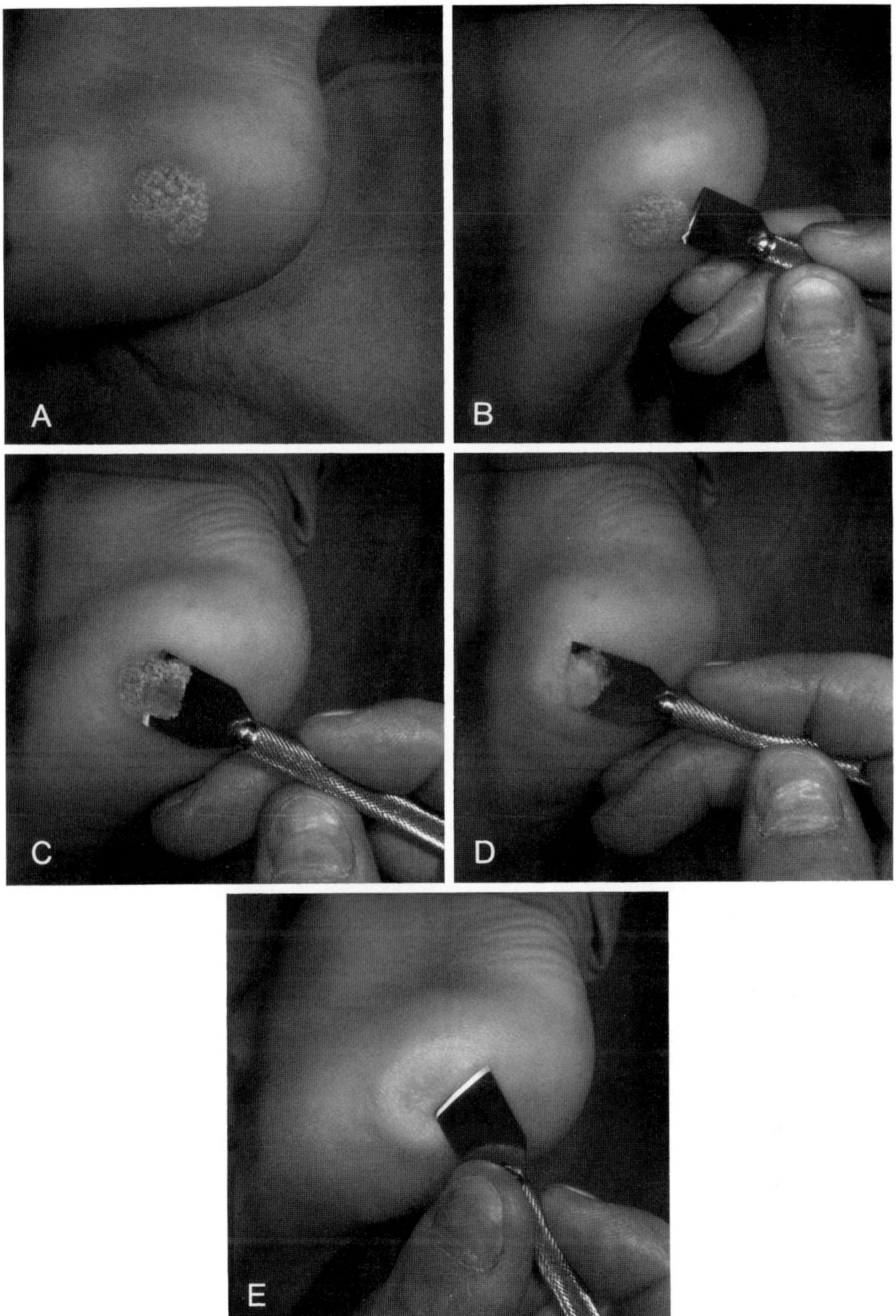

Figure 6.66. *A–E,* Mosaic verruca "planing" procedure.

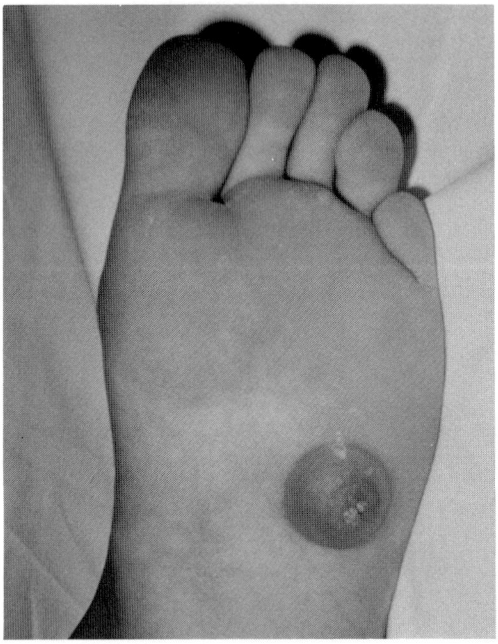

Figure 6.67. Liquid nitrogen destruction of verruca.

in a lanolin base. The area is debrided and eventually undergoes a liquefaction necrosis. In chronic cases, bismuth sodium triglycollamate (Bristrimate), an oral systemic bismuth therapy, was prescribed, 2 tablets, tid (adult). This dosage appears to stimulate and reinforce other processes being used in the treatment of warts. (A dark discoloration of the gums is one of the contraindications of the use of bismuth.)

Grady (84) used a high-speed drill with a steel burr to grind out plantar verrucas while the patient was anesthetized by infiltration of an anesthetic with epinephrine. Results in 20 patients were remarkably good, with a single failure attributed to the presence of diabetes.

Dry Ice Technique. In this procedure, the cartridge of carbon dioxide gas is released into a suitably sized plastic applicator as Dry Ice or carbon dioxide snow. The applicator, slightly larger than the wart, is held firmly over and surrounding the wart for 2 to 4 min until the wart is white, hard and frozen. Applying a warm, moist, gauze sponge allows for a rapid thaw and less discomfort. The part is covered by an adhesive protective dressing.

In about 7 to 10 days the patient returns for treatment. Typically the area appears as a bullous lesion that is removed and drained. The remaining ulceration repairs slowly and the results are good. This destructive measure has limited application as it is most effective only on the soft, nonweightbearing parts of the foot.

Kingland (85) discussed the treatment of 86 patients using cryotherapy. Sixteen warts were destroyed in one treatment, 24 in two treatments, 16 in three treatments, 22 in four treatments, 5 in six treatments and 1 in seven treatments. Goldman and Stillman (86) recommended Dry Ice followed by electrodesiccation as a painless treatment for warts.

Electrosurgery. The technique of electrosurgery is preceded by local anesthesia. The part is anesthetized with 1% lidocaine or other suitable injectable anesthetic. 1:100,000 epinephrine is desirable for hemostasis. A needle electrode on a short wave machine or other electrodesiccating and coagulating equipment is applied intermittently to the lesion by use of a foot pedal. The current emitted may be electrodesiccating or one that fulgerates or coagulates the tissue.

The operator starts at the periphery of the lesion working inward and, in one sitting, destroys the verruca by inserting the needle as it is sparked into the mass. The coagulum (necrosis) is either removed by sharp curettage or allowed to remain. If allowed to remain, the destroyed wart acts as an irritant to the underlying tissue. A liquefaction necrosis occurs, which can be evacuated in about 10 days. The remaining ulceration must be kept clean and treated as a third-degree burn.

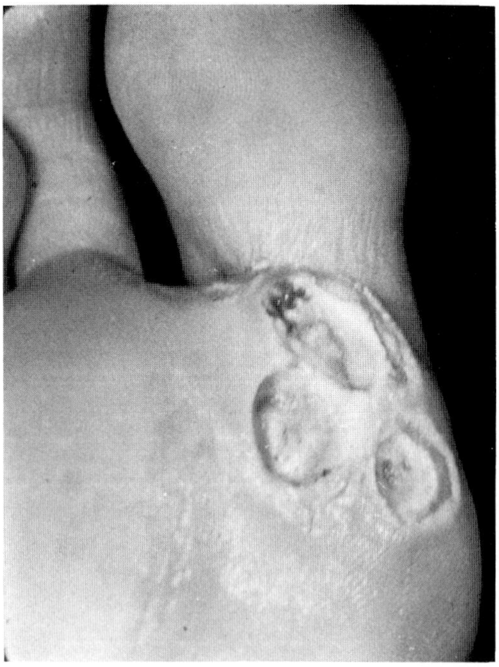

Figure 6.68. Chemosurgical removal of three plantar verrucas. Note crater-like destruction and removal of necrotic masses.

The technique of electrosection is handled the same way. The author uses a cutting loop electrode. The wire electrode can be carried about and underneath the verruca with a sweeping motion. The resulting ulcerative cavity must be treated as a third-degree burn and ulceration.

Superficial lesions may be dried or desiccated. Others are coagulated or cooked. Some masses are fulgerated or charred.

Injection Therapy. Injections of a local anesthetic directly into a verruca have been helpful. Needling of the lesion under local anesthesia has been described as successful. Smallpox vaccine has been used as another method, but is not recommended because of the possibility of adverse reactions. Vitamin A taken orally, 50,000 units bid, for several weeks has been advocated by some clinicians.

Injection of vitamin A, or injectable solutions of sclerosing or necrotizing agents intracapsularly, has been used successfully in the treatment of warts. Following local anesthesia, 0.3 to 0.5 ml of Steinberg's solution is injected intradermally. Cataldo (87) and others confirmed Steinberg's results. Steinberg (88) developed a technique using a solution of vitamin A palmitate, alpha tocopherol, sesame oil, polysorbate 80, and distilled water (Keramin).

Davidson and Schuler (89) report the treatment of 400 verrucas, including the single, multiple and mosaic varieties using a special curette. They claim an 8% recurrence with a 92% response to repeated treatment using a Dexmal Curette (Dittmar and Penn Instrument). Following local anesthesia, the instrument is used with a peeling motion to the white basal cell layer. Bleeders are electrocoagulated without destruction of viable tissue. Care must be instituted to remove two to three times the diameter of the lesion in its entire circumference. A topical enzyme antibiotic ointment is applied, and the area is dressed for the first 3 days, followed by weekly intervals. The new approach has been used by others for many years successfully. The new approach uses a "peeling" technique and an instrument that, according to the authors, will not damage viable tissue ring that is at the basal cell level, thus eliminating the possible scar incident to other surgical procedures.

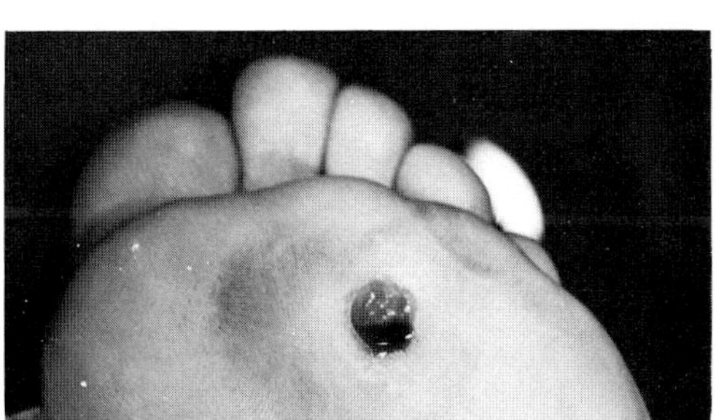

Figure 6.69. Verruca plantaris. One week postoperative excision packed with Gelfoam. Ulceration repairs by third intention.

Yale (90) recommended the injection of a solution containing Nupercainal, benzyl alcohol, quinine hydrobromide and physiological saline. Prolonged anesthesia was beneficial, but positive results were not as good as other chemotherapeutic measures. However, Stern (91) reported excellent results with the same formula, Quinocaine. Cramer (92) did preliminary studies with good results injecting parenzyme in oil.

Radium or x-ray therapy should be reserved for the recalcitrant wart. Ultrasoft x-ray therapy should be used judiciously, observing the usual precautions, dosage time, technique and good judgment.

A firm adherent fibrous connective tissue may develop at the site of radiation. Because radiation may be carcinogenic on the sole of the foot, the author advises less hazardous methods of removal for this common disorder.

Summary Results of Other Techniques. Curettage alone under local anesthesia has been most effective when carried out properly. A scooping motion from the periphery is effective. Weinstock (93) reports 87 cases with only 4 recurrences using this method.

Harris (94) applied concentrated phenol to warts following electrodesiccation with marked relief of pain and good results.

Gilbert and Williams (95) report an 18 month study on 100 patients with plantar verrucas treated with vitamin A (Keramin) injected into the lesion. Complete resolution occurred in 82% of the patients and relief of pain in 95%. If resolution did not occur in three to four treatments, injections were discontinued. Patients were able to return to work immediately.

Carpenter (96) injected local anesthetics with 1:50,000 epinephrine intradermally with excellent results. The needle is directed into the base of the verruca remaining within the capsule. He believes the intradermal pressure creates a pressure necrosis that destroys the mass. Sixty-one percent of the total number of warts were eradicated with a single injection, and 71% were rendered symptom-free. No more than three injections were administered in any of the cases.

Goodman (97) recommended liquid nitrogen for treatment of warts. He describes the skin reaction as a fuming sensation for a few hours, followed by a blister formation in about 3 days. Bullae should be opened if pressure builds up, but the smaller blisters will dry. Crusts drop off in about 3 weeks. Applications of liquid nitrogen may be used at 3-week intervals (Fig. 6.67).

Goldman and Palmero (98) obtained necrosis in warts by applying a heavy syrupy lotion prepared by mixing podophyllin 20%, trichloroacetic acid 25%, glycerin 25% and salicylic acid 30%.

Ormond (99) recommended the purified active principle of cantharides in a collodion tincture vehicle, Cantharone, in the treatment of intractable lesions involving the germinal layer of the skin. Cantharides are powerful vesicants that produce blisters. An acantholytic agent destroys the germinal layer of the skin by a selective process. The verruca is treated by direct application. The lesion is then covered with plastic tape. After 4 or 5 days, an aseptic bullous lesion develops. This is aspirated and should reveal a healthy base. At the first redressing the lesion looks like a blood blister; the second week a scab forms; about the third redressing, the scab comes off, leaving clean, healthy-looking skin. The part is kept clean, and a bandaid is applied for protection at each visit. Scar tissue is minimal, and healing is usually uneventful.

Locke and Zang (100) found that the jet spray injection of sodium tetradecyl sulfate combined with mepivacaine intralesionally was "effective, efficient and a convenient method for verruca therapy" in 78.7% of the cases treated.

Block (101) and Trapp (102) in separate studies, used ultrasound in verruca plantaris with a fair degree of success. Trapp concludes that ultrasound is effective on single warts and closely grouped multiple lesions. Mosaic warts are amenable to ultrasound, but require longer treatments. Weekly treatments are desirable. Block states that the "anti-inflammatory, antiviral effect of ultrasound has good therapeutic value in the management of plantar verrucas."

Falknor (103) used direct physical trauma in the form of needling to bring about dissolution of plantar warts. Insertion of the same needle used for local anesthesia about 60 times directly into the center and at the periphery of the wart produced good results with a minimum of pain.

Koenig and Horwitz (104) review the literature and present cases of bleomycin treatment of verruca plantaris. The authors utilize intralesional injections of 0.1% bleomycin sulfate. The significant success rate for eradication of verrucous lesions without subsequent scarring has shown this approach to be an effective treatment for plantar warts.

Keratoderma

Arsenical keratosis and keratoderma plantaris must be differentiated from plantar warts. A history of long-term use of arsenicals helps establish the diagnosis of arsenical keratosis. Keratoderma plantaris usually has a hereditary background. The lesions range from 1 to 3 mm in size and may be larger. They affect the palms, as well as the soles. These lesions manifest themselves as discrete hyperkeratotic papules. Their center is usually translucent. Friction and pressure seem to play a minor role in their development.

Keratosis palmaris et plantaris (Unna Thost) is reported by Fred et al., (105) as being a heredo-familial trait transmitted as a Mendelian dominant. Keratoses of the soles may be of systemic or local origin. The systemic disorder may be caused by such inorganic drugs as arsenic and gold or by an infectious systemic disease. The skin manifestations are usually generalized.

Superficial infections by *Trichophyton rubrum* may cause keratosis of the soles. Other keratoses may be idiopathic and present themselves as multiple, minute, punctate, hyperkeratotic skin lesions of unknown etiology.

Other hereditary plantar keratoses, in addition to keratosis palmaris et plantaris, include keratosis punctata, keratosis striata, mal de meleda, and Papillon-LeFevre syndrome. All of the hereditary keratoses affecting the plantar surface of the foot also affect the palms of the hands. (Fig. 6.70).

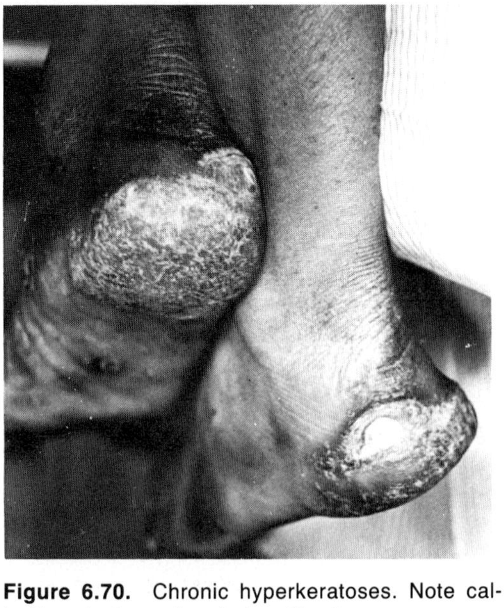

Figure 6.70. Chronic hyperkeratoses. Note callosities plantar and posterior of heal.

Grayson (106) reported a case of painful keratotic lesions on the palms and soles accompanied by papillomatous lesions of the buccal mucosa with opacities in the epithelium of the cornea. The combination is rare.

Treatment of keratoses varies with their etiology. Drug use is discontinued, and systemic disorders are diagnosed and treated by an internist. Irritating chemicals are avoided, and local treatment is instituted. Many emollient creams containing vitamin A are helpful. Lanolin may help soften the hyperkeratosis. Debridement by scalpel, sandpaper or diamond burrs may relieve discomfort. Salicylic acid in supersaturated solutions combined with a 30 to 40% tincture of benzoin may serve as a keratolytic.

Heiss and Gross (107) describe the successful clinical treatment of keratosis plantaris with topically applied vitamin A in 0.3% strength mixed in a base of petrolatum. Ammoniated mercury 10 to 20% may be helpful. Cocoa butter, mineral oil and a wide variety of emollients remove the scales. Exposure to sunlight has been recommended by some clinicians. Patients report relief of symptoms during warm weather.

Improvement of severe itching and scaling has been noted with the use of a betamethasone cream, Valisone, as an occlusive dressing. Cordran tape may be applied, removed in 12 hr, and reapplied to remove scales and keratotic lesions and to relieve itching and other symptoms.

Vance and Levy (108) note the occurrence of arsenical keratoses with a predisposition for the palms and soles. Relationships to the primary agent for treating syphilis, inorganic trivalent arsenic and industrial exposures in occupations using arsenic are established. Since the advent of antibiotics, it is reasonable to believe that the incidence of arsenic poisoning has diminished. Also, the growing attention to occupational hazards has sharply reduced its incidence.

The arsenical keratoses manifest as discrete amber-colored indurated keratotic papules. The palms and soles may appear thick and "leather-like." The toe and finger nails may demonstrate transverse white lines (Mee's lines). Subjective symptoms are minimal. The lesions may be slow growing, eczematoid or psoriasiform.

The diagnosis of arsenical keratoses is made by appreciation of the systemic symptoms and local skin lesions on the palms and soles, as well as histologic examination of the affected tissue. Blood chemistry may reveal thrombocytopenic anemia, basophilic stippling and eosinophilia depending on the severity and longevity of the symptoms. Loss of appetite, nausea, vomiting and marked diarrhea may cause sodium depletion. A hypoproteinemia may ensue with mild itching, joint pains and a variety of fatigue levels.

Microscopic examination reveals a hyperkeratosis of the skin and changes in the granular layer of a nonspecific nature. Parakeratosis is present with acanthosis and elongation of the rete pegs.

Sweat Gland Disorders

The two major disorders involving the sweat glands are hyperidrosis, an abnormal increase in perspiration, and anidrosis, an abnormal decrease in perspiration.

Both conditions are complicated by a variety of dermatologic lesions. The ability of the body to produce sweat and the ability of the sweat glands to deliver sweat are to be carefully considered in the treatment of these disorders.

Hyperidrosis is a functional disturbance of the sweat glands characterized by overactivity of the glands resulting in excessive perspiration (Figs. 6.71 and 6.72).

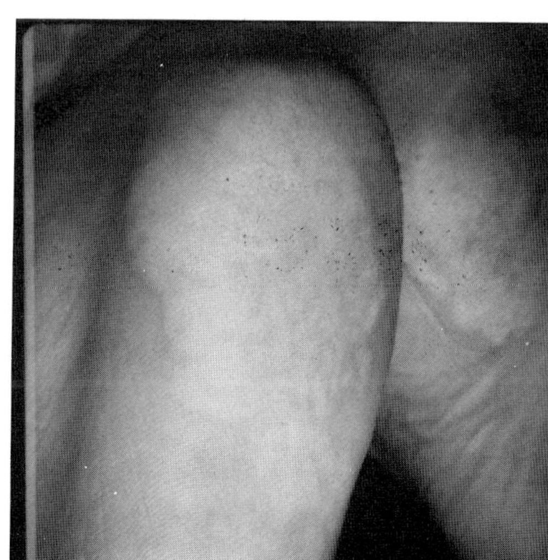

Figure 6.71. Hyperidrosis (pitted keratolysis). Note white spongy discoloration of skin on heels.

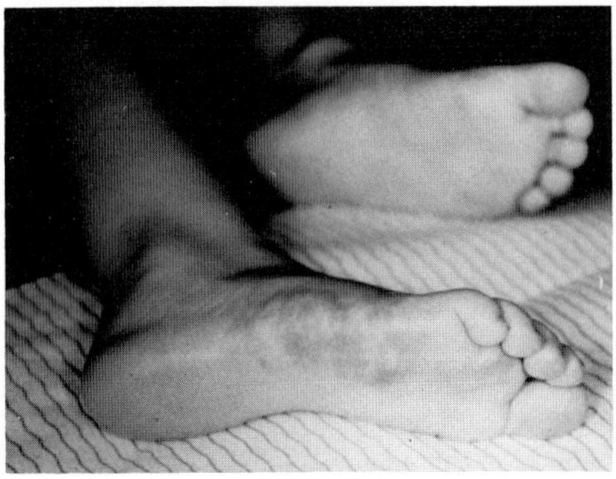

Figure 6.72. Hyperidrosis. Note moist, white to mild red macerated skin on soles of feet.

It is most commonly found in adolescents and in young adults. Extremely nervous individuals may perspire excessively when under mental strain. Violent exercise produces an overactivity of sudoriferous glands in normal individuals. Unbalanced diets and such systemic disturbances as tuberculosis and anemia cause excessive perspiration. Salicylates and excessive ingestion of fluids may result in increased perspiration. Hyperthyroidism and hypoadrenalism cause excessive perspiration. Many individuals with hyperidrosis as a result of the stress of ill-fitting footgear, occupational stress or imbalanced feet are relieved of this condition when the underlying cause is removed.

Under physiological conditions, sweating is associated with peripheral vasodilation. Failure of normal evaporation of perspiration may result in symptoms of hyperidrosis. Certain conditions are generally accompanied by excessive perspiration and are complications secondary to physiological or pathological bodily alterations. An acid reaction of pH 4.5 to 6.0 results from organic substances being secreted that yield organic acids on hydrolysis.

Bromidrosis is characterized by excessive perspiration with a fetid odor caused by saprophytic bacteria. The normal flora on cutaneous surfaces are the micrococci, diphtheroids and propionibacteria. Foot odor is caused by bacterial decomposition of skin secretions in the presence of moisture. The eccrine sweat combines with lipids and proteins, resulting in a decomposition of the sweat followed by digestion of the debris by diphtheroids and micrococci. Combinations of antiperspirants and antibacterial agents retard multiplication of bacterial flora. Caprylic and lactic acids on the skin have antibacterial properties (109). Rothman and Windhorst (110) feel that the organic acids on the skin have antifungal properties. Many times the odor is characteristic of certain dietary indiscretions with aromatic substances. The skin in some instances appears dry and even indurated when exposed to air allowing for evaporation of perspiration.

Chromidrosis is a rare condition characterized by a colored perspiration caused by abnormal constituents of sweat, bacterial action, chemicals in contact with the skin, synthetic materials in clothing and occupational stress.

Hematidrosis is a rare condition manifested by perspiration that is tinted by blood.

Hydrocystoma is a condition of elongation of the sweat glands or their ducts to form deep, noninflammatory papules resulting in tissue forming within the gland or duct that must be differentiated from verrucas.

Uridrosis is a condition of the sweat glands in which the excretion of urea in the sweat produces a urine-like smell in the perspiration.

A case of hidradenoma appearing as a gradual enlargement and a characteristic firm, round, subcutaneous mass on the plantar surface of the base of a third toe was reported by Steinhart (111). Brownstein and Shapiro (112). reported that 5% of sweat gland tumors were hidradenomas, and 4% were papillary syringocystadenomas. Winklemann and Wolf (113), following a study of 41 cases of hidradenoma, noted a 5% occurrence on the foot. In view of the varieties of this tumor, the podiatrist is cautioned to be suspicious of any subcutaneous or skin mass grossly exhibiting a mucoid, shiny and mildly lobulated appearance. This lesion is benign and should be submitted for microscopic differentiation.

Davis (114) studied the "differences in the wicking effect in sock materials as they relate to drawing away moisture from the foot surface to the outside of the socks during vigorous exercise periods." He measured the amount of moisture, the pH and skin temperature present on the foot before and after exercise in a variety of sock materials. Davis concluded that "the foot, in moderate temperatures to very hot, humid temperatures, kept cooler and drier during rigorous exercise in a sock containing 33% wool, 32% cotton and 35% nylon. In extreme cold, a thicker sock of 65% orlon, 25% cotton and 10% nylon knitted in a 'Birdwick' pattern gave fewer wrinkles and blisters to the athletes tested. The pH of the skin remained the same except in those athletes who had ankles strapped; the pH went to higher alkaline readings."

Treatment. Treatment of the conditions of abnormal perspiration is aimed at normalizing the functions of the sweat glands and depends on the general physical status of the patient. It includes treatment of systemic disorders by an internist and correction of local physiochemical problems. Surgical excision of "plugged" sweat ducts may be necessary. When systemic disorders are not a factor the following procedures may be used.

A patient with abnormal perspiration should wear hose capable of absorbing perspiration and yet with a weave wide enough to allow for evaporation of insensible perspiration. Lightweight woolen hose or good quality absorbent cotton hose should be worn. Synthetic substances, such as nylon and Orlon, do not allow for adequate evaporation of excessive perspiration and may cause the skin to become soggy, irritated, macerated and painful.

Poorly constructed and ill-fitting footgear is a common cause of excessive perspiration. Shoes constructed of plastic or rubber compounds allow for continued accumulations of perspiration on the skin and subsequent maceration and discomfort.

The following regimen has been used successfully to combat hyperidrosis and many of its complicating factors. The patient should bathe the feet daily in lukewarm water and a tetramethylthiuram disulfide- or hexachlorophene-containing bacteriostatic product. The skin should be patted dry, not rubbed. A suitable astringent should be applied between toes and over areas exuding increased perspiration. A 15 to 25% aluminum chloride tincture with isopropyl alcohol may be helpful. Tannic acid, 5% and 70% ethyl alcohol in solution, is mildly astringent. A 0.25 to 0.5% Formalin solution (properly scented) may be swabbed daily over the perspiring feet and toes to decrease the excessive perspiration.

Hyperidrosis and bromidrosis may be helped by the addition of a dusting powder. Useful prescriptions for these conditions are aluminum chloride 3%, salicylic acid 3%, alum 10%, talcum powder 84% dusted on affected parts tid; and tannic acid powder, boric acid powder, zinc oxide, equal parts of each dusted on the feet two to three times daily. Such commercial powders as Zeasorb medicated powder, BFI powder, Desenex, Efosorb, and Tinactin or Ammens foot powder are available.

Potassium permanganate soaks in 1:2,000 solutions, tid for 20 min, help decrease the activity of sweat glands and the multiplication of odor-forming bacteria. Burow's soaks 1:40 dilution is helpful.

In hydrocystoma, the firm papules are removed surgically. Care is exercised when removing the papule and its elongated sweat gland.

The use of sedatives and tranquilizers may be necessary in emotional and hypertensive patients. Effective drugs include chlordiazepoxide HCl, meprobamate (Equinil, Miltown, 200 to 400 mg three to four times daily), phenobarbital, and Benadryl. Anticholinergic drugs, such as methantheline bromide (Banthine), 50 to 100 mg taken orally three to four times daily; probantheline bromide (Pro-Banthine), 15 mg and 7.5 mg; and N-methylbromide of scopolamine (Pamine bromide), 2.5 mg taken orally qid may be helpful. Jenkins and Craft (115) advise Rubinul Forte 2 mg po tid for 1 week, followed by 2 mg po bid for 1 week continuing with the least amount of medication necessary to produce the desired response thereafter.

In a preliminary study, Davis (116) demonstrated the therapeutic potential of methenamine undecylenate for the treatment of hyperidrosis and bromidrosis. The controlled release of the active agents, formaldehyde and undecylenic acid, in effective but subtoxic concentrations provided relief of symptoms with very little skin irritation.

Hyperidrosis associated with small pitted and keratotic areas (pitted keratolysis) on the heel and along weightbearing areas of skin is not uncommon in the young adult. Treatment involves the use of topical Formalin in alcohol 20% interspersed with Whitfield's ointment (USP) as the affected areas dry. Patient self-regulation of the topical medication almost always produces a beneficial response.

Anidrosis is a skin disorder characterized either by diminished function of the sudoriferous glands or mechanical obstruction of the sweat ducts and pores, limiting the excretion of normal insensible perspiration and thereby causing dry skin (Figs. 6.73 and 6.74). The skin is dry, scaly and sometimes parchment-like. The nails are dry, split and sometimes thickened. The nail grooves become callused. Patients often complain of miliary helomas at sites of irritation, such as the medial aspect of the first metatarsophalangeal joint, at seams of hose and at pressure points caused by abnormal weight distribution on the plantar surfaces. Heels crack and fissures develop as a secondary problem. Ulcerations may result (Fig. 6.75). Plugging of sweat ducts may lead to the development of erythematous papules, vesicles and vesiculopustular lesions. Ichthyosis is a rare disease involving dysfunction of the sweat glands (Fig. 6.76).

The sebaceous secretion, sebum, which accompanies normal perspiration, is lessened with a malfunctioning of the sweat glands. The subcutaneous adipose is often diminished, and retention cysts may develop. Foot soaks avoiding excessive use of strong soap and hot salt water are useful. The disease may be aggravated or caused by diabetes, circulatory disturbances, a deficiency of vitamin A, hypothyroidism and congenital absence of the sweat glands. Feldman (117) states that "the cause of dry skin is due to a lack of water not a lack of oil or fat." Symptoms occur when the water content of stratum corneum falls below 10%.

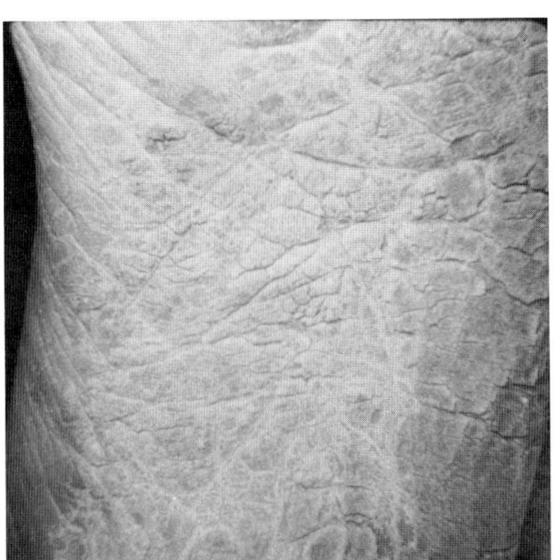

Figure 6.73. Idiopathic keratosis—sole is anidrotic and scaling.

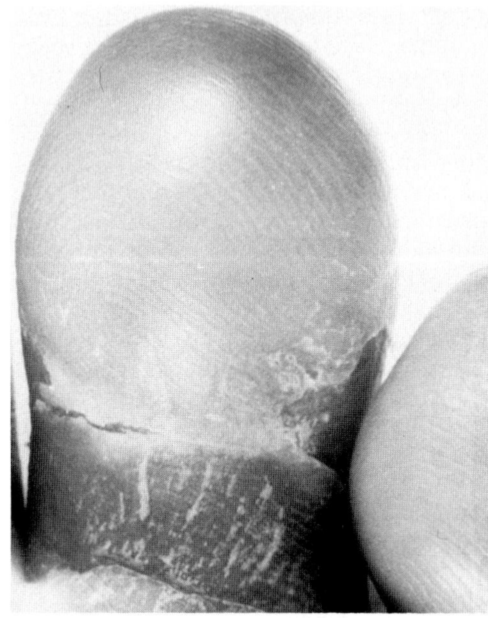

Figure 6.74. Anidrosis. Fissure plantar surface toe—secondary to dry skin.

Treatment. Excessive dryness of the skin must be treated both locally and systemically. The daily use of concentrated vitamin A in 50,000 to 100,000 U.S.P. units often improves the texture of the skin. The local use of emollient creams and moisturizing agents is suggested for maintenance of a healthy skin texture. Carmol (20% Urea) cream has been effective when applied after bathing. Lavin foot deodorant cream (zinc oxide base) applied at bedtime is reported to eliminate odor for 7 to 10 days. It is obvious that the skin must have proper application of moisturizing agents if the patient is to enjoy the comforts of supple skin. Correction of systemic, metabolic and endocrine disturbances often improves skin texture. In advanced circulatory problems, a sympathectomy has proven to be effective in some instances.

A breakdown of skin into fissures and ulcerations may hinder comfortable weightbearing and walking. Where fissures and ulcerations develop in anidrotic skin, it is advisable to use stimulating ointments or moisturizing agents. Fissuring of the skin is often relieved by application of tincture of benzoin compound. Use of heel cups (118) or plaster of Paris heel casts gives immediate relief and aids in repair of heel fissures.

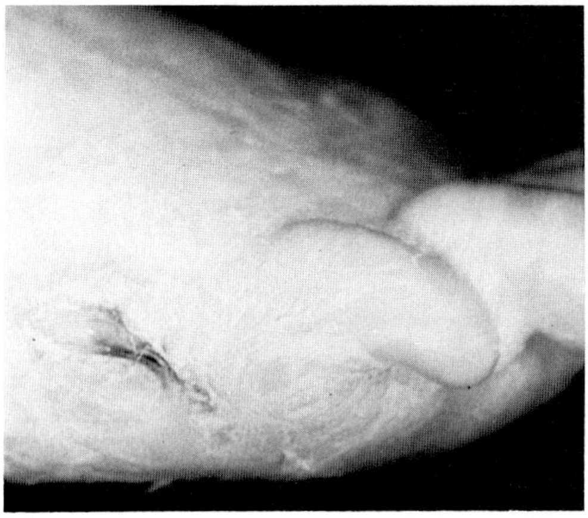

Figure 6.75. Ulceration in anidrotic skin, fifth metatarsal head.

Feldman (117, 119) recommends the use of a water-in-oil emulsion for dry skin, consisting of 50% water in a hydrophilic ointment base, Polysorb. Patients were advised to apply Polysorb hydrate once or twice daily according to the severity of dry skin.

Prentice and Brezak (120) recommend the use of hydrophilic water-in-oil emulsion either in a whirlpool bath or as a foot soak before treatment. It may also be used in the form of a spray for its prolonged aftereffect.

Boesenberg and Haas (121) used capsules of 50,000 U.S.P. units of natural vitamin A in a water-soluble base bid for several weeks. Results were especially promising in the 48 cases treated. Hyperkeratotic lesions regressed in 71.4% of fissured heels, in 58.3% of yellow clavi and 53.8% of senile keratosis. Oral treatment was supplemented by inunction of a vitamin A cream.

Sturtz (122) supported the use of oral vitamin A with hydrodispersant emollients or lipoidal baths. He cautioned against defatting the skin by using strong soap washings and recommended super-fatted soaps he calls "anti-dry soap."

Mulary and Urbach (123) used proteolytic debridement in severe hyperkeratosis of the palms and soles. The soles of the feet were soaked for 30 min in a 30% solution of commercial urea powder and water. The cutaneous horns and keratoses became white, translucent, slippery and soft. The hyperkeratoses were removed by scalpel until all thickened keratin was removed. This was repeated bid for 4 to 5 days. Rough spots were gently planed with a wire brush.

Small heel fissures may be excised and sutured successfully; however underlying tissues of the heel cannot be mobilized successfully. Free grafts provide only a temporary cover; hyperkeratosis may occur between the graft and normal skin. The thickness between the graft and plantar skin differs, and a keratin wall appears at the periphery. This scar is prevented by having the approximating edges of similar keratinized thickness. The fat and fascia must be about the same thickness, which is best accomplished by pedicle graft from plantar skin in an adjacent area.

Swanbeck (125) found that high concentrations of urea allowed for an increase in the uptake of water by the horny layer of the skin. Seven patients with ichthyosis were treated with urea cream, and 12 patients with atopic eczema were treated with combinations of urea cream and 1% hydrocortisone. Urea was found to be effective as a keratolytic agent and had the advantages of being nontoxic and nonallergenic.

Papa and Kligman (126) stated that in some cases return of sweating is affected by applying Scotch tape, and by pulling it off, the stratum corneum is cleared from the porokeratotic duct.

In senile keratosis or actinic keratosis the use of a 5% fluorouracil (Efudex) creates an inflammatory reaction and exfoliation of skin. Treatment lasts for 2 weeks, followed by a cessation of treatment to allow skin to clear. Results have been excellent in those cases that had previously been treated by desiccation with only fair results.

Dermatomycosis (Dermatophytosis)

The diagnosis of skin lesions of the feet cannot be made on the basis of clinical findings alone. It is necessary to evaluate itching, peeling, vesiculopurulent areas on the feet by direct microscopic slides

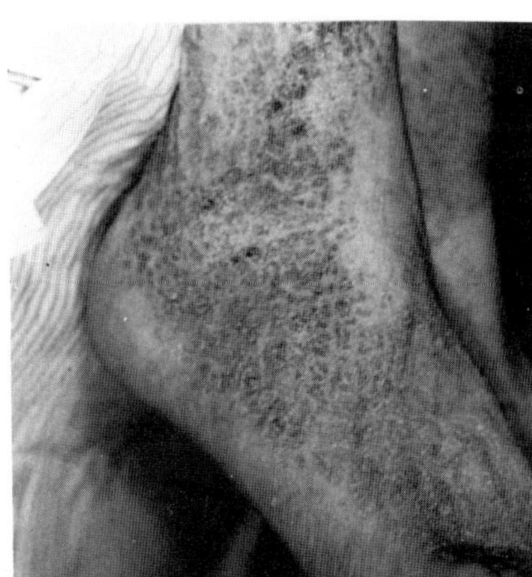

Figure 6.76. Ichthyosis. Note dry thick scales and crusts. Usually systemic and present to a variable degree all over the body.

and culture studies. Too often the presence of the classical clinical signs of tinea pedis is not confirmed by microscopic examination or culture. Potassium hydroxide (KOH) 10% slide preparation and Dermatophyte Testing Media (DTM) are excellent diagnostic aids. Positive cultures turn the media from yellow to red in 48–72 hrs and are 97% accurate. The podiatrist must differentiate between tinea pedis and a variety of skin disorders ranging from chronic eczema, psoriasis, nummular dermatitis, contact dermatitis, dermatitis medicamentosa and others (Figs. 6.77–6.84). Steinberg (88) noted a possible etiologic relationship between fungus infection of the human foot and rheumatoid arthritis through a complex antigen antibody effect.

Moisture, heat, dirt and alterations in pH on the surface of the feet create an ideal media for fungus growth. The normal range in pH of 4 to 6 is sufficiently acid to inhibit fungus growth. Kasdan (127), in an interesting study of the environment and fungal morphology of *Trichophyton mentagrophytes,* was led into an investigation of the enzyme systems of the granular and pleomorphic forms. His hypothesis that the pleomorph may well be the cause of chronic resistant cases of superficial mycotic infections is interesting, provocative and may well establish a treatment for permanent remission of symptoms.

Leyden and Klingman (128) discuss new concepts in pathogenesis of interdigital "athlete's foot." They provide an approach to the etiology and treatment

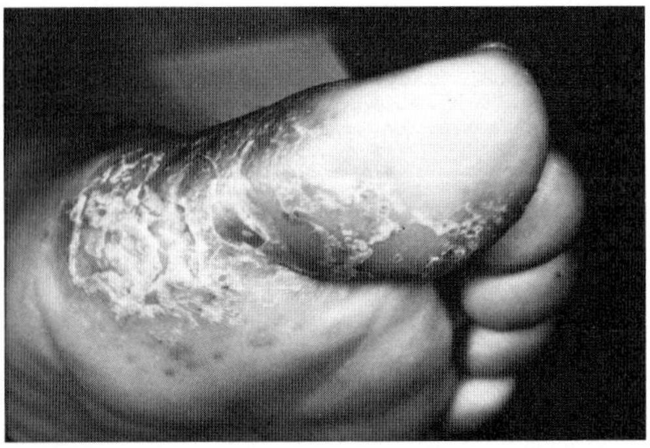

Figure 6.77. Psoriasis. Note silvery white imbricated scales.

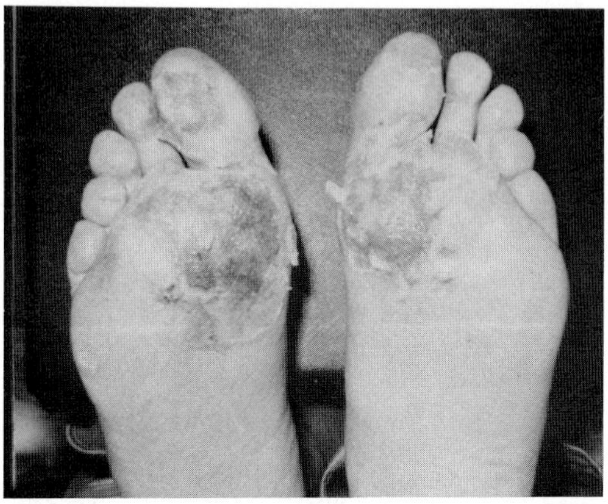

Figure 6.78. Mycotic and secondary bacterial infection.

that is based on maintaining the feet dry and free of moisture during the warmer weather and while performing sport activities. They acknowledge the invasion of the horny layers by dermatophytes, but recognize the normal resident aerobic diphtheroids as causing the wetness and maceration. They note an overgrowth of Gram-negative pseudomonas and proteus as responsible for the more serious cases of "athlete's foot." They blame the excess of moisture for the overgrowth of bacteria. They advise wearing sandals to enhance the evaporation of moisture. They state that perhaps the ideal would be a broad spectrum antibiotic and antifungal preparation. In conclusion, they state their agent of choice is aluminum chloride, which provides antimicrobial and drying action. However, the investigators shed very little light on the overall problem, nor does their resident bacteria concern provide anything new to the usual armamentarium of the podiatrist.

Interdigital tinea pedis usually begins with invasion of the horny layer by dermatophytes. Large numbers of normally resident aerobic diphtheroids cause the common wet, macerated type of "athlete's foot," whereas an overgrowth of Gram-negative organisms, such as pseudomonas and proteus, is responsible for the more serious cases. Drugs with broad spectrum antibacterial and antifungal activity may be helpful. The author's agent of choice, aluminum chloride, combines broad spec-

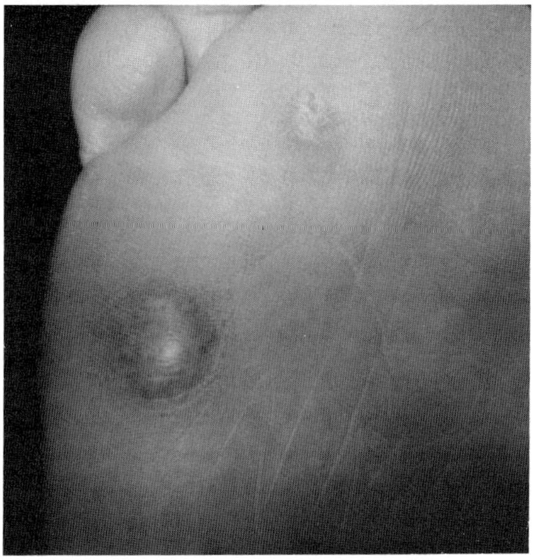

Figure 6.79. Acute mycotic bleb.

trum antimicrobial activity with chemical drying, a two-pronged attack. One should view drying as the decisive element; it is doubtful that any local treatment can permanently eradicate tinea pedis.

Hicks (129) noted that injections of trichophyton antigen into the skin of the unilateral affected leg with erythema nodosum and mycotic infection produced nodules similar to the erythema nodosum. He postulates that, whenever the etiology is obscure, erythema nodosum may be secondary to a mycotic infection. Griseofulvin orally appeared to correct both problems.

Levy (130) discussed the following signs and symptoms of fungal diseases of the foot that must be considered in a differential diagnosis: "contact dermatitis (shoes, socks, soaps, industrial materials, cosmetics), psoriasis, anidrosis, hyperidrosis, dysidrosis, intertrigo, erythrasma, lichen chronicus simplex, eczema, syphilis, systemic disease, pruritus, callus and others." Levy discussed the disease in reference to the etiology and levels of prevention and concerned himself with the agent, environment and host. He described three approaches to prevention: primary concerns, secondary therapeutic techniques and tertiary preventive approaches.

Treatment. There are a number of approaches in managing mycotic infections. First, the patient should avoid synthetic hose that prevent evaporation of insensible perspiration and should wear light-weight wool or loosely knit cotton instead. Feet must be bathed frequently in a hexachlorophene preparation and dried thoroughly, especially between the toes. Exposing the feet to sunlight is helpful. Other treatment depends on the type of fungus infection.

An acute eczematoid type of infection with blisters, crusts and scales, either primary or secondary to an old tinea, is treated with wet dressings of a dilute potassium permanganate solution about 1:12,000, an aluminum subacetate solution or Burow's solution in wet evaporating dressings to reduce inflammatory changes.

Maskin et al. (131), in a study of dermatophytosis from 1935 to 1954, point up the increase of *Trichophyton rubrum* as the cause of most dermatophytosis in this country.

Rothman and Windhorst (110) discuss tinea pedis as a source of infection in a family. A man with *T. rubrum* infection of the toes and heel placed his foot on the family toilet seat while treating his foot. His wife then acquired a tinea circinata of the left buttock. patients with tinea pedis must be warned of the contagious and autoinoculable characteristics of the infection.

Arancia and Montgomery (132), in discussing cutaneous moniliasis, say that "certain conditions of altered metabolism such as debilitation, obesity, diabetes mellitus, hyperidrosis, and pregnancy predispose to cutaneous infection." They conclude that effectiveness in treatment of moniliasis of the feet was 50% better when nystatin was used in combination with other drugs. Relapses did occur and the addition of

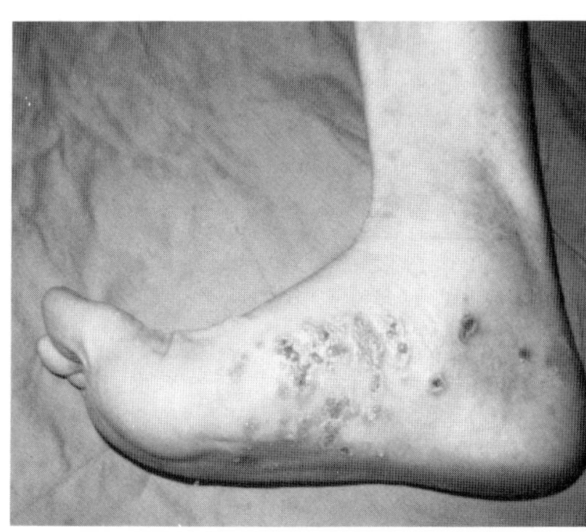

Figure 6.80. Actue mycotic infection with vesiculoserous dermatosis—positive microscopic examination and culture result.

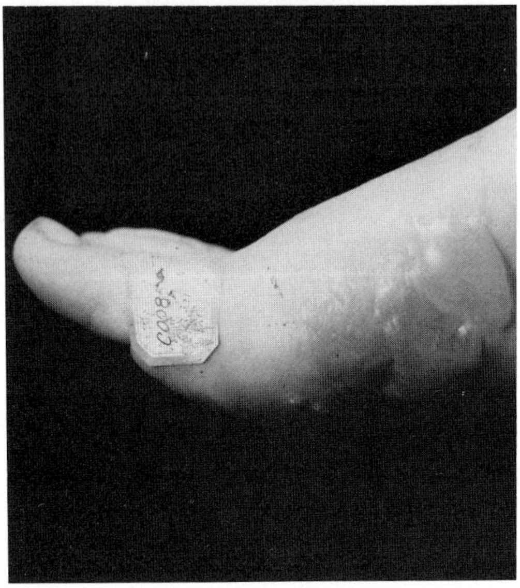

Figure 6.81. Large bullous lesion secondary to adhesive irritation. Differentiate from tinea. (Courtesy of D Mowbray.)

antibacterial agents to the nystatin shortened the course of therapy. Fluorohydrocortisone relieved erythema, burning and itching. Goldman and Unger (133) found that when *Candida albicans* is the causitive organism the specific drug nystatin results in permanent control of the infection.

Hirschberg (134) discussed a technique for destroying pathogenic microorganisms in footwear. The shoes and hose were placed in a nonhydrostatic polyethylene bag with a tablet containing trioxymethylene and hexahydrothymol (Zondex) as active ingredients. Hirschberg states that "95% of patients shoes tested before treatment contained spores of *C. albicans, T. gypseum,* aspergillus and *T. purpure.* After treatment with the fumigant for 24 to 48 hr, no evidence of the spores could be found on reexamination."

Walker (135) evaluated 1 to 2% copper sulfate solution iontophoresis. He stressed the local effect, the low toxicity of the solution, its fungicidal properties and its deterrent effect on chronic recurrent eczema or "id" reaction. The patient's tolerance at an average of 10 mA for 10 min is considered desirable.

Goldberg (136) showed that "clinically well feet seldom harbor pathogenic fungi and the shoes of these patients have little or no fungal elements."

Secondary reactions of cellulitis, lymphangitis and lymphadenopathy are treated with care to reduce sensitization from antibiotics. Systemic penicillin should not be used at this time for fear of sensitizing the patient. Wet dressings of sodium chloride as a warm physiological saline or dilute potassium permanganate soaks are helpful. Aspirin, 2 tablets q.4 h with rest and elevation reduces fever. Neomycin sulfate is the topical antibiotic of choice. Griseofulvin is best used when the condition is subacute and in a quiescent state.

The chronic mycotic infection is manifested by dryness and scaling. Acute flare-ups can be avoided by reducing the scratch-itch syndrome. Unsaturated fatty acids, such as undecylenic and proprionic acids, in creams or ointments may be used effectively to reduce the infection. The feet are kept dry. Undecylenic and/or propionic acid powders used regularly between toes, shoes and hose inhibit the growth of fungi.

Oral griseofulvin may be prescribed for mycotic infections. Careful observation of the patient for sensitivities and blood dyscrasias is recommended. Ultrafine griseofulvin, 320 mg or 500 mg taken once daily seems to be effective. Lindenberg (137) reported improvement in 25 of 28 cases studied under treatment with griseofulvin. Pruritus disappeared in 1 week. Minor headaches and occasional gastrointestinal disturbances were noted.

Gibbs (183) classified the clinical varieties of tinea pedis as 1) a dry scaly interdigital type; 2) dry scaly plantar type; and 3) vesicular type; dermatophytidic type. The dry scaly interdigital type presents erythrasma in the webs. It can be diagnosed by the reddish fluorescence of Wood's light even though cultures are negative.

The dry scaly plantar type of tinea pedis, usually resulting in a moccasin-like diffuse scaling, is pathognomonic of *T. rubrum* infection. Obviously, these lesions must be differentiated from primary irritant contact dermatitis. Unilateral vesiculation

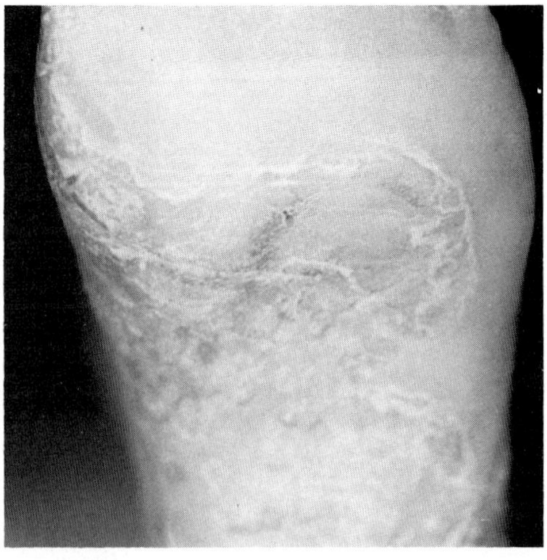

Figure 6.82. Psoriasis. Note silvery white imbricated scales. Lesions also on elbows and knees.

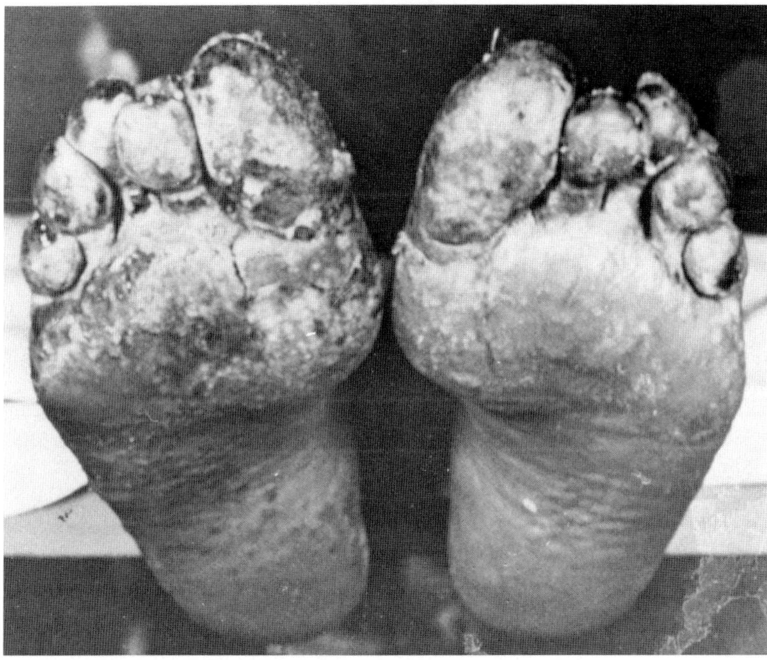

Figure 6.83. Exfoliative dermatitis secondary to sensitivity to man-made materials in shoes. Patch tests indicated to aid in differentiation from mycotic infection.

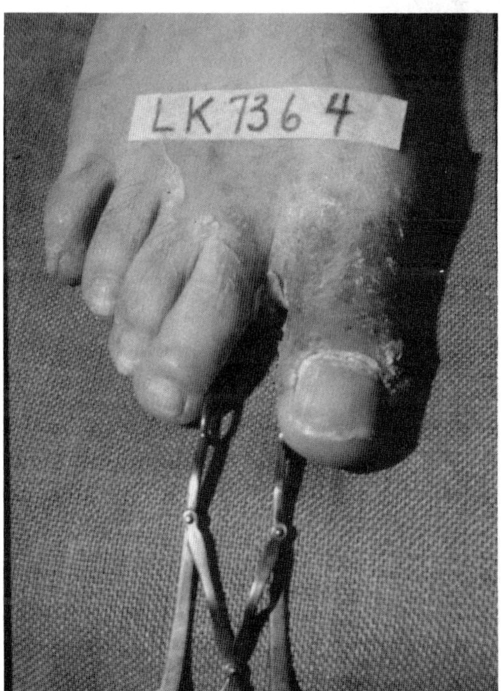

Figure 6.84. Dermatitis secondary to irritation of prescribed medication for mycotic infection. Acute inflammations of this type often damage the nail bed resulting in loss of toe nail. Note eponychium. (Courtesy of M Shapiro.)

probably has another cause than fungus. The vesicular type of tinea pedis may have to be differentiated from herpes zoster, which is severely painful. Mycotic infections are rarely painful unless secondarily infected.

The "id" reaction on the hands secondary to mycotic foot infections have to be differentiated from dysidrosis and pustular psoriasis. Fungi are not found in "id" lesions of the hands.

Apt (139) notes that the clearing of a primary lesion results in disappearance of the "id" reaction. Because the "id" lesion is sterile of fungi it is not desirable to use antifungal agents in treating it. Conant et al. (140) recommend treating the "id" reaction with warm, wet saline or boric acid compresses, soothing lotions and creams.

The ringworm organism excretes an allergen to which the tissue is sensitized or produces cytotoxic toxins affecting nonallergic skin. Apt hints that resistance or susceptibility may be genetically transmitted and that a high percentage of humans are naturally resistant to most dermatophytes.

Blank et al. (141) described the typical response of tinea pedis to griseofulvin as relief of itching and burning in 2 to 6 days. Cultures and microscopic examination become negative in 2 to 6 weeks as vesicles and scales disappear completely. Topical keratolytic agents aid in eradicating fungi from the skin of the feet. Haas and Boesenberg (142) reported a rate of cure or major improvement of 84% in the treatment of 30 patients with onychomycosis and dermatophytosis and with both diseases being treated concomitantly. Many patients had mixed culture responses, such as *T. mentagrophytes* and *T. rubrum* or *C. albicans.*

Ashur and Farrar (143) treated 104 patients with tinea pedis and 56 patients with onychomycosis using griseofulvin, 1,000 mg. daily. The infecting organism was *T. mentagrophytes, T. rubrum* or *Epidermophyton floccosum.* Ninety-one patients with tinea pedis were cured, and nine substantially improved. Of the patients with onychomycosis, 39 were cured and 5 substantially improved. Tinea pedis was usually cured in 2 months and onychomycosis within 12 months. Clinical side effects were mild and transient, and no pathological changes were noted following regular examinations of blood and urine.

The author has had excellent results in eradicating toenail mycoses by means of periodic (every 2–3 months) local surgical debridement and topical application twice daily of three drops of clotrimazole solution 1% (Mycelex, Lotrimin). Clotrimazole is effective against *Trichophyton, Epidermophyton,* Microsporin, and *Candida.* However, it is only effective if the mycotic infection has not progressed proximal to the lanula. If the mycotic infection has so progressed, the nail is avulsed. As the new nail grows, three drops of clotrimazole solution are applied morning and evening. In the rare instance that topical therapy is ineffective, a dose of 320 mg of griseofulvin ultramicrosize (Fulvicin P/G) after the large meal of the day is prescribed. Because of previous matrix cell damage from the mycotic infection, new nail growth may be abnormal in a significant percentage of cases. This new growth may manifest as hypertrophy or atrophy of the nail plate or involution of the sides.

Ganley (144) reported excellent treatment results in 38 of 50 patients with mycotic infections using solutions of tolnaftate (1%) (Tinactin). Tolnaftate is available in a solution, as a cream and as a powder for use bid. He notes disappointing results when pre-existing disease processes and associated illnesses exist. Results with this fungicidal agent in solution with a vehicle of butylated hydroxytoluene and ployethylene glycol have been good.

Stern and Fletcher (145) in a study of 131 patients found that Tinactin was the best treatment for acute and chronic tinea pedis.

Carpenter (146), in a 10-month controlled clinical study, noted clearing of the clinical signs of infection using tolnaftate in solution on lesions between the toes and on the dorsum. He suggests that local treatment is best combined with systemic griseofulvin if laboratory examination corroborates the diagnosis. According to his experience penetrability of tolnaftate is increased following a bath or foot soaks.

Ilowite (147) concluded that 1) dermatophytes cannot penetrate the stratum corneum unless irritation or maceration of the skin occurs, 2) disease ensues where tissue structure and function become deranged and 3) exposure to fungi plays a minor role in eliciting attacks of "athlete's foot."

Goldfarb et al. (148) noted few undesirable reactions in a group of 137 patients treated with from 0.25 to 3.0 g of griseofulvin per day. Therapy was discontinued when severe headache, persistent diarrhea or extreme fatigue occurred in rare cases. Despite relief of clinical symptoms, about one-third of the patients clinically cured continued to be mycologically positive on KOH slide examination.

Reiss and Kornblee (149), in a 5-year study of tinea pedis treatment, state that "the average duration of treatment of patients was 8 weeks for those infected with *T. rubrum;* 6 weeks for those with *T. mentagrophytes;* 7 weeks for those with *E. floccosum.*"

Estershon (150) noted in his study of 16 elderly patients with skin and nail mycotic infections that oral pulvule type ultrafine griseofulvin proved more effective, safer, and easier to administer than topical preparations. Cacciaglia et al. (151) review the literature and discuss ketocanazole therapy in the treatment of tinea pedis and onychomycosis. Ketocanazole, an imidazole derivative, is the first encouraging new oral and now topical antimycotic in 20 years. It has demonstrated usefulness against a variety of fungal diseases, including tinea pedis, when griseofulvin has failed.

Jones (152) suggested that incision areas are often protected, dressed and medicated to prevent infection, yet create the very media for the overgrowth of *C. albicans.* The treatment of choice following positive identification of the sterile vesicular lesions around a postoperative site is to remove occlusive dressings, use drying agents and medicate with drugs containing nystatin or amphoteracin B. Nystatin is provided in cream, ointment, powder, oral tablets and suspension form. Amphoteracin B comes in a cream, lotion and ointment.

In treating mycotic skin infections, the author recommends removal of all irritants, identification of the infecting organism and use of correct footgear. Local applications of tolnaftate, clotrimazole or clotrimazole and betamethasone dipropionate (Lotrisone) cream, or ciclopirox olamine (solution or powder) are effective, as are undecylenic solutions, creams and powders. Systemic griseofulvin, 320–500 mg daily, may be a necessary adjunct if local treatment is ineffective.

Other Dermatologic Lesions

Mycetoma pedis **(Madura foot)** (Fig. 6.85), a superficial mycosis, usually occurs in young adults and is characterized by a painful enlargement of the forefoot that is pitted and presents multiple discharging sinus tracts. Regional lymph glands may be swollen and necrotic with a discharge containing fungi. Often the lesions are deep, involving tendons, muscles and bone. The patient appears to have a markedly enlarged foot extending from an atrophic leg.

Treatment consists of incision and drainage of the sinus tracts followed by excision of the infected tissue. Skin grafts may be necessary. The drug of choice is chlortetracycline, 250 mg q. 6 h, together with diaminophenylsulfone, 50 mg daily for the first week and 100 to 250 mg daily during the second week. Oyston (153) described the lesions and the treatment in a study of 20 cases.

Multiple vesiculobullous lesions of the feet with intense pruritus in the presence of hyperidrosis may be **pompholyx (dysidrosis).** Ingestion of sensitizing food may be etiologic. Pompholyx may develop in the presence of epidermophytosis and often is incited by allergic and toxic manifestations. It is usually resistant to treatment.

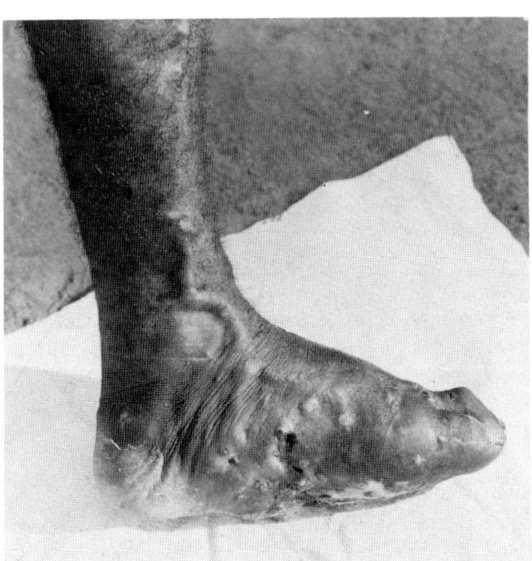

Figure 6.85. Madura foot. (Courtesy of Armed Forces Institute of pathology, #045-386-1.)

Haber and Wells (154) described a subcorneal pustular dermatosis of the soles. The vesiculopustular lesions failed to respond to bed rest, local application of superficial x-ray therapy and a variety of internal and topical drugs.

There was no evidence of fungus infection on microscopic examination and cultures. Bacteriologic cultures were sterile. The bullae were filled with neutrophiles, and the base appeared to undergo acantholysis. The great number of polymorphs under the stratum corneum produced a slight inflammatory reaction. No etiologic explanation has been given for this subcorneal lesion.

Treatment of bullous lesions includes draining. Cultures are prepared. Undecylenic acid compounds are applied, and the part is kept dry.

Atopic Dermatitis and Allergic Eczematous Contact Dermatitis

An eczematous eruption on the feet of a patient with a history of asthma, hay fever, urticaria or migraine headaches may be atopic dermatitis. Gibbs (155) defines atopic dermatitis of the adult type as dermatitis appearing on the feet as a circumscribed scaly area, especially on the toes, or lichenified plaques around the ankles, dorsa of the feet and instep (Figs. 6.86–6.88).

Contact dermatitis caused by shoes, hose, adhesive tape or other sensitizing materials or chemicals may primarily affect the dorsum of the foot, especially the skin overlying the hallux. It manifests as a scaling erythematous vesicular and bull-

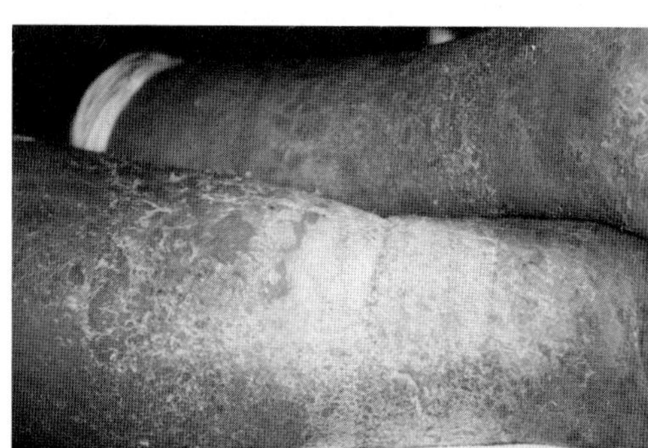

Figure 6.86. Eczematoid dermatitis—lichenification.

ous dermatosis that spreads to the dorsum of the adjacent toes. Secondary inflammatory reactions may develop from the itch-scratch syndrome. These include infections accompanied by hyperidrosis, cellulitis, lymphangitis and lymphadenopathy. The condition may be bilateral, and often a secondary id-like reaction may affect the hands. Pruritus may be severe, and the characteristic appearance may develop on any part of the foot that comes in contact with an irritant. Sensitizing agents may be the thermoplastic substances used in toe caps of shoes and the accelerators and antioxidants of rubber. People who perspire excessively are good candidates for this condition. It is believed that excessive moisture leaches some of the sensitizing agents from the shoe, causing them to act as an irritant of the foot.

The toxic agents that obviously cause urticaria are believed to do so by acting on the mast cells in the dermis. Lerner and Lerner (156) cite the triple response of Lewis in some allergic reactions as a red reaction caused by capillary dilation, a diffuse flare caused by arteriolar dilation and a wheal or local edema from transudates caused by increased capillary permeability. The release of histamine can be blocked by antihistamines. The antihistamines probably work by inhibiting cutaneous nerve fibers that cause pain and itching.

Cangialosi (157) reports two cases of aquatic contact dermatitis affecting the foot arising from contact with venomous marine organisms. The article delineates the marine and podiatric physiology involved, as well as pertinent biochemical, pharmocological and management aspects to be considered.

Young (158) describes the symptoms of winter pedal dermatitis in a series of 156 cases. The etiology is briefly discussed and related to contact with an irritant substance (contact dermatitis), hereditary predisposition (atopic dermatitis), aging skin through tissue loss (asteatotic eczema), possible low humidity changes and winter heating (winter eczema) and unknown etiology for psoriasis.

The author has been able to isolate causative agents by patch test despite

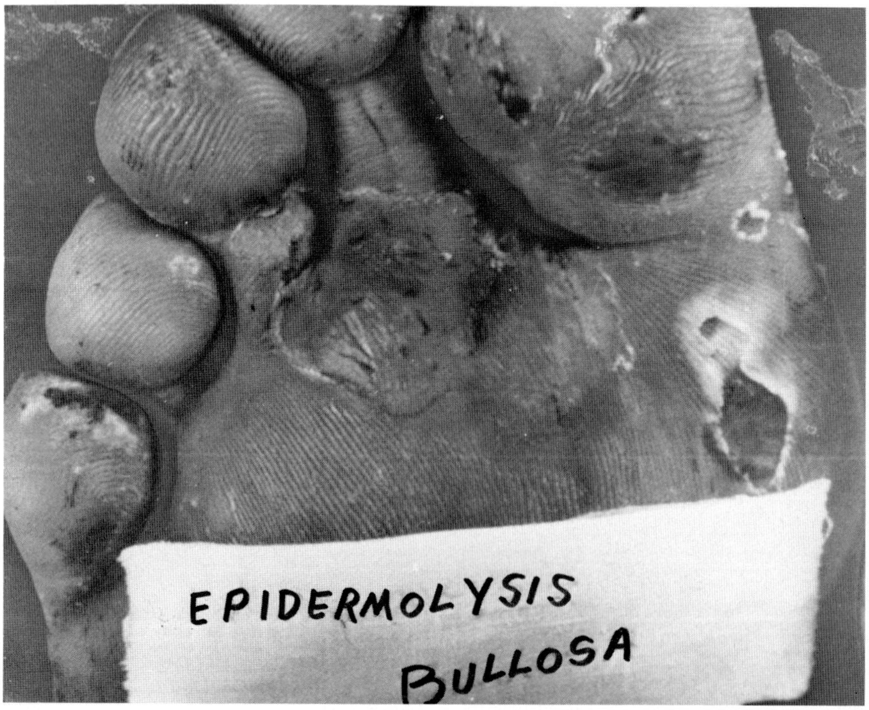

Figure 6.87. Epidermolysis bullosa. Note broken-down bullous lesions and excoriations from scratching.

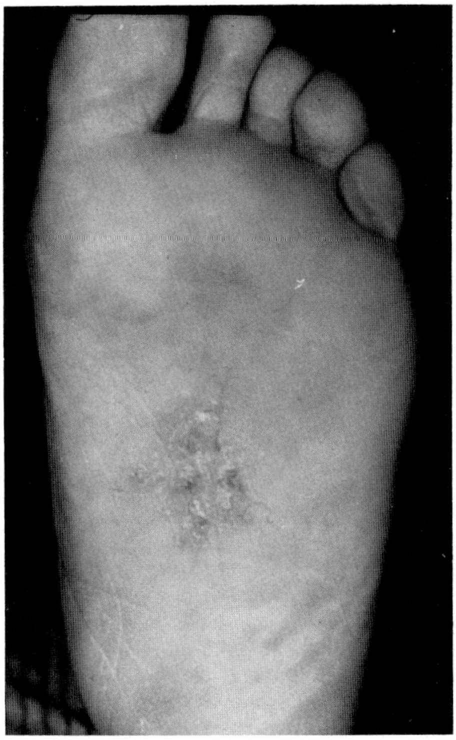

Figure 6.88. Atopic dermatitis.

varying opinions as to that test's efficacy (Fig. 6.89). Shoe polish, shoe dyes, plastic heel seats and insoles have been found to be directly responsible for the dermatitis. Many patients are sensitized to the chemical used in tanning leather, synthetic linings in shoes and rubber cements used to make shoe parts adhere in the manufacture of shoes.

Hack (159) discusses the availability of hypoallergenic shoes for relief of sensitivity reactions to materials in the manufactured shoe. Oxidizers and accelerators normally used in the manufacture of rubber may be the irritant. "Fish glues or cereal pastes" may be used successfully. Only those shoes of vegetable tanned leathers should be used if available. Excessive perspiration must be controlled, and if chromates are etiologic, the doctor should consider uppers made of Corfam. The Alden Shoe Company makes a hypoallergenic shoe called "Derma-Pedic."

Treatment. Removal of the sensitizing agent is the first step in treatment (Figs. 6.90 and 6.91).

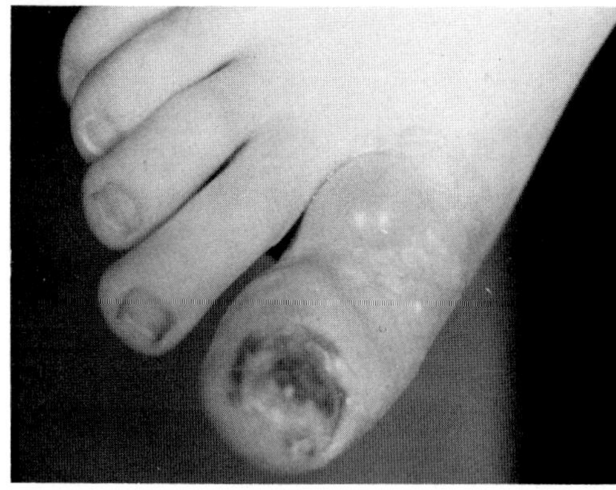

Figure 6.89. Contact dermatitis. Vesiculobullous lesions secondary to contact with "nonsensitizing" bandage. Patch test confirmed.

Burow's solution soaks diminish inflammatory changes and may reduce weeping. Antipruritic medications, such as calamine, hydrocortisone cream 0.5–1%, or other stronger steroid creams are indicated if itching persists. Soothing protective pastes and 1 to 3% Vioform in a suitable base are helpful. In the presence of secondary infection, topical applications of antibiotics and systemic broad spectrum antibiotics are essential. In the presence of severe allergic reactions, the author prescribes terfenadine (Seldane), 60 mg AM and PM or diphenhydramine (Benadryl), 50 mg capsules, 3 to 4 capsules daily for relief of itching. Tablets of methdilazine (Tacaryl HCl) are helpful to relieve pruritus. A methylprednisolone (Medrol Dosepak) may be necessary.

Kierland (160), in investigating pruritus, states that management comes with cure of the basic condition causing the pruritus. Pruritus may be severe in uremia even when the degree of nitrogen retention is slight. When little cutaneous re-

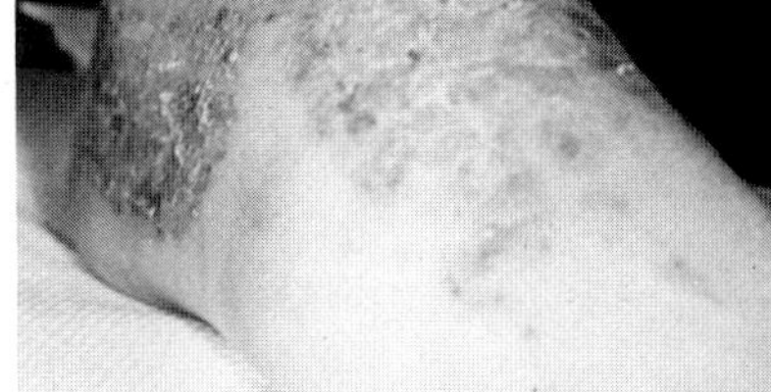

Figure 6.90. Contact dermatitis. Heel counter and tongue of shoe.

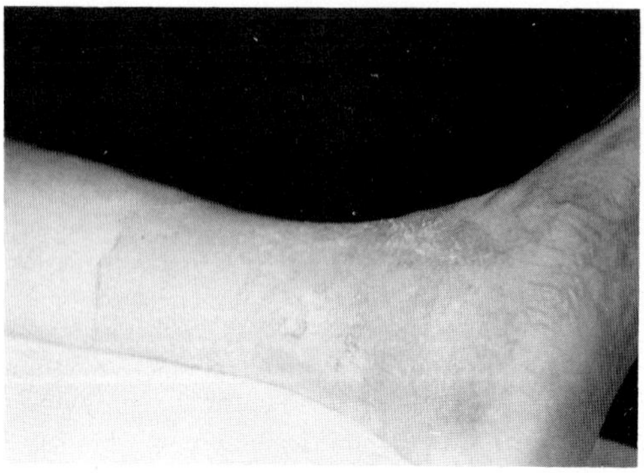

Figure 6.91. Contact dermatitis. Note line of dermarcation at upper end of stocking.

action is noted, the pruritis may be due to a systemic reaction.

Dermatitis therapy should begin with the simplest and mildest form of treatment. If successful, the treatment should not be changed.

Local treatment consists of cool or warm wet dressings, menthol in proper vehicles, 1 to 2% phenol in lotions, ointments or pastes. Steroids alone or in combination with antibiotics may be helpful.

Systemic treatment for pruritus may be disappointing. In urticaria, the itching may be relieved with antihistamines, such as Benadryl, 50 to 100 mg 3 to 4 times daily, dimenhydrinate (Dramamine), 50 mg tid, chlorpheniramine maleate (Chlortrimeton), 4 mg tid, or brompheniramine maleate (Dimetane), 4 to 8 mg. Systemic steroids should be used in only the most severe cases of skin lesions. Acetylsalicylic acid is helpful for relief of itching. Chloral hydrate does not increase itching and can be used effectively for nocturnal itching. Chlorpheniramine maleate (Teldrin), 8 and 12 mg spansules or capsules taken one on arising and one at night, often provides 24-hr relief from itching. The 8 mg spansule is suitable for children.

Vegetable-tanned shoes and inner linings or nonleather substitutes may be helpful when patients are sensitive to dichromate. Rubber insoles and dyes, fabrics that "bleed" and nickel sensitivity from eyelets may cause reactions in sensitive patients.

Weiner (161) described a dermatitis caused by shoes with plastic uppers and rubber soles. The impermeability of the material used in construction trapped excessive perspiration in the shoes causing the dermatitis.

In the treatment of such types of dermatoses as keratosis of the soles with a variety of skin manifestations, including crusts, scales, fissures, atopic lesions and dry and lichenified skin, the podiatrist may wish to use foot baths for their soothing and beneficial antipruritic and keratolytic effect. Aluminum subacetate, milk, potassium permanganate, tar, colloidal oatmeal in a starch-protein complex of oat grain in dispersible emollient oils, saline in physiological strengths and emollient oils or lubricating soaps may be used in baths (Fig. 6.92).

Franks (162) advises baths for treatment of patients with dermatitis to incorporate medication and for sedation of tense patients. The baths are helpful in removing crusts and debris.

Jillson (163) discusses the role of pathogenic and saprophytic fungi in causing allergic dermatitis. Intradermal skin tests are used to deter-

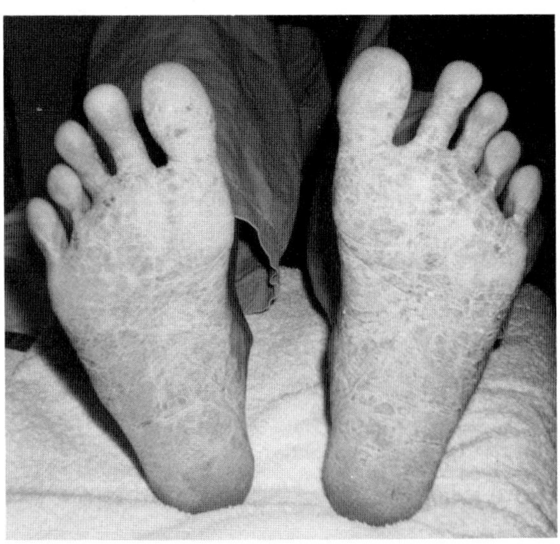

Figure 6.92. Idiopathic keratosis palms and soles in presence of ulcerative colitis.

mine the allergen. Treatment consists of avoiding the sensitizing molds in house dust, upholstered furniture mattresses, etc, followed by intradermal administration of dilute antigens in fixed amounts for desensitization. Extracts are injected twice weekly until the dermatitis has been cleared for several months. Booster shots can be given every 3 to 4 weeks while other dermatologic treatment continues.

Fisher (164) points out that most inexpensive shoes have a rubber thermoplastic toebox composed of scrap from old tires and girdles and the like. The rubber compound contains felt, turpentine, resin, rosin, styrene, asphalt and Carbowax as additives, as well as antioxidants and accelerators. He states that a satisfactory shoe should have a Celastic toebox made with cotton flannel impregnated with pyroxylin. The lining of all shoes may also contain rubber cement.

Trivalent chromic sulfate or hexavalent sodium dichromate used in tanning leathers is considered nonsensitizing. Fisher (164) found a 26% sensitivity to dichromate. Perspiration leaches chemicals from the leather.

Everall and Truter (165) could not find any basis for an antigen-antibody reaction in contact dermatitis. Existence of antibodies in epidermal hypersensitivity has not been proved, nor are there antibodies in the serum.

Following a study of adhesive tape as an irritant, Ignatoff (166) came to some interesting conclusions. The formula used in the manufacture of adhesive tape is physiologically acceptable. He states that adhesive tape reactions in ascending order of frequency are allergic, bacteriologic, chemical and mechanical. He found that less than 1% of patients exposed to adhesive tape have an allergic response. The improper application of adhesive tape accounts for the mechanical reactions.

Montgomery and Brezak (167) treated the pruritus of contact dermatitis, atopic eczema and neurodermatitis on the feet with good results by using a 3% Vioform-1% hydrocortisone preparation in a cream, lotion or ointment.

Schamberg et al. (168) treated 510 patients with a variety of dermatoses with a topical steroid and a placebo. They found that "steroid therapy is effective in only a limited number of selected dermatologic patients, and is dependent on the degree of inflammation, its location and other factors."

Reyer (169) described four cases in which adhesive tape applied to the feet to relieve strain resulted in a sensitivity over a period of months that ultimately affected the periorbital skin. It was believed that pathogenic amounts of tissue protein metabolites in the circulation after relief of the spasm and painful feet resulted in this pathology.

The symptoms of atopic dermatitis are controlled by use of topical preparations, such as Burow's solution, aluminum acetate, Dalibour solution or Buro-Sol, applied to dry weeping lesions to reduce inflammation. Betamethasone valerate or dipropionate (Valisone, Diprosone) cream and ointments relieve itching and reduce inflammatory changes. Flurandrenolone cream and ointment (Synalar) 0.05%, also with neomycin (Neo Synalar) or as a lotion or cream in half-strength (0.025%), or desoximetasone (Topcort) cream are also helpful in controlling symptoms. Hydrocortisone cream or lotion with or without neomycin in 0.5–1% relieves itching and helps control secondary infection.

Psoriasis is characterized by silvery-white imbricated scales overlying an erythematous base (Figs. 6.93 and 6.94). The nails often have a characteristic grayish-white discoloration with pitting and subungual hyperkeratotic debris.

Pathognomonic of the disease is the presence of deep redness with overlying white scales on the elbows and knees. Small bleeding points (Auspitz Sign) observed upon removal of a psoriatic scale are also pathognomonic. Pustular psoriasis occasionally develops on the feet and especially around the toenails.

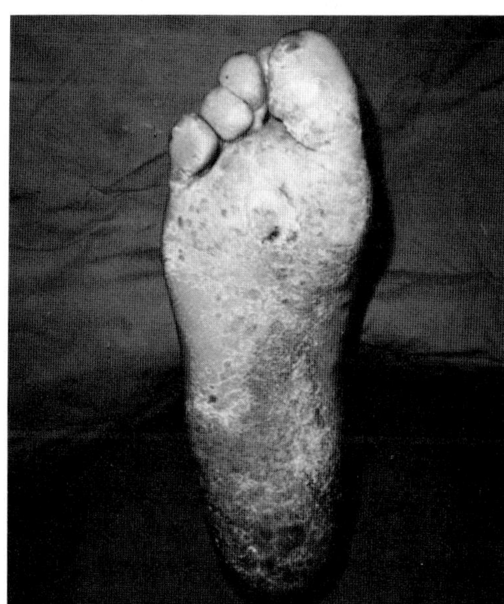

Figure 6.93. Pustular psoriasis—silvery white imbricated scales with interspersed seropurulent vesicles.

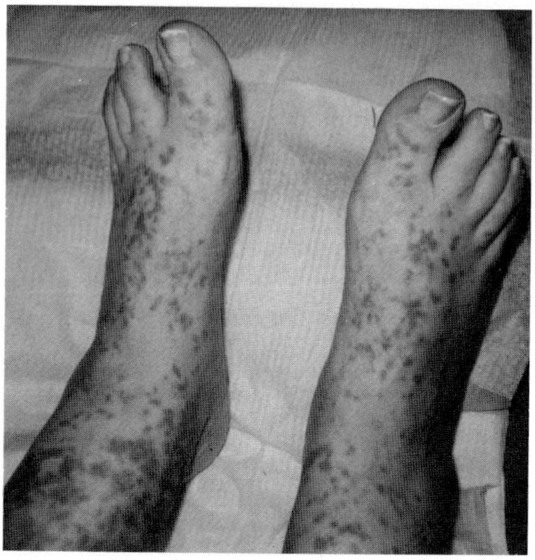

Figure 6.94. Purpuric spots—idiopathic. Must differentiate from psoriasis or rose spots secondary to peripheral vascular disease.

Treatment for psoriasis has been discouraging to the patient and doctor alike. However, research has been conducted at 16 medical centers in the United States confirming the effectiveness of a photochemotherapeutic treatment for psoriasis. 1,308 patients with severe psoriasis were treated two to three times weekly with an orally administered drug called 8-methoxypsoralen, followed by carefully controlled exposure to a specially constructed high-intensity, long wave ultraviolet light source. Melski et al. (171) noted that 88% of those patients under treatment were cleared and only 3% failed to clear. One percent dropped out of the study due to treatment complications, and 8% dropped out for other reasons. The treatment induces and maintains a temporary remission of psoriasis.

Whitfield's ointment (USP) is helpful in removing the scales associated with chronic psoriasis. Steroid ointments and creams, e.g., betamethasone valerate (Valisone) or betamethasone dipropionate (Diprosone), applied bid or tid are effective in controlling the psoriatic lesions. (See Chapter 13, Podiatric Treatment).

Lichen planus (Fig. 6.95). may occur on the soles of the feet, although that area is not the usual site. It is characterized by flat-topped, violaceous, polygonal papules. The lesions are discrete, but may coalesce to form plaques. They commonly occur around the ankles, and when they develop on the soles, they must be differentiated from mycotic infections.

Treatment may be by tincture or ointment serving as a keratolytic and antipruritic reducing agent. A tar tincture, such as rectified oil of birch tar, 10 g, alcohol (U.S.P.), 50 g; ether q.s. ad 100 g; or a hydrophilic petrolatum ointment containing epithelial cell cytotoxic substances, such as podophyllum in 0.25%, 0.5% or 1% strengths, may prove effective if treatment is exercised with care. Hyperkeratoses may regress, and itching is usually relieved.

Exfoliative dermatitis (Fig. 6.96) is an indurated erythema of the skin that progresses to lichenification and scaling. The skin is warm, and the patient experiences chills and fever. The skin itches, and the palms and soles may peel with fissuring. Hair loss and nail changes may follow an acute episode in middle-aged and elderly patients. Previous eczemas and ingestion of drugs may be etiologic. Systemic steroids are generally helpful.

Erythrasma is a bacterial infection of the skin most commonly manifested in the foot as an intertriginous affliction of the toe clefts. It is characterized by fissur-

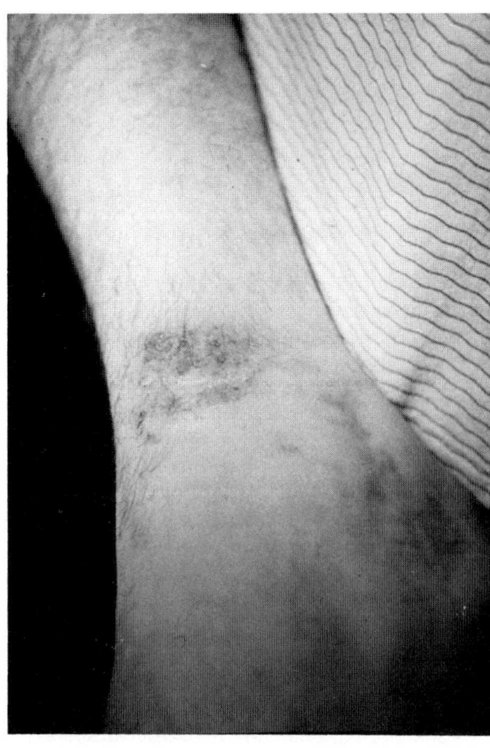

Figure 6.95. Lichen planus.

ing, scaling and maceration between the toes but is not caused by fungus or *Monilia*.

Sarkany et al. (172) noted that 23% of 109 normal subjects examined presented symptoms of erythrasma. Temple and Boardman (173), in an examination of 371 university students with Wood's light, found a 14.3% incidence of erythrasma. Bacteria were cultured from 50 of the 53 specimens examined. Clinical findings demonstrate dry, irregularly shaped, fine, red to brown scales with coral red fluorescence seen under Wood's light and by electron microscopic examinations. Smears demonstrate the presence of Gram-positive rods and filaments with granules; corynebacterium minutissimum.

Treatment. Erythromycin, especially the propionyl ester of erythromycin, (Ilosone, Erythrocin), 250 mg qid for 5 days, proved to be the drug of choice. Topical applications of soothing soaks, powders and creams are justified in controlling the symptoms. Brown (174) approves of topical applications to relieve pruritus, but has not seen beneficial results with topical antibiotics. Ointments containing phenol, menthol, camphor, salicylic acid or tar in low percentages are effective in relieving the itch.

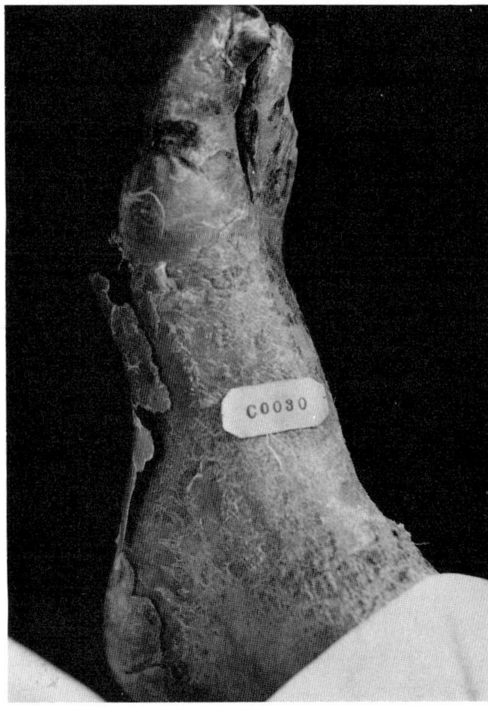

Figure 6.96. Exfoliative dermatitis—unknown etiology. Note indurated erythema and lichenification with scaling. (Courtesy of D Mowbray.)

Black Heel—Pseudochromidrose Plantaire

Kirton and Price (175) report on 49 cases of plantar pseudochromidrose as described by Baze and co-workers from 1962 to 1964. The unusual complaint consisted of a small black patch on the back or side of the heel occurring predominantly in girls between the ages of 12 and 22. Some of the spots were circular or oval with minute round dark spots and some scattered granules of pigmentation. The condition is generally unilateral with only a single lesion occurring on a foot. The keratotic tissue can be reduced often without bleeding.

Histochemically the lesion gives a positive reaction of peroxidase, benzidine and hemochromogen, proving the presence of hemoglobin. Pigment is present in the sweat ducts. Often the lesion undergoes complete spontaneous resolution and is painless. Removing trauma is essential for cure. According to Wilkinson (176), the lesion has been confused with a melanoma.

Cutaneous Herniations (pizeiogenic papules) have been described by Galinski (177) as "fatty subcutaneous tissue passing through a defect of the connective tissue into the fascial layer of the dermis." These fat herniations are not uncommon and are rarely painful. Galinski describes a unilateral case in a patient, age 27. The author has seen these papules in children as young as 6 years old and in individuals in their sixties and seventies. There seems to be a predisposition for their formation in overweight individuals and in those people who wear open-backed footgear. The multiple herniations on the medial, lateral and posterior of the heels measure 0.3 to 1.0 cm in diameter on weightbearing and disappear at rest. The lesions are easily compressed. No treatment is necessary. In the rare instance of associated discomfort, a Tuli, M/F heel cup or firm heel-countered shoe may be used for relief.

Neurodematitic Reaction (Neurodermatitis)

Sachs et al. (178) describe a neurodermatitic reaction as a "pathologic process and not a disease" (Fig. 6.97). They stated that the reaction involves both the cutis and the epidermis. The epidermis is acanthotic, somewhat regular and with very little evidence of swelling. The middle and upper layers of the dermis present thickened walls of the arterioles and small arteries. A focal infiltration of small round and connective tissue cells is found around the vessels.

Clinically the neurodermatitic reaction resembles other dermatoses, especially nummular eczema, which differs only in the presence of an intraepidermic vesicle. An exudative inflammatory process exists in both conditions. However, discoid chronic dermatosis presents a cellular infiltration of the productive type.

Sachs et al. (179) classify nummular eczema as a form of neurodermatitis. It has been described for years as a coin-shaped patch with a vesicular border and clearly pigmented center. The lesions occur on the dorsum of the hands and feet.

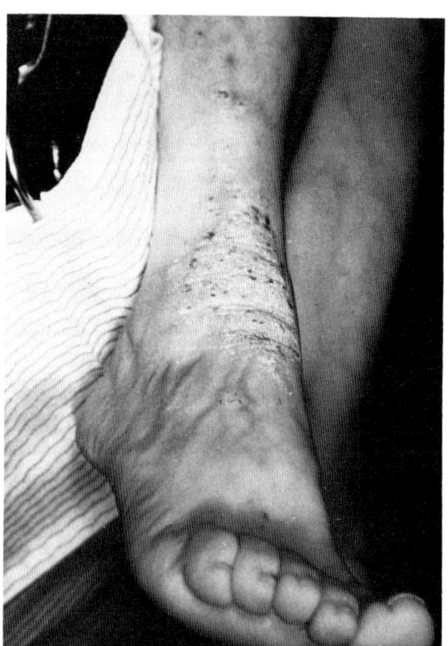

Figure 6.97. Neurodermatitis. Note location anterior of ankle; elevated, angular margins with excoriations.

The vesicles are small and never enlarge to the size of a bulla. Itching is common and scarring never occurs.

Patients with neurodermatitis tend to be quite anxious and may present with other psychological overlay disorders, including gastric ulcer, blepheritis or ulcerative colitis.

Treatment. Removal of the etiology of the itch-scratch cycle is often difficult. Referral to a psychologist or psychiatrist for consultation is sometimes necessary. Occlusive topical steroid dressings, such as betamethasone dipropionate (Diprosone), covered with plastic wrap, then affixed with nonallergenic paper tape and covered further with a cotton sock, are helpful. Because the sleeping patient has a tendency to scratch, excoriate and aggravate the affected areas with the toenails of the opposite foot, both feet should be covered with cotton socks while the patient sleeps. Oral antihistamines, such as terfenadine (Seldane), 60 mg bid, are helpful.

Scars and Keloids

Scars and hypertrophic scars occur along an incision line. Keloids progress beyond the area of skin incision.

Scar tissue on weightbearing surfaces may result from injury, lacerations, operative incisions and multiple, minimal trauma by irritants in footgear. Repair of lacerations on weightbearing areas often causes scar tissue, with a tendency for proliferation of keratoses producing painful callosities. Surgical excision of lesions on weightbearing sites, such as verrucas under the head of the first, second or fifth metatarsal, may carry a possibility of scar tissue formation. Ragged cuts or irritations from irregularities in shoes can produce scar tissue. Blacks more readily develop heavy elevated scars or keloids. Scars often develop following the electrocoagulation of plantar skin lesions (Fig. 6.98).

Treatment. Removal of the source of irritation occasionally diminishes the size of a scar. Dermabrasion, when properly performed, is effective. Blau (180) recommends skin planing, which provides uniformly excellent results. This technique is followed by use of 2% panthenol cream (Panthoderm) for several months. Generally, excision of the mass with careful fine sutur-

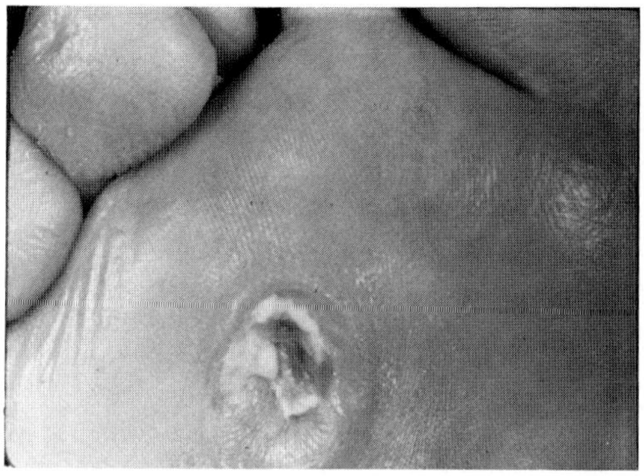

Figure 6.98. Surgical ulceration with keloid formation following electrocoagulation of plantar wart. A "collar button" type keloid is developing.

ing or the use of Steri-Strips to coaptate tissue minimizes scar tissue. Carbon dioxide snow has been useful. Bichloroacetic and monochloroacetic acid may destroy some scars and allow for a better repair of the affected tissue. Inunction of vitamin A and D cream helps maintain the integrity of the skin.

Dermabrasion may be very useful in removing scars, tissue pigments and helomas. Some benign superficial nevi, vascular nevi and port wine stains may be abraded, as may keloids, keratoses, adenoma sebaceum and skin graft sites. Planing is contraindicated if scarring is slight. Equipment should include stainless steel brushes, burrs, serrated stainless wheels and heatless stones of proper sizes, an electric motor capable of 12,000 r.p.m., and ethyl chloride sprays. Antisepsis must be scrupulously observed because a totally aseptic technique is rarely achieved (Fig. 6.99).

Treatments are given at 4 to 6 week intervals as described below. Ethyl chloride, Dermafreeze or Dermathone is sprayed over the area to be treated. Luikart et al. (181) suggests freezing with dichlorotetrafluoroethane to eliminate hazards of explosion. An air blower is then played over the sprayed site, resulting in freezing hardness of the tissue.

The operative field should be limited to 1 to 1½ square inches to prevent early thawing and to guard against damage to previously abraded tissue. Abrasion should be up and down, rather than across. The field generally is bloodless and new skin regenerates.

Blau (180) uses Dermathone, which acts as an anesthetic and skin hardener. Following the planing procedure, tissue appears red, smooth and soft to the touch.

It is important to select carefully those patients amenable to plantar surgery. Remove pressure from the affected part. Follow surgical repair with 50,000 units of vitamin A daily, and anoint the affected part with lanolin cream or any emollient with a lubricating base.

Intralesional injections of corticosteroids into scars may reduce their size and prevent keloid formation. The usual dosage is 0.3 to 0.5 ml of the steroid. The author has found Celestone Soluspan to be especially effective in hypertrophic scars less than 3 months old.

The administration of drugs sublesionally or intralesionally promises to be of great help in the treatment of many skin disorders seen in podiatric practice. Helomas, tylomas, verrucas, psoriatic, contact dermatitic and other lesions may be amenable to this therapy.

Triamcinalone injected in combination with 2% lidocaine was suggested by Prentice (182). A concentration of 6.25 mg/ml was combined with lidocaine hydrochloride as the diluent. No more than 25 mg should be injected in a 7-day period. A disposable syringe with 25 to 26 G ⅜-inch disposable needle is used to inject into or beneath the lesion to a depth of 3 to 5 mm. Intractable psoriatic lesions appeared to undergo resolution with injections of the steroid. In Prentice's series of cases, good to excellent responses were noted in a variety of skin disorders, such as contact dermatitis, eczema, granuloma annulare, lichen planus, lichen simplex chronicus and psoriasis of local, generalized and pustular type.

Similar injections for plantar verrucas may be made using vitamin A, bismuth subtartrate, benzyl alcohol, lidocaine hydrochloride, and a variety of sclerosing agents.

Locke (183) described the techniques and use of injection of prednisolone 21 phosphate, a rapid-acting, freely soluble steroid for intralesional therapy. He recommended fanning the solution out beneath the lesion for best results in neurofibrous lesions, heloma molle, heloma dura and tylomas (Fig. 6.100).

Keratosis of the Soles (Fig. 6.101)

Ichthyotic dry scaling lesions may occur on the soles of the feet as a secondary dermatosis to chemical irritants. The appearance of the scales is not unlike that of ichthyosis, a genetically predetermined systemic dryness of the skin. Complete laboratory studies are indicated to rule out systemic disorders, and the local irritants are then sought out and removed. Treatment consists of local applications of keratolytic agents followed by local and systemic use of vitamin A.

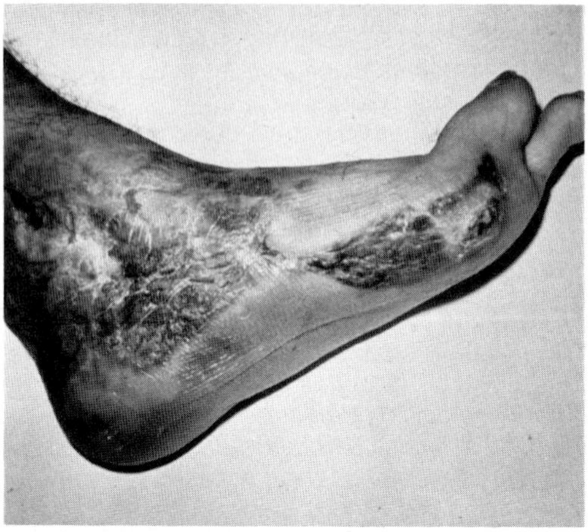

Figure 6.99. Skin graft broken down following surgery for extensive burns.

Foot and Ankle Ulcerations

Ulcerations may occur on the feet in debilitating disorders or neurotrophic or vascular disease (Table 6.2). Destruction of tissue occurs at points of pressure. Ulcerations may be due to the exciting factors of trauma due to ill-fitting footgear, faulty foot structure, abnormal foot posture and disturbed function. The common locations for ulcers are over the bony prominences, such as the posterior and plantar surfaces of the heels and the heads of the first and fifth metatarsals. Callused areas and helomas may break down from irritation, causing an ulceration that is often difficult to heal. Ulcers on the foot may also occur on the plantar surface beneath the heads of any of the metatarsals, the dorsal aspects of the toes and the distal tips and webs of the toes.

The location, shape, appearance and character of the ulcerative discharge are often suggestive of its etiology. Gangrene may occur at the tips of the toes, beneath the nail plate or on the plantar surface of the great toe and about the heels secondary to ulcerations. Areas of focal gangrene are quite small and are usually seen in diabetics, arteriosclerotics and in patients with certain blood dyscrasias. They are generally localized and self-limiting, but could potentially lead to widespread gan-

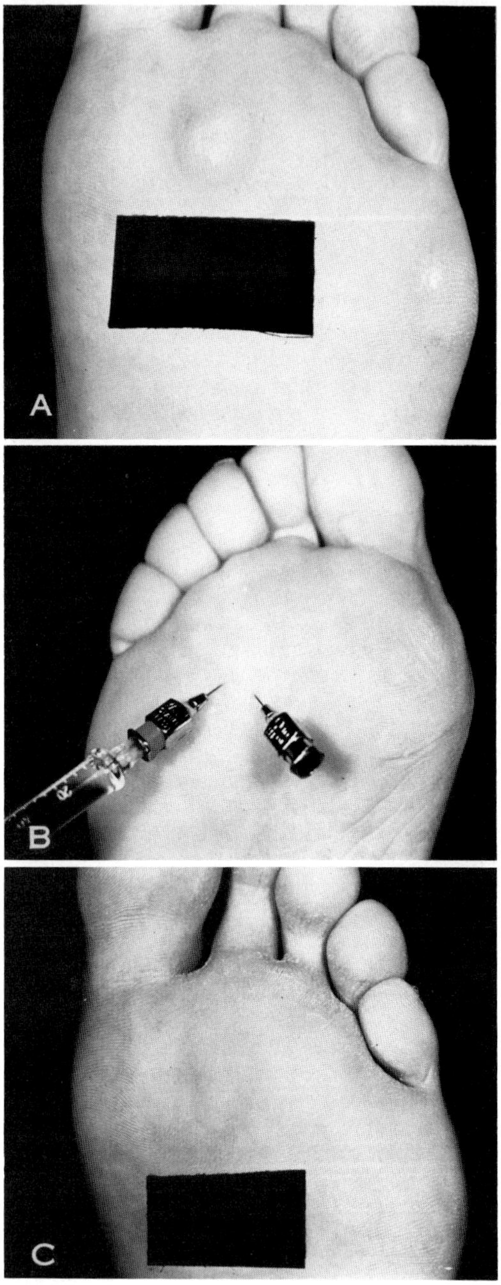

Figure 6.100. *A,* Intractable tylomas second and fifth metatarsophalangeal joints in male, age 34. *B,* Needle positions for plantar injections of the anesthetic and corticosteroid. *C,* Following three injections, lesion under the second metatarsophalangeal joint (one injection of 4 mg long-acting prednisone, two injections of 6 mg prednisone 21 phosphate, one injection lesion under fifth metatarsal head of 6 mg prednisone 21 phosphate). (Courtesy of RK Locke.)

grene. One must not confuse focal gangrene with a neurovascular heloma that may be painful but less dangerous. Gangrene of the heel, leg, and foot may result from trauma, burns and incisions in the presence of occlusive vascular disease.

Ulcers are usually caused by venous stasis, arteriosclerosis, thromboangiitis obliterans, impaired cutaneous sensation, neoplasms, arteriolar disease, fragility of small arteries and arterioles, infections and a host of other variables. They may occur secondary to trauma and infections (Fig. 6.103). Scheduled periodic prophylactic podiatric care is essential in the diabetic patient and those with peripheral vascular disease (184). Black and Simons (185) (1983) surveyed 100 diabetic patients regulated with oral hypoglycemics. The majority had neuropathy, had a diabetic relative and needed podiatric care.

Treatment. Fox (186) described a therapeutic regimen for treatment of ulcers that was designed to reduce or eliminate edema and control infection by means of oral therapy using a combination of diuretics and a suitable antibiotic. After bacterial culture and antibiotic sensitivity tests were conducted, an oral diuretic in proper dosage and a broad spectrum antibiotic were prescribed. Tetracycline, 1 g daily for 5 days, is the antibiotic of choice.

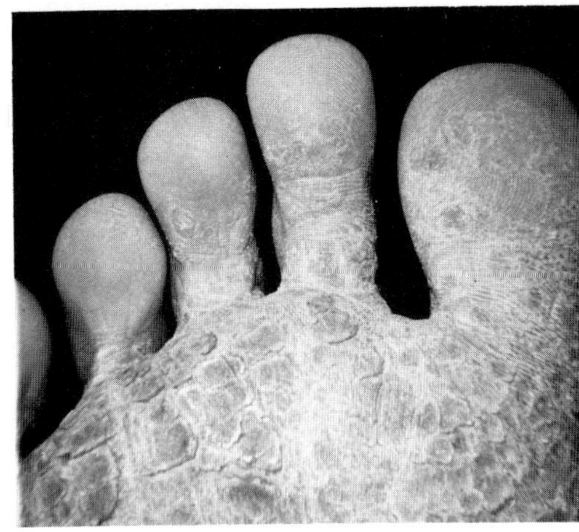

Figure 6.101. Keratosis of the soles.

The systemic treatment is augmented by local treatment of the ulcer. The ulcer is covered by sterile pads, and an elastic bandage is applied from the foot to just below the knee. After a week, an additional test is made to find the antibiotic of

Table 6.2.
Foot and Ankle Ulcer Classification[a]

1. Traumatic
   a. macrotrauma: laceration, missle wound, hematoma
   b. multiple minimal microtrauma: friction and pressure, biomechanical abnormality
2. Local infection: bacterial, fungal, viral, osteomyelitis
3. Neurotrophic: leprosy, syphilis, yaws, diabetes, syringomyelia, peripheral neuropathy
4. Pressure: decubitus, shoe, occupational, heloma, tyloma, bursa
5. Hysterical: neurotic, self-induced, neurodermatitis, local excoriation
6. Secondary: contact dermatitis, radiodermatitis, neoplastic, burns—radiation, chemical or thermal, frostbite, trench foot, lichen planus, insect bite—spider or snake, Cushing's disease, Azotemic hyperparathyroidism, psoriasis, benign skin tumor, malignant skin tumor (Fig. 6.99)
7. Vascular: arteriosclerosis obliterans, thromboangiitis obliterans, venous, hypertensive, phlebitic, livedo reticularis, hemophilia, chronic pernio, Raynaud's disease or phenomenon, chronic venous insufficiency, arteriovenous fistula, lymphatic
8. Systemic disease: diabetes, thalassemia, dysproteinemia, lichen amyloidosis, gout, deep fungus, tuberculosis, pretibial myxedema, porphyria cutanea tarda, erythema induratum, chicken pox, leukemia, anemia—pernicious, sickle cell, spherocytic, polycythemia vera (Fig. 6.102).
9. Collagen disease: rheumatoid arthritis, scleroderma, Reiter's syndrome, systemic lupus erythematosus, periarteritis nodosum, vasculitis, angiitis, polyarteritis, pyoderma gangrenosum.
10. Medication: local and systemic toxic reaction, acids, alkalis, halogens, ergotism, methotrexate

[a] Because of the multiple etiologies and varieties of ulcers affecting the foot and ankle, the author has attempted to formulate a classification system unique to podiatric medicine. The nature of foot and ankle ulcerations dictate that some ulcers will fall into more than one category.

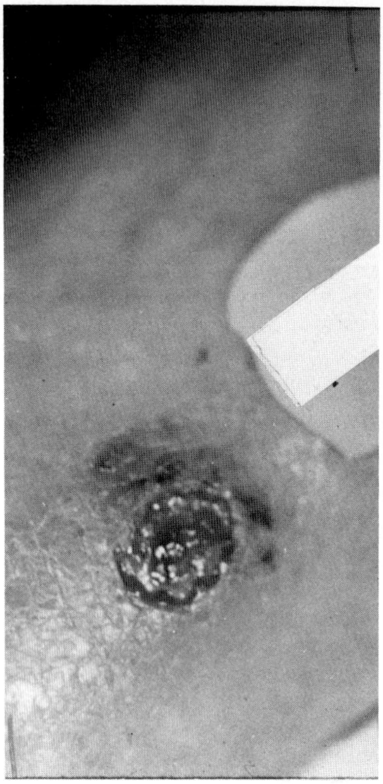

Figure 6.102. Ulcer secondary to pernicious anemia.

choice to attack the bacteria insensitive to tetracycline. After an additional 2-week period, potassium depletion is evaluated, and the continued use of the diuretic is reassessed. Henze et al. (187) noted that dietary zinc sulfate, 110 to 210 mg tid, promotes wound healing in the feet. Op-Site, a sterile adherent plastic dressing material, has been effective in treating noninfected foot ulcers. The wound must be kept dry and the dressing changed every 3 to 6 days.

Traumatic Ulcers

Ulcerations develop in devitalized tissues as a result of mechanical irritation, such as injudicious instrumentation, pressure from ill-fitting footgear, occupational stress, sudden severe injury or abnormal weight distribution. They are often complicated by circulatory and systemic disease, such as arteriosclerosis and diabetes. In studies by Dieter and Graziano (188), cultures of traumatic and stasis ulcers revealed offending organisms to be *Staphylococcus aureus*, beta-hemolytic *Streptococcus*, *Pseudomonas*, *Proteus*, *Aerobacter aerogenes*, paracolon bacilli, *Micrococcus* and yeast. Granuloma

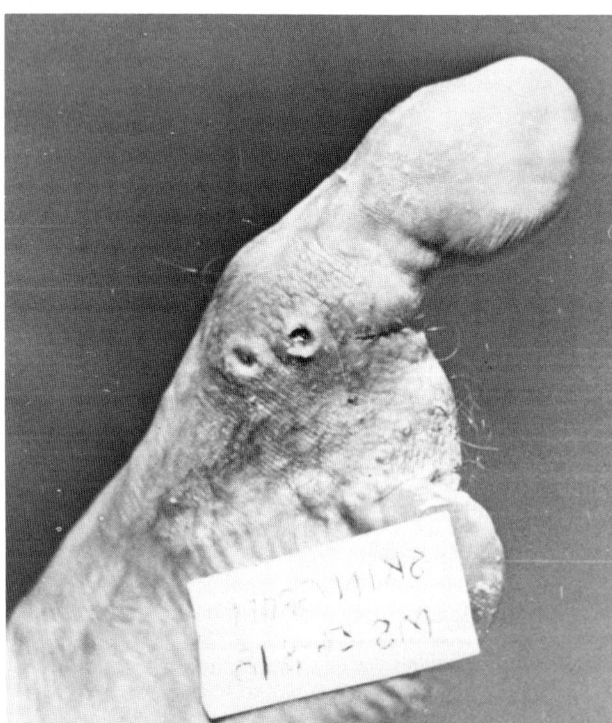

Figure 6.103. Amputation, skin graft and punctate ulcers.

pyogenicum may develop in an ulcer (Fig. 6.104).

Treatment. Remove the source of trauma and seek consultation for early treatment of complicating systemic disorders. Cleanse the ulcer with hexachlorophene or povidone-iodine solution, and debride devitalized tissue by careful instrumentation or by the use of animal or vegetable proteolytic enzymes. Walkes and Hazen (189) noted excellent clinical results with an im injection of aqueous trypsin (Parenzyme) in 44 of 53 cases. A collagenase ointment (Biozyme) or fibrinolysin and desoxyribonuclease ointment (Elase), and Panafil ointment seem to be helpful in combining antibacterial and proteolytic action in repair of some ulcers. Improve granulation and repair by use of stimulating antibiotic enzyme topical medication. Ultraviolet radiation is helpful.

If the ulcer is secondarily infected, do a sensitivity test and prescribe a systemic antibiotic and local medication to combat the offending organism. In the presence of anaerobic bacteria, lavage with hydrogen peroxide is indicated when redressed. When infection is present, it is necessary to repeat sensitivity tests as new bacteria take over in long-standing ulcerations.

Construct a foot or toe prosthesis to remove undue stress from the affected part, and have the patient wear an elastic bandage for adequate support. Immobilization by plaster cast aids in repair.

Stasis Ulcers (Figs. 6.105 and 6.106)

Congestive ulcers result from devitalization of the tissues and include ulcers caused by poor venous return and bedsores. The medial ankle, heels and toes are commonly involved.

Treatment. In varicose veins it is necessary to assist gravitational return of venous blood by elevation of the affected extremity, bed rest and use of elastic stockings or bandages. Ligation and stripping of incompetent veins may be necessary. Skin grafts may be required to close the ulcer. Nitrofurazone dressing is helpful in protecting skin graft.

Repair is aided by prescribing stimulating ointments, such as a 0.5% water-soluble chlorophyll derivative (Chloresium), which promotes healing and reduces wound odor. Chloresium in solution (0.2%) may also be used. Povidone-iodine solution wet dressings may be helpful. Garamycin, gentamicin ointment or cream, may stimulate repair. Occasionally, there is a need for IM injections of proteolytic enzymes to aid digestion of debris and to stimulate repair as suggested by

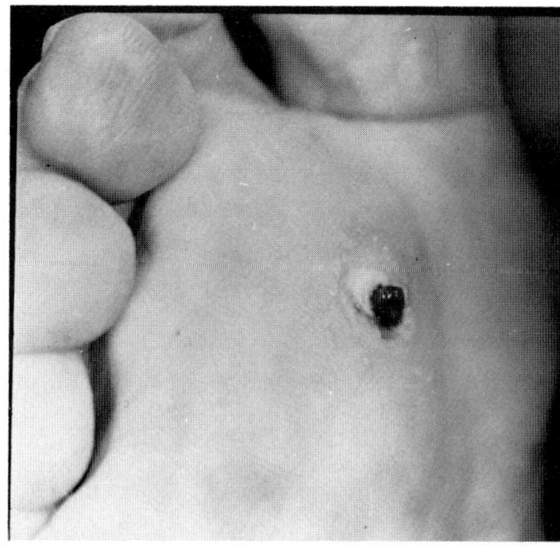

Figure 6.104. Granuloma pyogenicum developed in an ulcer secondary to trauma.

Corsaro (190). A colloidal solution of denatured proteolytic enzyme (Protamide), indicated in the presence of neuritis, is used as one ampule every 2 to 5 days.

McNerney (191), in a well-written article, concludes that "antibiosis should never be used to cover for poor surgical judgment or technique." Gram-negative infections have increased due to the improper use of penicillin for many years, resulting in a variety of resistant strains of bacteria. Antibiotics may be used on high-risk patients to prevent infection. However, good surgical judgment is essential in evaluating the necessity of surgical intervention. Topical antibiotics used postsurgically may result in a false sense of security where sterile technique has been broken. When surgery is anticipated and performed, one must have (1) a careful and thorough examination, (2) good judgment, (3) meticulous technique to minimize trauma, and (4) proper antibiosis based on sensitivity tests and cultures in the event of infection.

Sokolowski et al. (192) did a comprehensive overview of the therapeutics necessary in order to treat postoperative infections following podiatric surgery. This study provides an excellent review of the clinical criteria, laboratory studies and their interpretation and radiographic and surgical considerations. General principles and specific approaches to treatment are adequately covered by this article and are too lengthy for this text to review.

Stern and Shuman (193), in animal studies, conclude that, in contrast to high doses of systemically administered corticosteroids that delay wound healing, small dosages of soluble steroids such as dexamethasone injected locally

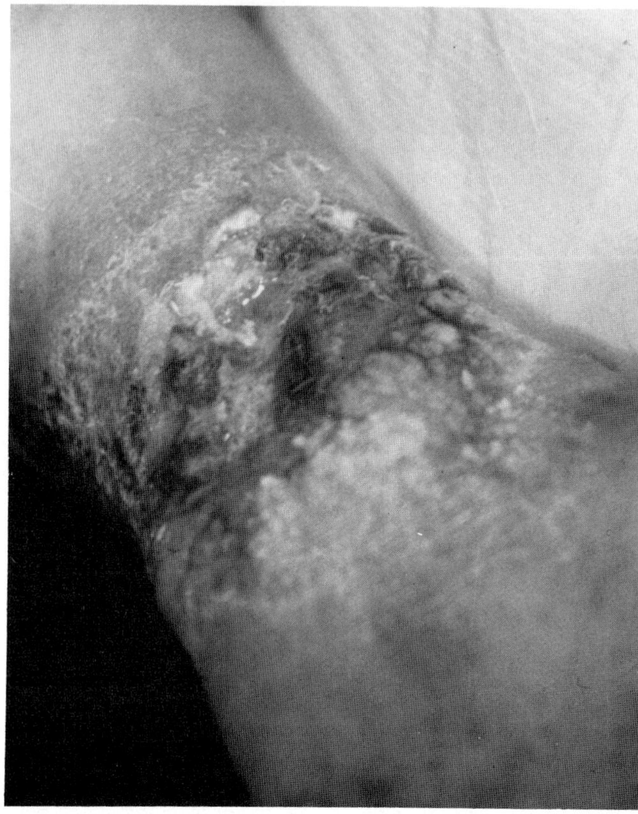

Figure 6.105. Stasis ulcer at ankle.

do not delay, but rather enhance would healing (some insoluble steroids appear to delay healing).

Hypertensive ulcers are found over the posteriolateral or anteriolateral aspect of the leg proximal to the ankle. Ulcer margins are irregular and ragged in appearance. Venous stasis skin pigmentation changes are usually absent. There may be a pale granulating base with surrounding cyanosis and necrosis. DP and PT pulses are usually palpable. These ulcers are extremely painful. Diagnosis is made by ruling out other etiologies and by careful clinical evaluation of the patient (194).

Treatment. Systemic treatment of the hypertensive ulcer is mandatory. Hyperbaric oxygen, thorazine, isoxuprine, and enzymatic debridement have been useful. Mechanical surgical debridement often causes an extension of the ulcer. Bacterial contamination should be controlled. Porcine skin graft dressings and Op-Site plastic dressings have been effective. If the ulcer is extensive, split or full thickness skin grafts may have to be utilized for closure.

Pyogenic ulcers may be caused by invasion of the tissues by pus-producing bacteria (Figs. 6.107 and 6.108). Unsterile instruments and careless antisepsis when treating simple skin lesions may cause pyogenic ulcers. In addition, these ulcers are often caused by breaking down of tissue from carbuncles, boils, pustules and acid therapy-destroying techniques. Extension to bone from infected ulcers is not uncommon, and radiographs may be helpful in establishing a diagnosis.

Treatment. Perform sensitivity test on bacterial flora in wound to determine the antibiotic of choice, which may include penicillin, cephalosporins, erythromycin, or tetracycline. Lincomycin (75 to 150 mg by injection) is suitable where secondary bone infection is noted and where sensitivity tests demonstrate its efficacy. Local debridement and application of antibiotic enzymatic medications are helpful. Warm saline

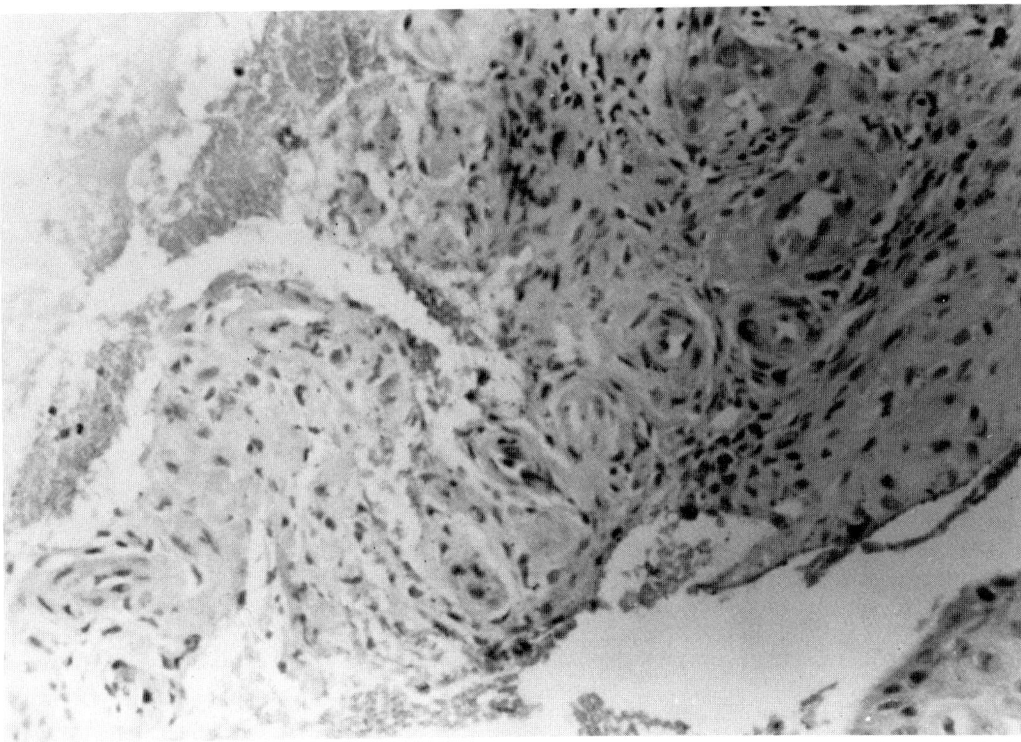

Figure 6.106. Photomicrograph of stasis ulcer showing ulceration of epithelium (*upper left*) and vessel walls that are thick and vessels dilated (*right*). Hemosiderin pigment not evident.

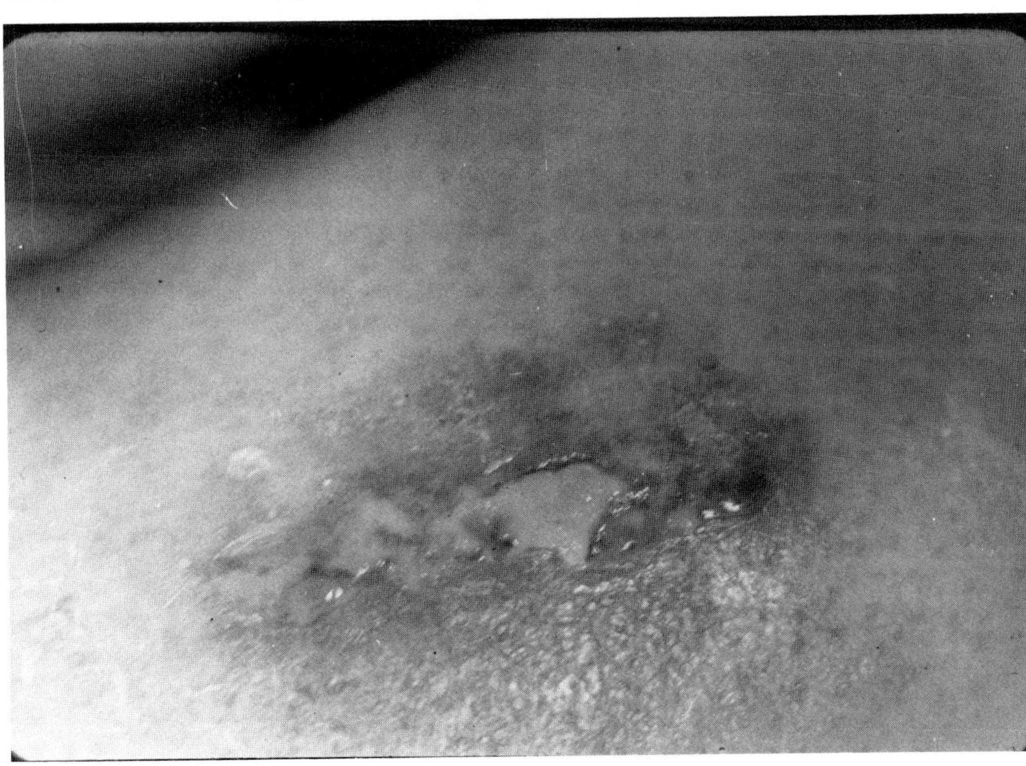

Figure 6.107. Pyogenic ulcer.

or povidone-iodine (Betadine) solution soaks facilitate drainage.

Trophic ulcers develop in peripheral neuritis, syphilis and tabes, diabetes, syringomyelia, leprosy, certain paralyses, peripheral vascular disease and other debilitating diseases (Figs. 6.109 and 6.110). Areas receiving great pressure and friction are usual sites for trophic ulcers. An x-ray examination is essential to rule out bone pathology.

Treatment. Remove pressure from affected part by the judicious use of felt, foam and pressure-sensitive rubber. Construct foot orthoses to relieve pressure.

Correct peripheral neuritis. Treat systemic diseases and peripheral vascular instability.

Bed rest with proper shielding of bony prominences may be beneficial (Fig. 6.111). Local and systemic antibiotics and enzymatic debridement may be necessary. Eisenberg (195) and Coleman et al. (196) recommend the application of a plaster cast for 3 weeks.

Schilansky (197) reviews the etiology, diagnosis, clinical course, and treatment of Hansen's disease (leprosy). Approximately 15 million people in the world have leprosy. The author describes a viable treatment program for pedal manifestations.

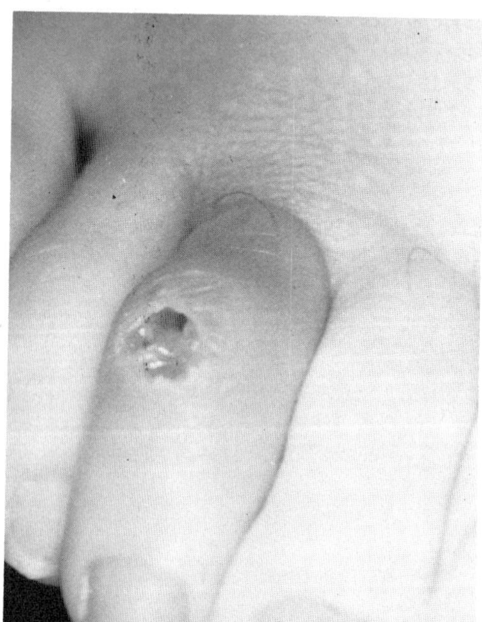

Figure 6.108. Pyogenic ulcer. Note swelling of the infected toe.

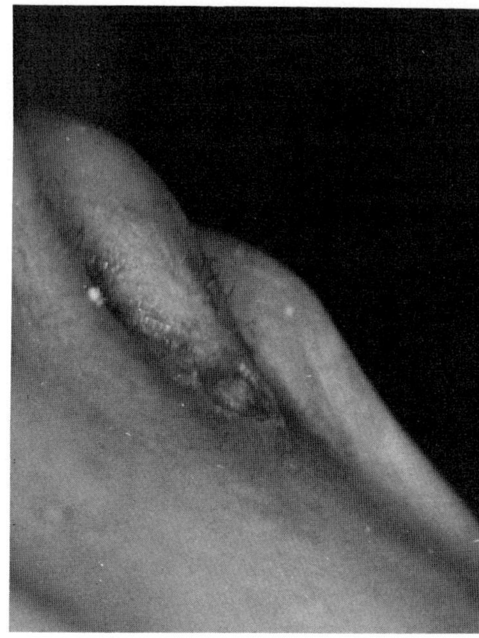

Figure 6.109. Trophic ulcer dorsum of toe. Exposed extensor tendon.

Specific ulcers are those caused by definite disease and are classified as syphilitic, diabetic, tubercular, arteriosclerotic and so forth (Figs. 6.112–6.114). Cohen and Shelley (198) described an ulceration due to Werner's syndrome in a male, age 30 with premature signs of senility, circumscribed hyperkeratosis of the soles, tightness of the skin over pressure points and local calcification of the skin.

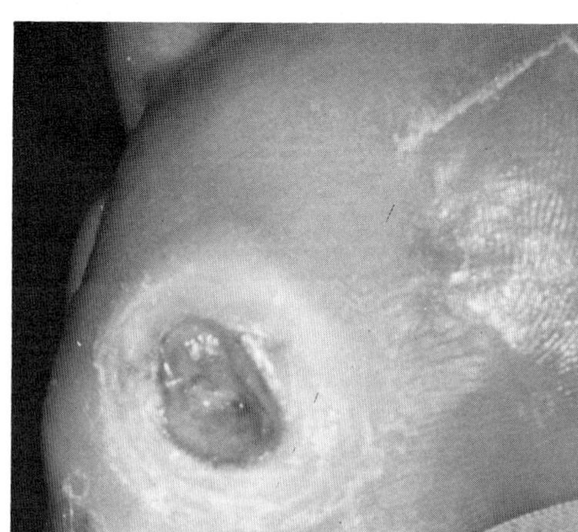

Figure 6.110. Trophic ulcer plantar surface of the first metatarsal head.

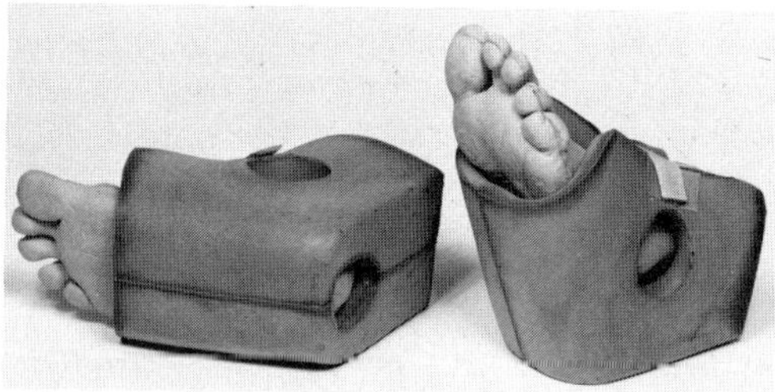

Figure 6.111. Protection device for prolonged bed rest. (Courtesy of Medical Plastics Laboratory.)

Treatment includes local measures to aid repair and control infection, as well as consultation with medical specialists for treatment of the systemic etiology. Large doses of vitamin B_{12} and specific medication for the etiologic basis are helpful in repair.

Malignant ulcers are caused by unintentional damage at the time of biopsy, excess radiation, metastasis from other malignant lesions and pressure of rapidly growing malignant tumors with destruction of tissue (Figs. 6.115 and 6.116).

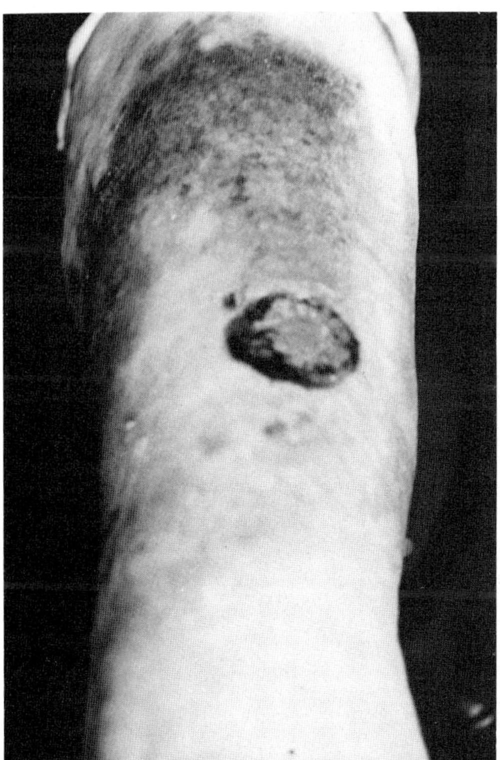

Figure 6.112. Luetic ulcer on extensor surface midthird of leg. Punched-out lesion with gray gummy base.

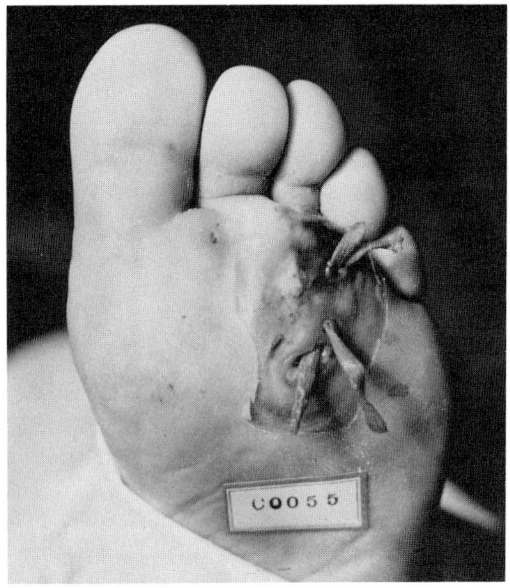

Figure 6.113. Diabetic ulcer. Drains in sinus tracts. (Courtesy of D Mowbray.)

Ulcers are shallow, cupped-out lesions of the surface tissue with either an irregular, smooth or elevated border. The surface may be sloughing, granulating or fungating. When the ulcer is on the plantar surface of the foot on a weightbearing area and penetrates to the bone, it is perforating. When it is adherent to the underlying tissues, it may be malignant.

Ulcers discharge serous or seropurulent fluids. Excessive hemorrhage may indicate the presence of a superficial arteriole or possibly a vascular malignancy; chalky discharges suggest sodium biurate crystals of gouty deposits. A caseous tissue discharge is usually of tubercular origin.

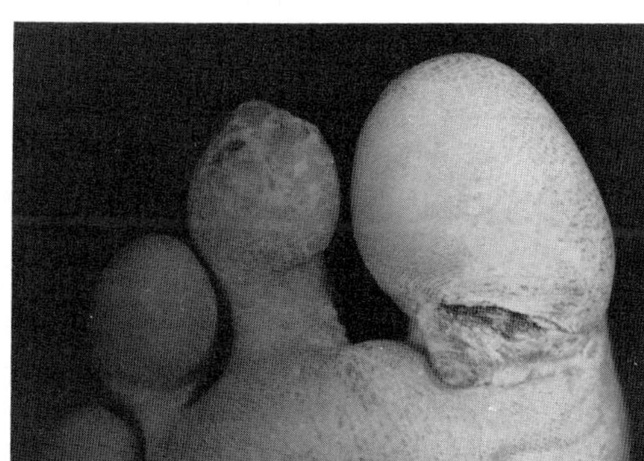

Figure 6.114. Arteriosclerotic ulcers.

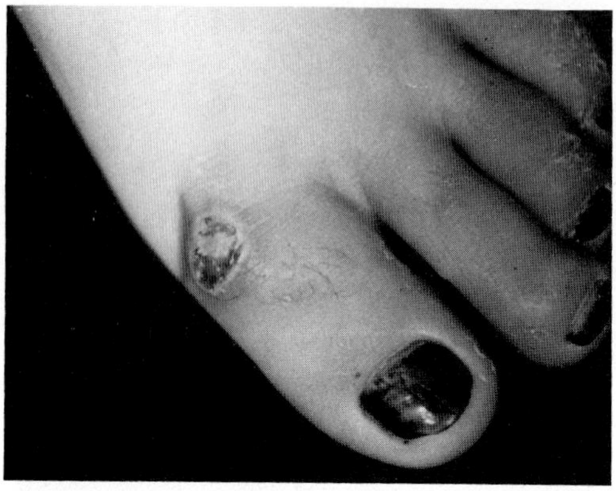

Figure 6.115. Neoplastic ulcer. (Nail discoloration caused by silver nitrate use in the treatment of onychomycosis.)

Deep, indurated, adhered ulcerations may be malignant. Marked evidence of infection around the ulcer may suggest pyogenic invasion. Sharply demarcated ulcers that are painless suggest a syphilitic origin. Marked circumscribed edema is the result of congestion.

Treatment. Limit the use of radiation on benign lesions because radiation can stimulate carcinogenesis. Early diagnosis and treatment of the underlying disorder are imperative. Surgical excision, radiation and chemotherapeutic techniques must be used early when biopsy is positive. Extensive ulcerations may require skin grafts to cover the surgical site.

Arterial perfusion with chemotherapeutic solutions is helpful in certain malignant lesions. Amputation at a high level including resection of regional lymph nodes may be lifesaving.

Varicose ulcers are common lesions occurring in the presence of varicose veins. Bluish discoloration of dilated tortuous veins surrounded by brownish-gray pigmentation of the skin encircling the ulcer is typical. The exciting etiologic factor is trauma to the vein or overlying tissue, such as a bruise, scratch or dermatitis over a dilated, decompensated vein.

Varicose ulcers are usually located on the medial side of the leg about 3 inches above the ankle. They have been observed covering two-thirds of the lower extremity and very often involve the feet. On the feet, lesions may be seen distal and anterior to the lateral or medial malleolus caused by trauma or friction from a stiff counter. Rarely is a varicose ulcer seen on the sole of the foot.

At first the ulcers may be pinhead in size and later extend around the entire limb. These superficial lesions give off a foul-smelling serous or purulent discharge. The surrounding pigmented skin is usually indurated in long-standing cases. A local phlebitis with purplish-red discoloration and numerous telangiectasias may be evident. The margins of the sore are usually irregular and rough, with a yellow surface and small pink granulations. Stagnation and congestion may cause the edematous tissues to become firm. Very often the discharge irritates the surrounding tissue, causing an eczema with intolerable pruritus, excoriation, fissuring and more ulcers.

Treatment. Early control of infection by antiseptic wet dressing of povidone-iodine (Betadine) solution and use of an antibiotic ointment are indicated. Judicious debridement of devitalized tissue by instrumentation and proteolytic enzymes may be necessary. Stimulate repair by using mild solutions of 5 to 15% silver nitrate. Destroy granulation tissue using silver nitrate stick 50%. A steroid cream may be used for inflamed noninfected varicose ulcers.

Oxycycline and hydrocortisone in a spray are helpful in controlling infection and moisture. Even

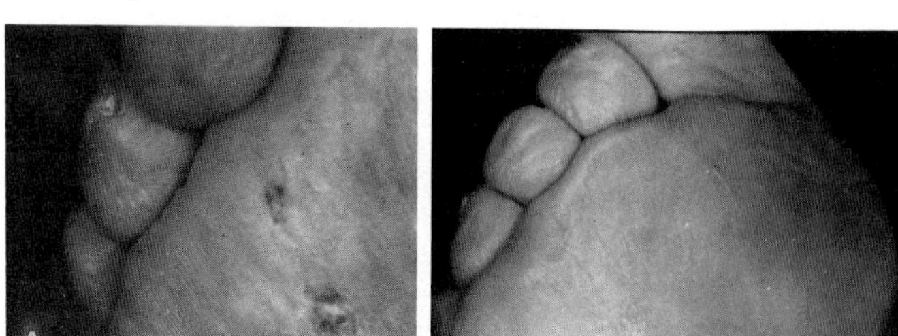

Figure 6.116. *A,* Malignant ulcers secondary to radiodermatitis following treatment of plantar warts in patient 82 years old. *B,* Malignant ulcers excised. Six months postoperative.

compression of limb by pressure bandages from behind the toes to below the knee or elastic stocking from behind the toes, with closed heel and of midthigh length, may be used.

A venous heart dressing may be helpful. Silver nitrate as indicated is used on the ulcer following mechanical or chemical debridement and control of infection. Stimulating ointments, such as ichthammol 10 to 20%, zinc oxide half-strength, or Scarlet Red Ointment may be applied. If the ulcer is infected, do a sensitivity test and prescribe accordingly. Enzymatic debridement, antibiotic ointments and nitrofurazone may be used topically. Systemic proteolytic enzymes are helpful early, as are systemic antibiotics of choice. Cover the ulcer widely with a sterile gauze pad. Use a 2-inch thick sponge rubber pad on gauze and compress firmly over the ulcer by bandaging. Elevate the extremity and apply an elastic bandage or elastic stocking. Change the dressing every 3 to 5 days.

Gelatin-like flexible compression casts are applied according to directions by the manufacturer (Gelocast bandages, Unna's boot). Bandages are changed weekly or more often if necessary.

Such activity as walking with compression dressings supplies a physiological environment. The contraction and expansion of leg musculature against the bandage provide a local hyperemia that aids in repair of the ulcer.

Saphenous ligations, geographic incisions, tying off or stripping of veins and injections of sclerosing agents may be used in recalcitrant cases. Skin grafts may be necessary where healing is stagnant.

Diabetic ulcers occur both in known and unknown diabetic patients on an area of the foot receiving abnormal trauma or friction (Fig. 6.117). The cause may be ill-fitting shoes or hose, irritating chemicals such as "corn remedies," extremes of heat and cold and the usual self-inflicted wounds resulting from injudicious instrumentation. Faulty weight distribution may cause abnormal pressure on certain parts of the foot.

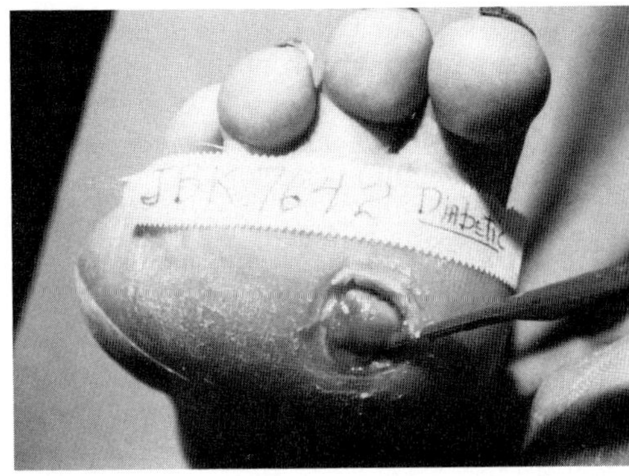

Figure 6.117. Diabetic ulcer. Note moist smooth base and undermining ulcer. (Courtesy of M Shapiro.)

The points receiving greatest pressure are the plantar surface of the first and fifth metatarsal head, other depressed metatarsal heads with superimposed luxation of the corresponding toe, the medial aspect of the first metatarsophalangeal joint and the lateral aspect of the fifth metatarsophalangeal joint, the posterior aspect of the heel, the borders of the toenails and the distal ends of the toes. Dribbon (199) describes the application and value of liquid crystal thermography as a diagnostic aid affording an early and specific indication of areas predisposed to tissue necrosis in patients with diabetes and with peripheral vascular disease.

The ulcer has a red margin, and the skin appears spongy. It is very slow and insidious in onset. Healing progress is usually discouraging while the margins appear undermined. A callus often overlies the ulcer on the plantar surface, and the discharge is serous and watery (Fig. 6.118). A

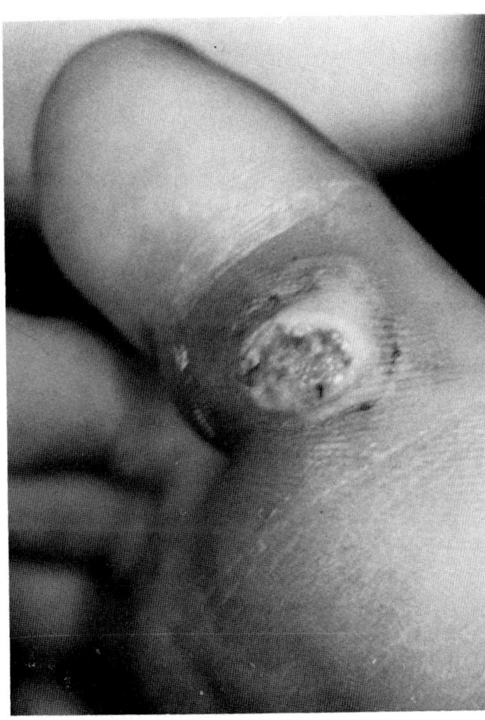

Figure 6.118. Diabetic ulcer with infection and cellulitis.

urinalysis, hemoglobin AIC, fasting blood sugar and a good case history confirm the diagnosis. The patient may be arteriosclerotic, and peripheral neuropathic symptoms are common.

Bernhard et al. (200) discuss incision and drainage, control of infection and rehabilitation for the uncommon medial, central, and lateral plantar space abscesses in the diabetic foot. Visser et al. (201), in their report concerning the diagnosis of osseous and soft tissue changes affecting the diabetic foot, discuss the importance of scanning techniques in differentiating cellulitis, osteomyelitis, osteolysis, neuroarthropathy, septic synovitis, and deep plantar abscess.

Goldenberg et al. (202) found that a patchy gangrene occurred in 40% of diabetic patients. This gangrene is often accompanied by a palpable and often strong dorsalis pedis and posterior tibial pulse, but exhibits other evidence of macrovascular disease and microangiopathy. The basement membrane of the capillaries is markedly thickened, but the direct etiology is obscure. There are many hypotheses about what causes the pathology. They range from faulty sugar metabolism and hydrostatic pressure to the vessel wall to adherence of platelets to the intima in a mass capable of restricting circulation.

The symptoms of diabetes and the local foot and leg manifestations are well known to the podiatrist. Only one or many symptoms may be found, as described elsewhere in this text under symptoms. The reader is referred to the discussion of cramping, intermittent claudication, ischemia, color changes on elevation and dependency, skin atrophy, specific ulcerations, infections, neuropathy and gangrene.

Many podiatrists have witnessed the patient who complains bitterly about an "ingrown toenail" and who exhibits an ischemia and sensory disturbances that appear nonspecific. The complexities of paresthesias and degrees of loss of pain sensation, together with the systemic symptoms of polyuria, polydipsia and polyphagia, should heighten the doctor's suspicion of an ischemic neuritis. This is often secondary to a microangiopathy characteristic of diabetes.

Much of the pathology is not definitive ultramicroscopically or chemically. Thus, the podiatrist must assume that certain visible gross changes are taking place despite the lack of laboratory confirmation. Consultation with the internist and peripheral vascular specialist is often necessary with mutual respect for the opinions of each. Absolute cooperation is necessary for good results and for avoiding complications of microthrombi, infection, necrosis and gangrene. Culture and sensitivity tests are mandatory, and infection must be treated with dispatch. Glycosuria and hyperglycemia must be treated early and wisely to avoid the development of infections, thrombi, possible embolus, coma and rapid deterioration of general bodily functions. Hunter (203) describes and discusses the use of sinography for determining the location, course and extent of sinus tracts found in the foot. This technique is accomplished by means of radio-opaque substance injection into the sinus tracts prior to radiography (Figs. 6.119 and 6.120).

According to Levin (184), diabetic patients are subject to many problems affecting the feet. Angiopathy is discussed in relation to the quality and quantity of pathology. Microvascular and macrovascular pathology affect the basement membrane of arterioles, capillaries and larger vessels. Levin notes that both the nondiabetic and diabetic patient seem to have similar

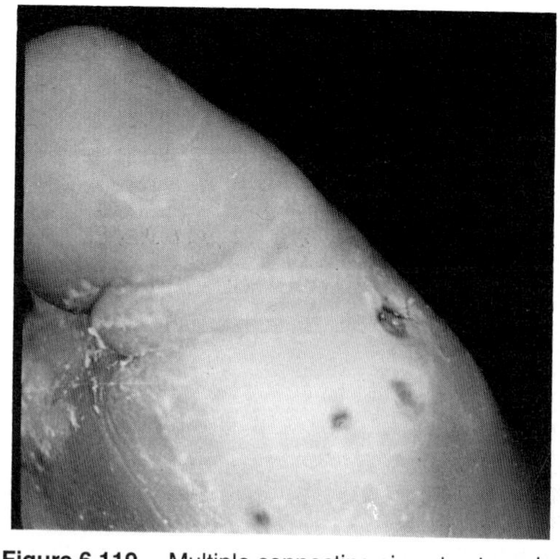

Figure 6.119. Multiple connecting sinus tracts undermining the skin in a diabetic patient.

changes in the vascular system. The difference is in the increased quantity of lipids and cholesterol in the intima and media of the diabetic vessels. These changes in the blood vessels occur more commonly and earlier in diabetic women than in diabetic men. Diabetic patients are more prone to infection and ultimate gangrene than nondiabetics. This is probably due to the bilateral atherosclerosis, which affects the peripheral vessels in the leg and foot more frequently in diabetics than in nondiabetics, who usually present with unilateral atherosclerosis of the femoral and iliac vessels.

Gordon and Oster (204), in a study of peripheral nerves in diabetic patients compared to nondiabetics, note a decrease in conduction velocity in diabetics under dietary control. They found an intermediate decrease in conduction velocity in diabetics on hypoglycemic agents, whereas those patients taking insulin presented the most marked decrease in peripheral nerve conduction velocities. In the presence of a lower extremity tourniquet on both diabetics and nondiabetics, the decrease in conduction velocity, distal to the tourniquet, was greater in the nondiabetics. It appears from this study that the diabetic in a chronic state of anoxia presents a limited nerve sensitivity.

Cohen et al. (205) found in a double-blind study of ten diabetic patients that vitamin B_6 (pyridoxine) 50 mg tid did not help the symptoms of diabetic neuropathy. However, the author has found a beneficial clinical response to 100 mg of vitamin B_6 taken three times a day for the subjective symptoms associated with diabetic neuropathy in the majority of cases. Clinical symptom response often takes longer than 3 weeks.

Helfand (206), in a comprehensive evaluation of pedal disorders in 123 diabetic patients, found 72.3% presented some form of traumatic or avascular hyperkeratotic lesion.

In diabetes mellitus, microangiopathy resulting from the proliferation of the endothelium of the intima and thickening of the basement membrane may occlude the lumen of the arterioles with atheromatous plaques. According to Defeo and Jay (207), the microthrombi are conducive to bacterial growth and secondary infection.

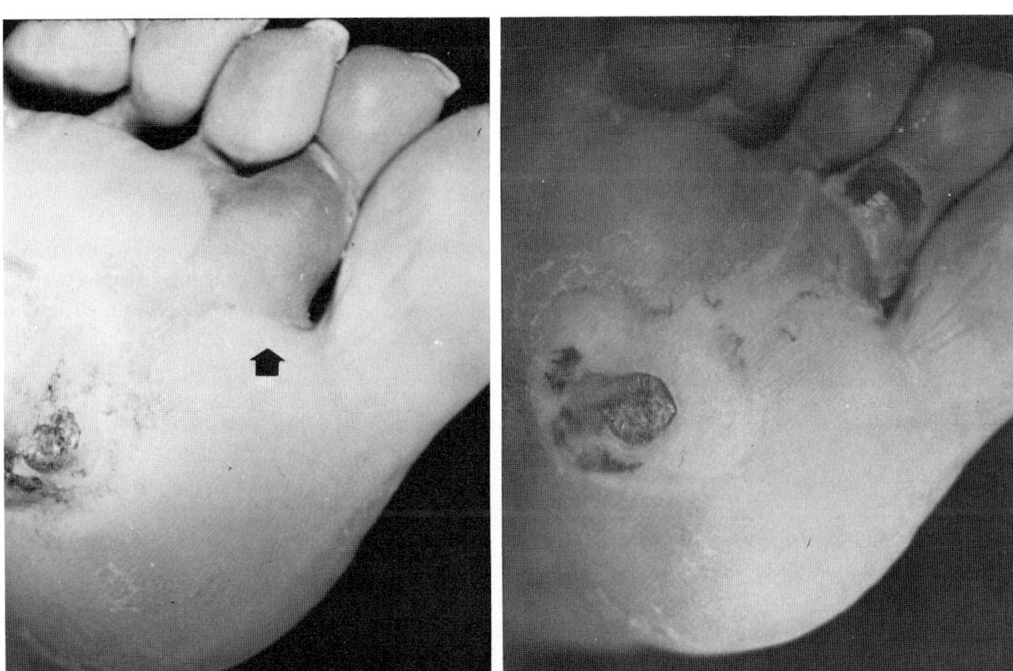

Figure 6.120. *Left,* Sinus tract in diabetic patients. Note infected tyloma and extension by way of least resistance distally to plantar surface of the second toe. *Right,* Incision and drainage of diabetic abscess.

Neurotrophic ulcerations are caused by abnormal pressure, as well as by anesthesia, according to Barrett and Mooney (208). They performed clinical studies that indicate sensory impairment was primarily noted along the distribution of the peroneal nerve. The loss of the ankle jerk seemed to be a conclusive factor in diabetic neuropathy. Unfortunately, the authors considered the shoe alone to be a major factor without too much concern for the biomechanical dysfunction secondary to structural foot changes.

The predominant organism in three diabetic foot infections was *Peptococcus magnus*, according to Sanderson (209). *P. magnus* was recovered in the blood culture of one patient and in two diabetics repeatedly in pure culture.

Effeney et al. (210) believed that transmetatarsal amputation is highly desirable in the presence of distal gangrene with no evidence of spreading infection. In their study of 25 patients, they found that their failures were younger and had a high incidence of diabetes and infections.

Wagner and Clarkson (211) provide a simple rationale for care of the dysvascular neuropathic foot. Either prevention or correction of deformities, or both, is of primary importance in the insensitive or poorly healing foot. Control of edema is necessary to achieve maximum healing potential.

Walden et al. (212) describe ten patients with pregangrenous and gangrenous toes in the presence of palpable peripheral pulses. Four patients had nonocclusive arteriosclerosis in large arteries; three had thrombocytosis and one had polycythemia vera; one had a monoclonal gammopathy and one was exposed to extreme cold 3 months before the onset of severe pain that preceded the gangrene. None smoked regularly, and those requiring amputation healed readily. Treatment of hematologic disorders and use of antiplatelet aggregating drugs were helpful. The investigators recommend the correction of the arteriosclerosis of large vessels to avoid thrombosis. Amputation is only advised when a definite line of demarcation develops between the healthy and necrotic tissue.

Karmody et al. (213) discuss the "Blue Toe syndrome," an indication for limb salvage surgery. They describe 31 patients in whom proximal lesions in the arterial tree were identified as probable sources of emboli causing the "Blue Toe syndrome." This syndrome consists of acute digital ischemia caused by microembolization to the digital arteries from a proximal source via a patent arterial tree, as evidenced by an otherwise well-perfused foot. It is closely analogous to the transient ischemic attacks of the brain and carries the same potential for serious tissue loss because of repeated embolic showers. The prompt delineation and eradication of the source are of prime importance, in addition to restoration of arterial continuity. Along with the other well-known features of chronic severe ischemia—that is, rest pain, gangrene, etc.—the "Blue Toe syndrome" is therefore an indication for limb salvage surgery.

Fifteen patients with peripheral atheroembolism were studied by Kwaan and Connolly (214). Transient foot pain may be the very earliest symptom of this condition. Gangrene commonly develops in the toes. Ankle pulses may be present on physical examinations. The authors demonstrate aortography showing proximal ulcerative plaques and digital arteriograms revealing the sharp cut-off pattern of an arterial embolus, providing diagnostic confirmation. Treatment consisted of endarterectomy or dacron graft interposition. Toe amputation was necessary in five patients with gangrenous toes.

Helfand (215), in a discussion of the common foot complications in the elderly diabetic patient, makes a simple and yet profound observation—one that podiatrists have observed and discussed for a few generations and yet have not fully accepted. He states, "A mirror of disease, the foot frequently becomes the focus of serious infection which can lead to significant disability, confinement and impairment." Helfand also says that a "total team provides an approach which does not segment the patient by anatomic or professional concerns."

Aside from the diabetic problem and its multiple complications, the podiatrist must recognize the necessity for strict controls on medication incompatibilities and their serious sequelae.

Treatment. The patient must be under an internist's care for diabetic control. Bacterial cultures and antibiotic sensitivity tests, identification of the bacteria and selection of the proper antibiotic and control of cellulitis are imperative. Footgear must be prescribed to support and accommodate the feet. Functional and structural deformities must be corrected, accommodated or protected by prosthetic devices.

Remove pressure from ulcerated areas by felt padding or accommodative removable orthoses or shields. A ripple-soled shoe may be used by cutting away the "ripples" on the spongy outer sole beneath the ulcer to protect the lesion. The ulcer is suspended between ripples.

A mild, wet dressing of saline solution (1 tablespoonful of table salt to each quart of water) or dilute povidone-iodine (Betadine) solution serves as a soothing, nonirritating antiseptic lavage, and an application of antibiotic enzyme ointments allows for proteolytic debridement. Judicious debridement of devitalized tissue may be necessary. Sterile loose dressings are applied and carefully observed for possible irritation.

Use necessary internal and local medication to stimulate circulation. Cyclandelate (3,3,5-trimethylcyclohexyl-mandelate) has proven to be helpful in diabetic and ischemic ulcers. Pentoxifylline (Trental) given orally in doses of 400 mg tid may be helpful. Trental is being prescribed currently for intermittent claudication to reduce blood viscosity by improving red cell flexibility. Systemic broad spectrum antibiotics may be necessary to control cellulitis. Instructions for diabetic foot care and cleanliness should be given.

Frank and Silver (216) found that ulcers in the presence of a neuropathy were best treated by excluding antibiotics and wet dressings. Instead they substituted a light cradle with a 25 watt bulb suspended 20 to 25 inches from the part and maintained at a temperature of 90°F.

Collens et al. (217) recommended dilute solutions of triiodide complex that release free iodine. The solution consists of 0.5 g of KI dissolved in 100 ml of water with 1.0 g crystalline iodine (I_2) added. They presented five cases in which gangrenous parts scheduled for amputation responded well to this treatment when the antimicrobial solution was used as wet dressing and injected into suppurating sinus tracts and sloughing tissue daily.

Rakow (218) recommends the use of the solution in a variety of ways, e.g., placing the iodine solution on a drain loosely packed into a sinus tract. It may also be applied directly into a tissue slough. A sterile pad may be saturated and sandwiched between two dry sterile pads, applied to the wound and allowed to release nascent iodine. Dressings should be changed daily. Rakow further notes in his experience that vasodilators and anticoagulants have not proved successful in treatment of diabetic ulcers.

Smith et al. (219), after studying the effect of electrical stimulation on wound healing in diabetic mice, propose that the proper practical application of direct electrical stimulation may be beneficial in the treatment of ischemic and diabetic ulcers in humans.

Sage and Doyle (220) reviewed 48 cases of diabetic ulcers treated with local surgical intervention to avoid higher amputation. Preoperative Doppler studies were performed in order to classify the diabetic ulcers as either ischemic or nonischemic. The success rate in the ischemic group (24 patients) was 25%, whereas the success rate in the nonischemic group (24 patients) was 83% healed.

Glasser and Barth (221) discussed diabetic wound healing and the use of topical insulin. Hanam et al. (222) studied the effect of topical insulin on wound healing in 41 diabetic and nondiabetic mice. Treatment regimens that included topical insulin provided better rates of wound healing than treatment regimens in which only base preparations or controls were used.

Ignacio et al. (223) present a study of 15 patients with extensive leg ulcers of at least grade III who were treated with topical oxygen. A 73.3% healing rate was obtained. Ulcers are classified into five categories (grades):

I. Small and superficial ulcers
II. Ulcers extending into the deep fascia, tendons and ligaments and into the superficial joints
III. Deeper and more extensive ulcers involving at least a quarter of the foot with a deep abscess or osteomyelitis
IV. Extensive involvement with gangrene of some portion of the foot
V. Ulcers involving at least half the foot, where amputation is strongly considered.

There are two distinct types of diabetic ulcer, i.e., the neurotrophic and the ischemic. Either of these ulcer types may be secondarily infected. Comparative x-rays of both feet should be performed. In order to keep the diabetic patient as fully under control as is possible, consultation with the treating internist is often necessary. Screening urinalysis, hemoglobin A1c and/or fasting blood sugar is indicated when there is a question of diabetic control.

The nondraining, noninfected neurotrophic ulcer should be protected from further trauma, surrounding keratosis and devitalized tissue should be debrided, and local enzymatic treatment should be initiated. If the ulcer is draining, aerobic and anaerobic culture and sensitivity tests should be performed and appropriate antibiotics prescribed. Foot soaks should not be prescribed as they tend to macerate tissue and lead to ulcer extension. Daily foot bathing in a dilute povidone-iodine (Betadine) solution is acceptable. If the ulcer is not healed within 6 weeks or if initial or follow-up comparative x-ray examination reveals neurotrophic changes (Charcot foot) and the patient had diminished and/or loss of sensation and nonreactive Achilles deep tendon reflex, the patient must be put at complete bed rest. If the ulcer is grossly infected with cellulitis and ascending lymphangiitis, the patient should be hospitalized and placed on appropriate iv antibiotics and diabetic control. Creatinine clearance testing prior to and during the use of aminoglycoside therapy is essential. Trough and peak serum concentrations should be monitored and serial audiograms are recommended prior to and during treatment.

If the diabetic ulcer is ischemic with skin and nail atrophy, poor capillary and venous filling time, feeble pedal pulses, and with rubor upon dependence, appropriate peripheral vascular examination, including x-ray examination of both feet, should be obtained; culture and sensitivity tests and appropriate antibiotics should be prescribed. If an infection is other than local, the patient must be hospitalized, appropriate intravenous antibiotics prescribed, and consultation obtained. Osteomyelitis must be ruled out. Excessive foot soaks tend to macerate tissue and are counterindicated. Warm whirlpool therapy leads to maceration, venous congestion and an exacerbation of the problem.

Perforating ulcers occur at points of pressure and usually in individuals between the ages of 40 and 60. They are characterized by a perforation from one tissue surface through to the opposite surface (Fig. 6.121).

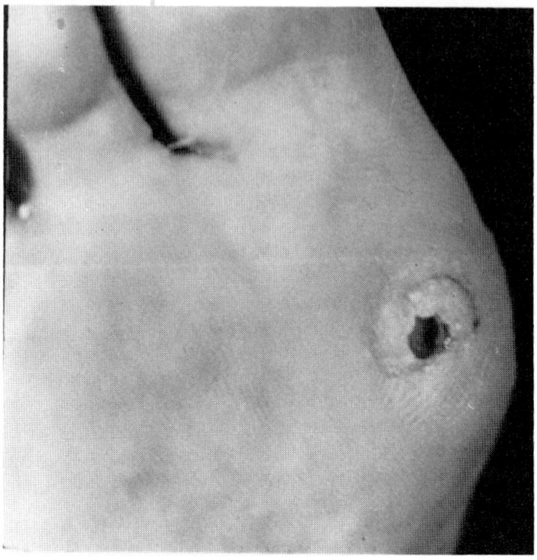

Figure 6.121. Perforating ulcer secondary to arteriosclerosis. Exposed flexor hallucis longus tendon.

Alcoholism, diabetes, syphilis and arteriosclerosis are the most common predisposing causes. Pressure from a heloma or tyloma over the first and fifth toes and their respective metatarsal heads and pressure and friction on the heel and ends of the toes are direct causes. The ulceration is deepseated, covered with a heaped-up callus and perforated by the avenue of a sinus through to the opposite skin surface, e.g., from plantar to dorsal.

It is believed that the combination of mechanical pressure, vascular instability and neurogenic disorders may cause perforating ulcers. A pathological degeneration of the dorsal root and ganglia in the lumbosacral area may be an etiologic factor.

Singer (224) discusses the surgical treatment of mal perforans. He concludes that mal perforans is a chronic foot ulcer commonly found in diabetic patients with neuropathy. Although it often responds to conservative measures, recurrence is frequent and brings with it the risk of spreading infection and serious destruction of tissues. If mal perforans exists beneath a metatarsal head, Singer suggests surgical excision of the metatarsal head or excision of the distal metatarsal and amputation of the affected toe to achieve long-term healing.

Treatment. Remove devitalized tissue mechanically and by enzymatic debridement, e.g., streptokinase-streptodornase (Varidase), fibrinolysin and deoxyribonuclease ointment (Elase) and neomycin, trypsin, chymotrypsin ointment (Biozyme).

The proper antibiotic ointment is determined by sensitivity tests. Identification of bacterial flora is mandatory. Insert Penrose drains and use warm saline dressings. This procedure may be followed by iodoform gauze packings. Protect the ulceration from trauma by judicious bandaging and foot orthoses or shields. McCarthy and Montgomery (225) recommend polyurethane occlusive dressings for dermal ulcers. The dressings are changed every 10 days, allowing optimal oxygenation of the healing ulcer beneath the dressing. The authors claim a sharp reduction in treatment time and expenditure during the therapy.

Consult the internist for treatment of the etiologic basis for development of the perforating ulcer, e.g., diabetes, arteriosclerosis or peripheral neuropathies.

Skin graft may follow wide excision of ulcer.

Bone disintegration at the distal ends of the toes resembling osteomyelitis is capable of "almost complete reconstruction," according to Pogonowska et al. (226).

Syphilitic ulcers are painless, typically gummatous lesions often found at the head of the first and fifth metatarsals (Figs. 6.122 and 6.123). The plantar surface of the hallux interphalangeal joint is a favorite site of many ulcers of all types. A usual location of the syphilitic ulcer is on the upper two-thirds of the thigh and the anterior surface of the leg. It may be perforating and have a cadaverous appearance.

The ulcers are pale grayish-white and are covered by a heavy parchment-like tissue. Often there are multiple lesions that coalesce with clearing on one side and destruction at the other. The edges are pigmented and depressed toward the center, and the resultant scar is thin and pliable. These ulcers have a punched-out appearance with sharply cut, undermined edges and a ragged base. They may be circular, semicircular or serpiginous in shape, and the margins are indurated and sharp.

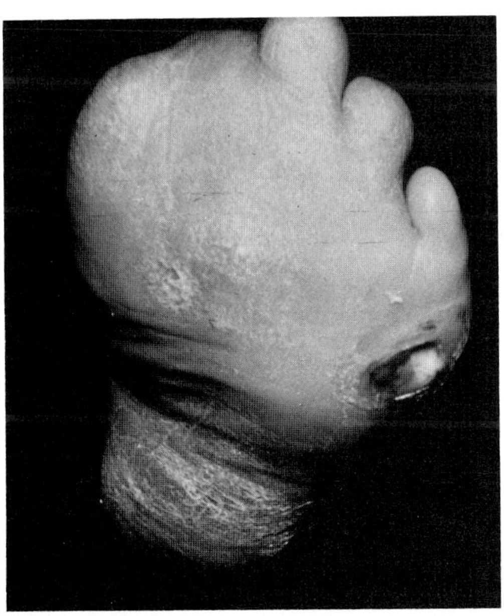

Figure 6.122. Charcot deformity with secondary syphilitic ulcer head of fifth metatarsal.

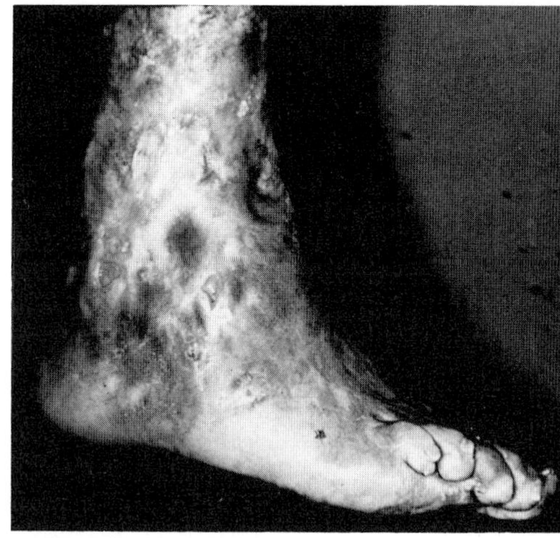

Figure 6.123. Syphilitic ulcers. Gummatous lesions on anterior of leg and dorsum of foot.

Very often a regional adenopathy; skin rashes of macular, papular and erythematous lesions; a positive VDRL test; and rapid healing with the therapeutic use of potassium iodide are characteristic of this type of ulcer, which can be treated in the same way as a perforating ulcer.

Tuberculous ulcers occur in tuberculous individuals with a history of tubercular abscess in the subcutaneous tissues and bone.

Objectively, the skin is undermined for some distance around the margins of the ulcer. The surface is pale, granulations are small and areas of caseation necrosis are characteristic. The discharge is thin and scanty, whereas the periphery of the ulcer is livid and mildly tender. No evidence of increase in temperature is noted. A biopsy may often provide the diagnosis of tuberculous ulcer.

Treatment. Systemic treatment of tuberculosis is mandatory. The patient should have bed rest. Daily foot baths in solutions of warm saline are helpful in preventing secondary infections.

Excision and curettage of necrotic bone with sterile dry dressings relieve the ulcers.

Infective ulcers affecting the toes, soles and the heels are the most common kind of ulcer found in the feet. A strong proprietary medicine for helomas and tylomas; injudicious cutting of corns, calluses, and nails; or unsterile debridement of a blister may cause an infective ulcer. This type of ulcer is the same as pyogenic ulcer. Objectively, the ulcer is small, deep and bounded by a heavy, tough, slowly growing skin. A purulent exudate is evident.

Treatment. Sensitivity tests of bacterial flora are indicated. Warm saline or povidone-iodine soakes may be helpful. Use of local medication and internal antibiotics depends on the type of bacterial invasion. Rest of the affected part and adequate systemic hydration aid in control and repair of the infected ulcer.

Hazan (227) suggested injectable trypsin as an adjunct to treatment with antibiotics. Inflammation is reduced readily by this method.

Luft (228) studied the reactions to parenteral enzyme therapy and made the following observations. "Trypsin and chymotrypsin, oral and parenteral, are excellent drugs for use in inflammatory conditions of the lower extremities." Luft further notes that allergic or anaphylactic reactions are not uncommon. These reactions were preceded by local swelling at the site of injection. The generalized reaction varies from malaise to severe anaphylaxis. Frequent signs are urticaria, respiratory distress, conjunctivitis, nausea, abdominal cramps and vomiting. Epinephrine 1:1000 should always be at hand for immediate use if a reaction occurs.

Local antibiotics, such as neomycin for Gram-negative bacteria and bacitracin for Gram-positive bacteria, or polymixin combined with chymotrypsin, streptokinase, ribonuclease and other proteolytic enzymes are helpful. Chymoral-100 is taken orally qid. Orenzyme or Papase may relieve swelling and inflammation associated with infected ulcers.

Fibrinolysin and deoxyribonuclease combined may be mixed with 50 to 100 ml or sodium chloride solution to make a solution for treatment of the infected ulcer. Strips of gauze are soaked in the solution, applied to the wound for about 6 hr and then removed along with the necrotic tissue. This procedure is followed until healthy granulations appear in the wound.

Ulcer Wound Healing. After the first 4 to 5 days, the wound undergoes a proliferative phase of fibroplasia with development of immature collagen and a mucopolysaccharide ground substance. This phase lasts about 2 weeks and is productive of considerable tensile strength.

The phase of maturation occurring about the third week involves a complex local metabolic remodeling of tissue in which the wound collagen fibers are remodeled. The tensile strength is gradually enhanced as the scar and narrowing hyperpermeable capillaries develop into a firm but healthier tissue. The usual normal rete ridging is altered during repair and produces a different type of union at the epidermodermal contact. This is distinguishable microscopically, but is grossly visible in the different character of scar tissue, as opposed to the true skin, in epithelial repair. It is believed to be the result of an immediate rapid mitotic division of the epithelial basal cells at the wound edges. It appears that an inhibiting factor, chalone, in the epidermis is lost, causing an uninhibited rapid mitotic division of cells stimulating repair.

Surgical injury stimulates fibroblasts in surrounding tissues and blood vessels to proliferate in great numbers, creating a biological machinery capable of producing mucopolysaccharides, collagen and elastin. This function is a precursor to the normal development of scar tissue. It is also believed that circulating monocytes might play a part in the development of fibroblasts.

The biochemistry of collagen formation, including the part played by the amino acids, the ribonucleic acid factors, iron and ascorbic acid, is beyond the scope of this clinical offering.

Healing depends on the physiological viability of vitamin C, adequate protein, sufficient fibroplasia, and synthesis of mucopolysaccharides, collagen and components of amino acids not clearly identified. Of course it is also necessary to have adequate circulation, sufficient oxygen tension, minimal systemic pathology and synthesized fibroblasts.

The inflammatory phase of healing may overlap the proliferative phase because there is little evidence of a clear line of delineation. The inflammation following a surgical incision brings with it a wound that is vascular and capable in a normal situation of cellular infiltration and the development of biochemical hemostasis. Debris and less virulent bacteria and their toxins are removed by macrophage invasion and polymorphonuclear leukocytes. Fibroblasts invade the would to assist in collagen formation. A fibrin clot is formed, and reactions occur involving glycoprotein chemistry. Migrating basal epithelial cells and strands of fibrin provide a central closing process of the wound at the dermal level. This process may take 4 to 5 days in the healthy noncontaminated wound. The collagen is immature at this stage of healing. Migliori and Kanat (229) examine the integrated system of wound healing, including an analysis of leukocyte function. Leukocyte dysfunction during the first phase of healing, as a result of disease, drugs, or improper surgical techniques, must be controlled or given special consideration by the surgeon.

McCarthy and Axler (230) provide interesting data concerning the efficacy of porcine xenografts and heterografts. Their study embodied standard light transmission, electron and scanning electron microscopic procedures. The porcine skin is similar to human skin and presents a stratum corneum graft with a keratinized layer that protects the underlying ulcer. The two skins have an affinity that protects the ulcer while it allows for proper drainage. The researchers note that epithelialization proceeds in centripetal fashion. Several excellent scanning electron microscopy photomicrographs provide observations of the efficacy of porcine grafts on the tissue and cellular level.

In a later clinical research project, McCarthy et al. (231) noted that a Gram-negative microbial population in an ulcer is incompatible with adequate repair in the presence of a porcine graft.

Toenail Disorders (Onychology)

Structure and Function of the Nails

The nails are horny, elastic, transparent tissue on the dorsal distal ends of fingers and toes formed by intimately adhered keratotic cells similar to the cells of the epidermis.

The nail proper is composed of a nail body that is convex on the outer side and concave on the under surface with a distal free edge and two lateral edges. The two lateral edges described anatomically are medial or tibial and lateral or fibular, respectively. The nail plate rests on the nail bed and is imbedded posteriorly into the dermis. The eponychium is a thin layer of skin overlying the proximal nail.

Below the eponychium, the matrix is thickened and raised in a series of longitudinal ridges. It is from this matrix tissue that the nail is developed, produced and grows forward. The matrix is pink in color and is a specialized, highly vascular tissue corresponding to the mucous layer of the skin. It is readily visible when the nail plate is removed.

Toenails protect the vascular anastomoses at the ends of the toes and are subject to trauma from ill-fitting footgear, local pathological processes and systemic disease. The nails are affected by the same pathology that affects the skin from which they are differentiated (Fig. 6.124).

Common Nail Disorders

Below is a glossary of terms used to describe common nail disorders.

I. Congenital
- *Anonychia:* absence of nail
- *Macronychia:* large, wide, broad nail
- *Micronychia:* unusually small nail
- *Pachyonychia:* thick, hard, often longitudinally striated nails (involves all nails) (Figs. 6.125 and 6.126)
- *Onychotropia:* nail atrophy
- *Polyonychia:* more than one distinct nail on a digit
- *Synonychia:* webbed toes with one nail
- *Onychoheterotopia:* nail growth other than in the usual place
- *Unguis incurvatum:* involuted nail

II. Acquired
- *Leukonychia:* white or white spotted nail; may be due to injury
- *Onychophosis:* callus in the nail groove; due to friction and pressure
- *Paronychia:* local soft tissue infection surrounding the nail
- *Onychia:* local medial or lateral and posterior nail infection
- *Onychocryptosis (Unguis incarnatus):* ingrown toe nail; due to obesity, shoe pressure, biomechanical abnormality or injudicious nail cutting
- *Onychogryphosis (Ram's horn nail):* thick tortuous nail; due to trauma or arterial insufficiency
- *Onychauxis (Club nail):* thick, long, hard overgrown nail; due to trauma, decreased arterial circulation, peripheral neuropathy or systemic disease
- *Subungual exostosis:* dorsal distal phalangeal exostosis resulting in a convex, thin, waxy nail
- *Onychophemia:* subungual hematoma or hemorrhage; due to trauma
- *Agnail:* ungua labia fissure; due to irritation
- *Onychophagia:* nail biting
- *Hapalonychia:* soft, thin, transparent nails; may be due to systemic illness
- *Koilonychia:* spoon nail with concave

surface; due to polycythemia vera, hypochronic anemia, thyrotoxicosis or an unknown cause

Onychoschizia: loosening of nail from nail bed; due to vitamin deficiency, eczema or trauma

Onychomadesis: spontaneous nail loss; due to chronic debilitating systemic illness

Onycholysis: separation of nail from nail bed; due to local contact allergy, tetracycline therapy, psoriasis,

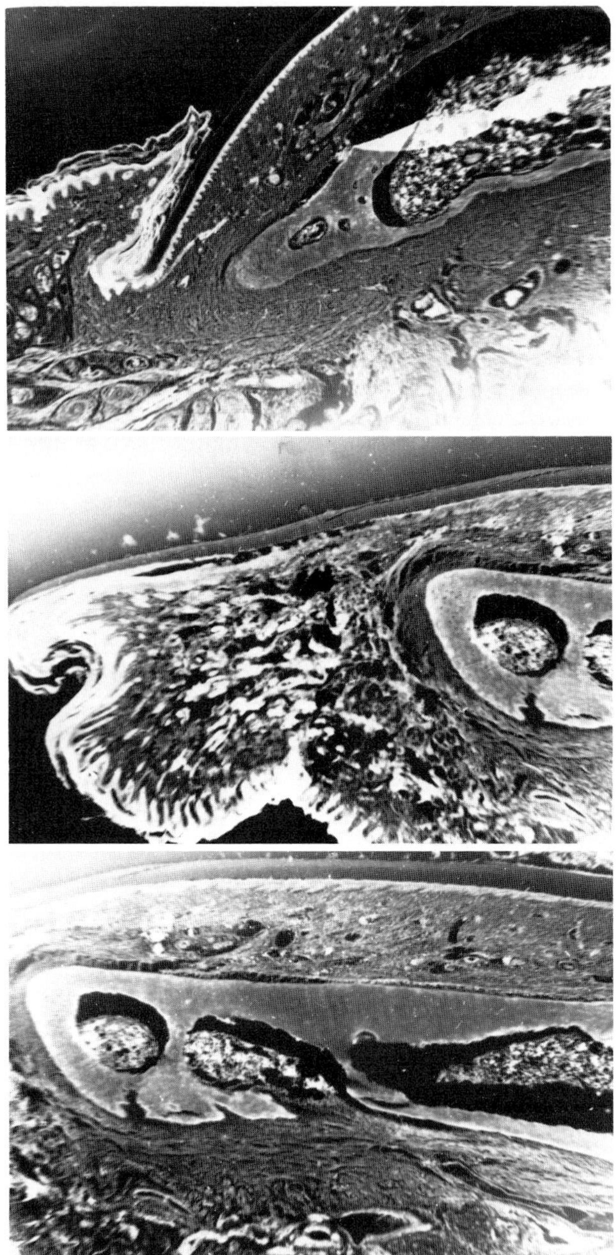

Figure 6.124. *Top,* Cross-section of the toenail. Note part of nail plate, lateral nail fold, papillary ridge of bed and a section of the phalanx. Full-term fetus, stillborn. *Center,* Longitudinal section of the toenail. Note that the plate has reached the distal end of the toe in this full-term fetus. *Bottom,* Most of nail body is observed. (Courtesy of CE Krausz.)

trauma, tabes dorsalis, hyperidrosis or hyperthyroidism

Hippocratic nails: club-like, thick, light gray to brown, convex from side to side and from the proximal border to the distal end; seen in pulmonary, kidney and cardiac disease

Onychoclavus: medial or lateral fifth toe nail groove callus; due to pressure and toe rotation

Onychomycosis: thick brownish-yellow superficial fungus infected nail

Pulsating nail: glomus tumor

Subungual Heloma: keratoma beneath nail; due to subungual bone lesion, friction and shoe pressure (Figs. 6.127 and 6.151)

Onychomalacia: soft nail; no known cause

Onychorrehexis: longitudinal splitting of brittle nail; may be due to trauma or arterial insufficiency

Beau's Lines: transverse grooves in the nail; due to interruption of nail growth from trauma, illness, disease or foot surgery

Mee's lines: transverse white lines in the nails; due to arsenic poisoning

III. Specific Disease Associated

Pityriasis: thick discolored nails; onychauxis

Psoriasis: thickened, white, sometimes yellow and lusterless pitted nails; onycholysis often seen

Hyperthyroidism: shiny, well-developed nails; may become soft from excessive perspiration

Hyperpituitarism: shiny, well-developed nails; may be convex

Eczema: thin, friable, fragmented nails

Ichthyosis: thick discolored nails; onychauxis

Scleroderma: thin atrophic nails

Rheumatoid arthritis: pitting during acute flair

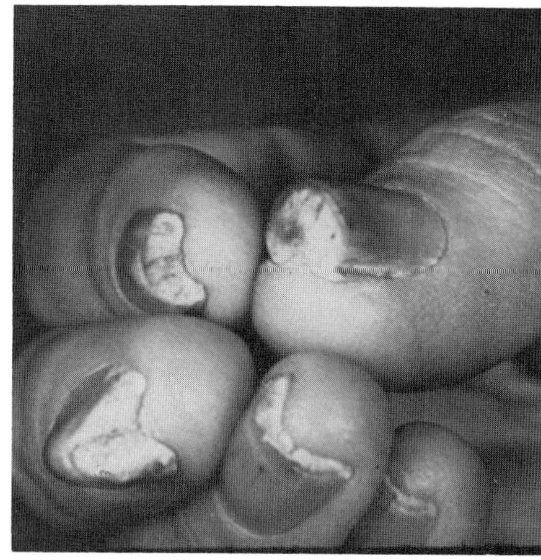

Figure 6.126. Pachyonychia, fingernails. (Courtesy of C Krausz.)

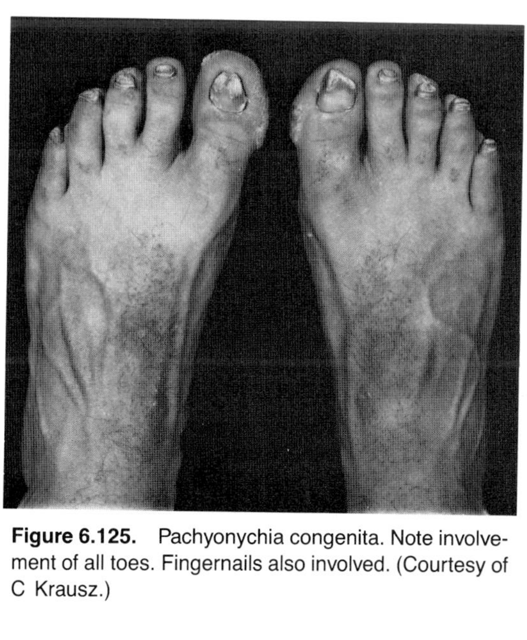

Figure 6.125. Pachyonychia congenita. Note involvement of all toes. Fingernails also involved. (Courtesy of C Krausz.)

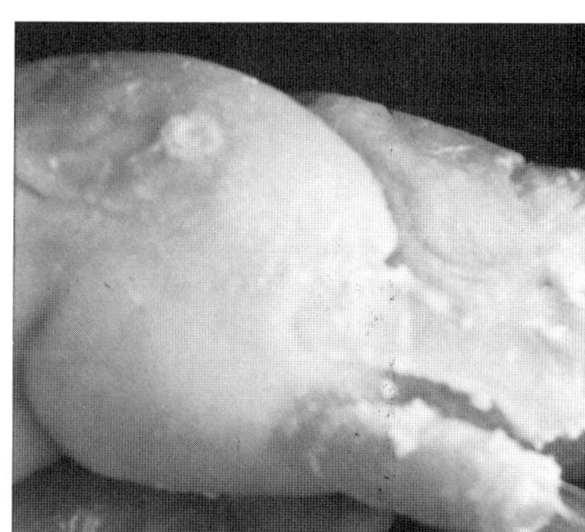

Figure 6.127. Cutaneous horn developing from nail bed and bulbous end of toe.

Osteoarthritis: dry, brittle nails with subungual keratosis
Lupus erythematosus: multiple paronychia
Lichen planus: thin, friable, scaling, fragmented nails
Anemia: Beau's lines, onychoschizia, onychomadesis and koilonychia
Arsenical poisoning: darkly pigmented nails or transverse white lines
Diabetes: onychogryphosis, onychauxis
Atherosclerosis: onychogryphosis, onychauxis
Avitaminosis: thin nails; Onychoschizia
Raynaud's disease: whitish, atrophic, loose nails
Buerger's disease: whitish, atrophic, loose nails
Syphilis: paronychia (early stage); onychauxis (late stage)
Tuberculosis: acute paronychia
Pemphigus: nail discoloration, pitting and transverse sulci
Elephantiasis: atrophic nails with raised distal borders
Hypothyroidism: brittle, thin, white-spotted, striated nails
Hypopituitarism: loss of lanula
Pulmonary disease: convex, club-like, thick, light gray to brown nails
Kidney Disorders: convex, club-like, thick, light gray to brown nails
Congenital Cardiac Disease: convex, club-like, thick, light gray to brown nails

Krausz (232) reported a nail survey of 10,900 podiatric patients with a total of 6754 nail disorders. This study indicates that at least 61% of those patients examined for podiatric problems had some nail disorders. The four most prevalent problems reported by Krausz were onychocryptosis, 1,765; onychauxis and onychogryphosis, 1,493; onychophosis, 1,334; and onychomycosis, 551. Each of these conditions may be a precursor to secondary infection and even subsequent loss of limb in the diabetic or the patient with peripheral vascular disorders.

Onychocryptosis is a condition in which the free edge of the nail has penetrated the periungual layers and has become embedded in the soft tissues. Usually the etiology involves trauma, a diseased nail, obesity, biomechanical abnormality, ill-fitting footgear or injudicious cutting of the nail. Occasionally the nail lip is hypertrophied and is forced into the nail edge; also occasionally a subungual exostosis elevates the center of the nail forcing the margins down. Secondary infection and profuse granulation are common. An ischemic hyperesthesia may develop at the site of greatest nail pressure in peripheral vascular disorders. The author has treated several infants from birth to 12 months old suffering from onychocryptosis.

A subungual heloma may develop at the distal third of the nail plate from trauma or pressure of a short shoe or a seam in an open-toed shoe. The nail plate appears discolored and is elevated from the excrescence in the nail bed. Pressure from the dorsum of the nail plate against the subungual mass produces pain.

Often the painful lesion is an onychophosis or callus in the nail groove. When a nail groove is callused, lateral digital pressure causes pain. A yellow, gray to white, hard, horny, flat or deep keratotic mass may be in evidence beneath the nail plate. Reduction of the callus by sharp curettage and advice on footgear are necessary.

Treatment of the ingrown toenail depends upon the extent of the pathology. X-ray examination of the affected toe is essential to rule out osteomyelitis (when infection is present), exostosis, osteochondroma or the presence of a foreign body. Unlike treatment in the past, therapy today is highly specialized and varies according to whether the condition is uncomplicated or complicated.

Uncomplicated onychocryptosis occurs when there is penetration of the nail groove or lip by an offending portion of an essentially healthy nail caused by injudicious cutting of the nail or by trauma to the lip. The lip may be forced into the nail by shoe pressure or by a blow, or the nail may be forced into the groove or nail lip. The resultant pressure on soft tissues may create a tyloma or heloma in the nail groove or along the side of the lip. A slight contusion or small ulceration or abrasion is very often found in these cases.

Treatment is aimed at relieving pressure. Ensuring the proper fit of shoes and hose is essential. Removing the offending portion of the nail by careful specialized techniques of splitting or sharp curettage may be necessary. Packing the nail groove as described below keeps the nail away from the traumatized tissues.

If a callus is present, the nail groove is packed with a 15 to 25% salicylic acid ointment and cotton. In 3 to 5 days and with judicious curettage, the tyloma and debris are removed. If necessary a new salicylic acid pack is applied. If the entire tyloma has been removed, care is taken to keep the nail free from the groove.

Packs are constructed from cotton, gauze, felt, Celastic, latex, resins, dental acrylic, adhesive plaster, plaster of Paris, foam rubber and a variety of other substances. Sulci protectors and toenail wiring have been used extensively in England with a degree of success (Fig. 6.128). All of these methods have been tested and proven to be effective in keeping the nail from penetrating the groove.

Sanders (233), Sivitz (234) and Mogull (235) cite the advantages of using acrylic to protect and pack nail grooves.

The pack is placed in the groove with or without a soothing ointment or cream. The packing material is placed underneath the lateral margin of nail to lift it up and away from the nail bed and groove. It is carried out along the cutting edge of the nail to separate the edge from the groove and nail lip. The packing is removed at intervals, and new packs are applied as needed.

If an ulceration is found in the nail groove, it is treated as necessary before packing. Goldy and Steinberg (236) have described the etiologic factors in multiple-infected onychocryptosis and stress the need for laboratory studies, bacteriologic evaluation and often complete physical examinations to clarify the etiology.

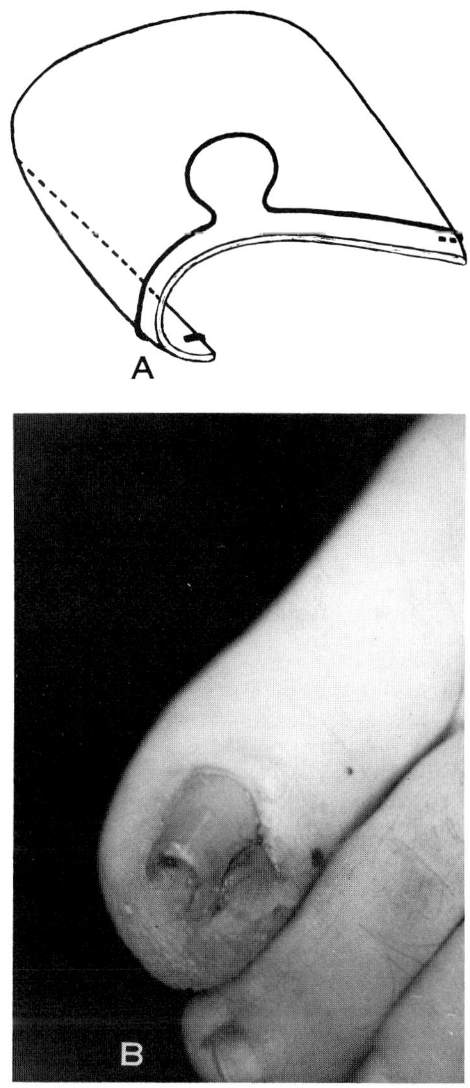

Figure 6.128. *A,* Toenail wiring for correction of ingrown toenail. (Courtesy of Ross Fraser.) *B,* Complicated onychocryptosis in which wiring would not be appropriate. Granuloma in nail groove overlapping nail border.

Complicated onychocryptosis requires all the skill of the professional. Multiple infections may be challenging. The pathology varies from deep ulcerations in the grooves, profuse granulations, granulomas, infections, paronychia, and distortion of the nail plate. Hypertrophy of the lips of the nail where the edges of the nail are incurvated at their margins and are incapable of being reversed may be a complicating factor, along with or secondary to other pathology.

The accepted treatment for complicated onychocryptosis is as follows.

Local anesthesia is produced by nerve block or field block. The podiatrist must be sure to remove a large enough section of the offending plate to allow for drainage. The nail plate is split by a nail splitter and/or straight-edged nail forceps directly back to the eponychium following the nail striations. The eponychium is elevated, and a nail splitter is carried back through the nail matrix. The splitter is forced back gently until all resistance is lost. The sectioned portion of the nail is freed from its attachments by a sharp nail splitter and is gently extracted with a hemostat. A drain may be inserted and analgesics and antibiotics prescribed for pain and to avoid inflammatory and infectious changes. Such wet dressings as dilute boric acid solution, saline, betadine, aluminum subacetate, potassium permanganate or nitrofurasone are indicated. Follow-up care may necessitate use of systemic or local antibiotics.

If profuse granulation is present, radical treatment, rather than use of palliative astringents and cauterizing agents, facilitates earlier repair. The author prefers to use a sharp tissue forceps when excising the profuse granulation and then to touch up the capillary bleeders with a concentrate of silver nitrate stick or electrocoagulating current. To leave the granulation prolongs postoperative care and slows down repair.

Radical Correction of Complicated Ingrown Toenail. When the nail is inverted from its base forward and is, in the judgment of the podiatrist, a chronic offender, radical surgical procedures should be attempted. Radical surgery consists of removing offending portions of the nail, nail bed and matrix. Plastic surgical repair of lip anomalies may also be necessary if the nail lips are chronically enlarged.

DuVries (237) describes the technique of removing a longitudinal wedge from the hypertrophied nail lip and suturing down the elevated enlarged lip without disturbing the matrix. The author has found this technique valuable in selected cases of hypertrophy of the unguilabia.

The Winograd Technique for Correction. In another technique (238) used for many years with good results, the nail is split back from the distal edge through the nail plate and matrix to isolate the offending portion of the nail. A scalpel is placed through the split of the nail and carried back through the eponychium down to the bone to about ¼ inch distal to the distal interphalangeal joint. It is then carried forward to and through the soft tissue at the distal end of the nail plate. A semielliptical incision is then carried from the proximal to distal end of the first incision to include the matrix, offending portion of nail and nail lip. The section removed should be wedge-shaped. The wound is debrided with special attention to removing all of the visible matrix. The margins are underscored and the tissues apposed for closure by sutures. Some operators suture only the posterior fold; others carry sutures through the entire wound including a single suture through the nail plate. If a suture is to be used through the plate, one must place a hole in the plate before attempting to force the suture needle through. Doing so facilitates better union and protects the nail from damage. Sutures are removed between 7 and 12 days postoperatively.

Because the need for sutures is questionable and their use in an avascular area results in considerable postoperative pain, the closure may be facilitated by use of Steri-Strips instead of suturing material. This technique is less painful, allows for more rapid healing and is most effective in minimizing scar tissue. The author has performed various modifications of the Winograd Technique to correct complicated ingrown toe nails in hundreds of cases. Results have been excellent.

However, the author prefers the technique developed by Frost (239) and described below.

The Frost Technique for Correction (Fig. 6.129). Under a 1 or 2% lidocaine toe block and with a tourniquet around the base of the toe, the nail is split longitudinally along its entire length by

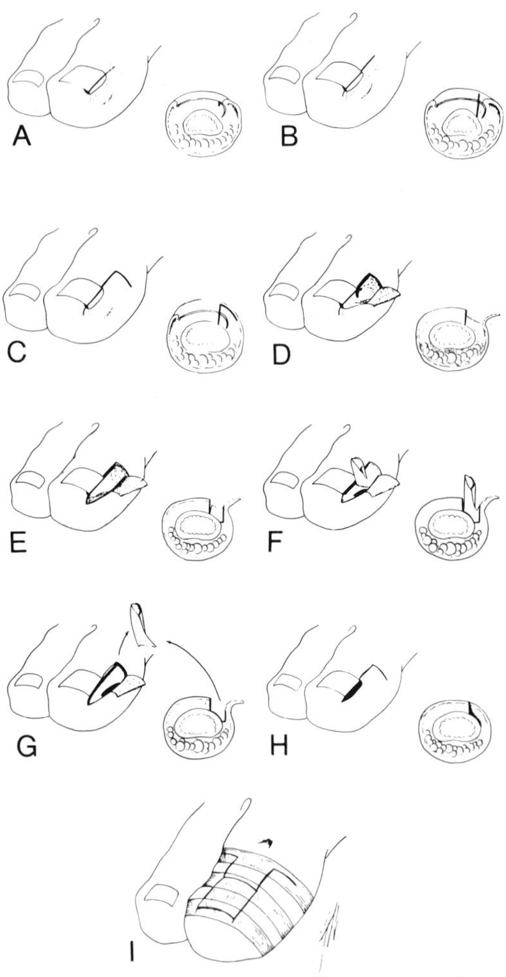

Figure 6.129. Frost technique. (Courtesy of Lawrence Frost.)

following a longitudinal ridge or striation just within the beginning of the arc and the incurvation as indicated by the solid and broken dark lines (Fig. 6.129A).

A scalpel is laid in this channel, and a vertical incision is made down to the phalanx for the entire length of the nail to about 1⁄16 inch beyond each end of the nail plate (Fig. 6.129B).

At the proximal end of this incision, another incision is made at right angles to it just beyond the proximal end of the nail and just through the skin down to the adipose tissue layer (Fig. 6.129C).

The corner of this skin triangle is grasped, and a scalpel is used to free it from the adipose tissue to form a full thickness skin flap (Fig. 6.129D).

With this flap retracted to one side, another longitudinal incision is made, as indicated by an additional black line (Fig. 6.129E), about 1⁄16 inch external to the edge of the nail and parallel to the first incision to the same depth. Nearing the tip of the toe, the depth of the incision is decreased, and the line of the incision is turned to meet the first incision.

The distal point of this segment is grasped with forceps, and an incision is made down to the phalanx. This segment of tissue is removed (Fig. 6.129F) from the dorsum of the phalanx by sharp dissection.

The nail root area is inspected for glistening white fragments of matrix that when found, are removed by sharp dissection (Fig. 6.129G).

The flap is repositioned (Fig. 6.129H), and the tourniquet is removed. Three Steri-Strips are applied (Fig. 6.129I). The area will bleed profusely for a short time, but in about 5 min a coagulum will form. A piece of Telfa, paraffin wax mesh or Adaptic is applied over the wound followed by three 2 × 2-inch gauze squares and a firm circular dressing of 1 inch Kling bandage or tube gauze anchored at the base of the toe by Fabco.

Patients are kept off their feet for 48 hrs., when the dressing, stiff with coagulated blood, is removed. They return for redressing in 10 days, at which time the Steri-Strips are removed. Cutout shoes are worn until regular shoes can be worn comfortably.

The author delivered a paper before the Military Society of Orthopedic Surgeons at West Point on the success achieved in keeping soldiers ambulatory by using a phenol-alcohol technique for correction of the ingrown toe nail. The technique described is a refinement of those utilizing phenol as originally proposed and reported by Boll (241), and improved by Nyman (242), Suppan and Ritchlin (243), Kleiman (244), Greene (245) and others who have also lectured on this effective method of toe nail surgery. Although the actual surgical approach varies with individuals, the objective—destruction of the matrix—is the same.

The chemosurgical technique described in 1970 to the Military Society of Orthopedic Surgeons with a report of 500 cases during a 2-year period has proved to be of tremendous value. The procedure, performed under local anesthesia on an ambulatory outpatient basis, is done in the face of local infection without the utilization of systemic antibiotics. With specific application to the military, soldiers treated with this technique are able to return to limited duty the same day and to full duty within 1 week.

The Phenol-Alcohol Chemosurgical Technique for Correction (Fig. 6.130). The procedure outlined below is for an infected ingrown toenail at the lateral aspect of the right hallux (Fig. 6.130A).

After preparation of the toe for surgery, anesthetize the hallux by field block utilizing about 1.5 ml of lidocaine (1 or 2%) plain. Apply a Penrose drain tourniquet at the base of the toe with the first hemostat. Use a sterile gauze (2 × 2 inches) between the tourniquet and the skin.

Split the nail distal to proximal beneath the eponychium following the linear nail lines approximately 1⁄16 to 1⁄8 inch medial to the lateral nail border. Excise the offending nail spicule with a hemostat clamped onto the entire spicule below the eponychium by rotating the hemostat toward the main nail body.

Curette the enlarged nail groove after excising the matrix below the eponychium. Excise any exuberant granulation tissue present with the toenail nipper.

Remove most of the cotton from a cotton applicator stick. Dip the tip of the stick into a bottle of 88% carbolic acid (phenol) without getting too much phenol on the tip. Apply the phenolated tip to the nail groove and matrix from distal to proximal beneath the eponychium for 1½ min taking care that the phenol does not run across the posterior nail wall (Fig. 6.130B). Remove the first applicator stick, sponge the area and apply the second applicator stick in the same manner for a period of 3 min (Fig. 6.130C).

Flush the surgical site with isopropyl alcohol.

Apply a Neosporin-G cream dressing to the surgical site utilizing two sterile gauze pads, 2 × 2 inches, and toe stockinet. Remove the tourni-

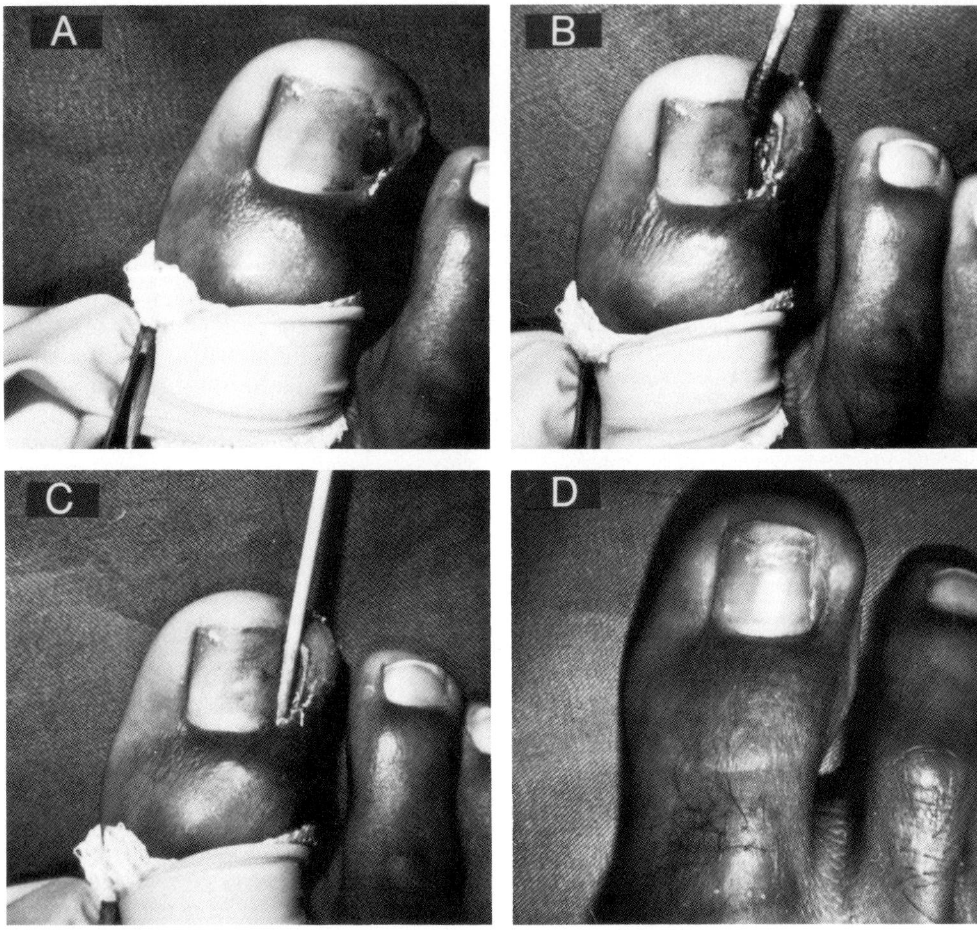

Figure 6.130. Phenol-alcohol technique for correction of ingrown toenails.

quet and apply ⅛-inch Fabco to the base of the toe to anchor the dressing.

There is very little postoperative discomfort. The patient is instructed to dissolve one tablespoon of salt in a quart of lukewarm water and soak the affected toe for 10 min bid. The dressing remains wet. Vinegar (acetic acid) or betadine solution soaks may be used. Vaseline may be used on the nail plate aspect of the offending nail border to protect the eponychium from the phenol as it is applied to the nail matrix area. When performing this procedure for a noninfected onychocryptosis, cortisporin otic solution (246) sulfamylon, silvadene or steroid cream, used to lessen the inflammatory response, may be substituted for neosporin. When exuberant granulation tissue has been excised, it is beneficial to pack the area with sterile gauze to facilitate drainage. Care must be taken to extirpate the nail matrix from distal to proximal with small nail cutters beneath the eponychium prior to sharp curettage.

After the performance of over 2,500 partial and total phenol-alcohol chemosurgical procedures for eradication of toenail matrix over the past 20 years, recurrence rate remains less than 3%. The author has encountered only one bone infection subsequent to performing this procedure for an infected ingrown toenail. Preoperative x-rays are important to rule out osteomyelitis or subungual neoplasm. Sterile gloves are not used. However, full sterile technique is used for other nail procedures requiring skin incision. Serous drainage lasts for an average of 2½ weeks after partial phenol-alcohol matricectomy and 3½ weeks after total great toe phenol-alcohol matricectomy. Nails that were locally infected before the procedure drain for a slightly longer period postoperatively. Prolonged drainage is caused by individual hypersensitivity to phenol, the use of too much phenol, matrix or nail spicule left in area, formation of an epidermoid inclusion cyst or indolent infection (Figs. 6.131 and 6.132).

The first redressing is done in 4 to 7 days. A

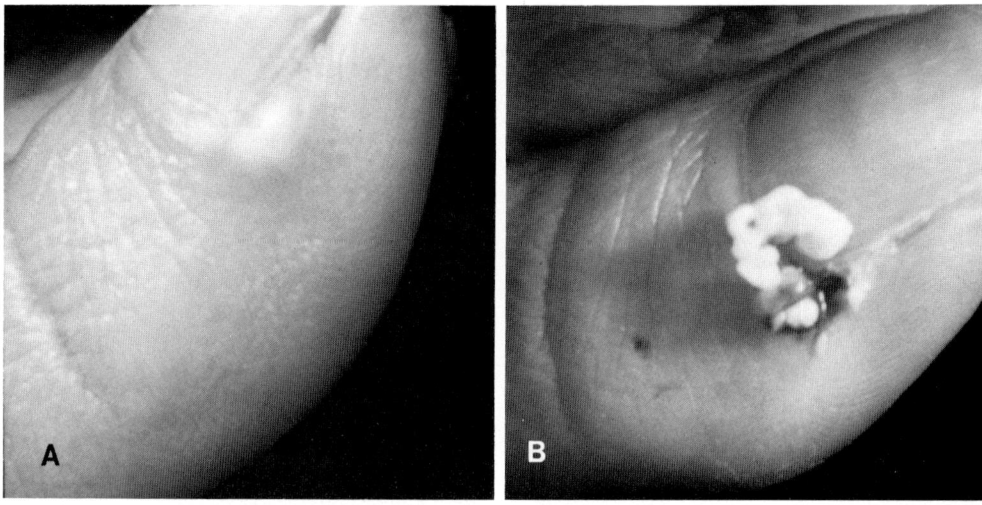

Figure 6.131. *A,* Epidermoid cyst postphenol correction of onychocryptosis. This is not an uncommon complication of any nail surgery procedure. *B,* Ruptured epidermoid cyst postphenol.

serous drainage, the result of the phenol producing a chemical burn, is noted and lasts from 2–5 weeks (two month's postphenol-alcohol, Fig. 130D).

It is imperative that fresh phenol be used and that the procedure be accomplished under strict hemostasis. Because of the phenol's neurolytic effect, a minimum of postoperative pain is experienced. If an infection exists the predominant organism cultured is staphylococcus coagulase positive. In infections caused by beta streptococcus, cellulitis has remained localized to the infected toe. Postoperative x-rays reveal no periosteal or subperiosteal changes. Care must be

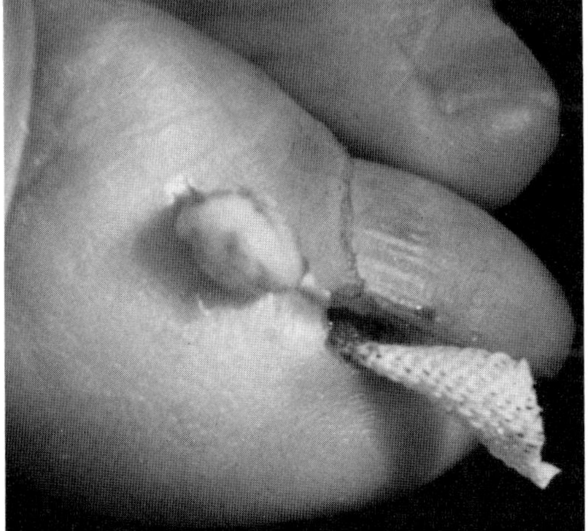

Figure 6.132. Epidermoid cyst. Gross specimen and drain in site of excision.

taken to avoid a chemical eponychia caused by the careless application and spread of the phenol. This would result in the formation of transverse lines in the form of sulci (Beau's lines) that progress forward with the growth of the nail.

Negative Galvanic Technique for Correction. Polokoff (247, 248), Rubin and Weiss (249) and Dyer and Cohen (250) report on the use of negative galvanism for correction of incurvated nails. Gardner (251) notes that there is little postsurgical pain, and rarely is there infection in this use of negative galvanism. The foot is prepared for surgery, and toe block or field block anesthesia is instituted. The offending border of the onychocryptosis is split from the distal end through the matrix. The offending nail border and matrix are gently removed, and hemostasis is affected by tourniquet or by digital pressure. A wet, warm saline-soaked, positive electrode, 4 × 4 inches, is placed on the calf, and a blunt sabre-shaped blade is fitted into a holder connected to the negative pole. The blade is placed in the nail groove and the negative current raised to 5 mA. The blade is worked along the nail groove and into the matrix area alternately for about 10 to 15 min. Hydrogen bubbles exude from the contact area of the needle. An ointment dressing is applied, and the wound is treated as a burn for a few days. Treatment is enhanced by enzymatic debridement of the necrotic tissue.

Electrocoagulation using a high-frequency current is also used to destroy matrical tissue.

Onychotripsy Techniques for Correction. Perrone (252) developed a nail matricectomy by use of a low-speed, high-torque air motor. He believes that the onychotripsy is accomplished with a minimum of surgical trauma and less pain when the air motor is used. The section of nail is removed by nail splitter (onychatome) under local anesthesia. A Busch burr is used in the chuck handpiece and placed in the eponychial envelope. Careful onychotripsy "erases" the nail matrix. One must develop a touch and feel of tissue through the burr and handpiece. The technique is rapid, and postoperative care is minimal. The site is kept dry and coagulum forms.

The Trephine Technique for Correction. Steinberg (253) introduced a new instrument and technique for surgical correction of ingrown toenail. The instrument has a trephine-like annular cutting head. In this procedure, the toe is anesthetized and prepared for surgery. A nick is made at the distal nail margin about ⅛ inch from its embedded border, and an incision is made at the junction of the posterior and lateral eponychium or the posterior corner of the nail. The incision should be extended to the tubercle at the base of the phalanx and angled slightly toward the affected edge of the toe. The incision is undermined by blunt section. The trephine engages the nick in the nail and is gently forced back in a boring fashion to include the nail, nail lip, nail bed, profuse granulations and fibrous connective tissue. The head of the instrument should advance to a point under the skin in the region of the matrix. The instrument is held perpendicular to the bone at this point, and the sharp edges at its end sever the tissues that are engaged in the trephine. These include the aforementioned tissues and the matrix.

Sterile sulfanilamide powder is dusted into the wound. The posterior section of the wound is closed by clip or Steri-Strips. The free edge of the nail in the wound is excised to remove a possible irritant from the site of wound healing.

A dry dressing is applied, and the usual measures for wound repair are followed. Healing is usually rapid. Steinberg reports success in 100 cases in 1956 and to date can record thousands of cases successfully treated in this manner.

Onychauxis and Onychogryphosis

Onychauxis or club nail is an overgrowth or hypertrophy of the nail in any or all of its dimensions (Fig. 6.133). The affected nail assumes a dirty brown, yellow, gray or black color, and the surface of the nail becomes horny and claw-like. The great toe is the most commonly affected either by trauma, fungus infections, pressure from ill-fitting shoes and hose, nutritional disturbances, psoriasis or circulatory disease. The nail bed may also be hypertrophied from the pressure of the thickened nail plate. Calluses and often helomas are found in the thickened nail bed beneath the free tibial, fibular and distal margins. Callused nail grooves may become extremely painful.

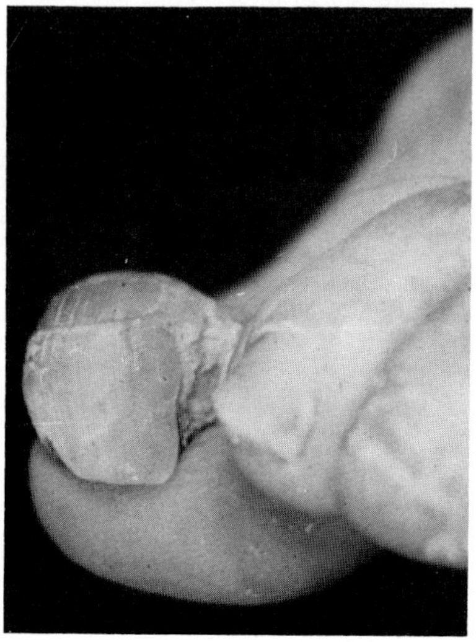

Figure 6.133. Onychauxis.

Onychogryphosis is a deformity of the nail accompanied by hypertrophy beginning at the matrix and extending either laterally, medially, forward and downward over the end of a toe, or upward and backward to press into the dorsum of the foot (Figs. 6.134–6.136). If the etiology is systemic, all the nails are involved; if it is traumatic, only one or two may be affected. The palliative and surgical treatment prescribed for onychauxis are suitable for onychogryphosis. It is usually necessary to reduce this type of nail with a suitable burr and utilize curettage to remove callus debris and straighten out the margins.

Palliative treatment consists of cutting, high-speed drill grinding and debridement of the nail under aseptic conditions. Surgical debridement of the hypertrophic nail may be necessary as often as every 4 weeks in the presence of arterial insufficiency, so as to prevent subungual pressure ulcer and an increase in morbidity. One must constantly be aware of the presence of septic subungual debris. The reduced nail and exposed nail bed are covered with an antiseptic analgesic and emollient dressing to relieve tenderness. Results are excellent. If the subungual tissue is callused or if a heloma is present, the use of a 25 to 40% salicylic acid ointment or

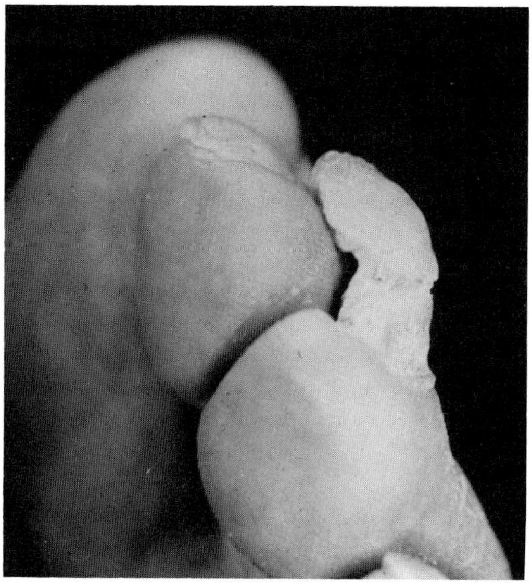

Figure 6.134. Onychogryphosis.

plaster applied for at least 3 days loosens the tissue for a better and more successful debridement at the next visit when the patient returns for curettage and further debridement. The use of the term *"routine care"* is to be condemned. Individual evaluation and treatment of hypertrophic nail conditions result in less morbidity.

Surgical treatment is instituted when circulation is adequate. Removal of the entire nail plate under nerve block anesthesia is often indicated. This is accomplished by using a flat or semicurved instrument and running it from side to side beneath the nail plate to separate the plate from the bed. Upon loosening the entire plate, it is easily separated under the posterior fold and extracted with a slight twist of the Allis forceps or hemostat. With the use of the phenol-alcohol technique the nail matrix is extirpated medially lateraly and posteriorly by means of a small nail cutter. The bed and posterior fold are swabbed first with 88% carbolic acid (phenol) for 3 min and then with isopropyl alcohol. Drainage is 3–4 weeks with this technique, but results are good (Fig. 6.137).

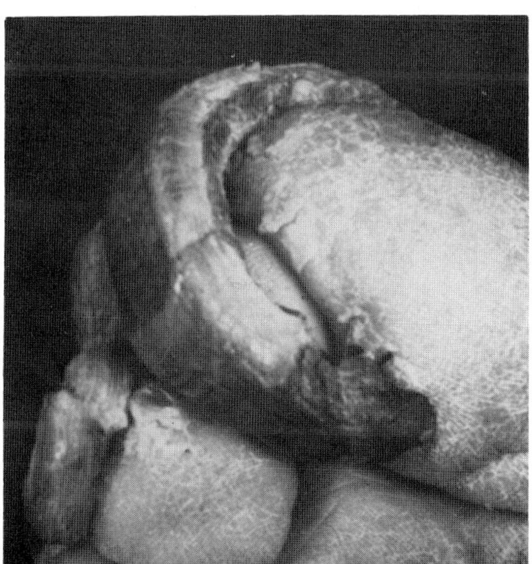

Figure 6.135. Onychogryphosis. Overlapping distal end of hallux causing pressure pain plantar surface of toe.

Another technique for radical removal of the nail plate entails removing the distal two-thirds of the distal phalanx of the toe together with the nail. Although this is effective, cosmetic results are poor.

Basically, the technique is as follows. Complete toe block anesthesia is effected. An incision is made starting at the level of the dorsal medial aspect of the toe about ¼ inch distal to the interphalangeal joint. The incision is carried forward below the medial nail lip, around the distal end of the toe to meet a similar incision from the lateral side. Another transverse incision is made over the dorsum of the toe to connect the incisions. The soft tissues, including the nail plate, nail bed, subcutaneous tissue and nail folds, are dissected back, staying close to the bone and removing the section as outlined above from ¼ inch anterior to the joint forward. The distal two-thirds of the distal phalanx are resected by bone forceps and rasped smooth. The plantar flap is brought up over the remaining bone and sutured.

Zadik (254) advocated obliteration of the hallucal nail bed without shortening the distal phalanx.

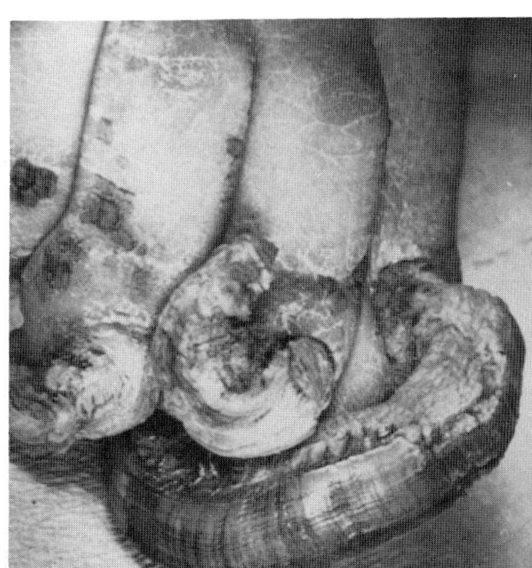

Figure 6.136. Onychogryphosis.

Kaplan (255) developed a technique to eradicate completely the club nail, minimize postoperative pain and provide a good cosmetic effect. Of over 500 cases that had been operated, 359 were followed, with not a single recurrence of the hypertrophied nail. Kaplan's technique is described below.

Following induction of anesthesia by complete toe block and adequate hemostasis, the handle end of a Bard-Parker scalpel is forced under the nail, separating it from the nail bed and removing it completely by blunt dissection. The site is given a complete surgical prep, and a tourniquet is applied. Two linear incisions about 1.5 cm in length are made on the medial and lateral aspects of the toe following the nail fold lines proximally to just short of the interphalangeal joint and including the posterior eponychium. The eponychial skin is sharply and superficially dissected back to expose the matrix. A third incision is made at the distal end of the toe joining the distal ends of the medial and lateral incisions connecting the nail folds. The distal end of the incised tissue is grasped by Allis forceps and dissected back on the distal phalanx to include the nail bed and matrix beneath the previously elevated eponychium. All loose tissue and bony exostoses are removed by bone rongeur, and the retracted eponychial flap is sutured back in place with one suture of 3-0 silk (nylon) on each side of the medial and lateral incisions.

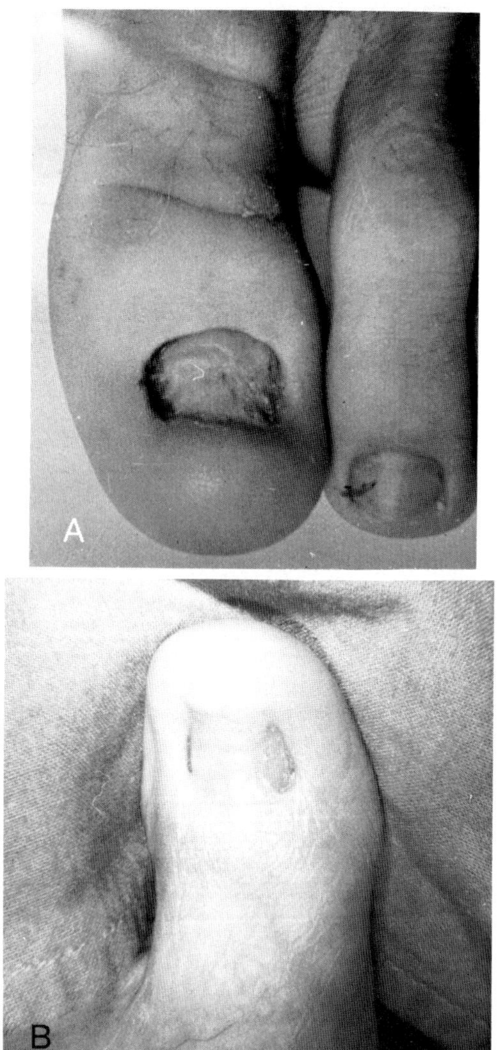

Figure 6.137. *A,* Excision of hallux nail in toto followed by phenol and alcohol. Postoperative result—5 months. *B,* Four years after total phenol-alcohol procedure.

Owens (256) described a technique for complete removal of onychauxis. The technique consists of a modified Winograd operation to excise the inverted medial and lateral margins of the nail. This is followed by total excision of the remaining nail plate and bed with the matrix back to the base of the distal phalanx on its dorsal surface. The flaps are sutured back to the lateral skin margins, and the center heals by third intention. The technique is similar to Kaplan's (255) but allows for excision of nail lips.

Jones (257) used a full-thickness graft from the dorsum of the foot to the denuded dorsal surface of the toe for closed postsurgical healing and no disfigurement of the hallux.

Whitney (258), following total avulsion of the nail plate, rescrubs the foot with hexachlorophene. Frost incisions are carried back from the nail grooves and laterally just proximal to the distal interphalangeal joints. Skin flaps are lifted back by sharp section to expose the medial and lateral aspects of the matrix. The central posterior fold is dissected back exposing the entire matrix. The total matrix is then excised by sharp section, and all remnants and bony irregularities are removed. The flaps are folded back and sutured with 4-0 silk (nylon). The end of the eponychial central flap is sutured to the nail bed. The entire operative site is carefully bandaged, following apposition of the tissues.

Porcine xenografts following total nail avulsion and phenol chemomatricectomy have been described by Elleby et al. (259) with an enthusiastic conclusion. Their results indicated that the graft adhered well without rejection in 90.6%, pain was absent in 85.9% and drainage significantly decreased in 75% of the 64 nail procedures performed. The authors attributed their successful results to "the strong fibrin-elastin bond formed between nail bed and graft, prevention of the usual exudate, increased tissue temperature and acidity, and the possibility of the residual Betadine solution used to prepare the graft."

In a scholarly review of the literature, Hatch and Pascente (260) provide a basis for establishing tetracycline and its associated photosensitivity as an etiologic basis for onycholysis. Treatment consists of removing tetracycline as a drug of choice and observing precautions relative to overexposure in sunlight.

Onychomycosis is commonly caused by *Trichophyton mentagrophytes, Trichophyton rubrum* and *Candida albicans,* and it may destroy the entire nail or cause secondary infections (Figs. 6.138 and 6.139). The clinical characteristics may vary from slight scaling in the lateral folds of the nail to thickening and opaqueness of the plate with the distal portions becoming powdery.

Pardo-Castello and Pardo (261) found that about 18% of nail problems are due to onychomycosis. White and Laipply (262) present 708 cases of onychomycosis studied microscopically. They conclude that the presence of spores or hyphae, especially in subungual keratin or the nail plate, is indicative of onychomycosis. Staining with the Periodic Acid-Schiff reaction technique revealed fungi twice as frequently as did other methods in their series (Figs. 6.140 and 6.141).

Fletcher (263) and others had difficulty in culturing for positive identification of fungus infections of the nail. Studies revealed that identification was possible through clinical observations: *Trichophyton gypseum,* circular white plaques with scaling; *T. rubrum,* dry, lusterless, scaling, streaked, raised from bed and epithelial debris under nail plate that is discolored brownish-yellow, with worm-eaten appearance spreading back to matrix; *C. (Monilia) albicans,* the only member of its genus that infects nails. Paronychia is the common sequela to *Candida* infection. The nail plate is soft and a light-colored yellow and white. The subungual tissue is moist and purulent. Re-

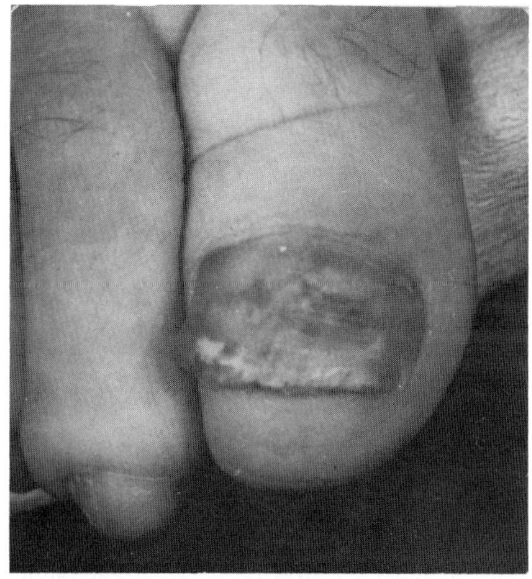

Figure 6.139. Onychomycosis. Brown, gray, yellow discoloration of hallux nails with subonychial debris was present.

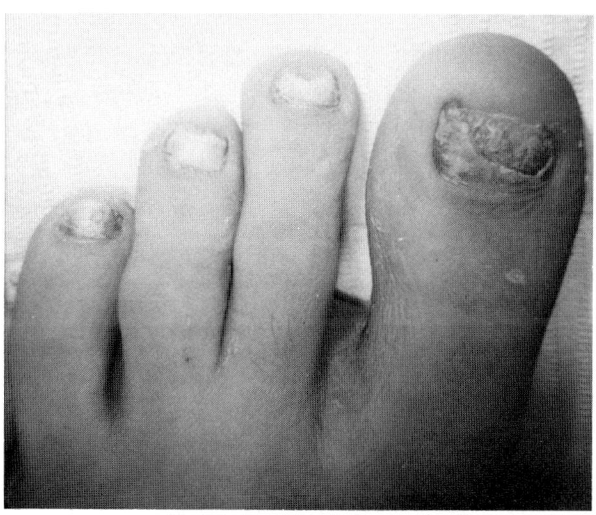

Figure 6.138. Mycotic toe nails.

moval of the nail plate often reveals an ulcerated nail bed.

Treatment of onychomycosis is most difficult. Perserverance on the part of both the doctor and patient is required for successful treatment. Reduction and removal of the objective nail pathology are essential for best results. Treatment may be either radical or palliative.

Palliative treatment is accomplished through surgical debridement, such as grinding, cutting and curettage of the gray, yellow-brown diseased nail tissue. Care must be taken not to inhale the resulting nail dust. Abramson and Wilton (264,

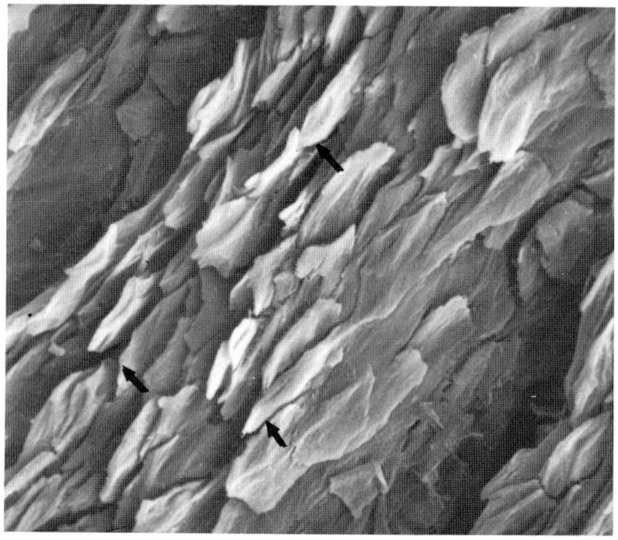

Figure 6.140. Mycotic hallucal nail (*T. mentagrophytes*). Cell boundaries (*arrows*) are arranged in basket weave formation and are well demarcated in this view of the free surface of the nail. Scanning electron micrograph × 100. (Courtesy of Luther Gilliam and Daniel J McCarthy, DPM, PhD, Veterans Administration Medical Center, Perry Point, MD.)

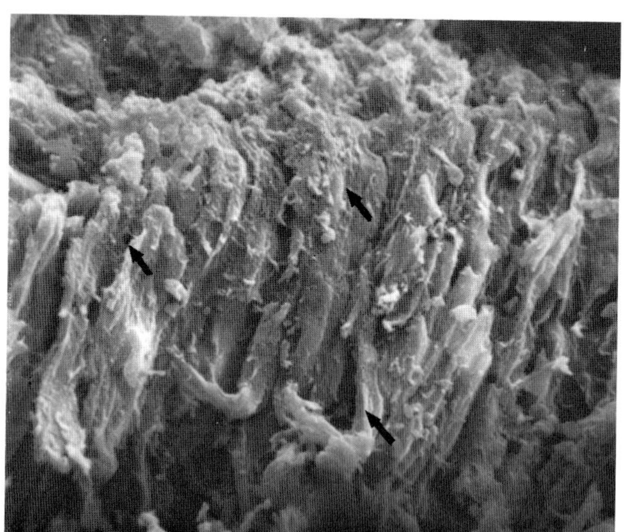

Figure 6.141. Mycotic hallucal nail in cross-section. Cell boundaries (*arrows*) are less well defined than those of the free surface of the nail, and cellular arrangement is poorly organized. It is interesting to note that no mycotic elements can be seen in this cross-sectional view. Scanning electron microscopy × 100. (Courtesy of Luther Gilliam and Daniel J McCarthy, DPM, PhD, Veterans Administration Medical Center, Perry Point, MD.)

265) report that 86% of the nail dust would reach the bronchioles and alveoli of the practitioner, and 31% could be expected to deposit in these areas. A 23% incidence of precipitin antibodies to *Trichophyton rubrum* in sera of podiatrists in practice from 1 to 15 years and a 29% incidence in those in practice 16 years or more were reported. Symptoms of coughing, asthma, conjunctivitis, rhinitis, hypersensitivity, and impaired lung function presented in podiatrists who were chronically exposed to nail dust aerosols. Destruction of the diseased nail by 40% salicylic acid is helpful. Fungicidal solutions and ointments are applied daily to the nail bed. Commonly used topical medications are borotannic complex, clotrimazole solution, tolnaftate solution, salicylic acid, undecylenic acid, sodium propionate and ammoniacal silver nitrate. Ultraviolet light may also be used. Periodic debridement by the podiatrist follows. Scheduled surgical debridement may vary from monthly to four times a year depending on the extent and degree of pathology, painful symptoms, vascular status, interference with ambulation, and incidence of recurring paronychias. Home care may consist of scrubbing the affected nails nightly with hexachlorophene followed by application of a fungicide. Antimycotic therapy for prevention of skin activity should be a part of the overall regimen.

More radical procedures consist of complete avulsion of the toenail and destruction of the matrix with concentrated phenol followed by use of penetrating fungicides on the nail bed. White (266), Bereston (267) and Peck and Klein (268), however, do not feel that use of fungicides alone have been effective.

Another technique of proven value is the debridement of the diseased nails as much as possible. The remaining nail is further reduced by the application of a 40 to 60% salicylic acid or 40% urea ointment. The acid is applied first by isolating the infected nail with adhesive; then the acid is placed in the aperture of the adhesive overlying the nail. The patient returns in 4 to 6 days and debridement continues, followed by additional acid treatment. When the entire nail plate is reduced and the nail bed appears pink, fungicidal therapy is administered in the form of undecylenic or proprionic acid compounds or a borotannic acid compound. Frequent changes of solution are desirable. Complete surgical removal of the nail plate and application of fungicidal solutions are also effective treatments (Fig. 6.142).

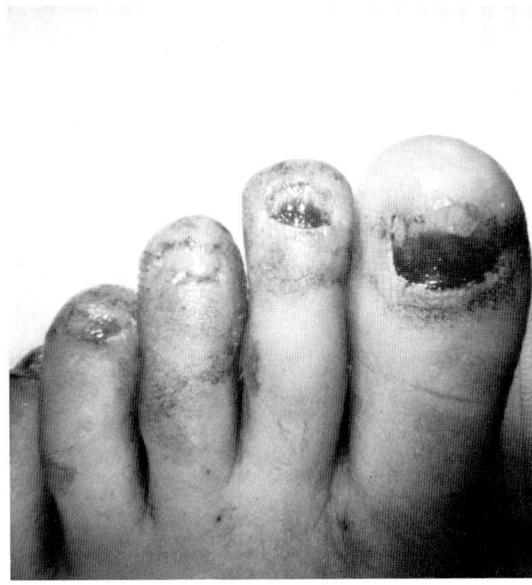

Figure 6.142. Total avulsion of mycotic toenails.

Hendler (269) describes the fungi most frequently infecting nail tissue. *T. gypseum* and *T. mentagrophytes* show the initial lesion as a white superficial patch on the posterior nail fold. This patch progresses to inflammation and destruction of tissues surrounding the plate and results in a yellow, lusterless, opaque and often friable nail. Subungual hyperkeratosis and dystrophic changes develop, but rarely is paronychia a complication. Infections of *T. gypseum* are difficult to treat successfully. Reducing the thickness of the nail periodically by using a high-speed drill followed by sharp curettage may be helpful. Adjunctive fungicides applied to the diseased nail daily prevent and often cure the condition.

In *Trichophyton purpureum* (*T. rubrum*), the lesion develops slowly and insidiously at the lateral border of the nail. Yellow and/or white streaks coalesce, and subungual hyperkeratosis is prominent. The plates become thin and brittle. An "id" reaction may develop. Paronychia is absent.

In *C. albicans*, onychia and paronychia are common. Pain may be slight to severe, with evidence of infection. The posterior fold is red and spongy to touch. On incision, seropurulent discharge may be noted. The nail plate may be elevated and loose, yet firm in texture. *C. albicans* often responds well to treatment.

Locke (270) discusses the etiologic basis for onychomycosis and establishes some interesting data. Predisposing factors causing onychomycosis are direct trauma, multiple minimal trauma and contamination by instruments. Short, narrow shoes may result in contact with infected shoe lining and leather.

Jaskoski et al. (271) established from 70 fungus specimens cultured on Sabouraud's agar that only 3 of 30 identified species were pathogenic; the remaining 27 were soil contaminants.

The hallux nail is the most commonly affected nail, yet the fourth and fifth toenails are often affected through trauma. Subonychial hemorrhage often acts as a culture media for fungi and should be avoided. Onychia and paronychia may be secondary infections where tinea pedis is the exciting factor.

Mogull (272) developed a technique of debridement of the infected nail and removal of infected nail borders followed by the construction of an acrylic nail plate. The color of the acrylic is matched to the nail, several serrations are made in the nail plate, and the acrylic is applied to conform to the shape of a new nail. Wet cellophane is placed over the new acrylic plate. When the acrylic is hardened the new nail is shiny. It can be buffed and shaped. An interesting observation by Mogull is that the new nail forming beneath the acrylic takes on a healthier look. The author has also observed this change in several cases where an acrylic nail plate covering a diseased nail for several weeks resulted in marked improvement of the diseased nail.

Ignatoff and Bleiberg (273) note that onychomycosis occurs in about 15% of all mycotic infections, although it often is the consequence of dermatophytosis. They found that the following procedure was most effective in treating onychomycosis. Thorough burring down of the infected nail should be accomplished. Occlusive dressings of 60% salicylic acid ointment should be applied weekly. After 4 to 10 weeks, debridement results in a clear, pink nail bed. A chemical compound with strong fungistatic qualities, a borotannic complex (Onycho-phytex) is applied bid. This topical medication consists of a molecular fusion of borates and tannates in a penetrating vehicle of ethyl alcohol. As the new nail grows, all dystrophic and diseased nail is removed.

According to the author's experience, debridement and curettage increased the rate of repair only when the judicious use of chemicals served as part of the treatment regimen.

In an unusual case of ocular keratitis accompanied by onychomycosis and corneal dystrophy, Spoor (274) reported that the attending ophthalmologist and dermatologist concluded that an allergic reaction keratitis was the etiologic basis for the eye problem. Griseofulvin was the medication of choice, and its continued use was necessary to prevent recurrence of the keratitis.

In a study of the treatment of 25 subjects with onychomycosis, Jaskoski (275) found that 76% either showed no improvement or the condition persisted. He ascertained from his study that more effective results are predicated on longer periods of treatment with borotannic complex combined with the use of oral griseofulvin.

Frost (276) described encouraging results in a series of 36 cases treated by atraumatic avulsion of the nail plate followed by daily use of a borotannic complex.

Goldberg (277) notes that clipping and abrasion enhances the process of recovery when using oral griseofulvin, 250 mg tablets qid.

Strahs (278), following thorough debridement of the nail bed, used a lacquer formulation of Chloranil in treating 25 cases of onychomycosis.

Feldman (279), Walker (280), Maibach and Kligman (281), Carpenter (282) Reiss and Kornblee (283) and Dix and Sloan (284) disagree as to the treatment time necessary to cure onychomycotic infections with oral griseofulvin. Dix and Sloan also conclude that the borotannic complex alone was more effective than when combined with griseofulvin orally.

Other Toenail Diseases and Deformities

Inflammation of the matrix may produce nutritional or trophic disturbances of the nail plate. These disturbances are evidenced by deep rubor behind the eponychium accompanied by swelling, elevated temperature and pain. Secondary infection resulting in destruction of the matrical cells may follow.

Treatment depends on the etiology. Whether multiple minimal trauma from footgear, sensitivity to allergens or invasion of bacteria are the causative agents, they must be sought out and treated.

Eczema. Generalized eczema may present dystrophic changes in the nails. The eczemas must be handled judiciously to prevent chronic deformities of the plate. Although the nail may become corrugated, if it repairs well the corrugations disappear. Deep discoloration, splitting and brittleness may occur. Paronychia and secondary inflammatory changes around the nail are often seen in acute eczematous states.

Treatment. Early incision and drainage are indicated in paronychia. The eczema is calmed by use of saline soaks, aluminum subacetate wet dressings and combinations of nystatin, neosporin and corticosteroid cream or lotions. Avulsion of the entire nail plate is indicated to facilitate drainage.

Onychia is an ulceration or inflammation of the matrix of the nail and is usually of bacterial origin. Psoriasis of the nail is also a common cause of onychia. Typical signs of infection are present to assist in the correct diagnosis. Treatment involves incision and drainage with the use of local antibiotics.

Paronychia, an inflammation of tissues around the nail, may be caused by trauma or by abrasions about the nail or in the nail grooves. It is pyogenic and often exhibits staphylococcus, streptococcus and colibacillus on examination. All the signs of infection and the lesion that becomes noticeable 24 to 36 hr after primary insult establish the diagnosis. Krausz (285) noted that in a series of 278 nail cases only 0.5% had the symptoms of paronychia. This percentage is based on screening patients with a variety of nail conditions. In the author's experience the percentage of infected nails that exhibit paronychia is much higher (Figs. 6.143–6.145).

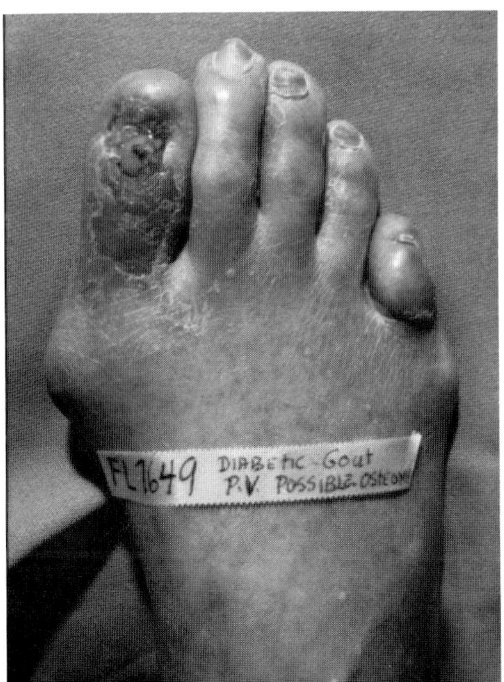

Figure 6.143. Diabetic ulceration hallux nail bed. Patient has high blood levels of uric acid with complicating gout. (Courtesy of M Shapiro.)

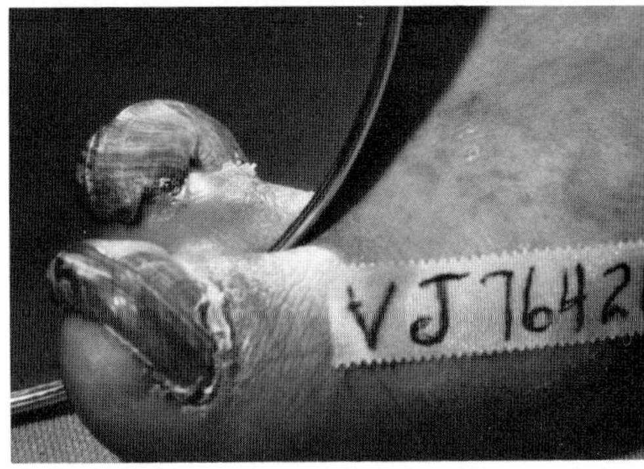

Figure 6.144. Onychogryphosis with complicating ulcer at nail margin. Cellulitis. (Courtesy of M Shapiro.)

Treatment. Paronychia is best treated by removing the entire nail plate to allow for drainage. The use of local antibiotics and wet saline dressings usually proves to be successful therapy. In cases of cellulitis and lymphadenopathy, a sensitivity test determines the type of antibiotic best suited to combat the infection.

Psoriasis (Figs. 6.146 and 6.147). Several nails may be affected by psoriasis. The nails become dry and lose their luster. The process usually starts at the distal margin of the plate and works back to the

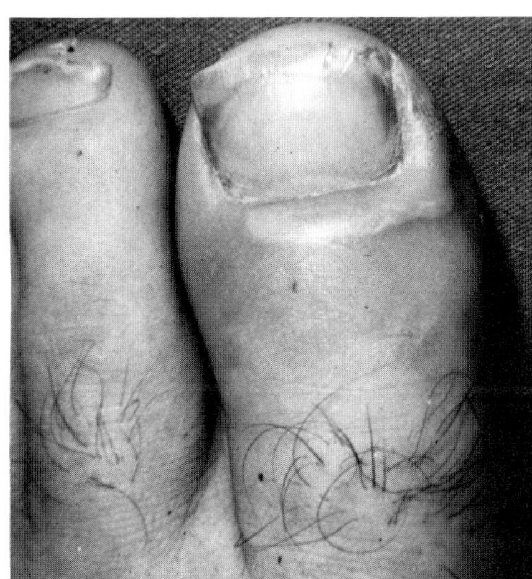

Figure 6.145. Pyogenic paronychia.

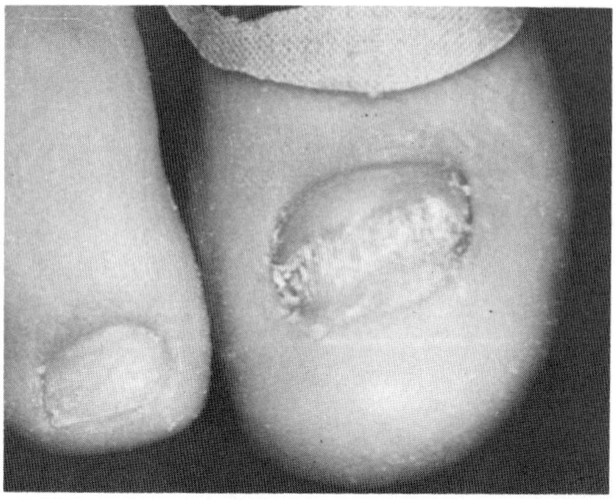

Figure 6.146. Psoriatic toenails. Note distal margin irregularity.

nail matrix with the formation of thick, friable yellowish-brown, corneous material between the nail plate and bed. Small, circular, "thimble-like" pitting concavities develop at the loose margins of the nail plate. These pits and grooves result from previous damage to the matrix from the psoriatic inflammation. Discoloration of the nail bed, onycholysis and subungual keratosis develop from the nail bed or hyponychial involvement in advanced psoriatic nail disease (286). Psoriatic arthritis may affect the interphalangeal joints in the presence of severe skin disease and psoriatic nails.

The nail becomes separated from the nail bed and may break, split or fall off. In mild cases accompanied by typical psoriatic skin lesions, small punctiform depressions in the nail plate are noticed early. There is a decrease in the growth potential. Generally, the patient presents skin lesions on the extensor surfaces of the elbows and knees. A red base appears with an overlay of silvery-white imbricated scales.

Palliative treatment for psoriasis of the nails may be advisable. Grinding the nails down by high-speed drill and removal of debris by curettage are beneficial. Scheduled surgical debridement may vary from monthly to four times a year depending on the extent and degree of pathology, painful symptoms, vascular status, interference with ambulation, and incidence of recurring paronychias. The application of fungicides to prevent secondary mycotic infection is advisable. Applications of mineral oil, cod liver oil and vitamin A cream keep the nail plate smooth following periodic debridement. Very often the treatment of choice is total excision of the nail plate without matricectomy so that a better nail may develop or total matricectomy.

Onychophosis. Johnson (287) described onychoclavus as being a special type of onychophosis occurring on the tibial or fibular edge of the fifth toenail. An onychophosis may develop in any of the nail grooves as a secondary complication of shoes with pointed toes or from pressure of deformed nail margins. Onychophosis or callused nail groove is commonly found at the medial aspect of the hallux nail. This is a common source of medial great toenail pain. It is not uncommon for a patient with medial hallux nail groove callus to complain of paresthesias and/or overt anesthesia at the distal medial aspect of the great toe secondary to a pressure neuritis. This condition is also commonly seen in the pres-

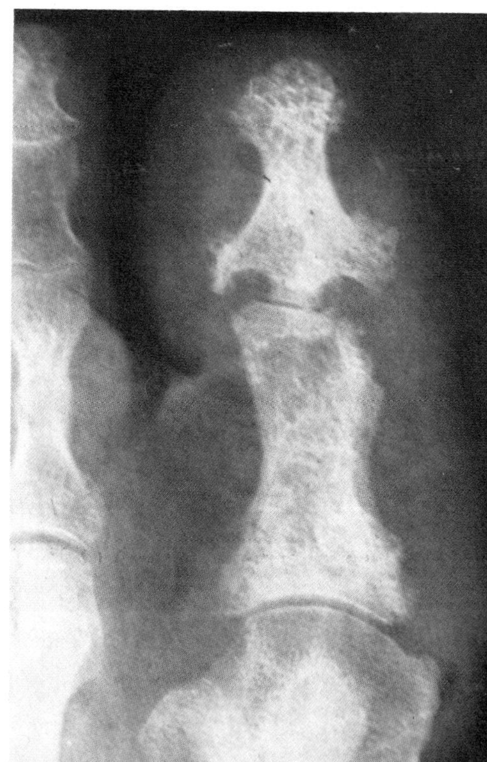

Figure 6.147. Psoriatic arthritis. (From FO Gamble and I Yale. *Clinical Foot Roentgenology.* Baltimore, Williams & Wilkins, 1966.)

ence of onychocryptosis, tight footgear and abduction eversion deformity of the hallux. Johnson notes the rotation of the fifth toe on its long axis resulting in trauma of weightbearing on the dorsolateral aspect of the nail. A clavus develops at the nail margin receiving the pressure of weightbearing from a tight shoe. The distal interphalangeal joint is hammered or flexed. The lesion is a very gray to brown, circumscribed, waxy-looking mass.

Treatment. A conservative treatment is reduction of the excrescence, repeated application of a 25% salicylic acid ointment, subsequent debridement of the remaining clavus and proper shielding. A sinus tract may develop in the nail bed at the site of a clavus. A radical or surgical approach that sacrifices the nail and the distal phalanx may be necessary (Fig. 6.148).

Exostoses are removed at the margins of the middle phalanx. This removal is accomplished by two elliptical incisions around the nail distally and dorsally placed to provide a plantar flap and total removal of the matrix, nail plate, clavus and distal phalanx.

Subungual Granuloma Pyogenicum. Ross (288) notes that granuloma pyogenicum, when described by others, has been located at the margins of the nails (Fig. 6.149). When it occurred under the nail plate it was usually described as onychia. Comparative studies suggest the correct terminology should be subungual

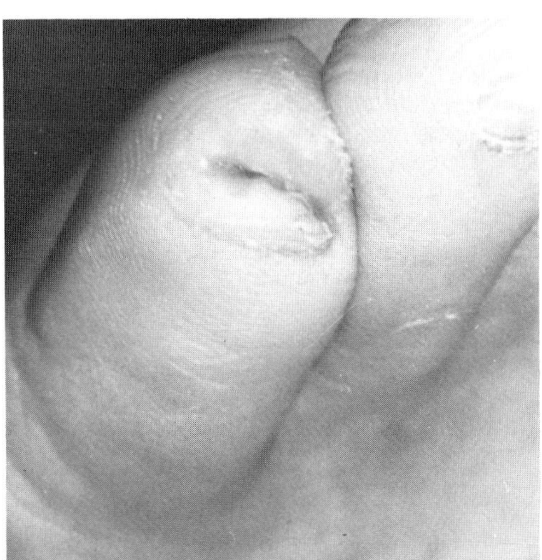

Figure 6.148. Sinus tract distal end of nail bed.

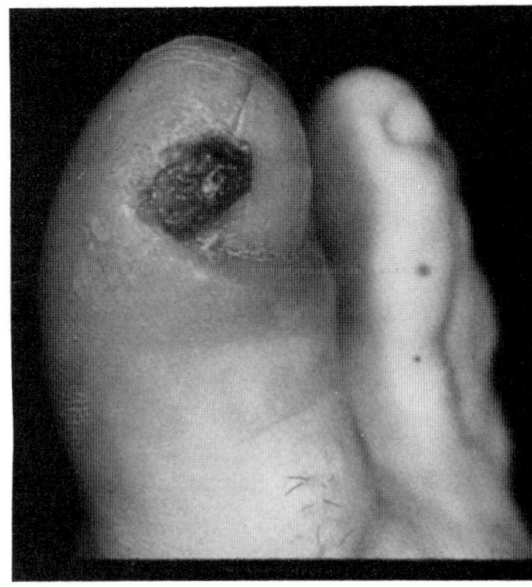

Figure 6.149. Granuloma—onychocryptosis.

granuloma pyogenicum. Das Gupta (289) records 34 cases of subungual melanoma that were operable, and Eichenholtz and De Angelis (290) demonstrated squamous cell carcinoma with invasion to the bone following old subungual infections.

The author has seen hundreds of cases of subungual granuloma pyogenicum secondary to multiple minimal trauma, direct trauma to the hallux nail and injudicious debridement of subungual debris. Often a subungual exostosis is an etiologic factor.

Treatment of this soft pedunculated mass of moist, vascular, often infected tissue is performed under local anesthesia. The nail plate and necrotic tissue are removed by sharp section, and the base is cauterized with an electric needle or silver nitrate concentrate. If an exostosis exists, this should be removed.

Subungual hematoma, from overt trauma or multiple minimal trauma, can be quite painful. By incising the nail plate with a high-speed drill or nail nipper, the hematoma may be drained with subsequent relief of pressure and pain. When the subungual hematoma affects the sublunular space, the nail almost always will go on to future spontaneous avulsion. Whenever there is damage to nail matrix, the patient must be forewarned that nail deformity or involution may result.

Digital Calcinosis in Nail Sulcus. Frost (291) reports a case of digital calcinosis at the proximal end of the great toe fibular nail sulcus. The nail was mildly incurvated. The mass was a small, hard, immobile nodule covered by an adherent cornified, yellowish epithelium. Dorsoplantar and mediolateral x-ray views revealed a nodular calcified mass lateral to the middle-third of the distal phalanx. Pathologically the bone was arranged in a circular fashion and represented a calcification of a previously existing cyst structure. No cartilage matrix was recognized. This condition could represent local ossification as a result of trauma, trichinosis, epidermoid cyst, periungual fibroma (Fig. 6.150) or foreign body. Excision is the treatment of choice.

Subungual Exostosis (Figs. 6.151–6.153). The presence of an elevated nail plate with or without discoloration, a thickening of the nail bed and pain on digital pressure may be evidence of a subungual exostosis. Subungual heloma, inclusion cyst, granuloma, ulceration, glomus tumor or enchondromas and intramedullary cysts must be ruled out by careful clinical, laboratory and radiographic examinations (Figs. 6.154 and 6.155). It is believed that most subungual exostoses represent an ossifying form of fibrocartilaginous metaplasia caused by multiple minimal trauma.

Treatment. Surgical excision is the treatment of choice. Toe block anesthesia is induced, and an elastic tourniquet is applied for hemostasis.

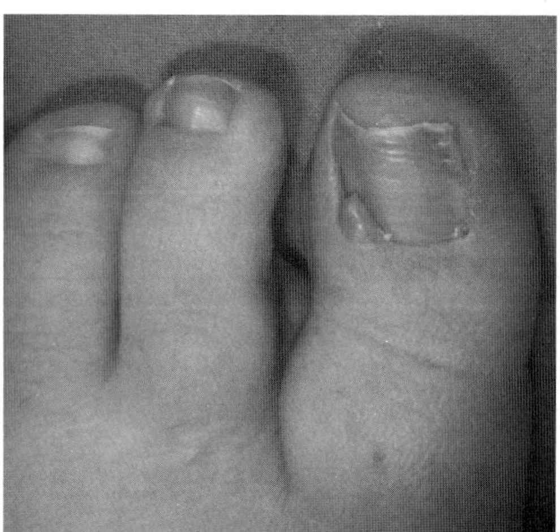

Figure 6.150. Periungual fibroma.

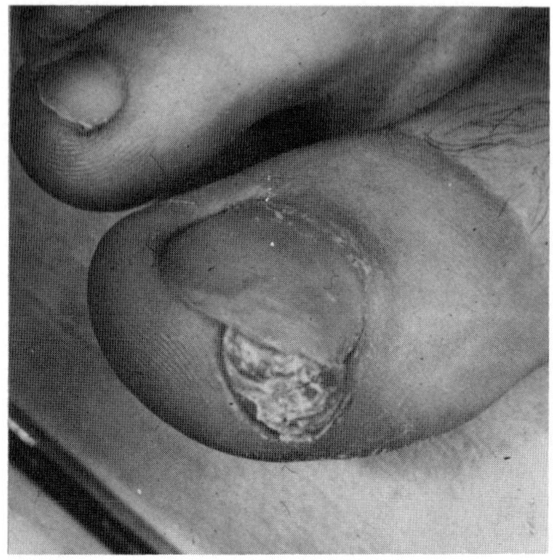

Figure 6.151. Subungual heloma overlying exostosis.

The affected nail plate is gently separated from the nail bed with a minimum of trauma, and the exostosis is exposed. This exostosis is removed with bone forceps and curettage. A sterile dressing of antibiotic ointment is applied, and the wound is allowed to granulate in with subsequent redressings of stimulating ointments. On occasion a complication of all nail surgery may result in the development of an inclusion cyst (Fig. 6.154).

Sandel (292) believes the fishmouth type of incision to be too traumatizing, resulting in sloughing and occasional gangrene. However, the author has used this procedure without incident for many years.

Wichman (293) describes a simplified version of subungual exostectomy. Following the usual sterile preparation for surgery, a transverse incision about ¼ inch long is made at the distal end of the toe. The dorsal surface of the phalanx is explored blindly by inserting a ⅛ inch wide dental chisel to chip off prominent surfaces. This procedure is completed using a cross-cut rasp to file the bone smooth. Bleeding is encouraged to flush out the wound. The patient is ambulatory, and no sutures are necessary. Similar approaches have been used by Polokoff and Probber with excellent results. Their raspostectomy and osteotripsy techniques have provided good to excellent results in hundreds of cases.

Toenails and Systemic Disorders

Dermatitis Exfoliativa. In dermatitis exfoliativa, nail lesions are common. The nails become deformed and thickened, lose their color and develop underlying hyperkeratosis. The nail loosens and may

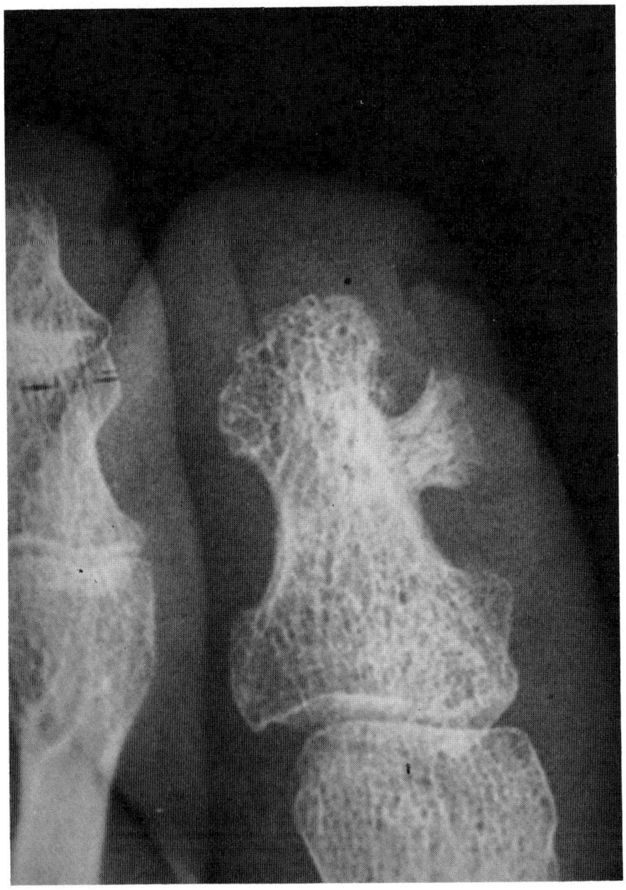

Figure 6.152. Subungual exotosis. (From FO Gamble and I Yale: *Clinical Foot Roentgenology.* Baltimore; Williams & Wilkins, 1966.)

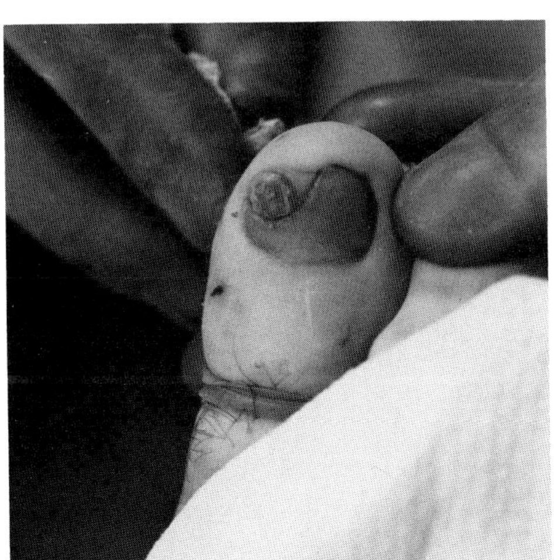

Figure 6.153. Subungual exostosis. Note overlying excresence. (Courtesy of D Mowbray.)

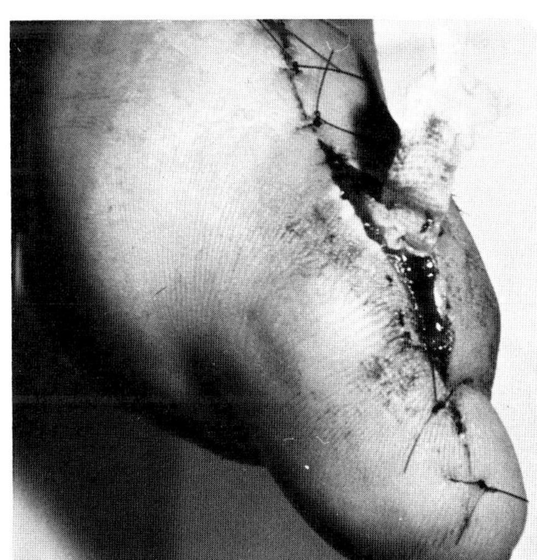

Figure 6.154. Inclusion cyst. Complication of nail surgery. Excision of inclusion cyst.

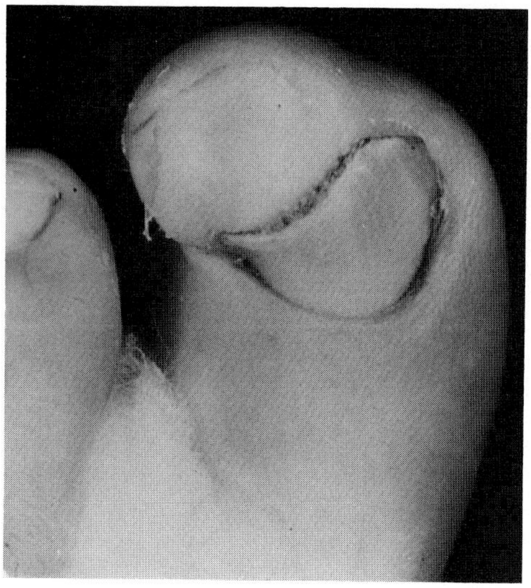

Figure 6.155. Chondroma distal end of hallux.

be lost completely. The thickened nail is reduced by drill, scalpel or sharp curettage. Emollient creams are prescribed to maintain the texture of the skin.

Ichthyosis. In ichthyosis a marked hyperkeratosis develops under the nail, the periungual tissue is scaly and the nail plate is often deformed. Onychauxis and onychogryphosis with discoloration are common. Debridement and vitamin A by topical application are indicated.

The matrix is radiosensitive and becomes thinned, friable, discolored and atrophied with injudicious overexposure to radiation. The surrounding skin may be pigmented, wrinkled and atrophied as in ichthyosis. A history of treatment by x-ray therapy should differentiate the problem.

Pemphigus. In pemphigus the changes taking place in the skin affect the growth of the nail. Dystrophic changes, discoloration, pitting and transverse sulcus formation may result from inflammatory changes, edema and faulty nutrition around the matrix. Contact dermatitis caused by sensitivity to detergents or nail polish may cause thickening of the nail, brittleness and cracks. Oils, tar and greasy substances may cause discoloration.

Transverse lines in an atrophic nail that is shiny and bent over the ends of the fingers and rarely on the toes is seen in **sclerodactylia.** This must be differentiated from trauma-induced lines.

Elephantiasis. In elephantiasis, the skin is thick, corneous and hyperkeratotic. The nails develop a raised, free border atrophy and become otherwise deformed with spicules implanted in the nail bed. The color varies from gray through brown to black. Curettage and reduction of nail borders by drill help prevent secondary infections.

Syphilis, being the great imitator that it is, may produce almost any objective characteristic to which nails are heir. The nail plate often presents Beau's lines, and infections in the adjacent tissues are common. Early treatment by an internist, however, reduces the possibility of permanent nail damage and other sequelae of advanced syphilis.

Onycholysis, or separation of the nail from the nail bed, is seen in tabes dorsalis tetracycline therapy, and hyperthyroidism and may also occur from trauma, psoriasis, contact allergy and hyperidrosis. The distal nail plate gradually separates from the nail bed and progresses proximally, resulting in a white nail caused by air entering the subonychial space.

Koilonychia is characterized by a thin lusterless nail plate with central bending in spoon-like fashion and usually occurs in cases of hypochromic anemia. Stanley (294) states that it also accompanies thyrotoxicosis and may develop in certain occupations exhibiting toxic reactions. It is not found in severe pernicious anemia. Cases have been found where koilonychia has responded to correction of an underlying polycythemia vera. Bergeron and Stone (295) report a suggestion of autosomal dominant genetic transference affecting males and females alike in a study of 12 members of a family. The presence of secondary infection requires excision of offending borders of the deformed nails.

Black nails are the result of subungual hemorrhage and should be differentiated from melanocytic and pigmented changes in the nail bed and matrix (Fig. 6.156). Higashi (296) noted that most pigmented changes in the nail were due to an increase in the number of melanocytes caused by such factors as inflammation, irradiation and metabolic disturbances.

Bodine (297) described **subungual coagulum** as a dark red mass with vertical dark lines running along the long axis of the nail caused by multiple minimal trauma and capillary fragility. Often following trauma, a massive hemorrhage lifts the nail plate up from the bed. Early release of pressure by drilling an opening through the nail plate is indicated, and repair is then usually uneventful. Failure to drain the blood may result in an accumulation of a dark blood clot that serves as an excellent focus for bacterial and mycotic infection.

The presence of pigment and an ulceration in the nail bed must be differentiated from a subungual melanoma by biopsy and histologic examination (298).

Beau's Lines. Beau's line, a transverse indentation or elevation of the nail, may present subsequent to any disease process interfering with the nail growth, e.g., digital surgery, circulatory disorder or severe systemic illness. In Raynaud's disease or other vasospastic and circulatory disturbances, Beau's lines may be seen on a cyanosed nail plate. The cyanosis remains; distortion and atrophy of the nail take place, and gangrene eventually destroys the tissue.

Anemia and Vitamin Deficiency. Grayish, thinned nails with longitudinal striations may be due to anemia. The symptoms subside with appropriate treatment with folic acid and vitamin B_{12} or with iron therapy, and the blood picture improves. Brittle, ridged and furrowed nails may improve with administration of vitamins B_{12} and D.

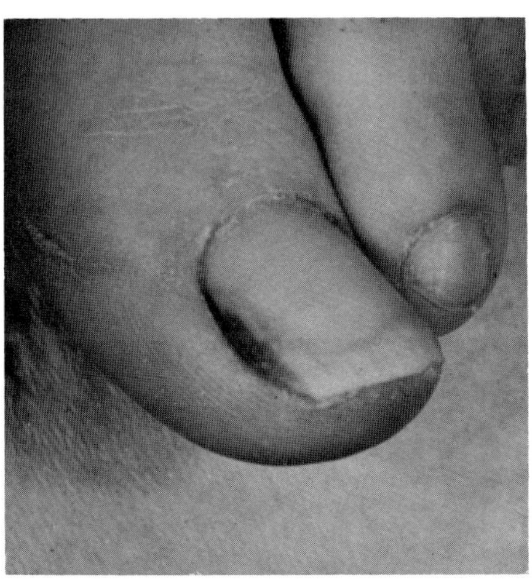

Figure 6.156. Pigmented nevus at nail border.

Endocrine Disorders. The hypothyroid myxedematous patient may present brittle, thin, white-spotted, striated nails in addition to the typical dry, scaly skin. Adequate systemic treatment by an internist relieves podiatric symptoms.

A loss of lunula is noted in hypopituitary disease. Hypogonadism may produce a watch-crystal type or thinned, transparent nail plate. Patients with hyperthyroidism or hyperpituitarism exhibit shiny, well-developed nails. In hyperthyroidism the nail plate may become soft from excessive perspiration. Hyperpituitarism may result in the nails appearing convex from side to side and from proximal to distal edges.

Onychotropia is a diminution in the normal development of the nail in size, thickness or texture. The nail may appear thin, brittle, pitted in the center or spoon-shaped and is often separated from the nail bed. Paronychia or onychia may cause vascular or nutritional disturbance to the matrix, causing onychotropia. Inflammatory skin disorders, nervous disease, trauma and constitutional disorders may be etiologic. The nail may develop a longitudinal split, such as in cerebral paralysis, tabes, syphilis, tuberculosis, congenital familial dystrophy, thyroid disease, circulatory disease and chemical poisonings. Systemic treatment may be necessary, and local palliation prevents infection.

Anonychia is a congenital absence of matrix and complete lack of development of a nail plate (Fig. 6.157).

Pulmonary diseases, kidney disorders or congenital cardiac problems may cause Hippocratic nails that are club-like, thick, light gray to dark brown in color and convex from side to side and from the proximal border to the distal end.

Arthritis. The nails may pit in acute rheumatic disturbances and in chronic psoriatic arthritis. A dry, brittle nail with subungual keratosis is seen often in chronic osteoarthritis.

Quincke's pulse is alternate redness and pallor of the nail plate produced by the capillaries in the nail bed. Heat increases this pulsation. Blanching occurs with

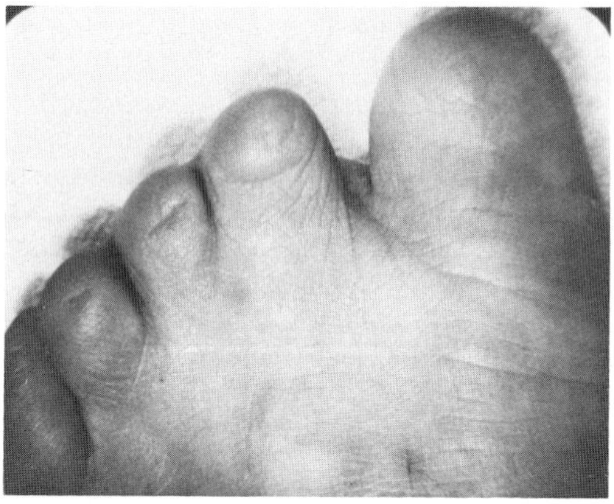

Figure 6.157. Congenital anonychia.

each diastole of the heart. When this pulse pressure is so great as to be visible, one must consider the possibility of aortic valvular insufficiency, rheumatic heart disease or arteriovenous fistula, and the patient should be referred to an internist for diagnosis and treatment.

Raynaud's Disease. In vasospastic arterial disease, the cuticle is widened and the nail fold thinned. There is a blending of the nail fold, cuticle and nail plate that returns to normal after sympathectomy. Severe ischemia is the usual cause of extremely painful nails that are not deformed. Treatment is aimed at the etiology and pathology, and surgical intervention is frowned upon in vasospastic disorders (299).

References

1. Stoughton RB: *The Human Integument, Normal and Abnormal. The Skin as an Organ of Protection.* Washington, DC, AAAS Publication no. 54, 1959.
2. Sano S, Kuroda M, Miyazawa I: Some biochemical aspects on pathological keratinization. Glycogen, pentose, hexasamine and beta-glucuronidase in normal and pathological horny layers. *Kobe J Med Sci* 11:1–12, 1965.
3. McCarthy DJ, Habowsky JE: Structural variability of the dermo-epidemal interface of skin of the human foot as related to function. *J Am Podiatry Assoc* 65:450–464, 1975.
4. Conrad NL: Some experiments involving modifications of fungus culture media. *J Am Podiatry Assoc* 51:121–125, 1961.
5. Gamble FO, Yale I: *Clinical Foot Roentgenology,* ed. 2. Huntington, NY, R Kreiger Publishing Co, 1975.
6. Bonavilla EJ: Histopathology of the heloma durum: Some significant features and their implications. *J Am Podiatry Assoc* 58:423–427, 1968.
7. Penneys NS, Fulton JE, Weinstein GD, Frost P: Location of proliferating cells in human epidermis. *Arch Dermatol* 101:323–327, 1970.
8. Pinkus H: Examination of the epidermis by the strip method of removing horny layers. I. Observations on thickness of the horny layer, and on mitotic activity after stripping. *J Invest Dermatol* 16:383–386, 1951.
9. McCarthy DJ, Habowsky JE: A cytological survey by strata of skin in heloma durum using electron microscopy. *J Am Podiatry Assoc* 62:239–249, 1972.
10. Freed JB: Histologic post mortem evaluation of bone hyperplasia accompanying digital clavus. *J Am Podiatry Assoc* 59:467–472, 1969.
11. Gibbs RC: Skin and nail changes in the elderly foot. *J Am Podiatry Assoc* 65:471–474, 1975.
12. Sansone RE: Parallel strip padding for weight stress distribution and redirection. *J Am Podiatry Assoc* 60:193–198, 1970.
13. Deffinger TL: Neuroma accompanying heloma durum. *J Am Podiatry Assoc* 52:27–32, 1962.
14. Sivitz SC: A new resilient plastic for orthodigital prosthetics. *J Natl Assoc Chirop* 47:172–175, 1957.
15. Polokoff M: Lesser toe latex shield made with tubular gauze. *J Am Podiatry Assoc* 48:432–433, 1958.
16. Streiker FB: New uses of chymotrypsin in podiatry. *J Am Podiatry Assoc* 51:713–717, 1961.
17. Acker I: Subcutaneous implantation of a soft tissue substitute for the relief of heloma. *J Am Podiatry Assoc* 54:623–625, 1964.
18. Kaplan EG, Kashuk K: Disclaiming the myth of use of epinephrine local anesthesia in feet. *J Am Podiatry Assoc* 61:335–340, 1971.
19. Steinberg MD, Block P: The use and abuse of epinephrine in local anesthetics. *J Am Podiatry Assoc* 61:341–343, 1971.
20. Austin DW: New concepts of etiology and treatment of helomata. *J Natl Assoc Chirop* 40:1927, 1950.
21. Jacobs J: Mobilizing adhesions with negative pressure. *J Am Podiatry Assoc* 50:116–117, 1960.
22. Locke RK: Arthritides and allied disorders as factors in everyday chiropody practice and their treatment. *J Natl Assoc Chirop* 46:756–777, 1956.
23. Locke RK: Corticosteroid injections therapy in the foot. *J Am Podiatry Assoc* 48:505–511, 1958.
24. Ashur M, Farrar R: Griseofulvin in the treatment of tinea pedis and onychomycosis. *J Am Podiatry Assoc* 51:103–108, 1961.
25. Cameron DJ: A new rapid and prolonged acting steroid for intraarticular inflammatory disorders. *J Am Podiatry Assoc* 56:317–319, 1966.
26. Levy SE: A controlled evaluation of subdermal corticosteroid injections. *J Am Podiatry Assoc* 48:403–407, 1958.
27. Silverman A, Arancia L, Steiner J: The place of an intradermal vitamin A injection in routine

management of helomata. *J Am Podiatry Assoc* 48:408–413, 1958.
28. McCain LR: Transplantation of the flexor digitorum brevis in hammertoe surgery. *J Am Podiatry Assoc* 48:233–235, 1958.
29. Polokoff M: Raspostectomy—Reduction of exostosis and hypertrophied condyles with files and rasps. *J Am Podiatry Assoc* 52:599–602, 1962.
30. Perrone MA: Nail matricectomy by onycho--tripsy with airmotor. *J Am Podiatry Assoc* 60:92–93, 1970.
31. Levin B: Heloma surgery. *J Am Podiatry Assoc* 48:244–245, 1958.
32. Austin DW: New concepts of etiology and treatment of helomata. *J Natl Assoc Chirop* 40:1927, 1950.
33. Locke RK, Strauss H: The reduction of post operative pain and edema in foot surgery through local instillation of corticosteroids. *J Am Podiatry Assoc* 54:703–708, 1964.
34. Kaplan EG: A new approach to the surgical correction of overlapping toe. *J Am Coll Foot Surg* 3:24–25, 1964.
35. Subotnick SI: Digital deformities, etiology and treatment. *J Am Podiatry Assoc* 65:542–555, 1975b.
36. Wheeless JV: Porokeratosis of mibelli. *Arch Dermatol* 100:381–382, 1969.
37. Mullens E: An effective treatment for heloma neurofibrosum. *J Natl Assoc Chirop* 46:772–774, 1956.
38. Hall V: An improved method for the injection of Keramin in the treatment of heloma neurofibrosum. *J Am Podiatry Assoc* 48:97–98, 1958.
39. Trice EW: A new hypothesis on the etiology of heloma milliarc. *J Natl Assoc Chirop* 45:28 29, 1955.
40. Kleiman MA: Treatment for heloma milliare. *Footprints Fla Podiatry Assoc* 4:1, 1958.
41. Locke RK: Shoe sponging—A new adjunct in treatment of plantar excresences. *Chirop Rec* 25:105, 1942.
42. Kurtz CM, et al.: Syndaclylization: A surgical approach to heloma molle. *J Foot Surg* 23:407–409, 1984.
43. Woolf WH: Eradication of the problem plantar keratoma. *J Am Podiatry Assoc* 74:163–167, 1984.
44. Balkin SW: Silicone injection for plantar keratoses. *J Am Podiatry Assoc* 56:1–11, 1966b.
45. Spence WR, Shields M: Prevention of blisters, callosities and ulcers by absorption shear forces. *J Am Podiatry Assoc* 58:428–434, 1968.
46. Sansone RE: Parallel strip padding for weight stress distribution and redirection. *J Am Podiatry Assoc* 60:193–198, 1970.
47. Polokoff M: Removable shield for lesions about head of fifth metatarsal. *J Am Podiatry Assoc* 57:566–568, 1967.
48. Roven MD: A latex forefoot device with threefold action. *J Am Podiatry Assoc* 48:417–418, 1958.
49. Amberry T: Sesamoid surgery of the great toe. *J Am Podiatry Assoc* 45:9, 1955.
50. DuVries HL: New approach to the treatment of intractable verruca plantaris. *J Am Podiatry Assoc* 44:26, 1954.
51. Henenfeld M, Walkes MH: A modification of the DuVries plantar condylectomy. *J Am Podiatry Assoc* 50:24–27, 1960.
52. Henenfeld M, Walkes MH: Subluxations of the metatarsophalangeal joints. *NY State J Podiatry* 20, 1959.
53. Bronston G: A soft tissue approach for plantar lesions. *J Am Podiatry Assoc* 57:331–332, 1967.
54. Balkin SW: Liquid silicone for plantar keratoses, case reports. *J Am Coll Foot Surg* 5:114–115, 1966a.
55. Balkin SW: Silicone augmentation for plantar calluses. *J Am Podiatry Assoc* 66:148–154, 1976.
56. Levine LA: Collectomy: Lesser metatarsal neck resection. *J Am Podiatry Assoc* 62:447–458, 1972.
57. Weinstock RE: Surgical judgment in metatarsal surgery for elimination of intractable plantar keratosis. *J Am Podiatry Assoc* 65:979–987, 1975.
58. Steinberg MD, Taub J: Porokeratosis plantaris discreta. Lecture delivered to the American Society Clinical Pathologists, Los Angeles, 1969.
59. Michota RS, Peridiue RL, Mason WH: A clinical report of 60 cases of porokeratosis plantaris discreta. *Curr Podiatry* 26:6–12, 1977.
60. Weisfeld M: Understanding porokeratosis plantaris discreta. *J Am Podiatry Assoc* 63:138–144, 1973.
61. Kipping H: A case of eccrine poroma. *J Bull Millard Fillmore Hosp Buffalo NY* 9:95–97, 1962.
62. Okun MR, Ansell HB: Eccrine poroma. *Arch Dcrmatol* 88:561–566, 1963.
63. Tanenbaum MH: Eccrine poroma. *Am J Surg* 31:603–604, 1965.
64. Gibbs RC: Differential diagnosis of plantar verrucae. *J Am Podiatry Assoc* 59:90–92, 1969.
65. McConaly JG: Common warts: Immunity as a result of therapy. *Cutis* 17:301, 1976.
66. Carrel JM, Davidson DM: Topical immunotherapy of recalcitrant verrucae. *J Am Podiatry Assoc* 63:283–296, 1973.
67. McCarthy DJ: Alterations in the morphology of dermo-epidermal interface of pedal verrucae as revealed by scanning electron microscopy. *J Am Podiatry Assoc* 66:505–514, 1976.
68. Goodheart CR: *An Introduction to Virology.* Philadelphia; WB Saunders Co, 1969.
69. Almeida JD, Howatson AF, Williams HG: Electron microscope study of human warts, sites of virus production and nature of inclusion bodies. *J Invest Dermatol* 38:337, 1962.
70. Lyell A, Miles JA: The Myrmecia, a study of inclusion bodies in warts. *Br Med J* 1:912, 1951.
71. Mendelson CG, Klingman AM: Isolation of wart virus in tissue culture. Successful reinoculation into humans. *Arch Dermatol* 83:559–562, 1961.
72. Yale I: *Podiatric Medicine,* ed 2. Baltimore, Williams & Wilkins, 1980.
73. Kuflik EG: Cryosurgery for cutaneous lesions. *Curr Concepts Skin Dis* 6:15–18, 1985.

74. Woolf WH: Capillary tube acid applicator for verrucae. *J Am Podiatry Assoc* 49:18–20, 1959.
75. Churney AM: Moles, warts and birthmarks. *Pediatr Clin North Am* 8:249–252, 1961.
76. Lieberman H: An empirical treatment for mosaic verrucae. *J Am Podiatry Assoc* 50:737, 1960.
77. Levy SE: A controlled evaluation of subdermal corticosteroid injections. *J Am Podiatry Assoc* 48:403–407, 1958.
78. Lerner L: Management of plantar verrucae via excision and curettage. *J Am Podiatry Assoc* 49:11–14, 1959.
79. Bornstein B: Effects of oral chymotrypsin on surgical sequelae. *J Am Podiatry Assoc* 53:349–351, 1963.
80. Antahades LM: Refrigeration anesthesia in the surgical excision of a plantar verruca. *J Am Podiatry Assoc* 53:662–663, 1963.
81. Suppan RJ, Besterman G: Curettage and chemocautery for verrucae. *J Am Podiatry Assoc* 53:265–268, 1963.
82. Buske EG: Local parenteral and oral bismuth therapy for verrucae. *J Am Podiatry Assoc* 53:269–271, 1963.
83. Smernoff R: A new treatment for verruca. *Curr Podiatry* 18:12, 1969.
84. Grady ED: A simple method of removing plantar warts. *Gen Practitioner* 25:89, 1962.
85. Kingland HD: Cryotherapy in treatment of verrucae. *J Am Podiatry Assoc* 52:435, 1962.
86. Goldman L, Stillman L: Combined cryotherapy and electrodesiccation in the management of verrucae. *Podiatry Q* 2:16–19, 1963.
87. Cataldo E: Experience with local vitamin A injection in the treatment of helomata and verrucae. *J Am Podiatry Assoc* 49:203–206, 1959.
88. Steinberg MD: Observations on the possible etiologic relationship between fungus infection of the human foot and rheumatoid arthritis. *J Natl Assoc Chirop* 46:589–592, 1956.
89. Davidson MR, Schuler BS: Skin curette and the treatment of plantar verruca. *J Am Podiatry - Assoc* 66:331–336, 1976.
90. Yale I: A new injection technique for the treatment of verrucae as proposed for practice in the armed forces. *NY State J Podiatry* 3:7–9, 1941 and 4:12–13, 1942.
91. Stern J: Quinocaine injection therapy for verrucae. *J Am Podiatry Assoc* 51:413–415, 1961.
92. Cramer LL: Parenzyme injection for plantar warts. *J Am Podiatry Assoc* 48:526–528, 1958.
93. Weinstock B: An evaluation of the curettage treatment of plantar verrucae. *J Natl Assoc Chirop* 47:67–68, 1957.
94. Harris L: Combined electrodesiccation and chemosurgery for plantar verrucae. *J Am Podiatry Assoc* 56:160–161, 1966.
95. Gilbert RS, Williams MJ: Local injection of vitamin A (Keramin) for plantar verrucae. *US Armed Forces Med J* 10:843–847, 1959.
96. Carpenter WE: Results of a four-year study of injection therapy in the treatment of plantar warts. *J Am Podiatry Assoc* 51:407–409, 1961.
97. Goodman JM: Liquid nitrogen therapy of warts and other skin lesions. *Can Med Assoc J* 82:628–630, 1960.
98. Goldman L, Palmero J: A podophyllin lotion for warts. *Arch Dermatol* 84:505–506, 1961.
99. Ormond CS: Cantharone, a cantharidin tincture as a useful agent in treating intractable plantar lesions. *J Am Podiatry Assoc* 52:427–430, 1962.
100. Locke RK, Zang K: Controlled intralesional deposition of a sclerotic in verruca therapy. *J Am Podiatry Assoc* 59:377–384, 1969.
101. Block I: Treatment of verruca plantaris with ultrasound. *J Am Podiatry Assoc* 57:330–331, 1967.
102. Trapp B: Ultra-sound in verruca plantaris. *J Am Podiatry Assoc* 57:326–329, 1967.
103. Falknor G: Needling—A new technique in verrucae therapy. *J Am Podiatry Assoc* 59:51–52, 1969.
104. Koenig RD, Horwitz LR: Verrucae plantaris—effective treatment with bleomycin: Review of the literature and case presentations. *J Foot Surg* 21(2):108–110, 1962.
105. Fred HL, Geisler RG, Berry W, Eiband JM: Keratosis palmaris et plantaris. *Arch Intern Med* 113:866–871, 1964.
106. Grayson M: Corneal manifestations of keratosis of plantaris and palmaris. *Am J Ophthalmol* 59:483–486, 1965.
107. Heiss HB, Gross PR: Keratosis palmaris et plantaris treatment with topically applied vitamin A acid. *Arch Dermatol* 101:100–103, 1970.
108. Vance CE, Levy L: Recognizing arsenical keratosis. *J Am Podiatry Assoc* 66:91–94, 1976.
109. Pillsbury DM, Shelly WB, Kligman AM: *Dermatology.* Philadelphia, WB Saunders Co, 1956.
110. Rothman SKG, Windhorst D: Tinea pedis as a source of infection in the family. *Arch Dermatol* 75:210–271, 1957.
111. Steinhart AN: Combined papillary syringocystademoma and hidradenoma, a case study. *J Am Podiatry Assoc* 67:659–660, 1977.
112. Brownstein MH, Shapiro L: The sweat gland adenomas. *Int J Dermatol* 14:397, 1975.
113. Winkelmann RK, Wolf K: Solid-cystic hidradenoma of the skin, clinical and histopathologic study. *Arch Dermatol* 97:651, 1968.
114. Davis JA: A study to determine the relative absorbibility and wicking effect of certain major sock materials on perspiration of the human foot. *J Am Podiatry Assoc* 11:1051–1057, 1975.
115. Jenkins WM, Craft CW: Management of idiopathic plantar hyperidrosis. *J Am Podiatry Assoc* 73:475–480, 1983.
116. Davis AN: A new dermatologic agent for hyperidrosis and bromidrosis—A preliminary report. *J Am Podiatry Assoc* 50:901–906, 1960.
117. Feldman B: Dry skin: Its cause and treatment. *J Am Podiatry Assoc* 18:191–194, 1958.
118. Ignatoff W: Dermatology in geriatrics. *J Am Podiatry Assoc* 48:183–188, 1958.
119. Feldman B: Dry skin—A further report. *J Am Podiatry Assoc* 49:257–258, 1959.
120. Prentice H, Brezak S: An investigation of a water- miscible oil preparation for topical treatment of podiatric dermatoses. *J Am Podiatry Assoc* 48:197–200, 1958.
121. Boesenberg C, Haas M: Vitamin A as an anti-

keratinic factor. *J Am Podiatry Assoc* 49:255–256, 1959.

122. Sturtz H: The management of excessive dry skin. *Ind State Podiatry J* 24, 1959.
123. Mulary DH, Ubach F: Proteolytic debridement of hyperkeratoses of palms and soles. *Arch Dermatol* 78:758, 1958.
124. Yale I: Podiatric Medicine, ed 2. Baltimore, Williams & Wilkins, 1980.
125. Swanbeck G: A new treatment of ichthyosis and other hyperkeratotic conditions. *Acta Dermatol Venereol* 48:123–127, 1968.
126. Papa CM, Kligman AM: Mechanisms of eccrine anidrosis. I. High level blockage. *J Invest Dermatol* 47:1–9, 1966.
127. Kasdan PR: The environmental effects on the morphology of three strains of *Trichophyton mentagrophytes,* and a study of two of their enzymes. *J Am Podiatry Assoc* 60:109–115, 1970.
128. Leyden JJ, Kligman AM: Interdigital athlete's foot: New concepts in pathogenesis. *Postgrad Med* 61:113–116, 1977.
129. Hicks JH: Erythema nodosum in patients with tinea pedis and onychomycosis. *South Med J* 70:27–28, 1977.
130. Levy LA: Prevention of fungal infections of the feet (a comprehensive approach). *J Am Podiatry Assoc* 67:361–363, 1977.
131. Maskin IL, Taschdjian CC, Franks AC: Etiology of dermatophytosis. *Arch Dermatol* 75:66–69, 1957.
132. Arancia BS, Montgomery R: The management of cutaneous moniliasis with Nystatin. *J Am Podiatry Assoc* 49:1–5, 1959.
133. Goldman L, Unger L: A comprehensive treatment for monilial infections of skin and nails. *J Am Podiatry Assoc* 49:371–373, 1959.
134. Hirschberg S: A "missing link" in the treatment and control of epidermophytosis. *J Am Podiatry Assoc* 49:14–17, 1959.
135. Walker MH: An evaluation of some clinical data in the treatment of tinea pedis with copper sulphate iontophoresis and some fungicidal preparations. *J Am Podiatry Assoc* 49:303–311, 1959.
136. Goldberg HC: Laboratory re-evaluation of fungus growths in shoes, socks and skin. *J Am Podiatry Assoc* 49:433–437, 1959.
137. Lindenberg LM: Treatment of tinea pedis and tinea unguium with griseofulvin: Preliminary report. *Curr Podiatry* 8:11, 1959.
138. Gibbs RC: Pitfalls in differential diagnosis and treatment of tinea pedis. *J Am Podiatry Assoc* 60:125–128, 1970.
139. Apt AC: Mycology—Some immunological considerations. *J Am Podiatry Assoc* 57:515–517, 1967b.
140. Conant NF, Smith DT, Baker RD, Callaway JL: *Manual of Clinical Mycology.* Philadelphia, W B Saunders Co, 1971.
141. Blank IH, Smith JG, Roth FJ, Zaias N: Griseofulvin for the systemic treatment of dermatomycoses. *J Am Med. Assoc* 171:2168, 1959.
142. Haas M, Boesenberg C: Treatment of onychomycosis and dermatophytosis with griseofulvin. *J Am Podiatry Assoc* 50:814–817, 1960.
143. Ashur M, Farrar R: Griseofulvin in the treatment of tinea pedis and onychomycosis. *J Am Podiatry Assoc* 51:103–108, 1961.
144. Ganley JV: An effective topical fungicidal agent for use in podiatry. *J Am Podiatry Assoc* 56:121–124, 1966.
145. Stern J, Fletcher T: Anti-tineal effectiveness of a new topical agent. *J Am Podiatry Assoc* 56:162, 1966.
146. Carpenter WE: Tolnaftate, its effectiveness in pedal mycosis, a preliminary report. *J Am Podiatry Assoc* 56:541–546, 1966.
147. Ilowite NH: Experimental production of tinea pedis. *J Am Podiatry Assoc* 57:120–122, 1967.
148. Goldfarb NJ, Rosenthal SA, Bock A, Borota A, Dick L, Qurnari D, Fraser C: Dermatomycosis treated with griseofulvin. *Antibotic Ann* 7:693–700, 1959–1960.
149. Reiss F, Kornblee L: Common mycotic infections of the lower extremities. *NY J Med* 63:548–556, 1963.
150. Estersohn H: An effective oral antifungal for chronic infections in the aged. *J Am Podiatry Assoc* 56:117–119, 1966.
151. Cacciaglia G et al.: A review of the literature of Ketocanazole therapy in the treatment of tinea pedis and onychomycosis. *J Foot Surg* 23:420–423, 1984.
152. Jones CL: The cutaneous virulence of Candida albicans of the foot. *J Foot Surg* 7:22–24, 1968.
153. Oyston JK: Madura foot: A study of twenty cases. *J Bone Joint Surg* 43B:259–267, 1961.
154. Haber H, Wells GC: Subcorneal pustular dermatosis of the soles. *Br J Dermatol* 71:243–245, 1959.
155. Gibbs RC: Some dermatoses based upon allergic mechanisms: Special implications for podiatry. *J Am Podiatry Assoc* 5:209–214, 1967.
156. Lerner MR, Lerner AB: *Dermatologic Medications,* ed 2. Chicago, Year Book Publishers, 1960.
157. Cangialosi CP: Aquatic conduct dermatitis (report of two cases). *J Am Podiatry Assoc* 73:21–24, 1983.
158. Young CR: Common winter dematoses of the foot. *J Am Podiatry Assoc* 63:563–570, 1973.
159. Hack M: The shoe in contact dermatitis. *J Am Podiatry Assoc* 66:408–412, 1976.
160. Kierland RR: The problem and treatment of pruritus. *Rocky Mt Med J* 55:44–49, 1959.
161. Weiner E: Dermatitis of the feet due to wearing of impermeable shoes. *J Am Podiatry Assoc* 50:545–547, 1960.
162. Franks AG: Dermatologic use of baths. *Am Practitioner* 9:1998–2000, 1958.
163. Jillson OF: Allergic dermatitis produced by pathogenic and saprophytic fungi. *Ann Allergy* 15:11–24, 1957.
164. Fisher AA: Some practical aspects of the diagnosis and management of shoe dermatitis. *Arch Dermatol* 79:267–274, 1959.
165. Everall JD, Truter EV: New approach to the problem of epidermal contact hypersensitivity. *Arch Dermatol* 75:428–436, 1957.

166. Ignatoff WB: Reactions to adhesive tape. *J Natl Assoc Chirop* 46:749–755, 1956.
167. Montgomery RM, Brezak S: Topical use of vioformhydrocortisone in podiatry. *J Am Podiatry Assoc* 48:364–366, 1958.
168. Schamberg IL, Askovita SI, Greenberg M: Critical evaluation of the effects of steroid lotions on inflammatory dermatoses. *Arch Dermatol* 78:490–499, 1958.
169. Reyer WA: Periorbital dermatitis following adhesive tape strapping of the lower extremity. *Ann Allergy* 15:144–149, 1957.
170. Catanzariti AR, et al.: Epidermolysis bullosa. *J Am Podiatry Assoc* 74:222–228, 1984.
171. Melski J, Tannenbaum L, Parrish J, Fitzpatrick TB, Blrivh HL, et al.: Oral methoxsalen photochemotherapy for the treatment of psoriasis. *J Invest Dermatol* 68:328–335, 1977.
172. Sarkany I, Taplin D, Blank H: Erythrasma—common bacterial infection of the skin. *JAMA* 177:130–132, 1961.
173. Temple DE, Boardman CR: Incidence of erythrasma of the toewebs. *Arch Dermatol* 86:518–519, 1962.
174. Brown J: Erythrasma and identification with Wood's light. *J Am Podiatry Assoc* 60:322–323, 1970.
175. Kirton V, Price W: Black heel. *Trans St John Hosp Dermatol Soc* 51:80–84, 1965.
176. Wilkinson DS: Black heel as minor hazard of sport. *Cutis* 20:393–396, 1977.
177. Galinski AW: Cutaneous herniations. *J Am Podiatry Assoc* 60:128–129, 1970.
178. Sachs W, Miller CS, Gray MB: Neurodermatic reaction. *Arch Dermatol Syph* 54:397–407, 1946.
179. Sachs W, Sachs PM, Young AW: Nummular eczema. *Skin* 3:103–108, 1964.
180. Blau SH: Surgical skin planing. *J Am Podiatry Assoc* 49:202–203, 1959.
181. Luikart R, Ayres S III, Wilson JW: Surgical planing of the skin, dichlorotetrafluoro-ethane as a freezing agent. *Calif Med* 84:151–154, 1956.
182. Prentice H: Sublesional administration of corticosteroids; a new technique with broad applications in podiatry. *J Am Podiatry Assoc* 51:791–800, 1961.
183. Locke RK: Local injection of combined dexamethasone 21-phosphate-lidocaine in non-articular foot disorders. *J Am Podiatry Assoc* 53:510–514, 1963.
184. Levin ME, O'Neal LW: *The Diabetic Foot*, ed 3. St. Louis, C.V. Mosby Co, 1983.
185. Black JR, Simons JV: The foot health status in diabetics regulated with oral hypoglycemic agents. *J Am Podiatry Assoc* 73:569–572, 1983.
186. Fox DB: A new approach to the treatment of leg ulcers. *Br Med J* 2:1370–1373, 1962.
187. Henzel JH, DeWeese MS, Lichti EL: Zinc concentrations within healing wounds. Significance of postoperative zincuria on availability and requirements during tissue repair. *Arch Surg* 100:349–357, 1970.
188. Dieter RA, Graziano JL: Proteolytic enzyme—Antibiotic preparations in the treatment of stasis ulcers. *Clin Med* 77:20, 1970.
189. Walkes M, Hazen M: Parenzyme in podiatry. *J Podiatry* 2:9–13, 1957.
190. Corsaro JA: Ulcers and injection therapy. *Footprints Fla Chirop Assoc* 4:2, 1958.
191. McNerney JE: The use of prophylactic antibiotics in foot surgery. *J Am Podiatry Assoc* 66:840–846, 1976.
192. Sokolowski K, Smith SD, Weil LS: Therapeutic approaches to major postoperative infections in podiatric surgery. *J Am Podiatry Assoc* 65:522–541, 1975.
193. Stern SF, Shuman A: The effect of locally administered corticosteroids (soluble and dissoluble) on the healing times of surgically induced wounds in guinea pigs. *J Am Podiatry Assoc* 63:374–382, 1973.
194. Rude T: Hypertensive leg ulcers. *J Foot Surg* 23:134–138, 1983.
195. Eisenberg LA: Physiologic rest though a rigid immobilization in the treatment of foot problems. *J Am Podiatry Assoc* 51:485–487, 1961.
196. Coleman, WC, et al.: The total contact cast. A therapy for plantar ulceration on insensitive feet. *J Am Podiatry Assoc* 74(11):548–552, 1984.
197. Schilansky MM: Hansen's disease and its pedal manifestations. *J Am Podiatry Assoc* 73:389–392, 1983.
198. Cohen W, Shelley WB: Ankle ulcer or Werner's syndrome *Arch Dermatol* 87:86–89, 1962.
199. Dribbon BS: Application and value of liquid crystal thermography. *J Am Podiatry Assoc* 73:400–404, 1983.
200. Bernhard LM, et al.: Plantar space abscesses in the diabetic foot: Diagnosis and treatment. *J Foot Surg* 23:283–290, 1984.
201. Visser HJ, Jacobs AM, et al.: The use of differential scintigraphy in the clinical diagnosis of osseous and soft tissue changes affecting the diabetic foot. *J Foot Surg* 23:74–85, 1984.
202. Goldenberg S, Alex M, Joshi RA, Blumenthal HT: Non-atheromatous peripheral vascular disease of the lower extremity in diabetes mellitus. *Diabetes* 8:261, 1959.
203. Hunter WN: Sinograph-evaluation of fistulous lesions of the foot. *J Foot Surg* 22:97–99, 1983.
204. Gordon V, Oster C: *J Am Osteopath Assoc* 75:515, 1975.
205. Cohn KL, et al.: Effect of pyridoxine (Vit. B_6) on diabetic patients with peripheral neuropathy. *J Am Podiatry Assoc* 74:394–397, 1984.
206. Helfand AE: Hunting diabetics by foot. *J Am Podiatry Assoc* 64:399–406, 1974.
207. Defeo WT, Jay RM: Osteomyelitis associated with peripheral vascular disease secondary to diabetes mellitus. *J Foot Surg* 15:159–165, 1976.
208. Barrett JP, Mooney V: Neuropathy and diabetic pressure lesions. *Orthop Clin North Am* 4:43, 1973.
209. Sanderson PJ: Infection of the foot with peptococcus magnus. *J Clin Pathol* 30:266–268, 1977.
210. Effeney DJ, Lim RC, Schecter WP: Transmetatarsal amputation. *Arch Surg* 112:1366–1370, 1977.
211. Wagner WD, Clarkson TB: Effect on regression

potential of atherosclerosis produced by intermittent or continuous hypercholesterolemia. *Atherosclerosis* 27:369–381, 1977.
212. Walden R, Cedar R, Mozes M: Gangrene of toes with normal peripheral pulses. *Ann Surg* 185:269–272, 1977.
213. Karmody AM, Powers SR, Monaco VJ, Keather RP: Blue toe syndrome, an indication for limb salvage. *Arch Surg* 111:1263–1268, 1976.
214. Kwaan JH, Connolly JE: Peripheral atheroembolism: An enigma. *Arch Surg* 112:987–990, 1977.
215. Helfand AE: Common foot complications in the elderly diabetic. *J Am Podiatry Assoc* 67:406–408, 1977.
216. Frank IH, Silver AG: Diabetic foot lesions—Preliminary report on a method of healing. *J Am Podiatry Assoc* 52:596–598, 1962.
217. Collens WS, Vulahos E, Dobkin GB, Neuman E, Rakow RR, Altman M, Siegman F: Conservative management of gangrene in the diabetic patient. *JAMA* 181:692–698. 1962.
218. Rakow RB: The treatment of necrotic lesions in the diabetic patient. *J Am Podiatry Assoc* 57:412–421, 1967.
219. Smith J, et al.: The effect of electrical stimulation on wound healing in diabetic mice. *J Am Podiatry Assoc* 74:71–72, 1984.
220. Sage R, Doyle D: Surigical treatment of diabetic foot ulcers: A review of forty-eight cases. *J Foot Surg* 23:102–111, 1984.
221. Glasser J, Barth A: Diabetic wound healing and the case for supplemental treatment with topical insulin. *J Foot Surg* 21:117–121, 1982.
222. Hanam SR, Singleton, CE, Rudek W: The effect of topical insulin on infected cutaneous ulcerations in diabetic and nondiabetic mice. *J Foot Surg* 22:298–301, 1983.
223. Ignacio DR, Pavot AP, Azer RN, Wisotsky L: Topical oxygen therapy treatment of extensive leg and foot ulcers. *J Am Podiatric Med Assoc* 75:196–199, 1985.
224. Singer A: Surgical treatment of mal perforans. *Arch Surg* 111:964–968, 1976.
225. McCarthy D, Montgomery B: Polyurethane in the management of ulcerating lesions of the lower extremities. *J Am Podiatry Assoc* 73:1–9, 1983.
226. Pogonowska MJ, Collins LC, Dobson HL: Diabetic osteopathy. *Radiology* 89:265–271, 1967.
227. Hazan M: Proteolytic enzymes in podiatry. *J Am Podiatry Assoc* 50:207–208, 160.
228. Luft S: Reactions to parenteral enzyme therapy. *J Am Podiatry Assoc* 50:209–210, 1960.
229. Migliori V, Kanat IO: Surgical considerations in wound healing. *J Foot Surg* 23:337–381, 1984.
230. McCarthy DJ, Axler DA: The efficacy of porcine skin grafts for treating non-healing cutaneous ulcers. Part II. Microanatomical studies. *J Am Podiatry Assoc* 68:86–95, 1978.
231. McCarthy DJ, Axler DA, Terleckyj B, Kwasnik R, Novicki D, Culliton P: The efficacy of porcine skin grafts for treating non-healing cutaneous ulcers. *J Am Podiatry Assoc* 68:141–151, 1978.
232. Krausz CE: Nail survey (1942–1970). *Br J Chirop* 35:117, 1970.
233. Sanders SC: Acrylic nail groove protector by brush technique. *J Am Podiatry Assoc* 45:23–24, 1955.
234. Sivitz SC: Acrylic resins: A preliminary report on the use of self curing plastic resins in nail groove therapy. *J Natl Assoc Chirop* 43:34–39, 1953.
235. Mogull P: Uses of methyl methacrylate in the treatment of inverted nails. *J Natl Assoc Chirop* 44:35, 1954.
236. Goldy H, Steinberg M: Etiological factors in multiple infected onychocryptosis. *J Natl Assoc Chirop* 46:769–771, 1956.
237. DuVries HL: Hypertrophy of unguilabia. *Chirop Rec* 16:11, 1933.
238. Winograd AM: Modification in technique of operation for ingrown toenail *JAMA* 92:229, 1929.
239. Frost LA: Surgical correction for the incurvated nail. *Curr Med Digest* 29:119–121, 1962.
240. Yale JF: The phenol-alcohol technique for correction of ingrown toenail. Address to Military Society of Orthopedic Surgeons, at West Point Military Academy, New York, 1970.
241. Boll OF: Surgical correction of ingrown nails. *J Natl Assoc Chirop* 35:8–9, 1945.
242. Nyman SP: The phenol-alcohol technique for toenail excision. *J Natl Assoc Chirop* 5:2, 1956.
243. Suppan RJ, Ritchlin JD: A non-debilitating surgical procedure for "ingrown toenail." *J Am Podiatry Assoc* 52:900–902, 1962.
244. Kleiman MA: Some observations concerning the phenol-alcohol nail technique. *Footprints Fla Podiatry Assoc* 19:6, 1964.
245. Greene AA: A modification of the phenol-alcohol technique for toenail correction. *Curr Podiatry* 13:20–25, 1964.
246. Anton-Athens V, Ketai DL: Use of cortisporin otic solution in phenol nail surgery. *J Am Podiatry Assoc* 75:31–33, 1985.
247. Polokoff M: Negative galvanism in nail surgery. Lecture to Chiropodists Society of New Jersey, February, 1944.
248. Polokoff M: Negative galvanic procedure for Morton's neuralgia. *J Am Podiatry Assoc* 51:31–36, 1961a.
249. Rubin LM, Weiss SG: Complete nail eradication utilizing galvanic current. *J Am Podiatry Assoc* 54:401–403, 1964.
250. Dyer AM, Cohen MF: A report on the use of negative galvanic current for the correction of incurvated nails. *J Natl Assoc Chirop* 45:21–22, 1955.
251. Gardner P: Negative galvanic current in the surgical correction of onychocryptotic nails. *J Am Podiatry Assoc* 48:555–560, 1958.
252. Perrone MA: Nail matricectomy by onychotripsy with airmotor. *J Am Podiatry Assoc* 60:92–93, 1970.
253. Steinberg MD: A simplified technique for surgery of ingrown toenails. *Surgery* 36:1132–1137, 1954.
254. Zadik FR: Obliteration of the nail bed of the great tow without shortening the terminal phalanx. *J Bone Joint Surg* 32B:6, 1950.
255. Kaplan EG: Elimination of onychauxis by surgery. *J Am Podiatry Assoc* 50:111–113, 1960.
256. Owens RE: Surgical correction for onychauxis.

J Am Podiatry Assoc 52:591–593, 1962.
257. Jones CL: Skin graft following avulsion of nail, a preliminary report. *J Am Podiatry Assoc* 55:191–193, 1965.
258. Whitney AK: Total matricectomy procedure. *J Am Podiatry Assoc* 58:157–159, 1968.
259. Elleby DH, Weil LS, Sorto LA, Smith SD: The use of porcine xenografts on nail beds following total nail avulsion and phenol chemomatrixectomy. *J Foot Surg* 16:85–91, 1977.
260. Hatch DJ, Pascente RW: Photo-onycholysis associated with tetracycline. *J Am Podiatry Assoc* 68:172–177, 1978.
261. Pardo-Castello V, Pardo OA: *Diseases of the Nails*, ed 3. Springfield, IL, Charles C Thomas Co, 1960.
262. White CJ, Laipply TC: Diseases of the nails: 792 cases, clinical microscopic findings with resume of newer therapeutic methods. *Ind Med Surg* 27:325–327, 1958.
263. Fletcher TJ: Nail fungus—The problem and its management. *J Am Podiatry Assoc* 49:311–314, 1959.
264. Abramson C, Wilton J: Inhalation of nail dust from onychomycotic toenails. Part I, Characterization of Particles. *J Am Podiatric Med Assoc* 75:563–567, 1985.
265. Abramson C, Wilton J: Nail dust aerosols from onychomycotic toenails. Part II, Clinical and Serological aspects. *J Am Podiatric Med Assoc* 75:631–638, 1985.
266. White C: Diseases of the nails. *Postgrad med* 8:43, 1950.
267. Bereston ES: Diseases of the nails. *Clin Med* 57:238, 1950.
268. Peck S, Klein G: *Therapy of Dermatological Disorders*. Philadelphia, Lea & Febiger, 1951.
269. Hendler SS: Management of onychomycosis. *J Am Podiatry Assoc* 44:57–60, 1954.
270. Locke RK: Onychomycosis. *J Am Podiatry Assoc* 45:15–28, 1955.
271. Jaskoski BJ, Jacobs JF, Carr DL: Some mycotic problems in a podiatry clinic. *J Am Podiatry Assoc* 52:825–828, 1962.
272. Mogull P: Acrylic nail plate and onychomycosis. *J Natl Assoc Chirop* 47:401–402, 1957.
273. Ignatoff WB, Bleiberg J: A new therapy for onychomycosis. *J Am Podiatry Assoc* 48:359–363, 1958.
274. Spoor HJ: Onychomycosis and corneal dystrophy. *Arch Dermatol* 95:427–428, 1967.
275. Jaskoski BJ: Treatment of onychomycosis in a foot clinic. *J Am Podiatry Assoc* 59:230–233, 1969.
276. Frost L: Onychomycosis—Treatment by avulsion and onychophytex. *J Am Podiatry Assoc* 50:283–287, 1960.
277. Goldberg HC: Clinical observations on the use of griseofulvin by mouth in fungus diseases. *J Am Podiatry Assoc* 50:290–291, 1960.
278. Strahs R: Treatment of onychomycosis with a lacquer formulation of chloranil. *J Am Podiatry Assoc* 52:508–509, 1962.
279. Feldman B: Griseofulvin in podiatry. *J Am Podiatry Assoc* 50:292–296, 1960.
280. Walker MH: Report on griseofulvin. *J Am Podiatry Assoc* 50:297–303, 1960.
281. Maibach EI, Kligman AM: Short-term treatment of onychomycosis with griseofulvin. *Arch Dermatol* 81:733–734, 1960.
282. Carpenter WE: Preliminary results of a study to develop a treatment regimen for onychomycosis. *J Am Podiatry Assoc* 52:343–347, 1962b.
283. Reiss F, Kornblee L: Common mycotic infections of the lower extremities. *NY J Med* 63:548–556, 1963.
284. Dix R, Sloan B: An evaluation of a local and oral medication in the treatment of onychomycosis. *J Am Podiatry Assoc* 56:450–454, 1966.
285. Krausz CE: A nail survey of 4,600 patients. *J Natl Assoc Chirop* 40:5–11, 1950.
286. Zaias N: Psoriasis of the nail. *Arch Dermatol* 99:567–579, 1969.
287. Johnson AV: Onychoclavus, a fifth toe problem. *J Am Podiatry Assoc* 52:436–438, 1962.
288. Ross SB: Subungual granuloma pyogenicum. *J Natl Assoc Chirop* 45:17–18, 1955.
289. Das Gupta T: Subungual melanoma; 25 years review of cases. *Ann Surg* 161:545–552, 1965.
290. Eichenholtz SN, DeAngelis C: Squamous-cell carcinoma of the nail bed. *JAMA* 191:1080–1083, 1965.
291. Frost L: Digital calcinosis—A case report. *J Natl Assoc Chirop* 47:71–73, 1957.
292. Sandel RK: Unilateral multiple glomus tumors. *J Am Coll Foot Surg* 4:130, 1966.
293. Wichman B: Subungual exostoses and nail border problems. *J Am Podiatry Assoc* 57:521–522, 1967.
294. Stanley WJ: Koilonychia and polycythemia vera. *Med Illus* 10:399–400, 1956.
295. Bergeron JR, Stone OJ: Koilonychia: A report of familial spoon nails. *Arch Dermatol* 95:351–353, 1967.
296. Higashi N: Melanocytes of toenail matrix and nail pigmentation. *Arch Dermatol* 97:570–574, 1968.
297. Bodine G: Subungual coagulum. *J Am Podiatry Assoc* 57:377–378, 1967.
298. Pack GT, Oropenza R: Subungual melanoma. *Surg Gynecol Obst* 124:571–582, 1976.
299. Baran R, et al.: *Disorders of the Nail and their Management*. St Louis, C V Mosby, 1984.

Suggested Readings

Abramson DI: *Vascular Disorders of the Extremities*, ed 2. New York, Harper and Row, 1974.

Adam JE: Exfoliative dermatitis. *Can Med Assoc J* 99:661–666, 1968.

Apt AC: Diagnostic mycology, an introduction. *J Am Podiatry Assoc* 57:271, 1967a.

Ashby BS: Primary carcinoma of the nail bed. *Br J Surg* 44:216, 1956.

Balu S: Surgical planing for skin lesions of the foot. *J Natl Assoc Chirop* 47:277–278, 1957.

Barre JA, Masson P: Anatoma—clinical study of certain painful subungual tumors (tumors of the neuro-myoarterial glomus of the extremities). *Bull Soc Franc de Dermat et Syph* 31:148–159, 1924.

Bart RS, Andrade R, Kopf AW: Cutaneous horns. A clinical and histopathologic study. *Acta Derm Venereol* 48:507–515, 1968.

Bartlett RW: A conservative operation for care of so-called ingrown toenail. *JAMA* 108:1257, 1937.

Berlin S: *Skin Tumors of the Foot: Diagnosis and*

Treatment. Mt. Kisco, NY, Futura Publishing Co, 1974.

Bhutani LK, Kanwar AJ, Singh OP: Porokeratosis of mibelli with unusual features. *Dermatologica* 155:296–300, 1977.

Biberstein H: Immunization therapy of warts. *Arch Dermatol Syph* 50:12, 1944.

Blank IH: Protection against the invasion of bacteria and fungi. Symposium AAAS, December, 1970.

Bodian EL: Oral treatment of dermatomycosis and onychomycosis with griseofulvin. *Int Rec Med* 173:85–87, 1960.

Bowler CW: Nail techniques. *Br J Chirop* 32:85–87, 1967.

Burns AE (ed): Digital Surgery. Clinics in Podiatry. Philadelphia, WB Saunders, Co, 1986.

Cacciaglia GB, Reigelhaupt RW: Effectiveness of lasers on plantar papillomas: A preliminary study. *J Foot Surg* 24:71–75, 1985.

Carpenter WE: An evaluation of injectable vitamin A concentrate in the treatment of corns and calluses. *J Am Podiatry Assoc* 52: 120–121, 1962a.

Carter RT: Verruca, some impressions from a study of 118 cases. *J Am Podiatry Assoc* 59:336–339, 1969.

Chagas CP: Carcinoma of the nail matrix. *Brazil Medico* 233, 1921.

Clarke BF, Dillanger KA: Surgical treatment of ingrown toenail. *Surgery* 21:919–924, 1947.

Collins HL: Surgical nail flap operation. *Clin J Chirop Podiatry Pedic Surg* 9:220, 1937.

Conrad NL: Response of various fungi to specialized media and some chemical irritants. *J Am Podiatry Assoc* 55:109–112, 1965.

Costello JA, Costello JO: Chronic ulcerations of the lower extremities, differential diagnosis and treatment. *J Am Osteopath Assoc* 55:732–735, 1956.

Davies RR, Everall JD, Hamilton E: Mycological and clinical evaluation of griseofulvin for chronic onychomycosis. *Br J Med* 3:464–468, 1967.

DeCarlo R: Sinuses. *Chirop Rec* 18:3, 1935.

Dell JM: Demonstrations of sinus tracts, fistulas and cavities by lipoidal. *Am J Roentgenol Radium Ther* 61:223–231, 1949.

Dixon M: Keratosis palmaris and plantaris (a case report). *J Am Podiatry Assoc* 56:376–377, 1966.

Dockery GL (ed): *Dermatology of the Lower Extremities*. Clinics in Podiatric Medicine and Surgery. Philadelphia, WB Saunders, Co, 1986.

Drummer B: Keramin injection in the treatment of helomata. *J Am Podiatry Assoc* 48:99–101, 1958.

DuVries HL: Hypertrophy of the unguilabia. *Chirop Rec* 17:33–35, 1934.

DuVries HL: Ingrown toenail. *Chirop Rec* 27:155–159, 1944.

Emmert C: Operations for ingrown nail. *Arch F Klin Chirop* 11:268–277, 1869.

Engman MF Jr, Mook WH: Melanotic whitlow. *Arch Dermatol Syph* 1174, 1931.

Epstein E: Shoe contact dermatitis. *JAMA* 209:1487, 1969.

Everett MA, Alston HD: Griseofulvin therapy of superficial cutaneous mycoses. *J Okla Med Assoc* 52:793–795, 1959.

Evison G, Price CHG: Subungual exostosis. *Br J Radiol* 39:451–455, 1966.

Faris I: Foot lesions in diabetic patients: pathogenesis and management. *Med J Aust* 1:628–633, 1977.

Feder H, Feder J: Penetration of topical steroids. *J Am Podiatry Assoc* 58:388–390, 1968.

Fleck CJ: Verruca plantaris. *Chirop Rec* 17:95–99, 1934.

Frohlich H, Frons W, Cedar T: A reliable topical antifungal for podiatry. *J Am Podiatry Assoc* 57:177–178, 1967.

Frost L: Root resection for incurvated nail. *J Natl Assoc Chirop* 40:19, 1950.

Gibson SH, Montgomery H, Woolner LB, Brunsting LA: Melanotic whitlow (subungual melanoma). *J Invest Dermatol* 29:119–129, 1957.

Gottlieb MM, Gottlieb JJ: The permanent removal of nails by avulsion and chemical cauterization. *Chron Podiatry* 3:17–18, 1953.

Graham HF: Ingrown toenail. *Am J Surg* 6:411, 1929.

Greenberg W: Hereditary callosities. *J Natl Assoc Chirop* 46:327–328, 1956.

Grolich H, Irons W, Ceder E: A reliable topical antifungal for podiatry. *J Am Podiatry Assoc* 57:177, 1967.

Gull K, Trinci AJ: Griseofulvin inhibits fungal mitosis. *Nature* 244:292, 1973.

Gumport SL, Harris MH, Kopf AW: Diagnosis and management of common skin cancers. *Amer Cancer Soc Prof Educat Publication* no 3373–P.E., 1975.

Holmes JG: Diagnosis of ringworm. *Lancet* 2:62–63, 1956.

Howard WR: Ingrown toenail, its surgical treatment, *NY Med Surg J* 57:579–581, 1893.

Hutchinson R: The treatment of warts by viral interference. *Practitioner* 204:700, 1970.

Jablon VA: Epithelioma. *Chirop Rec* 20:232–234, 1937.

Jarrett A, Spearman RIC: The histochemistry of the human nail. *Arch Dermatol* 94:652–657, 1966.

Johnson SAA, Tuura JL: Glyceryl triacetate (triacetin) as a fungicide. *Arch Dermatol* 74:73–75, 1956.

Kalish SR: Iatrogenic, corticosteroid-induced acrodermatitis chronica atrophicans. *J Am Podiatry Assoc* 63:8–11, 1973.

Kalkera KH, Caruoto J: The evaluation and treatment of diabetic foot ulcers. *J Am Podiatry Assoc* 72:491, 1982.

Keyes EL: Surgical treatment of ingrown toenail. *JAMA* 102:1458, 1934.

Kilberg AJ: Surgical treatment of onychocryptosis. *Clin J Chirop Podiatry Pedic Surg* 7:222–224, 1935.

Kleger SJ, Feldman B: Larva migrans. *J Am Podiatry Assoc* 56:324–325, 1966.

Knox JM, Spiller WF: Eccrine poroma. *Arch Dermatol* 77:726, 1958.

Knudsen EA, Amdrup E: Verrucae vulgaris et plantaris treated with ultrasoft x-rays. *Acta Derm Venereol Scand* 35:379–389, 1955.

Kozak GP, et al.: *Management of Diabetic Foot Problems*. Philadelphia, W B Saunders Co, 1984.

Kozie LJ, Ballard R, Buividas A: A clinical evaulation of diphemanil methylsulfate in the treatment of hyperhidrosis. *J Natl Assoc Chirop* 47:398–400, 1957.

Laurence KR: Treatment of verrucae with smallpox vaccine. *J Am Podiatry Assoc* 61:12–19, 1971.

Layman CW: Use of liquid oxygen in dermatology. *Minn Med* 29:151–152, 1956.

Levey M: Formaldehyde and vitamin A in treatment of verrucae. *Curr Podiatry* 7:14, 1958.

Lloyd-Davis RW, Brill GC: The etiology and management of ingrown toenails. *Br J Surg* 50:592–597, 1963.

Louie TJ, Bartlett JG, Tally FP, Gorbach SL: Aerobic and anaerobic bacteria in diabetic foot ulcers. *Ann Intern Med* 85:461–463, 1976.

Luciano CS: Verruca plantaris. *J Am Podiatry Assoc* 67:858–869, 1977.

Mackee GM, Capallaro AC: *X-ray and Radium in the Treatment of Diseases of the Skin*, ed 4. Philadelphia, Lea & Febiger, 1946.

Madden JJ: Inflammatory disorders of skin of the feet. *JAMA* 124:743–747, 1944.

McCarthy DJ: A morphogenic and histochemical analysis of pressure-prone verrucae of the human foot. *J Am Podiatry Assoc* 67:377–387, 1977.

McCarthy DJ, Habowsky JEJ: Alterations in skin morphology in heloma dura utilizing maceration technique for examination of epidermal-dermal interface. *J Am Podiatry Assoc* 62:303–307, 1972.

McCarthy, DJ (ed), Montgomery, R (assoc. ed): *Podiatric Dermatology*, Baltimore, Williams & Wilkins, 1986.

McCarthy DJ, Rusin J: The implications of ultrastructural alterations induced by cryocautery in pedal verrucae. *J Am Podiatry Assoc* 67:312–327, 1977.

Michael CA: Pruritus, what it is and some suggestions for management. *J Am Podiatry Assoc* 52:432–435, 1962.

Montgomery RM, Montgomery AH: Common hyperkeratotic lesions of the foot. *JAMA* 124:756–761, 1944.

Ney GG: An operation for ingrowing toenails. *JAMA* 80:374, 1923.

Norton A: Nail disorders, a Review. *J Amer Acad Dermatology* 2, 1980.

Ottley CM: Glomus tumor. *Br J Surg* 29:387–391, 1942.

Overcast VC: Curetting verrucae with minimum hemorrhage. *J Natl Assoc Chirop* 47:187, 1957.

Pack GT, Adair FE: Subungual melanoma differential diagnosis of tumors of the nail bed. *Surgery* 5:47–72, 1939.

Perry GM: Molluscum Contagiosum—A case report. *J Am Podiatry Assoc* 54:32–33, 1964.

Polokoff M: Ingrown toe nail and hypertrophied nail lip surgery by electrolysis. *J Am Podiatry Assoc* 51:805–808, 1961.

Rakow RB: The treatment of necrotic lesions in the diabetic patient. *J Am Podiatry Assoc* 57:412–421, 1967.

Robin GM: A typical callus—A case report. *J Am Podiatry Assoc* 60:212–213, 1970.

Roenigk HH, Young RR: Leg ulcers. New York, Harper and Row, 1975.

Rogachefsky H, Rosenthal SA, Litt JZ, Baer RL: Trichophytin reaction after exposure to dermatophytes. *Arch Dermatol* 74:606–609, 1956.

Ronchesi F: Nail in lichen planus. *Arch Dermatol* 91:347, 1965.

Rowe L: Granuloma pyogenicum differential diagnosis. *Arch Dermatol* 78:341–347, 1958.

Rubin L: Intraepidermal squamous cell carcinoma of the nail bed. *J Am Podiatry Assoc* 63:195–196, 1973.

Samitz MH: Cutaneous lesions of the lower extremities in the diagnosis of systemic disease. *J Am Podiatry Assoc* 65:556–567, 1975.

Samitz NH: *Cutaneous Disorders of the Lower Extremities*, ed 2. Philadelphia, J. B. Lippincott Co, 1981.

Schwartz L, Peck SM: The patch test in contact dermatitis. *J Natl Assoc Chirop* 36:7–16, 1946.

Scott MJ, Costello MJ, Simuango SA: Keratosis punctata palmaris et plantaris. *Arch Dermatol* 64:301, 1951.

Sharpe A: Pathology of traumatic callus and heloma. *J Natl Assoc Chirop* 33:6–10, 1943.

Shatin H, Reisch M: Dermatitis of the feet due to shoes. *Arch Dermatol Syph* 69:651—666, 1954.

Sherman LH: Complicated onychocryptosis. *J Natl Assoc Chirop* 29:11–17, 1939.

Spencer F, Sage R, Graner J: The incidence of foot pathology in a diabetic population. *J Am Podiatric Med Assoc* 75:590–592, 1985.

Stalbach JJ: The nail plate—A key to diagnosis. *Chirop Rec* 22:184–187, 1939.

Stern J: Quinocaine injection therapy for verrucae. *J Am Podiatry Assoc* 51:413–415, 1961.

Strivastave KP, Kersarwani RC: Management of trophic ulcers in leprosy patients. *J Indian Med Assoc* 67:250–252, 1976.

Surman OS: Hypnosis in the treatment of warts. *Arch Gen Psychiat* 28:439, 1973.

Taub J, Steinberg MD: Porokeratosis dermatopathological entity. *Int J Dermatol* 9:83–90, 1970.

Temple DE, Boardman CR: Incidence of erythrasma of the toewebs. *Arch Dermatol* 86:518–519, 1962.

Vandenbos KQ, Bowers WF: Ingrown toenail: A result of weight bearing on soft tissues. *US Armed Forces Med* J 10:1168–1173, 1959.

VanScott EJ, Reinertson RP, McCall CB: Prevalence, histological types and significance of palmer and plantar nevi. *Cancer* 10:363, 1957.

Vernon S: Ingrown toenail, operation by electrosurgery. *Am J Surg* 42:396–397, 1938.

Waddell WA: The common corn clinically considered. *Can Chirop* J Summer Issue: 29–37, 1948.

Walker MH: A study of griseofulvin as related to tinea pedis. *J Am Podiatry Assoc* 51:112–122, 1961.

Weisfeld M: Understanding porokeratosis plantaris discreta. *J Am Podiatry Assoc* 63:138–144, 1973.

White CJ: Disease of the nail. *Chirop Rec* 32:115–119, 1949.

White CJ, Laipply TC: Diseases of the nails. *Chirop Rec* 41:6–7, 1958.

White RR, et al.: Management of wounds in the diabetic foot. *Surg Clin N Amer* 64:735–742, 1984.

Whitney AK: An illustrated labiomatricectomy procedure. *J Am Podiatry Assoc* 57:169–172, 1967.

Winograd A: The surgical treatment of ingrown toenail. *JAMA* 102:1458, 1934.

Woolf WH: Verruca: Its possible relationship to other neoplasms. *J Am Podiatry Assoc* 52:893–898, 1962.

Yale JF: Phenol-alcohol technique for correction of infected ingrown toenail. *J Am Podiatry Assoc* 64:46–53, 1974.

Yontef R: Treatment of dermatomycoses with griseofulvin. *J Med Soc NJ* 738–740, 1959.

Young R: Differential diagnosis of leg ulcers In Spittell JA, Jr (ed) *Clinical Vascular Disease* and Best AN (ed): *Cardiovascular Clinics*. Philadelphia, F A Davis Co, 1983, pp 172–173.

7

Skin and Soft Tissue Tumors and Cysts

The lesions discussed here are those that can be tentatively interpreted by clinical examination and later corroborated by laboratory study. Tumors and cysts involving bone are beyond the scope of this text, and the author recommends the study of *Clinical Foot Roentgenology* (1) for their interpretation.

All masses removed from the foot should be properly evaluated clinically and macroscopically and by microscopic examination. Careful history taking is essential if full appreciation of the pathology is to be realized.

There are exciting physical, chemical and biological factors that precede the development of tumors. Tumors are autonomous new growths that must be differentiated from inflammatory disorders, regenerative processes and repair mechanisms. They may be progressive and unlimited in their growth.

DuVries (2) differentiates benign from malignant tumors by noting that benign tumors have a capsule; if they are removed, they should not recur. Their blood supply is generally poor, and they do not adhere to adjacent tissue. Their outline is smooth, even or regular, and they do not metastasize. The cells of benign tumors are adult; growth is slow, and their influence on life is negligible. Malignant tumors have the opposite characteristics: they are composed of embryonic cells and can be fatal if not removed in their early development.

Nickel (3) states that, if malignancy is suspected, primary surgical excision is the treatment of choice. An operation may be too late if the patient must wait for a microscopic report. Malignancy may be presumed if a nodular elevation develops on a flat mole and there is crusting and oozing, if there is satellite pigmentation, if a red halo develops around a nevus, or if there are spontaneous bleeding and accelerated growth. Nickel also notes that malignant melanomas may show none of these changes, and thus he strongly recommends biopsy of all treated lesions. Excisional biopsy is the biopsy of choice in most foot lesions. Disposable biopsy punches are available in 2, 3, 3.5, 4 and 6 mm sizes.

Levene et al. (4) studied the relationship of pressure to the dissemination of melanoma. Five hundred eleven lesions of the foot were seen at Christie Hospital, Manchester, England. Melanomas commonly found in females all appeared in the arch areas of the foot, whereas squamous cell carcinomas and hyperkeratotic lesions were on the metatarsal and heel areas. Angiomas extended from plantar to dorsal areas. The squamous cell lesions were more common in males. Berlin (5) in an exhaustive study reviews 67,000 foot tumors and lesions. The 25 most commonly reported benign lesions, in order of occurrence, were verruca, Morton's neuroma, porokeratosis, neuroma, inclusion cyst, ganglion cyst, exostosis, squamous cell papilloma, fibroma, pyogenic granuloma, dermatofibroma, nevi, digital mucous cyst, plantar fibromatosis, junctional nevi, lipoma, hemangioma, leiomyoma, neurofibroma, rheumatoid nodule, eccrine poroma, gouty tophi, digital fibrokeratoma, giant cell tumor of tendon sheath and nodular subepidermal fibrosis.

Foreign Body Granuloma. When a minute foreign body penetrates the skin—as frequently occurs in the feet—an initial overlying lesion of hyperkeratosis may develop (Fig. 7.1). The lesion becomes nodular, resulting in pain that requires complete removal for relief. Very often the granulomatous lesion is enveloped by a firm fibrous capsule, resulting in a cystic degeneration.

Treatment. The treatment of foreign body granuloma is aimed at removing the foreign body and the pathological tissue surrounding it. This may be accomplished by the use of field block anesthesia with Xylocaine 1% and 1:100,000 epinephrine and by completely excising the entire granulomatous mass including its capsular attachments. The gaping space is closed with sutures followed by the use of compression bandages.

Granuloma Pyogenicum. These lesions commonly occur at the margins of the nails or in the nail grooves and on nail lips. However, they may develop at any site on the foot (Figs. 7.2 and 7.3). These lesions resemble an infected angioma, but are differentiated by their soft red to brownish color and vascular, sharply demarcated, pedunculated and sessile growth. Growth is rapid. These granulomas are caused by irritation of the skin, an offending portion of nail, or self-inflicted trauma. Entrance of staphylococci into a small opening is thought to be the causative factor. Sensation may vary from severe pain to painlessness. The granulomas bleed readily and often suppurate with no tendency to heal. The lesions measure from the typical 1 cm to 4 or 6 cm in size. Estershon and Stanoch (6) present a literature review and two case reports of granuloma pyogenicum.

Treatment of pyogenic granuloma consists of early correction of the localized infection with local or systemic antibiotic therapy and excision of the granulomatous mass. Healing is enhanced by removing an associated offending portion of the nail to diminish continued irritation. In most instances it is advisable to use toe block anes-

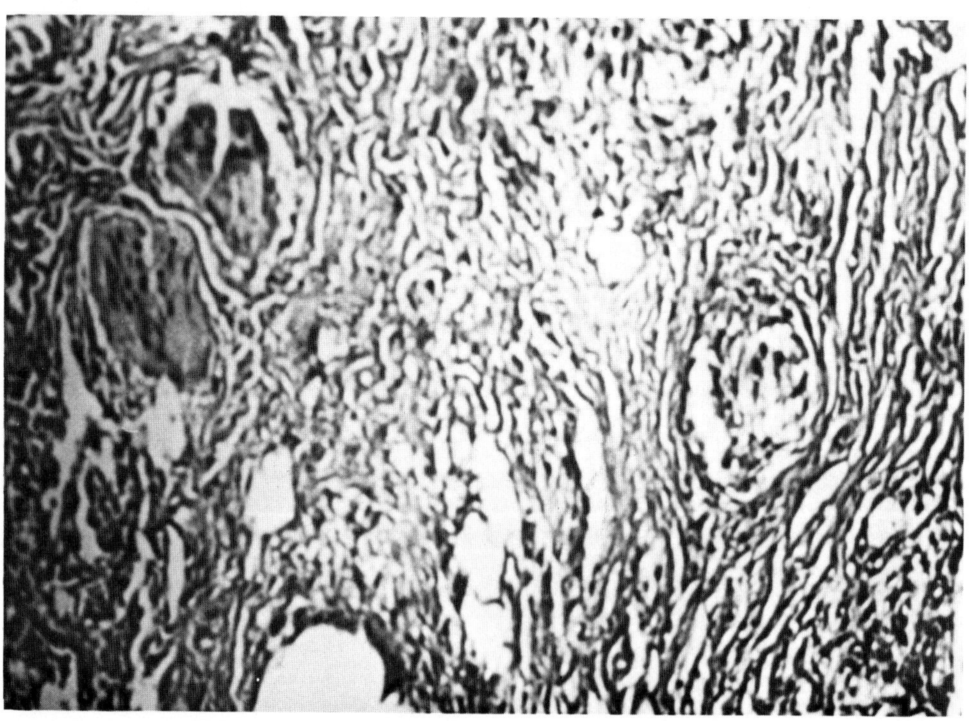

Figure 7.1. Foreign body granuloma. Note crystalline material. Foreign body giant cells visible with about 22 and 19 nuclei showing, respectively. Note collagen surrounding cells.

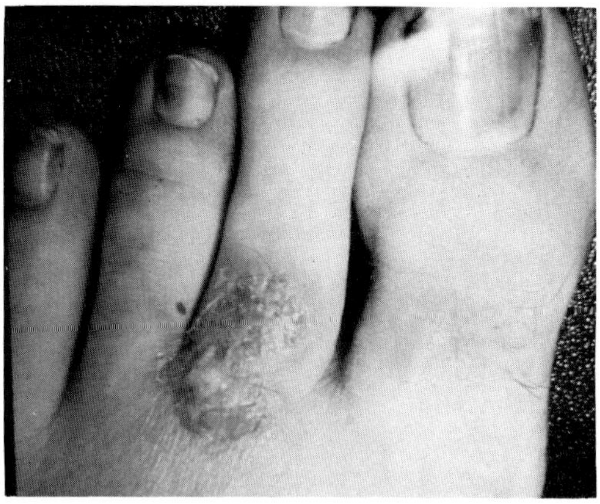

Figure 7.2. Granuloma pyogenicum. Slightly elevated moist red granulation tissue on the dorsum of the second toe.

thesia followed by removal of one-third of the offending border of the toenail. This is accomplished in a deft manner to minimize the trauma to the nail bed and the posterior nail fold. Complete excision of the granulomatous mass is followed by either electrocautery of the granulomatous base or the use of a silver nitrate stick while the patient is still under anesthesia. Treatment is continued in an effort to resolve the proliferation of the previously irritated cells.

Benign Multiple Acanthoma. Steinberg (7) calls attention to a condition that he calls "benign multiple acanthoma," which is found in multiple recurrent ingrowing toenails in young people. He reports cases to substantiate his findings and cites the following diagnostic criteria: persistent recurrence involving two or more toes; bulbous tissue formation on the distal nail flap, usually on both sides of the toe; mucopurulent exudate with a characteristic biopsy; little or no deformity of the matrix; familial tendency; less pain than from the usual ingrown nail; and firm tissue that does not bleed as freely as granulation tissue.

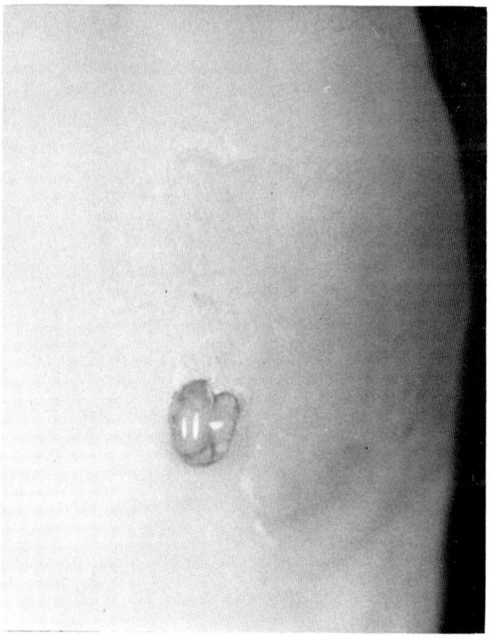

Figure 7.3. Granuloma pyogenicum on the plantar surface of the foot.

Treatment. Toe block anesthesia is instituted, and the offending border of the nail including the bulbous formation on the distal nail flap is removed. The patient is placed on saline soaks to calm down the inflammation and to cleanse the mocopurulent exudate from the affected part. This procedure is then followed by the use of electrodesiccation on the affected part or the application of a silver nitrate stick to diminish the activity of the cells. If mucopurulent exudate persists, culture and sensitivity tests are made to aid in selecting proper medication.

Profuse Granulation. A self-inflicted nail groove infection or irritation of the nail lip by a poorly cut or developing nail may result in abrasion of the nail lip or groove causing a superficial ulceration. With further irritation the tissue reacts with excessive proliferation and profuse granulations enveloping the nail border. These granulations are bright red, shiny, raw, oozing vascular tissues. They form a granuloma when left alone and untreated.

Treatment. Profuse granulations are best removed under local anesthesia. The excision of the entire granular mass plus the application of silver nitrate to the base is indicated. The patient should be followed at intervals of 3 to 5 days to determine whether the profuse granulations are under control. If there is any evidence of the development of granulation tissues, the presence of a foreign material or irritant should be suspected. Removal of a foreign body or matrical tissue in the nail groove is mandatory for correction of this disorder.

Granuloma Annulare. This dermatosis, commonly found in children, generally involves the dorsum of the feet, although it can occur on any part. An annular nodular lesion, red-brown in color, may enlarge by peripheral spread.

The center clears as the margin spreads. This condition is otherwise asymptomatic and is frustrating to treat. Politz and Miller (8) report an atypical case of subcutaneous granuloma annulare of the foot with a review of its histopathology.

Treatment. Intralesional injections of triamcinalone have been helpful. Often lidocaine injections and even biopsy result in clinical cure. Vitamin D may increase the activity of the lesion. Silver et al. (9) found that trauma to the lesion appears to be followed by involution. When lesions occur in other parts of the body, the patient is referred to a dermatologist for treatment. A psychogenic etiology must be considered.

Kamalam et al. (10) on two occasions isolated *Cryptococcus laurentii* from a granuloma on the foot and leg of a 40-year-old man. The bacteria were found in groups in the dermis and inside giant cells. Epitheloid cells were infiltrating the subdermis and cutis. Treatment consisted of amphotericin B infusions followed by antituberculosis medication.

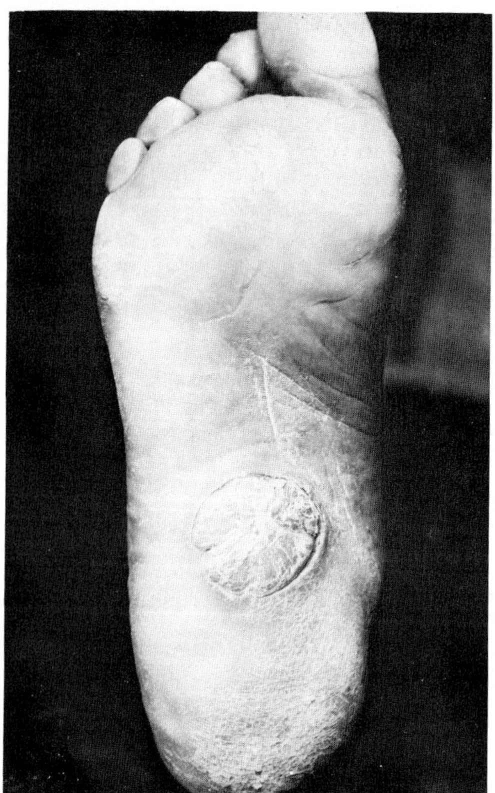

Figure 7.4. Nodular subepidermal fibrosis. (Courtesy of M Blass.)

Rheumatoid Nodules. Rheumatoid nodules may develop on the Achilles tendon or in periarticular tissues. They may adhere to bone periosteum or fibrous, ligamentous, tendonous and synovial sheaths. Palisading fibroblasts covered by a collagenous capsule surround a central necrotic area in the rheumatoid nodule (11). The underlying rheumatoid arthritic process is generally advanced when subcutaneous nodules develop. Commonly painless, rheumatoid nodules occur in approximately 25% of cases of rheumatoid arthritis. Pseudorheumatoid nodule (rheumatoid nodulosis), which is rarely found in an adult, may be a precursor to rheumatoid arthritis. These lesions occur dorsally without clinical symptoms of the disease and are similar to rheumatoid nodules and granuloma annulare histopathologically (12). Rheumatoid nodules must be differentiated from cysts, fibromas, lipomas, tophi, bursae, fibrosarcoma, and a variety of skin and subcutaneous masses (13). If they are painful, interfere with function or continually ulcerate, rheumatoid nodules should be excised. It is often unnecessary to remove a rheumatoid nodule after excision of an associated bony prominence.

Nodular Subepidermal Fibrosis. These benign lesions include the dermatofibroma, histiocytoma and sclerosing hemangioma (Fig. 7.4). They are hard, firm nodular lesions found in the dermis and attached firmly to the epidermis. The overlying skin has a shiny, red-brownish appearance and is often scar tissue secondary to a scratch, bite or other irritation of the skin. Steinberg described a plugged duct porokeratotic cyst that must be differentiated from a verruca and a nodular subepidermal fibrosis lesion (dermatofibroma). A moat at the dermatofibroma's circumference is one of the differential features, and it is histologically different from the verruca and the plugged duct porokeratotic cyst.

Treatment is surgical removal of the nodule.

Fibroma. A fibroma is a firm, benign, nodular, clearly circumscribed and palpable mass of fibrous connective tissue capable of developing in any tissue derived from mesenchyme (Figs. 7.5–7.12). Histologic examination corroborates the clinical impression. A fibroma may be found in combination with several tissues, such as in a neurofibroma, fibrolipoma and angiofibroma.

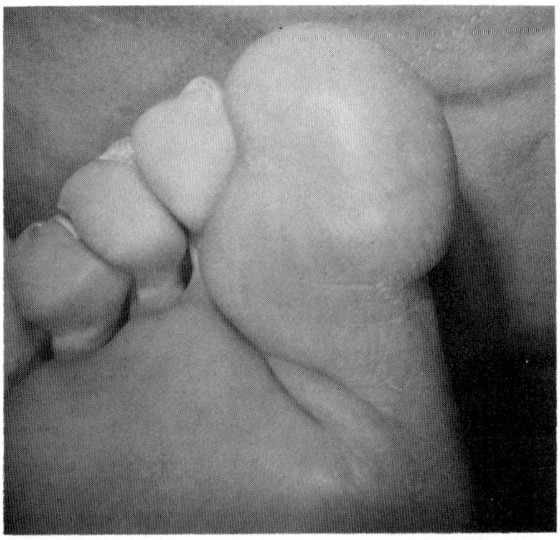

Figure 7.5. Calcified fibroma distorting shape of hallux. Mass is firm, indurated, movable and cool to the touch.

Beckett and Jacobs (14) review two cases of recurring digital fibrous tumor of childhood described by Reye in 1965. This condition is considered a distinct entity among the juvenile fibromatoses; it involves only the digits, recurs frequently following surgical excision without metastatic spread and demonstrates the distinct histopathlogical finding of intracytoplasmic inclusion bodies within proliferated fibroblasts.

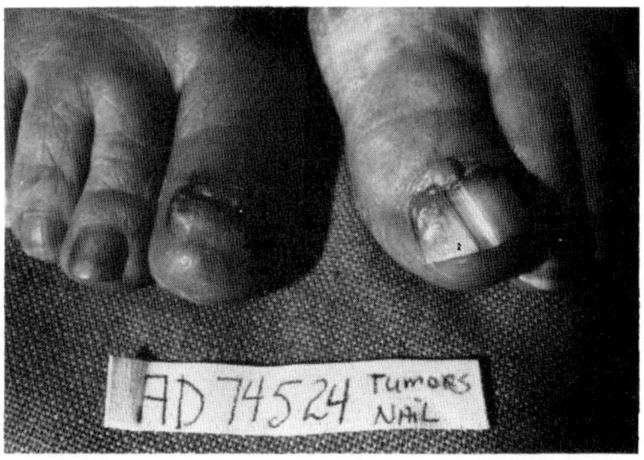

Figure 7.6. Ungual fibromas damaging growth and development of hallux nail. (Courtesy of M Shapiro.)

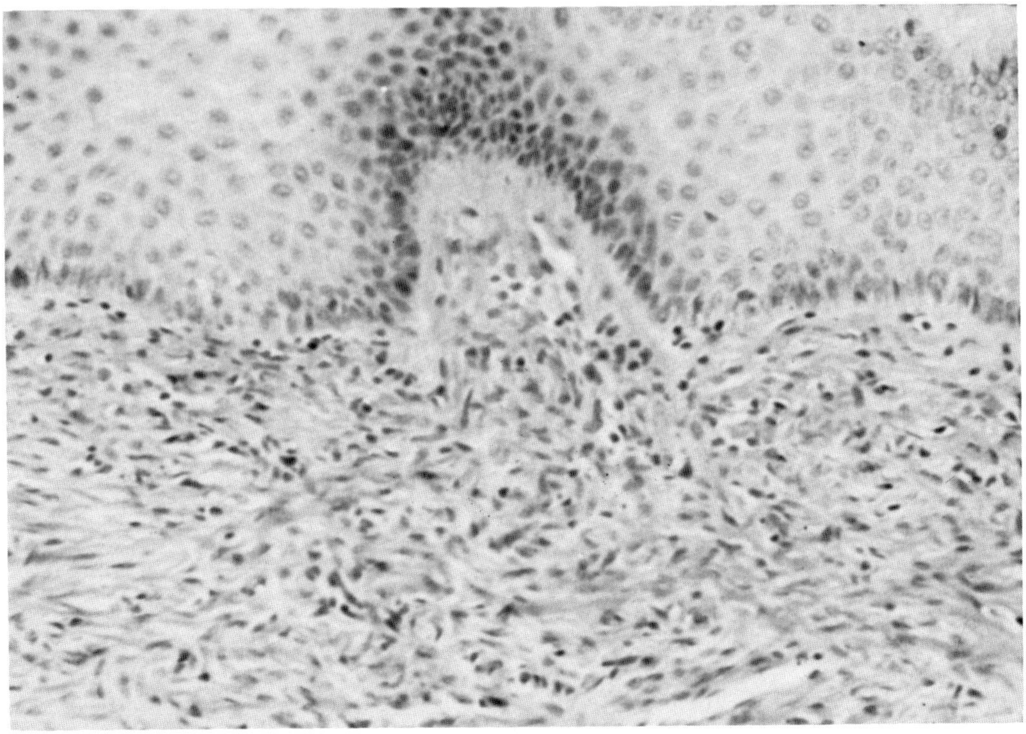

Figure 7.7. Photomicrograph of dermatofibroma. Note the proliferation of fibrolasts and capillaries pushing up the epidermis and distorting the basement membrane.

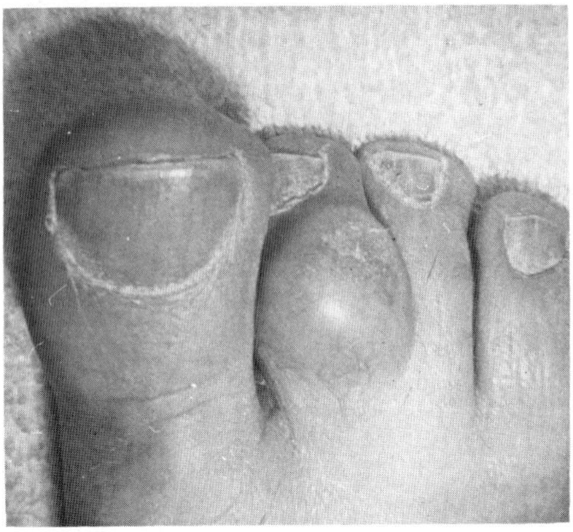

Figure 7.8. Fribroma.

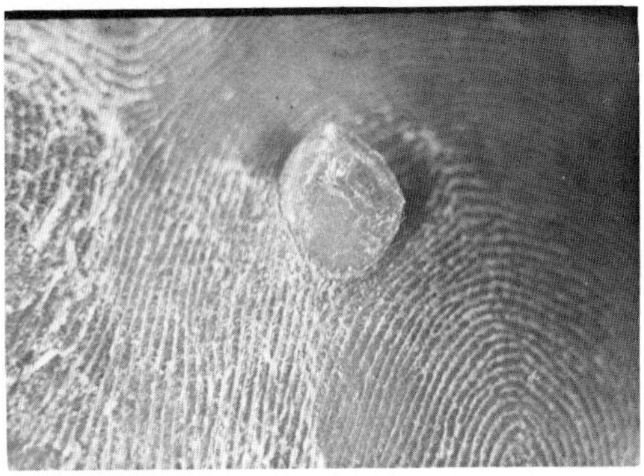

Figure 7.9. Fibroma, plantar surface.

Lerman and Winarick (15), in a study of the literature and a case of acquired digital fibrokeratoma on the distal aspect of a third toe, agree with the conclusions of Verallo (16), who mentions six cases occurring on the toes. Heretofore, most le-

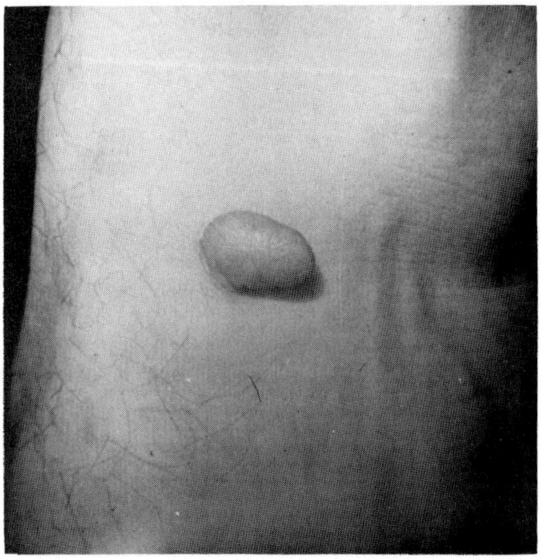

Figure 7.10. Fibroepithelioma, dorsum of the foot. Firm, fibrous, elevated mass about 0.7 cm in diameter with smooth shiny capsule.

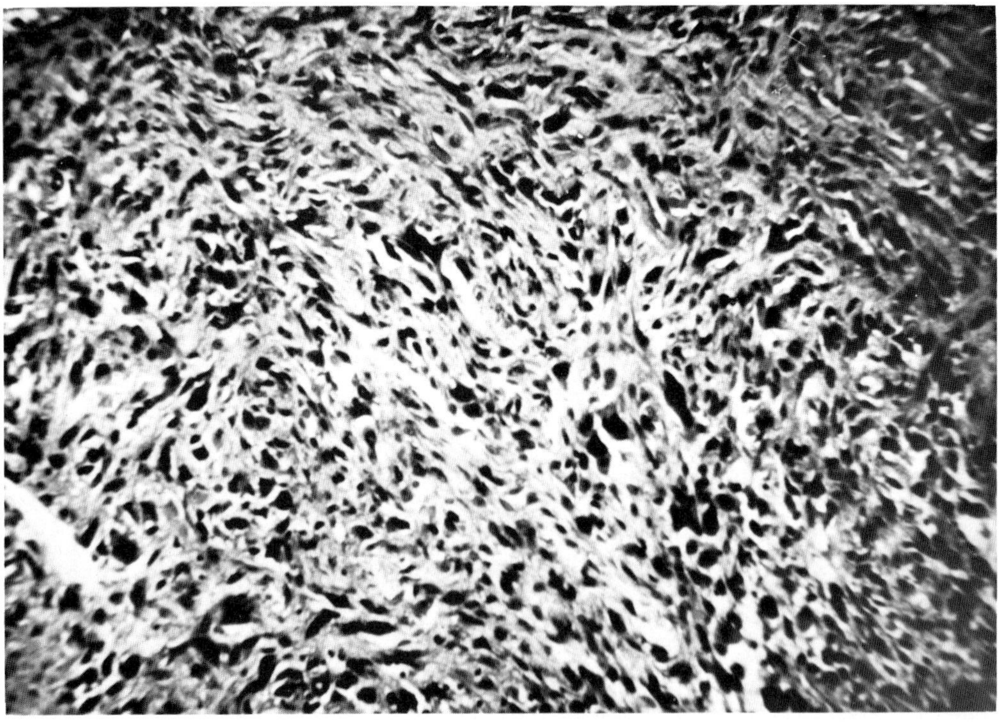

Figure 7.11. Plantar fibroma. Dense fibrous stroma with dark-staining nuclei and little collagen replacement.

sions described were located on the fingers. Following excision, the base of the lesion was electrodesiccated. A differential diagnosis must consider a supernumerary digit that of course, would be present at birth; trauma as an etiologic factor; the epidermal growth of a cutaneous horn without a dermal core; a fibroma simplex over bony prominences, or a subungual fibroma with its characteristic tuberous sclerosis. These articles conclude that there is no relationship between the acquired digital fibrokeratoma and tuberous sclerosis.

Toth (17) describes the presence of a Vater-Pacini corpuscle under the second metatarsal area that is manifested as an oval-shaped movable mass accompanied by burning, tenderness and sometimes pain.

Plantar fibromatosis is usually associated with the medial slip of the plantar fascia. However, the lesions, which may be solitary or in a linear cluster, are associated with the middle and lateral plantar fascial slips as well. Most of these lesions seen by the author have been associated with the medial slip of the plantar fascia in light-skinned males in their thirties or forties. Heavy alcohol consumption seems to be a predisposing factor. Palmar fibromatosis is often present. The rare lesion occurring in younger individuals must be differentiated from fibrosarcoma.

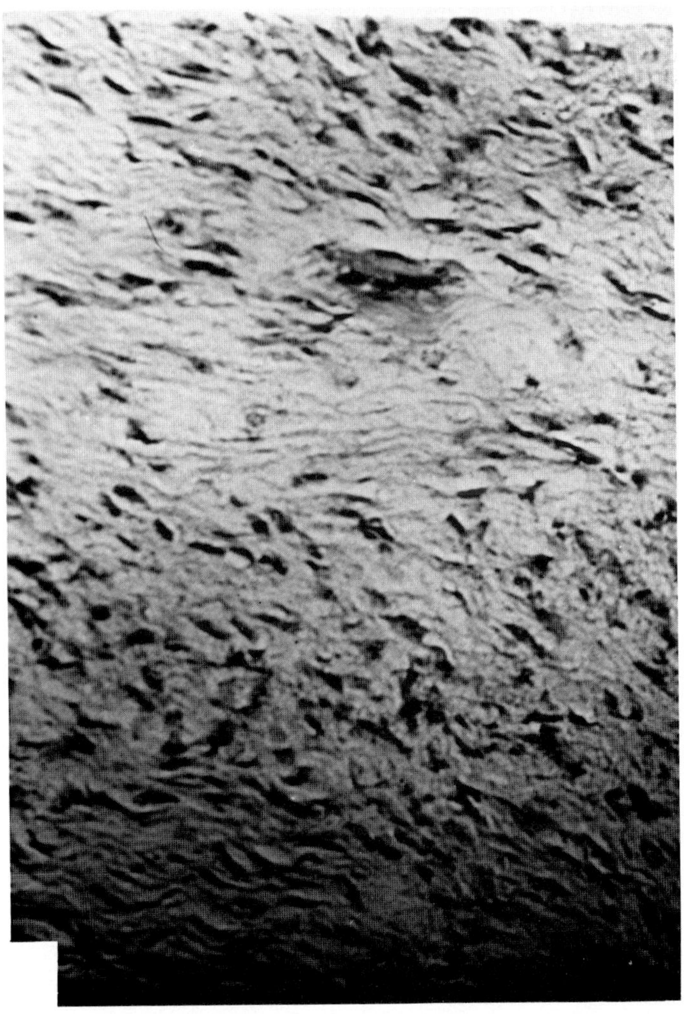

Figure 7.12. Fibroma. Old areas of cellularity have been lost and replaced with collagen. This lesion was removed after having been present for many years.

Treatment. Solitary skin and/or soft tissue fibromas should be excised taking care to include all pathological tissue. Rarely are intralesional steroid injections and removal of mechanical stress effective treatment options for plantar fibromatosis. In the majority of cases, the entire plantar fascial strip and associated lesions must be excised. Care must be taken to dissect carefully the plantar fascia away from the intrinsic musculature and not to interfere with the plantar neurovascular structures (19). One ml dexamethasone (4 mg/ml) is placed around the plantar fascial remnants. Deep sutures are not used. Rather, a running continuous 3-0 dexon or vicryl subcutaneous suture is utilized, followed by interrupted 5-0 monofilament stainless steel wire skin sutures. An adaptic or betadine-soaked sterile gauze pressure dressing is applied. A 1-week decreasing dose of oral steroid is prescribed. The patient is kept nonweight bearing on crutches for 4 weeks after 1 week of elevation. Skin sutures are removed in 3 weeks. A soft accommodative foot orthotic device is used 6 weeks postsurgery. The author has had three recurrences in 12 cases over the past 20 years. These may be attributed to insufficient tissue removal, premature weightbearing, and/or not using intra-and postoperative steroids.

Lipomas. These are soft lobulated masses of enlarged lipoid cells with an increase in fibrous stoma (Figs. 7.13–7.15). The size of a lipoma remains constant and does not enlarge as does a bursa that has been irritated and inflamed.

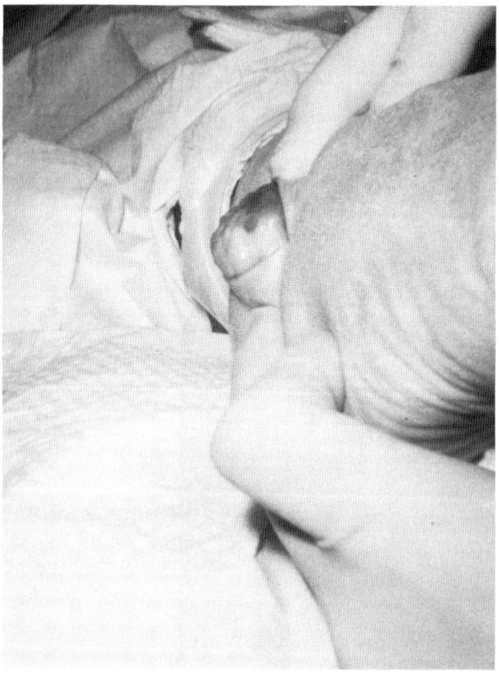

Figure 7.13. Large lipoma beneath lateral malleolus. Not to be confused with normal fat pad deposition seen in overweight individuals.

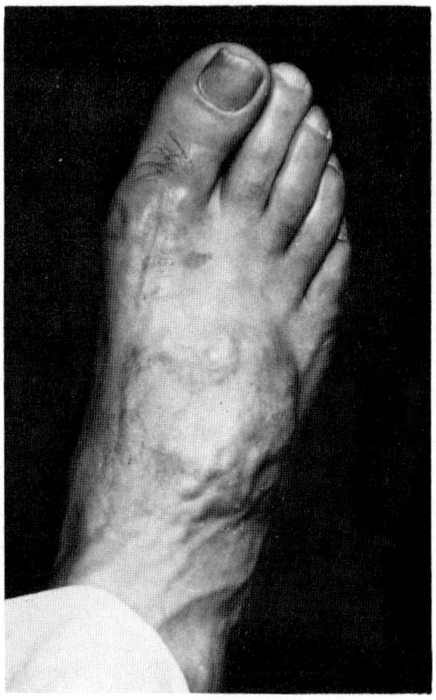

Figure 7.14. Diffuse lipoma. (Courtesy of D Mowbray.)

Treatment. The large lipomatous mass commonly seen beneath the lateral malleolus in women in their fifties and sixties is a normal anatomical variant and should rarely be removed. Other lipomas, if painful or disfiguring, should be excised.

Keloids and Hypertrophic Scars. Keloids are large, heavy scars commonly occurring in dark-skinned peo-

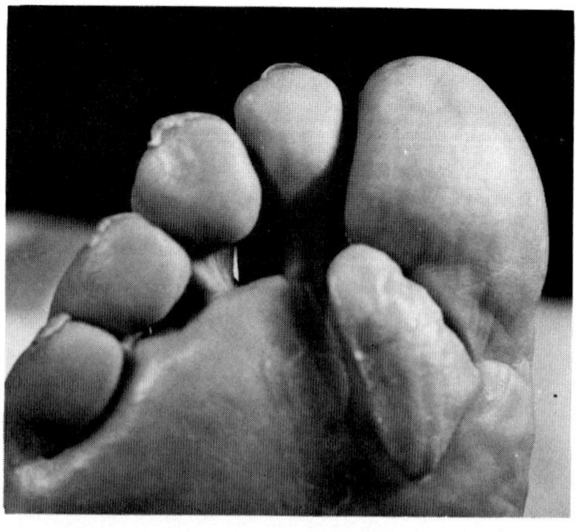

Figure 7.15. Fibrolipoma. (Courtesy of D Mowbray.)

ples and those with Group A blood type. Daniels (19) notes that keloids form beyond an incisional site, whereas hypertrophic scars do not. The scars stand out from the skin and are composed of large amounts of fibrous connective tissue simulating benign tumor formation (Figs. 7.16–7.18). The scars are disfiguring and commonly affect function when occurring on parts that normally are freely movable. Callus tissue often develops in scar tissue, causing pain on pressure. The author has seen several keloids develop following destruction of plantar warts by electrodesiccation. The resultant lesion becomes an intractable plantar keloidal keratosis.

Treatment. Injections of triamcinalone 10 to 40 mg/ml have been recommended at weekly intervals (19). The author has found a total of four intralesional injections of dexamethasone (4 mg/ml) given one every other day to be effective in early keloid or hypertrophic scar formation within 6 weeks of surgery or laceration. Intralesional steroid injections do not seem to be effective in lesions over 3 months old; older lesions usually have to be excised. Dorsal keloids predispose to shoe irritation and abrasion. At the first sign of hypertrophic scar or keloid formation, a topical steroid cream applied tid and ultrasound treatments are of benefit. The use of a decreasing dose of systemic steroids for 1 week, as well as an intradermal injection of dexamethasone at both sides of the incision site, seems to be effective as a deterrent to recurrence. Suberythematous doses of radiation and penicillamine have been reported to be of help in suppressing collagen maturation. On occasion, the use of Dry Ice over the affected part can result in destruction of the keloid and the removal of the hyperplastic scar tissue. Scars may also be removed by the use of a negative galvanic current. Some investigators have noted that the injection of vitamin A into the keloid has resulted in relief of pain and eradication of the scar. Periodic reduction by 40% salicylic acid plaster is effective when combined with other treatment as outlined above. Monochloroacetic acid has proven successful in the slow destruction of keloids.

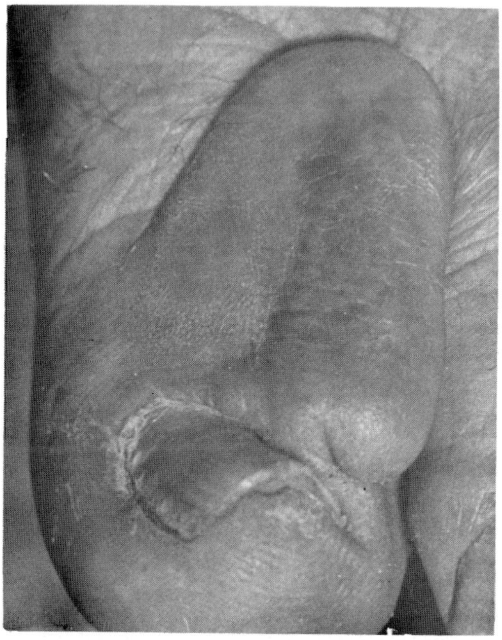

Figure 7.16. Keloid on hallux.

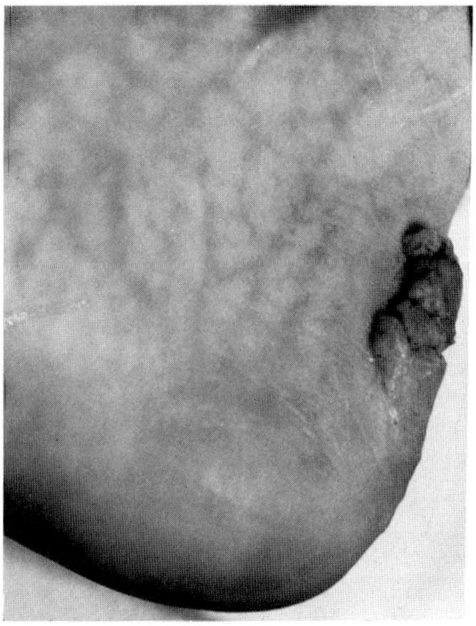

Figure 7.17. Keloid, posterior of heel. (Courtesy of D Mowbray.)

Benign Hemangioma. This lesion may be found in the skin, subcutaneous tissues, skeletal muscles, or tendon sheaths, bones or joints. Deep-seated hemangiomas may cause considerable pain, but when they are superficial they remain painless until irritated by extrinsic factors. Hemangiomas vary in size from a few millimeters to the involvement of a complete extremity. The foot is the most frequent site for angioneuroma or glomus tumors. Kaposi's sarcoma frequently originates in the feet and should be differentiated from hemangioma.

The classification of the various types of hemangioma has been difficult because of their different growth rates, histiologic appearance, and confusing etiologies. Bernhard et al. (20) discuss the clinical and pathological findings, operative technique and differential diagnosis of hypertrophic hemangioma and hemangiopericytoma, two vascular tumors uncommonly found in the foot. Oughterson and Tennant (21) categorized vascular tumors in three groups. The first group consists of the vascular malformations, such as arteriovenous fistula; vascular nevi; arterial, venous and lymphatic angiomas; and vascular blastomas (Fig. 7.19). The second group is made up of the glomus tumor and angioneuromyomas. The third group consists of Kaposi's idiopathic multiple hemorrhagic sarcoma.

The nevi of vascular growths may vary in size from a few millimeters to large, tumorous masses. Combinations of vascular growths may result in marked distortion of the lower extremity.

Treatment of hemangiomas depends on the location and degree of involvement. Treatment may vary from simple destruction through chemosurgical techniques or electrosurgical procedures to the extensive destruction or removal of the diseased parts by radical surgical intervention. Radiation may also be used.

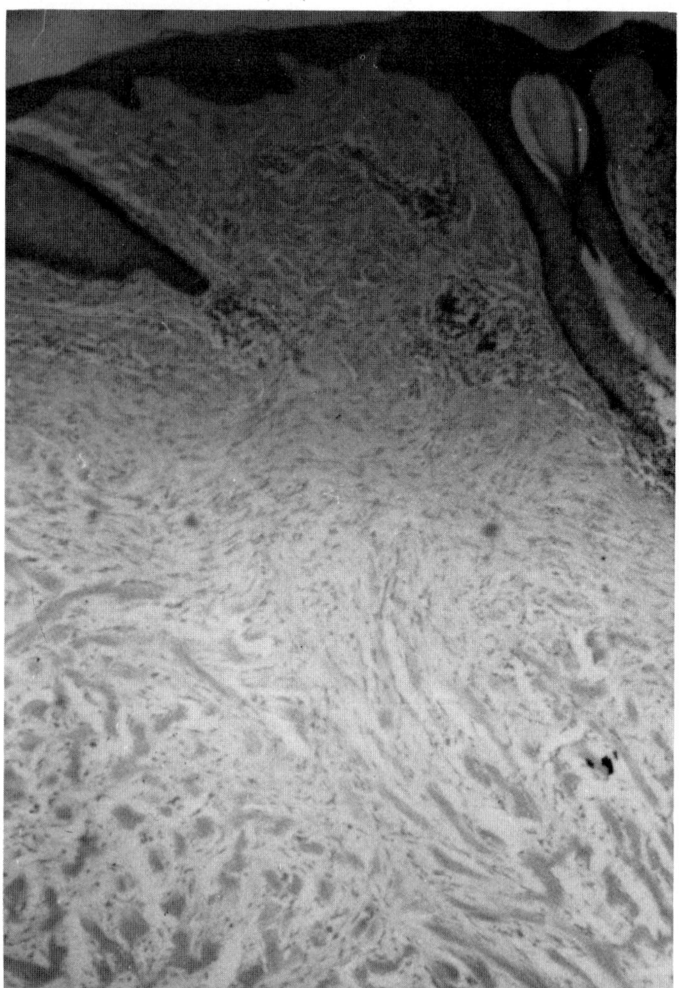

Figure 7.18. Photomicrograph of a keloid; hypertrophic fibrous reaction; bundles of collagen fibers in subcutaneous tissue.

Cutaneous Mucous Cysts of the Toes. The author (22), in a review of the literature and his experience with the diagnosis and treatment of cutaneous mucous cysts, described the lesion as follows: "Cutaneous mucous cysts are soft or fluctuant, rounded or oval, translucent lesions which sometimes are reddish in hue occurring on either side of the midline, over the distal interphalangeal joints of the fingers and toes. They range in size from 3 to 12 mm in diameter . . . In their early state they are covered by a thin, smooth, shiny epidermis. Older lesions may be verrucous in appearance. A straw-colored viscid material may ooze from a ruptured lesion . . . only to fill again without obliteration in 2 to 4 weeks. They commonly occur closer to the toe nail than to the joint (Figs. 7.20–7.22).

Cutaneous mucous cysts must be differentiated from inclusion cysts, sebaceous cysts, fibromas, ganglia, knuckle pads over joints, Heberden's nodes, xanthoma or giant cell tumors of the tendon sheath, blebs, verrucas, helomas, vesicles or bullae due to friction, osteochondromas, rheumatoid nodules, periungual abscesses and hemorrhagic blebs.

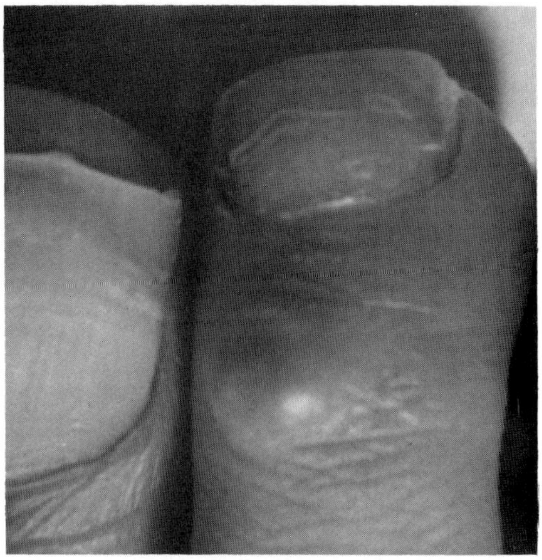

Figure 7.20. Cutaneous mucous cyst in a 40-year-old white male.

Treatment. The refractory nature of these lesions to intralesional steroid therapy and the poor surgical results reported in the literature make the eradication of these lesions difficult. It would seem that a better treatment is needed (22). Complete excision of these lesions, including distal interphalangeal joint dorsal capsule, is necessary for eradication. If adequate skin is not

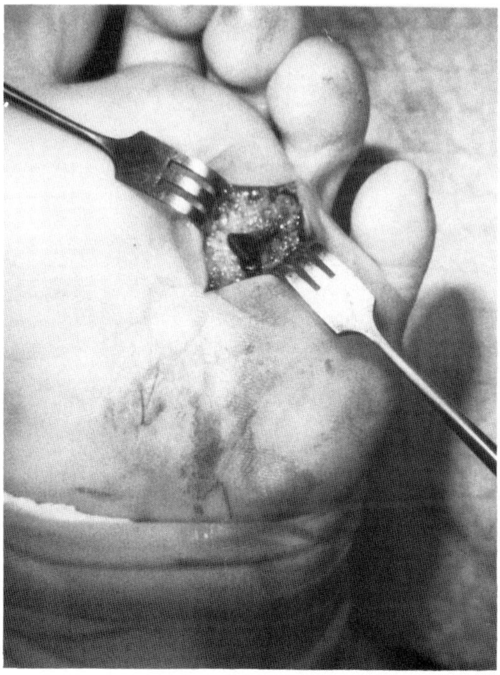

Figure 7.19. Varix.

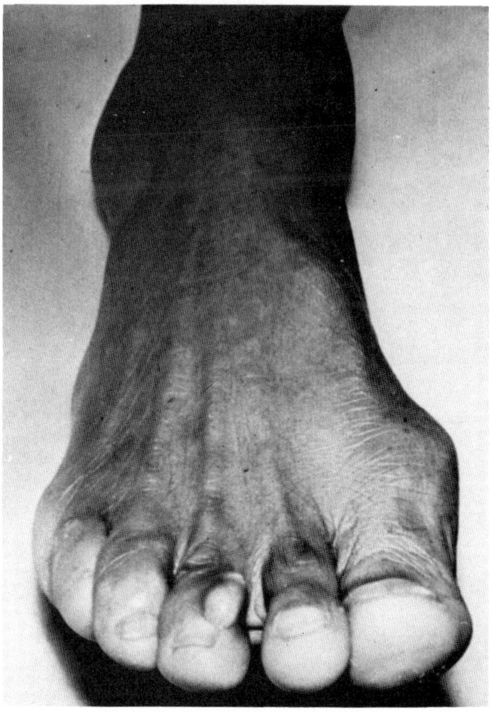

Figure 7.21. Cutaneous mucous cyst, third toe.

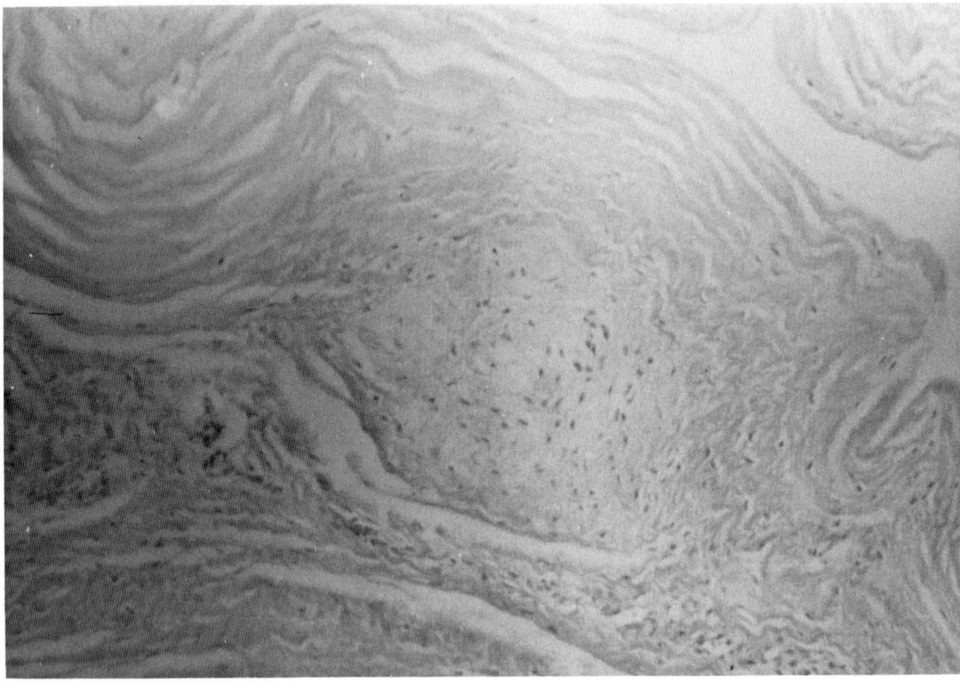

Figure 7.22. Microscopic structure of cutaneous mucous cyst in the late stage of evolution. Cyst has ruptured, and remnants of the cyst wall are obscured.

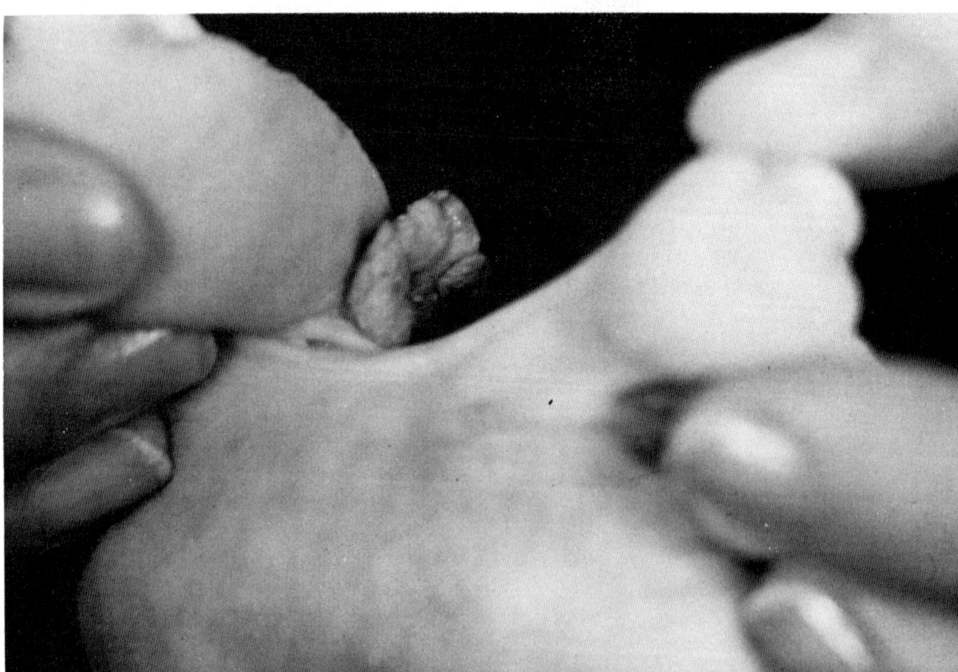

Figure 7.23. Interdigital hemangioma.

available for closure, middle phalangeal head excision or full thickness skin graft (taken from the dorsolateral aspect of the same foot) is indicated.

Hemangioma Simplex. These lesions are elevated and often pedunculated with an irregular surface and a varied color from bright red to dark red (Fig. 7.23).

It is essential to evaluate these lesions both microscopically and macroscopically.

Politz (23) and Cox (24) describe hemangiomata on the toes and heel, respectively. Berlin (25) reported a comprehensive review of these lesions on all areas of the foot. An important factor to consider aside from surgical excision is the differential diagnosis based on clinical and pathology studies. Yet of greater significance is the appreciation of pain that brings the patient to the podiatric surgeon for relief. The authors are in agreement that discomfort is primarily the result of the pressure of the mass in an enclosed area with very little areolar tissue. The toes, lateral aspect of the heel and tumors overlying bony prominences are subject to greater discomfort than other anatomical sites.

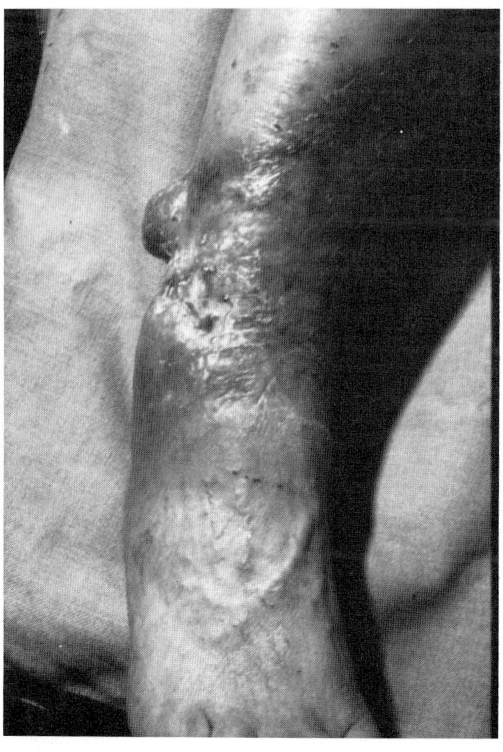

Figure 7.24. Giant hemangioma. (Courtesy of M Shapiro.)

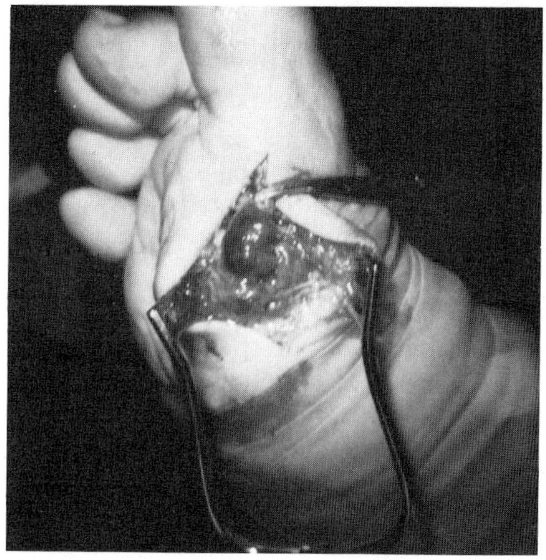

Figure 7.25. Excision hemangioma.

Treatment. If the lesion shows evidence of rapid growth or the development of hemorrhage, it is imperative that it be removed. Removal is accomplished by wide excision and closure with fine suturing material. Compression dressings are applied.

Cavernous Hemangiomas. These growths are typical of hemangioma simplex on a larger scale (Figs. 7.24–7.26). The color varies from red to cyanotic blue, depending on the size and depth of the lesion. Cavernous lesions are connected by vascular channels to the deeper blood supplies. Sometimes only a trace of blue is seen beneath the superficial skin over a wide area. They are spongy tumors, elevated and purplish-red. They are fully developed and do not undergo involution as do many growths noted at birth.

Treatment. The podiatric surgeon can allow these lesions to go untreated unless the patient complains of some discomfort. If removal is necessary, great care should be taken because of the ability of these lesions to spread into the adjacent tissues and the deeper blood vessels. Radiation may shrink the lesion sufficiently to give adequate relief.

Angioblastoma. Despite their malignant clinical and histologic appearance, angioblastomas do not metastasize. These vascular tumors are nodular and are red or bluish-red. Multiple lesions are often present. The larger lesions often ulcerate and become locally invasive and destructive.

Treatment consists of wide surgical excision of the lesion and adequate microscopic evaluation to differentiate it from Kaposi's idiopathic multiple hemorrhagic sarcoma.

Glomus Tumors. These tumors are commonly found in the extremities beneath the finger and toenails (Fig. 7.27). They are composed of muscle, nerve and vascular tissue and originate from the neuromyoaterial glomus in the nail bed. The tumor is red or bluish-red and is found in sites where granulomatous tissue development frequently occurs. Glomus tumors are small and can be diagnosed clinically by their slow growth and characteristic color with loss of normal color reaction beneath the nail. The glomus tumor is often painless, but can be extremely painful, with pain radiating back into the foot. There may be very little evidence of pathology despite severe pain. As pain increases, it varies from a stabbing to burning and excruciatingly sharp pain often out of proportion to the size of the lesion. Plotnick (26) states that the tumor may pulsate and skin temperature may increase.

Sandel (27) described unilateral multiple glomus tumors occurring in the fourth intermetatarsal space and one posterior to the cuboid on its inferior surface. Surgical excision and microscopic examination corroborated the clinical appearance of glomus tumor. Sandel states, "The cardinal point to remember in diagnosing glomus tumor is that its pain is far in excess of any other condition normally found in the part under consideration."

Freed (28) described a glomangioma that appeared on the mediodorsal aspect of the fourth toe. It presented itself clinically as a small, freely movable, sessile-shaped, subdermal mass. The tumor develops from the end organ of the arteriovenous anastamosis. Marked hemodynamic effects may accrue. Freed notes that the prompt removal of the entire glomus

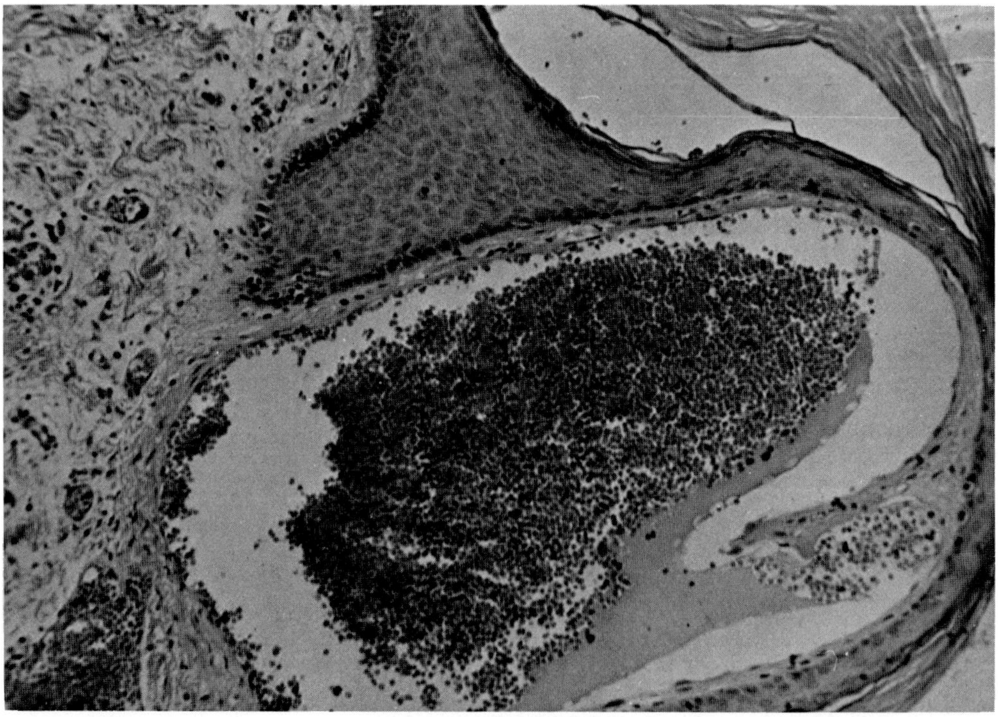

Figure 7.26. Microscopic structures of hemangioma. Vascular channel filled with blood. Channel lined with one layer of cells.

plexus produces intermediate relief of the severe pain.

Microscopic examination of glomus tumor reveals a well-encapsulated lesion. The growth must be differentiated from pyogenic granuloma and profuse granulations so common about the nail groove and lips.

In a scholarly dissertation on glomus tumors of the foot, LaPorta et al. (29) reviewed the literature and described the surgical excision of the benign mass. Of significant interest is that glomus tumors do not always occur beneath a nail plate. The glomus body is an arteriovenous anastamosis surrounded by a plexus of nerves. Glomus tumors have occurred on many internal organs and in the papillary dermis of palmar and plantar skin, as well as in subungual tissue.

Microtrauma is believed to be etiologic, especially beneath toenails. A differential diagnosis may run the gamut of ridiculous to simplistic, such as a subungual hemmorhage. Because of the many potential causes, the podiatrist must be fully aware of the potential hazard of gross error in diagnosis.

The glomus body is aptly described by LaPorta et al. (30) as a local regulator of blood with little or no effect on systemic circulation. It allows blood to flow to the venules during relaxation and to the dermal capillaries during contraction. The local circulation is affected by alterations in thermal and atmospheric conditions that are generally present in the human foot.

The glomus tumor is generally compressible and grossly appears spherical, measuring about 2 to 8 mm in size. They commonly occur in young adults, but have been removed in patients in their fourth and fifth decades. Care must be taken to remove the entire mass, and histologic examination is mandatory.

Treatment consists of wide excision of the lesion often followed by the use of electrodesiccation to the base. It is essential that all glomus tumors or suspected lesions be examined microscopically. A radiograph of the toe to rule out a subungual exostosis is helpful. If there are bone changes involving the distal phalanx, it is often good judgment to remove the entire nail, the tumor, nail bed and the distal third of the distal phalanx.

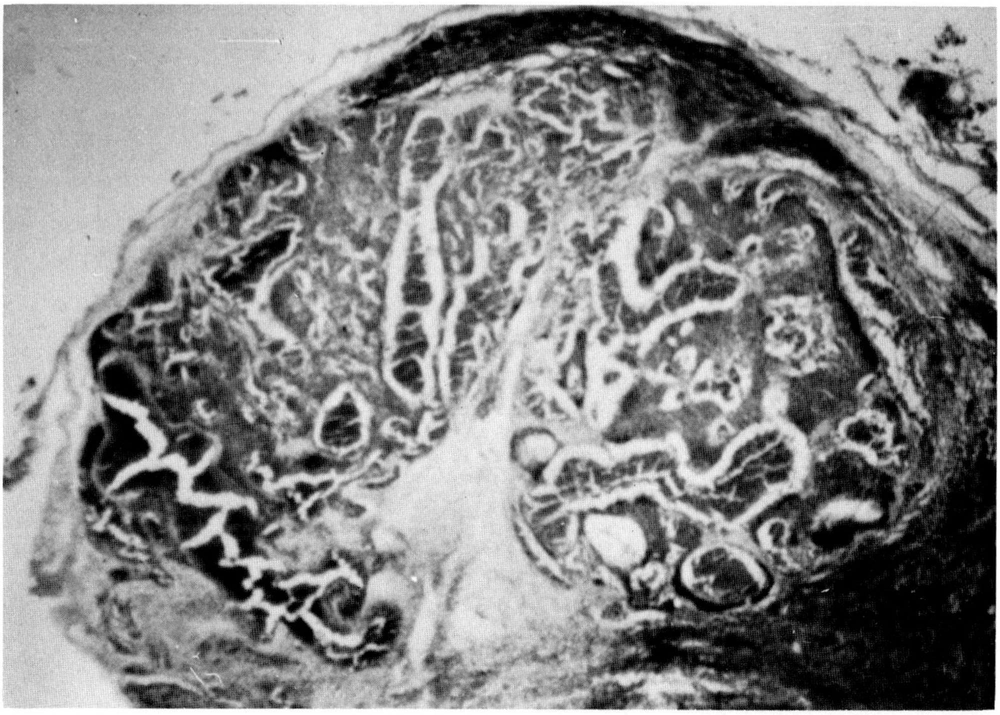

Figure 7.27. Photomicrograph of glomus tumor. Small vascular channels are surrounded by glomus cells.

Sebaceous Cysts. Clogging of the passage of sebum as it exudes from the sebaceous gland results in the formation of a sebaceous cyst. The growth is circumscribed in the dermis and encapsulated by a dense, shiny, white, fibrous tissue containing a cheesy, soft material. They are rarely found on the foot.

Treatment. The surgical excision of a sebaceous cyst is the only successful treatment for these lesions. Semielliptical incisions are made around the suspected lesion. The lesion is followed down to its origin in the dermis and subcutaneous tissue to which it may have extended. The adjacent tissue is explored for additional lesions. Closure is made in the usual manner; however, if the sebaceous cyst is large, closure should be effected with subcutaneous sutures prior to skin closure. Compression bandages are indicated.

Inclusion Cysts. These cysts may originate from embryonic misplaced epidermoid tissue or foreign body implantation. The walls of these cysts are firm and often contain hair, nail, matrix or other foreign bodies (Figs. 7.28–7.35).

The author has surgically removed shiny, white firm inclusion cysts beneath deep-seated tylomas. On several occasions the small cyst was removed from the deep-seated excrescence commonly called heloma neurofibrosum. These lesions occur very often on the ball of the foot beneath areas of extreme pressure and irritation. It is not unusual to find more than one mass in and about the affected part. Inclusion cysts are a common postsurgical complication following nail surgery, arising 2 to 6 months after radical excision of an ingrown toenail. The tissue beneath or adjacent to the previous skin incision scar becomes red, elevated and often pointed.

Treatment. Incision and drainage followed by excision of the entire white glistening capsule are the treatment of choice.

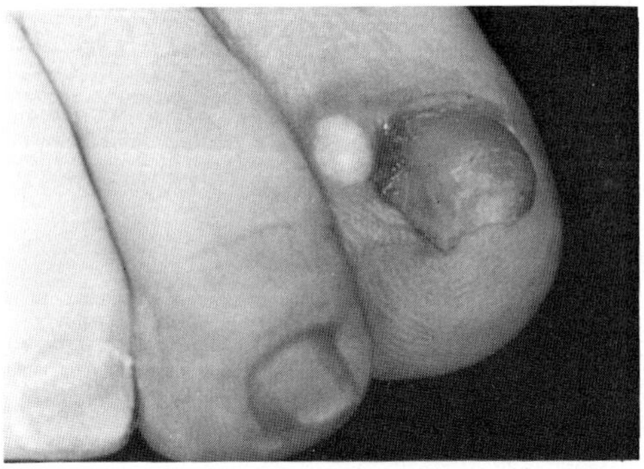

Figure 7.28. Inclusion cyst.

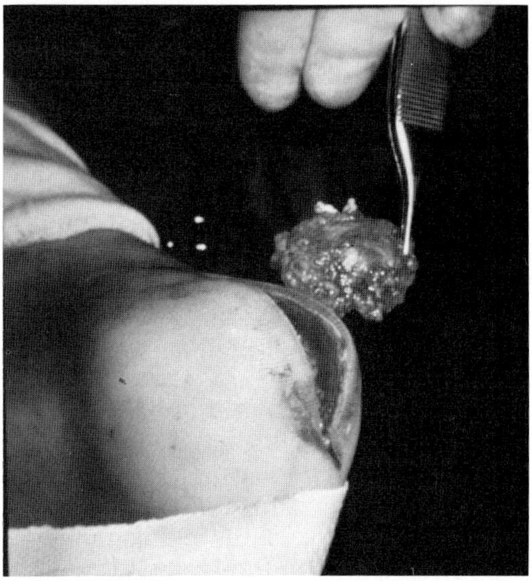

Figure 7.29. Epidermoid inclusion cyst removed from heel.

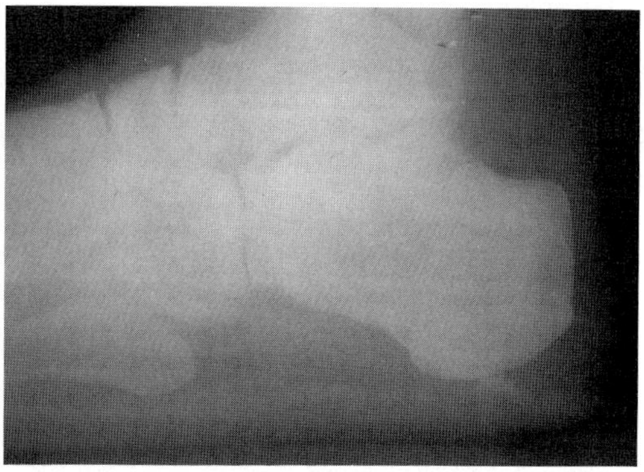

Figure 7.30. Calcified epidermoid inclusion cyst on the heel.

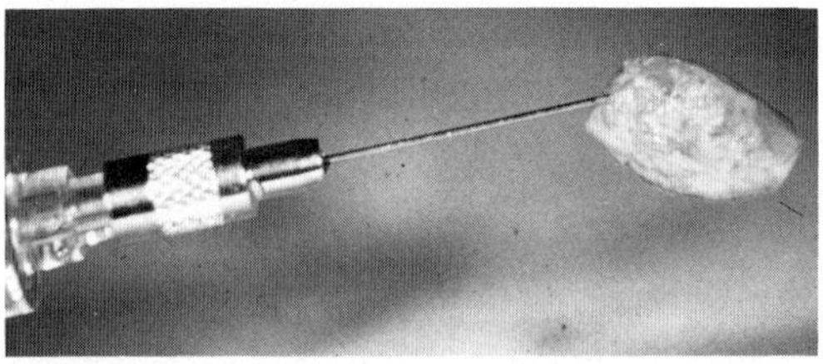

Figure 7.31. Inclusion cyst surrounded by reactive fibrosis due to chronic irritation of connective tissue.

Kaposi's Sarcoma. Kaposi's idiopathic multiple hemorrhagic sarcoma is most common in males and occurs on the dorsal and plantar surfaces of the feet (Figs. 7.36–7.38). The initial lesion is a soft and vascular rare malignant tumor thought originally to be caused by trauma. As the growths enlarge, they coalesce to form red, reddish-brown or bluish-black lesions that become indurated and often mildly hyperkeratotic. The vascular nodules may involute and leave atrophic pigmented scars. The slow development with remissions and exacerbations may be bilateral and symmetrical and often spreads to involve the lymph glands, spleen, liver

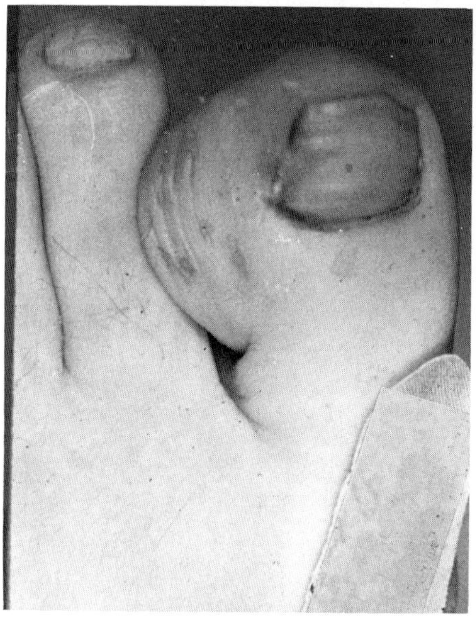

Figure 7.32. Epidermoid inclusion cyst. Lateral aspect of the left hallux.

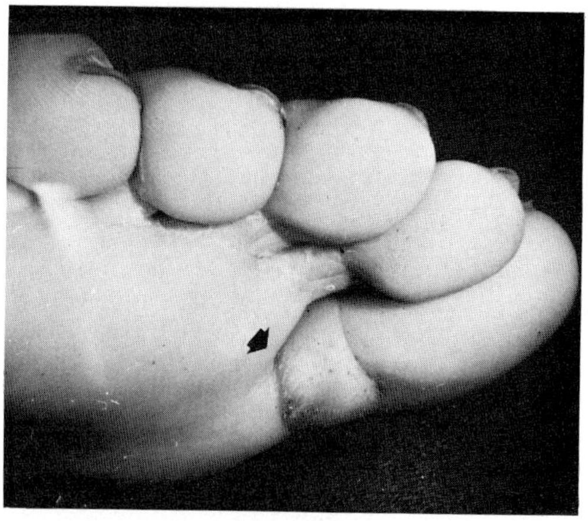

Figure 7.33. Epidermoid inclusion cyst.

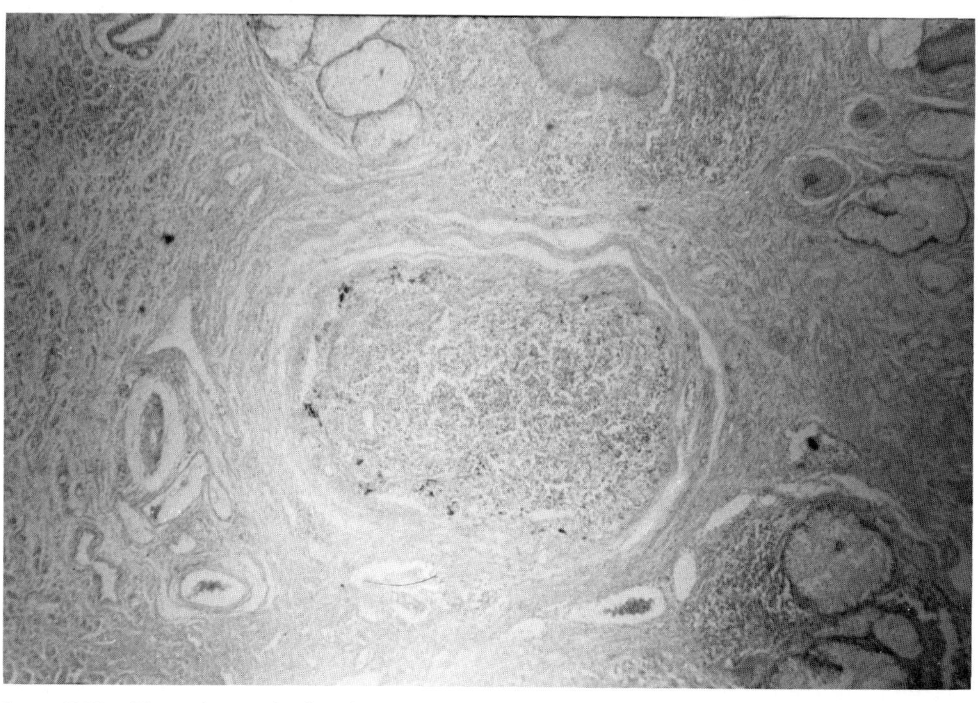

Figure 7.34. Photomicrograph of epidermoid inclusion cyst. Infected, only original wall remains identifiable.

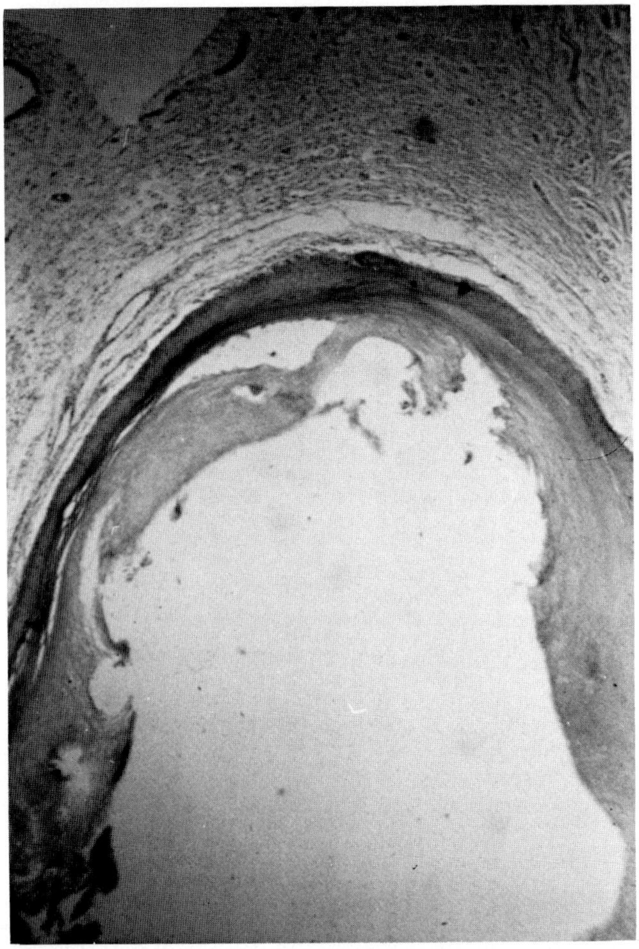

Figure 7.35. Photomicrograph of epidermoid inclusion cyst. Basement membrane is intact, and the squamous elements are easily recognized and maturing in an orderly fashion. Desquamated squamous cells are noted in the center.

and lungs. The extremities may become swollen, hard and distorted, presenting pigmented, atrophic scars. Patients usually die within 2 to 10 years after onset. Early detection before it spreads to the vital organs may save the patient's life, as Kaposi's sarcoma in its early stages is radiosensitive. A progressive form of Kaposi's sarcoma is found in male homosexuals (31). Foot lesions may be the first indication of acquired immune deficiency syndrome (AIDS).

Yale and Yale (32) discuss two cases of Kaposi's sarcoma. In one of these cases the sole of the foot presented several nodules. One of the lesions was 2 cm in diameter, with a large fungating mass overlying a smaller, malodorous, necrotic base. Me-

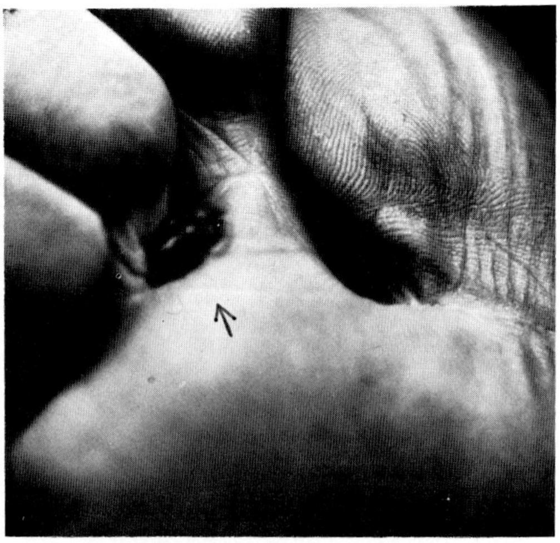

Figure 7.36. Kaposi's sarcoma.

dial and posterior to this lesion were lesions of 1 cm and 0.5 cm diameters with rough corrugated surfaces and dark red bases. Both of these lesions were elevated. Another lesion, 1.5 cm in diameter, was elevated and red-purple in color with a smooth surface.

Treatment of Kaposi's sarcoma is complete excision of the sarcomatous masses. Removal of the lesions does not cure the condition, but very often can relieve discomfort, especially if the lesions have developed on the weightbearing surfaces of the foot. Consultation with an internist is mandatory.

Nevi. The surface of a nevus is smooth, and the growth consists of small, dark pigmented red vascular dilations.

It is essential to remove nevi that show evidence of itching, crusting, increase in pigment or size, elevation, ulceration or rapid growth and hemorrhage. Wide excision and the careful utilization of plastic surgical techniques are essential. It is wise to have all lesions so removed evaluated microscopically by a pathologist. According to Ferguson (33), there is evidence that 50% of malignant melanomas arise from pre-existing nevi. Heller (34) notes that it is good prophylactic medicine to remove nevi on the foot where they are subject to multiple minimal repeated trauma.

Pigmented nevi should be carefully observed for evidence of growth. Davis (35) has stated that when these lesions become cancerous they are the most dangerous of all malignancies. When deeply pigmented and on an area of friction, it is wise to remove the growth to prevent metastasis because transformation of a mole into a melanoma may be very subtle. Commack (36) described five types of nevi.

1. Intradermal nevus (Fig. 7.39)—smooth, papillary, hairy and variously pigmented; they rarely occur below the knee.
2. Junctional nevus (Figs. 7.40 and 7.41)—flat, pea-sized, slightly raised, hairless and pigmented tan to black; they occur below the knee, and most melanocarcinomas are thought to arise from them.

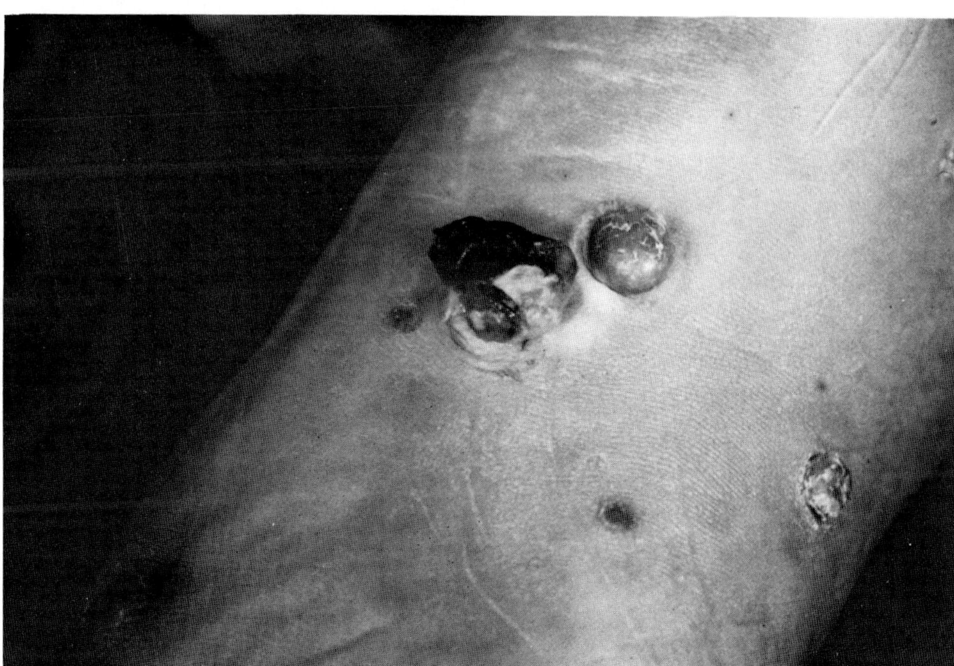

Figure 7.37. Kaposi's sarcoma.

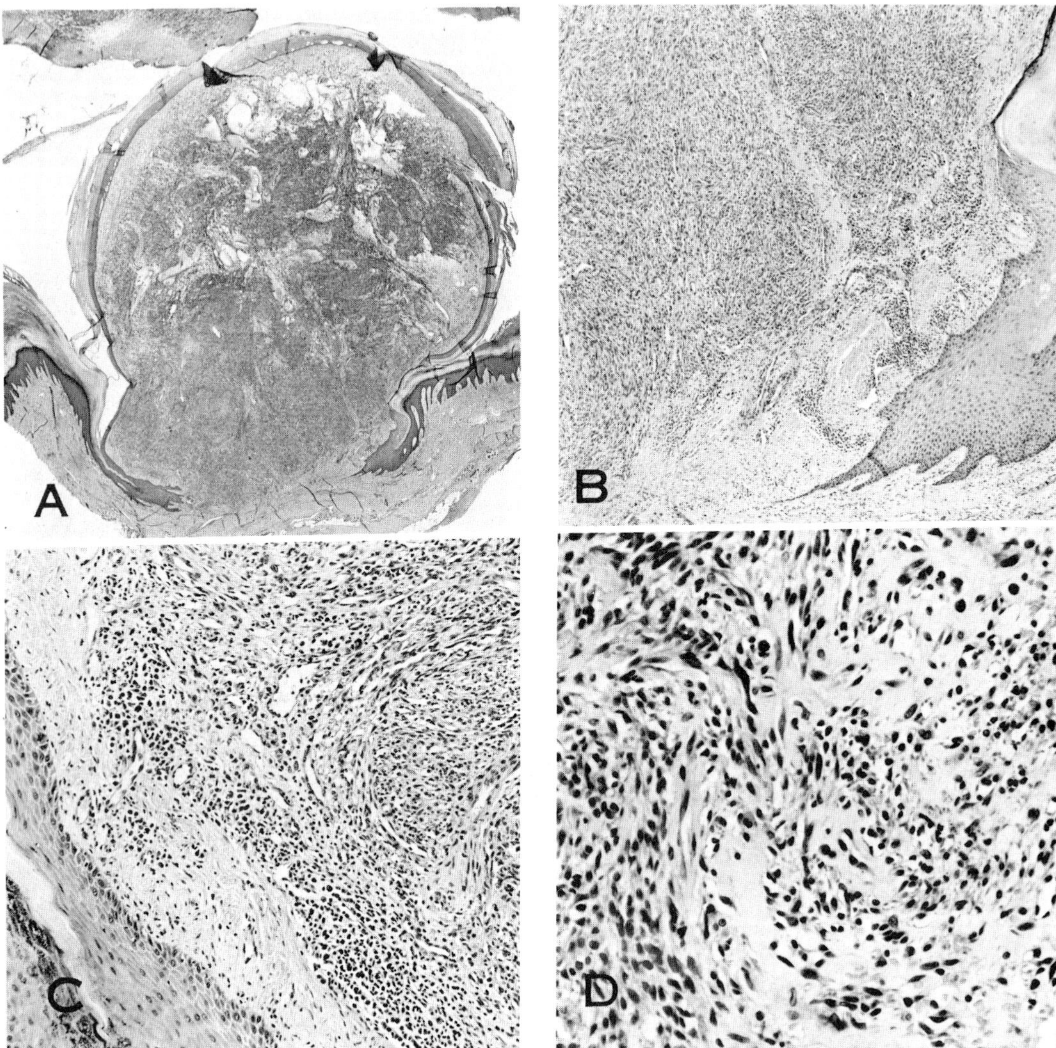

Figure 7.38. Photomicrographs of Kaposi's sarcoma. *A,* Note polypoid nature of the lesion, which is unusual for Kaposi's sarcoma. Many dilated vascular spaces are present in the edematous stroma. This is usually seen secondary to trauma. Thin, pale relatively acellular stroma completely surround tumor and separate it from the epidermis. No tumor in epidermis. *B,* Hypercellular sarcomatous pattern, *upper left.* Below this, a fibrous reaction and chronic inflammatory infiltrate. *Lower right,* Hyperblastic rete pegs. *C,* Note somewhat whorled pattern suggesting fibrosarcoma, *upper right.* Large vascular spaces of tumor; chronic inflammatory infiltrate with plasma cells; fibrous stromal reaction. *D,* Fibrosarcomatous appearance, *lower left.* Capillary spaces and vascular clefts; cellular stroma.

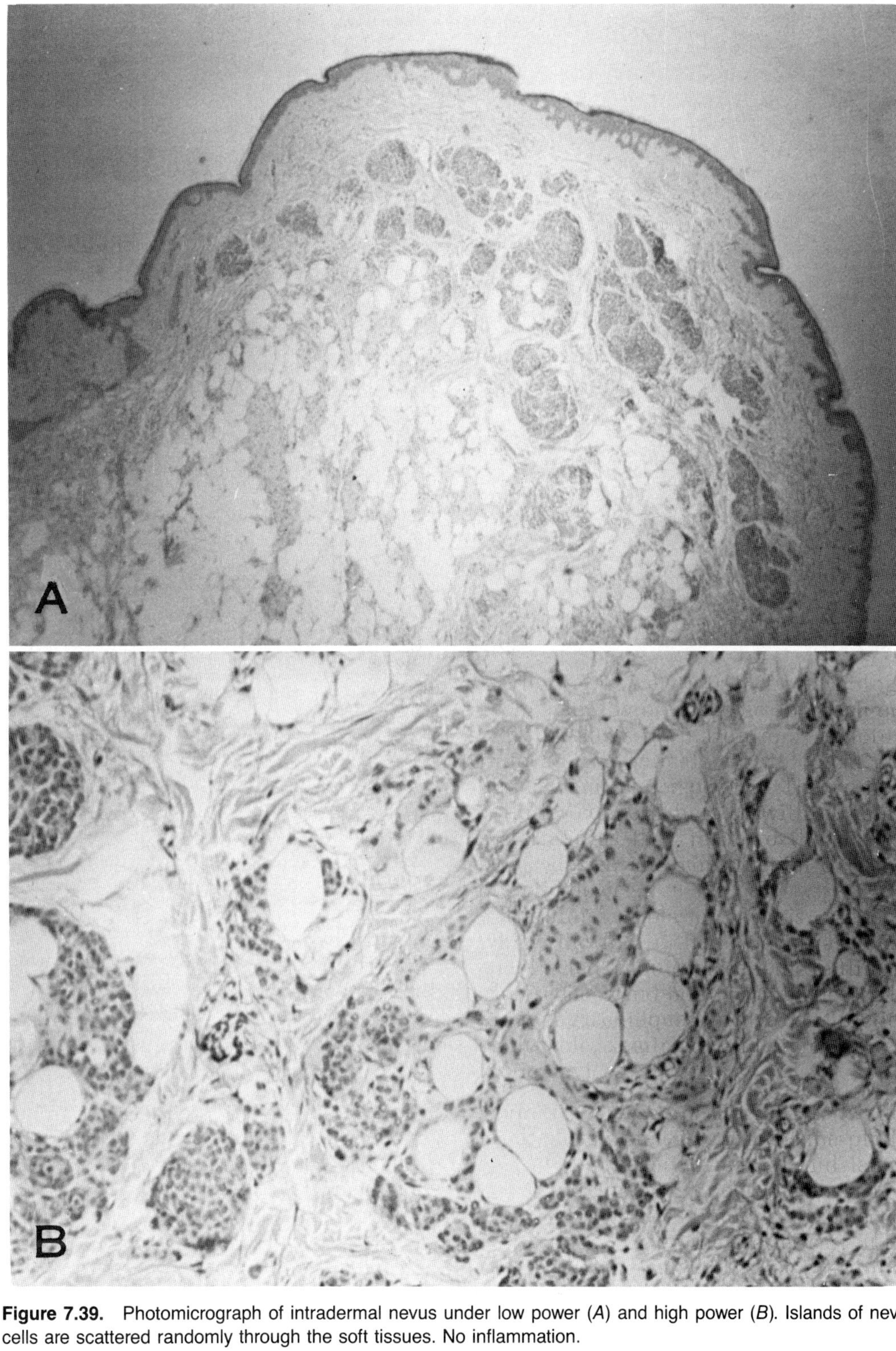

Figure 7.39. Photomicrograph of intradermal nevus under low power (*A*) and high power (*B*). Islands of nevus cells are scattered randomly through the soft tissues. No inflammation.

3. Compound nevus (Figs. 7.42 and 7.43)—a combination of intradermal and junctional nevi; is potentially dangerous.
4. Juvenile nevus—follows a benign course.

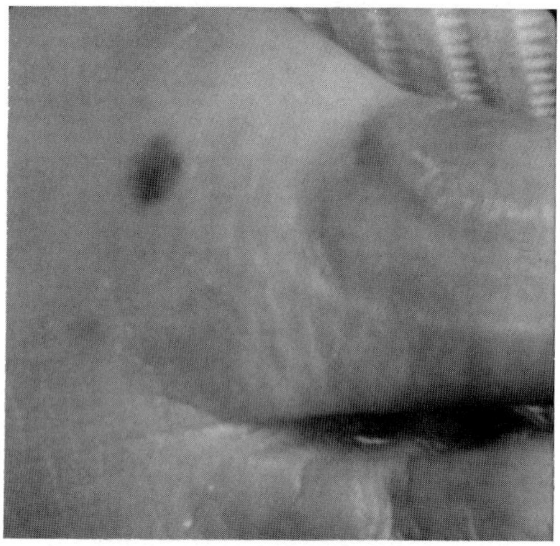

Figure 7.40. Junctional nevus.

5. Blue nevus (Figs. 7.44 and 7.45)—rarely becomes malignant and appears as a blue-black, flat or hemispherical elevated asymptomatic mass.

Treatment. Junctional nevi, occurring on the foot, ankle, or toes, should be widely excised. When there are changes in color or size or if they are located in an area subject to irritation, other nevi should also be excised.

Malignant Melanoma. According to Pack (37), about 15% of melanomas occur on the feet, and about 8% occur around the nails (Figs. 7.46–7.49). These tumors are usually pigmented, but may be nonpigmented. Pack states that 9% occur on the soles. Walker and Cunningham (38) present a case of malignant melanoma and describe proper diagnostic procedure.

The original growth may spread by development of nodules in an erythematous area in the periphery, surrounding the lesions. The peripheral lesions often enlarge and may metastasize to distant parts of the skin, the lymph glands, the lungs or the liver. The tumor is nodular with a broad,

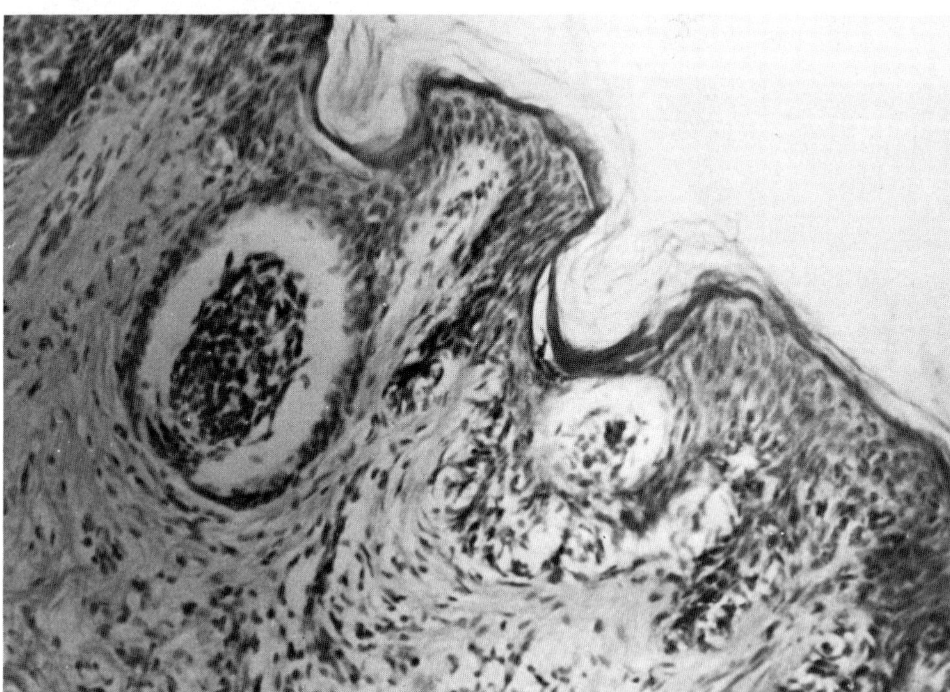

Figure 7.41. Photomicrograph of junctional nevus. Blurring of the basement membrane by marked proliferation of nevus cells.

pedunculated base. The growth may ulcerate and be covered by serous or seropurulent exudates.

The "melanotic whitlow" elevates the nail and is often difficult to differentiate from glomus tumors, subungual exostoses and profuse granulations. The great toe is the common site for all of these lesions. Observation of the nail plate in typical melanoma discloses pigmentation at the periphery of the suspicious lesion. The lesion beneath the elevated nail may be a black, well-demarcated, fungating, ulcerated tumor.

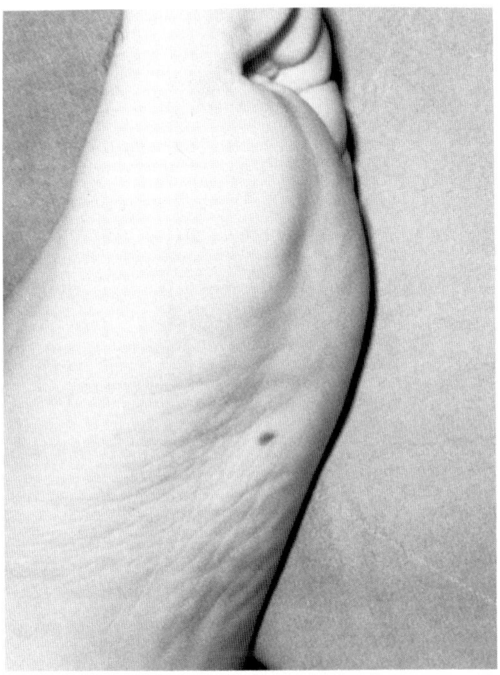

Figure 7.42. Compound nevis.

Malignant melanoma is rare. However, nail bed lesions that appear flat, eroded or ulcerated and black, brown, blue or red, with evidence of extension to regional lymphatics and the vascular system, do occur. A variegated color is pathognomonic. They may be superficially invasive or deeply invasive. The podiatrist's index of suspicion must be high in order to recognize a subungual amelanotic melanoma. The possible masking of symptoms after chemosurgical (phenol-alcohol) nail matrix procedure provides a difficult diagnostic task. When normal healing does not take place after partial or complete nail avulsion or chemosurgical procedure, biopsy is indicated.

A lentigo maligna melanoma is a melanoma variant that is flat and colorful, ranging from brown to black, tan, red, or blue. They spread and often develop an elevated nodule in an old plaque. The nodule rarely presents a surrounding hyperpigmentation.

Mihm et al. (39) presented early clinical signs and a color atlas of cutaneous malignant melanoma. Early detection was emphasized for lesions presenting variegated colors of red, white and blue. The authors considered shades of blue as the most ominous. The nodular type of lesion is generally smooth and may appear "bluish-black, bluish-grey or bluish-red." The superficial spreading type frequently presents a notched border that is irregular. The

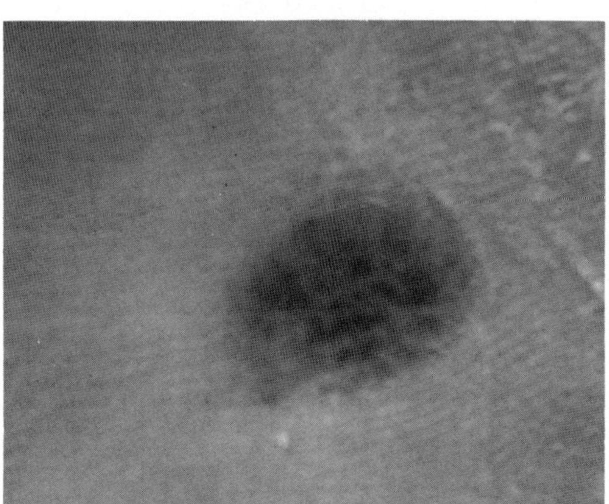

Figure 7.43. Compound nevus.

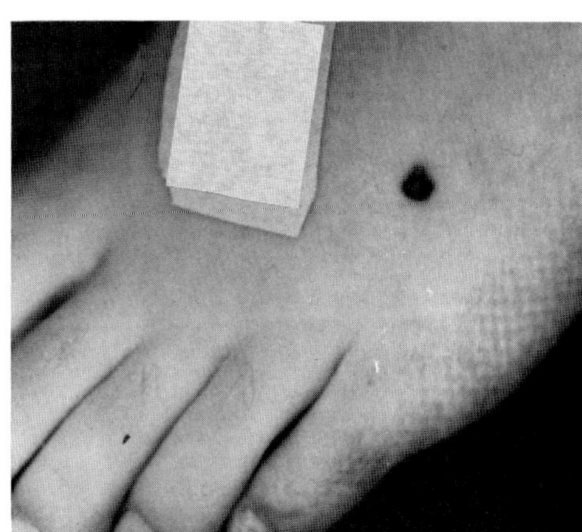

Figure 7.44. Blue nevus.

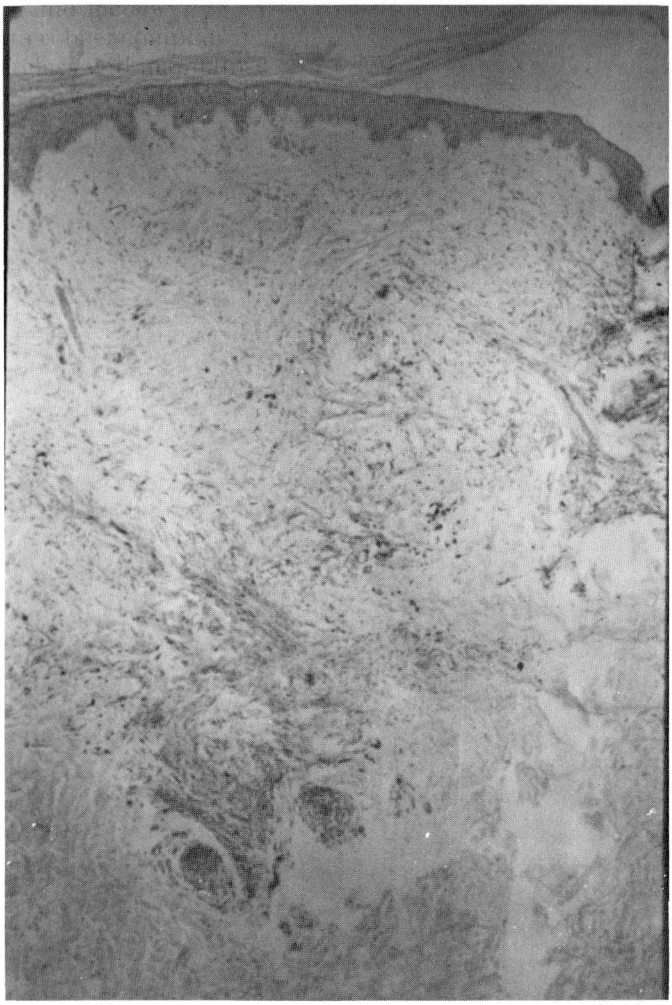

Figure 7.45. Photomicrograph of blue nevus. Common cellular nevus deep in the subcutaneous tissues. Fibroblastic proliferation.

surface may be irregular in the superficial but smooth in the nodular form.

Treatment of melanoma is wide radical excision with adequate closure or skin graft. Proper microscopic examination is essential in order to establish a diagnosis. Regional lymph nodes are excised or radiated. If there is evidence of an extension of the lesion or metastasis, x-ray therapy may be of benefit.

Carcinoma. Primary carcinomas are uncommon on the feet. Although the lesion is commonly believed to be caused by mechanical pressure, friction and old skin lesions and scars, there is no evidence to

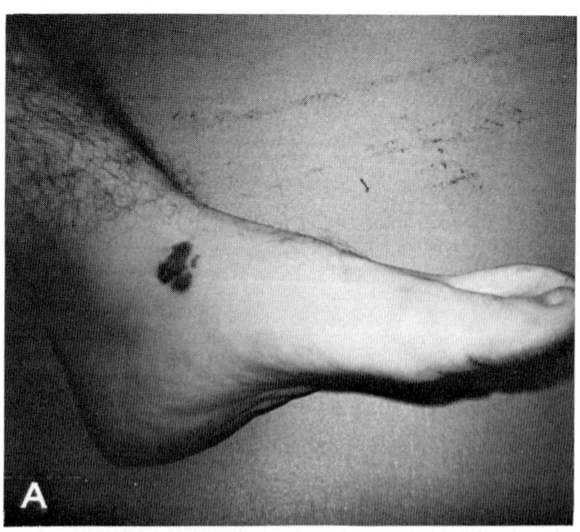

Figure 7.46. Malignant melanoma.

suggest formation of carcinoma from helomas or tylomas.

Keratoses as precursors to carcinoma develop from sun, wind irritants and lowered resistance of the skin. Scars from burns or lupus erythematosus are etiologic. Carcinomatous lesions may develop in chronic ulcers and at sites of benign tumors that have been irritated or irradiated.

According to Gumport et al. (40) *basal cell carcinoma* is the most common form of skin cancer (Figs. 7.50 and 7.51). Its incidence is greatest in fair-skinned Caucasians with light eyes and hair. Though metastasis is rare and the feet are said to be an uncommon site, the presence of characteristic lesions must heighten the podiatrist's suspicion. The nodular basal cell lesion appears as an umbilicated ulceration with a raised firm wax-like pearly border. A superficial lesion may appear to be multiple, with a central erythema and overlay of a dry, crusted skin plaque.

Careful examination and early biopsy are necessary when suspicion is heightened by ulcerations of unknown etiology that fail to respond to conventional treatment. The author has seen several radiation-treated plantar lesions that have developed into skin cancer. Ultraviolet irradiation and exposure to coal tar products may prove to be the exciting factor in the etiology. The podiatrist must carefully evaluate and/or biopsy any firm cutaneous nodule or subcutaneous mass before performing radical excision. It is also wise to

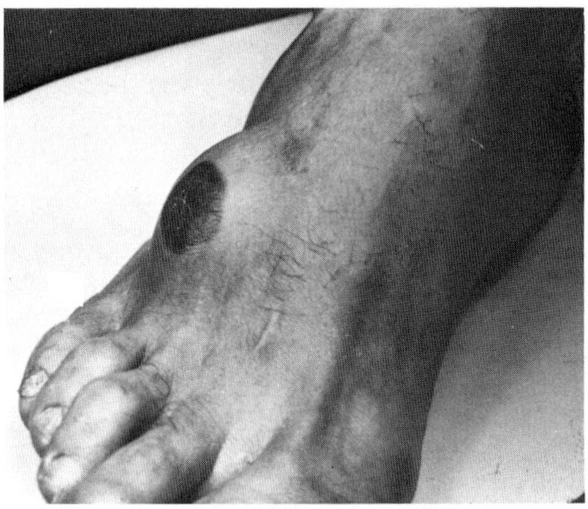

Figure 7.47. Malignant melanoma. Malignancy manifest by rapid growth, indurated swelling and firm mass that is adherent to underlying tissue. Skin is pigmented overlying mass with evidence of central necrosis.

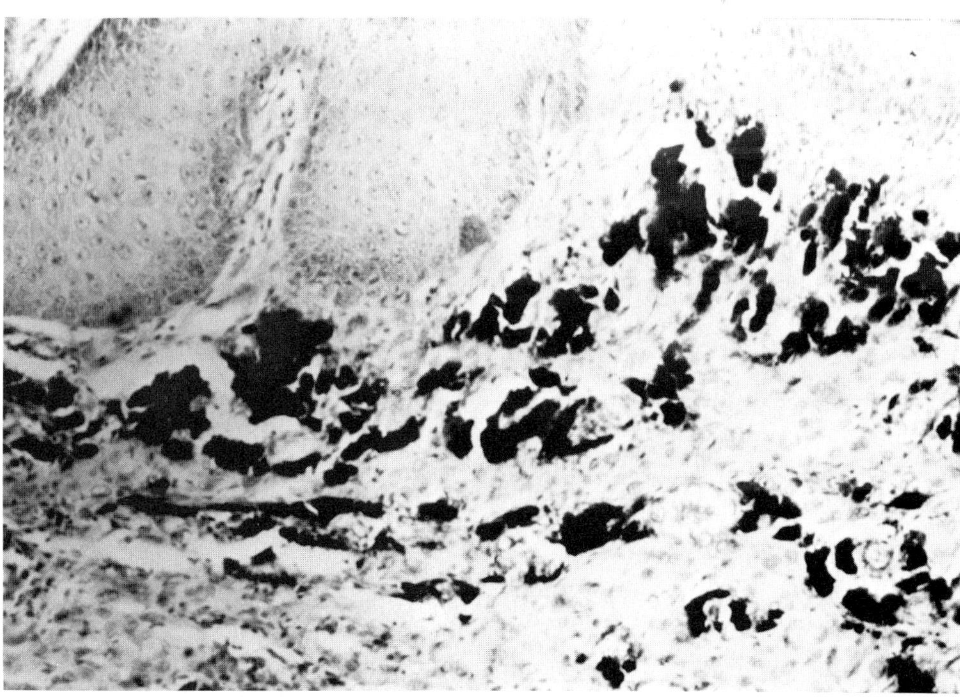

Figure 7.48. Photomicrograph of malignant melanoma. Note unusual heavy melanin deposit.

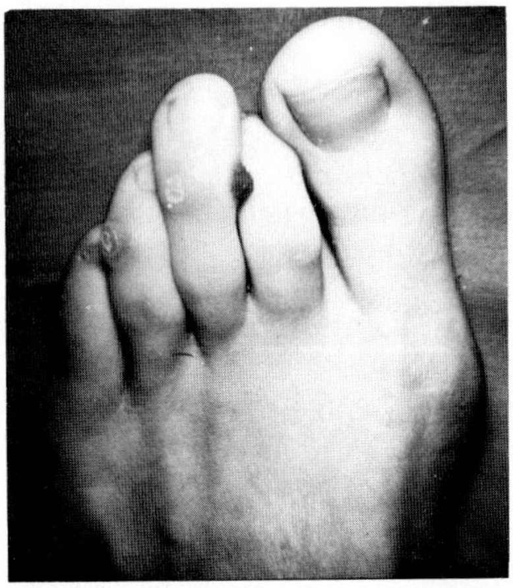

Figure 7.49. Black elevated verrucoid lesion on the medial aspect of the third toe. Occasional bleeding suggests the need for early excision and microscopic study. Excrescences on the dorsum of the third and fourth toes due to pressure from ill-fitting hose and shallow toebox shoe.

biopsy any mole occurring on the foot that changes color or spreads rapidly, whether it be pigmented or nonpigmented, with an irregular surface or border and bizarre shape.

Jacobs and Block (41) describe a case of basal cell carcinoma on the plantar aspect of the heel. They note that because this area of the body is not exposed to sunlight, which is believed to be a common etiologic factor, it presents an additional challenge to diagnosis. The characteristic staining of a large nucleus gives the tumor a basophilic appearance. Grossly, these lesions bleed readily and are small and crater-like.

Early carcinomatous lesions may be indurated nodules with a dry parchment-like surface. A verrucous-like hyperkeratosis may develop slowly, and ulcera-

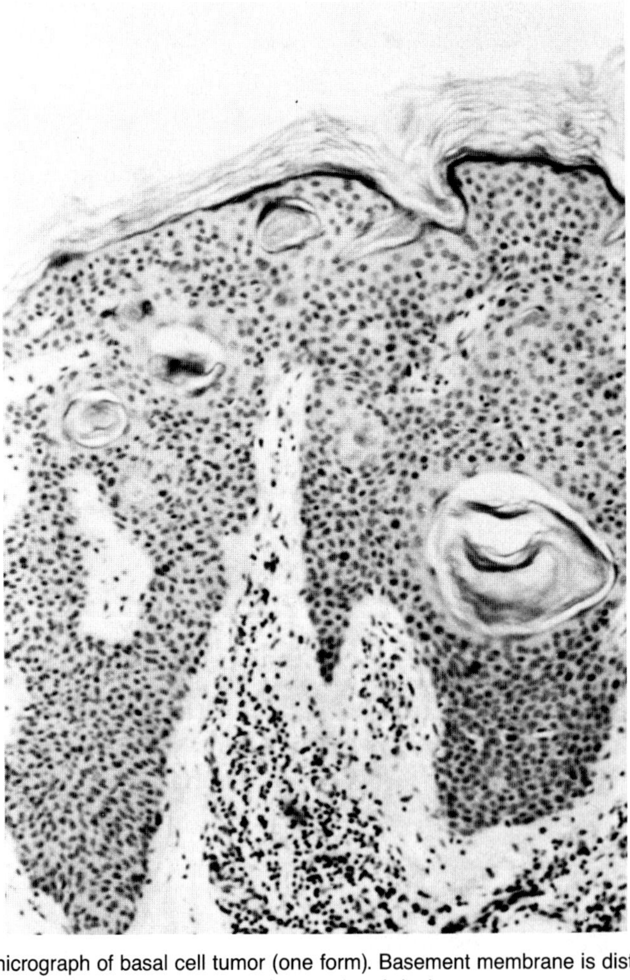

Figure 7.50. Photomicrograph of basal cell tumor (one form). Basement membrane is distorted. Cuff of lymphocytes in the upper dermis is commonly the result of secondary irritation.

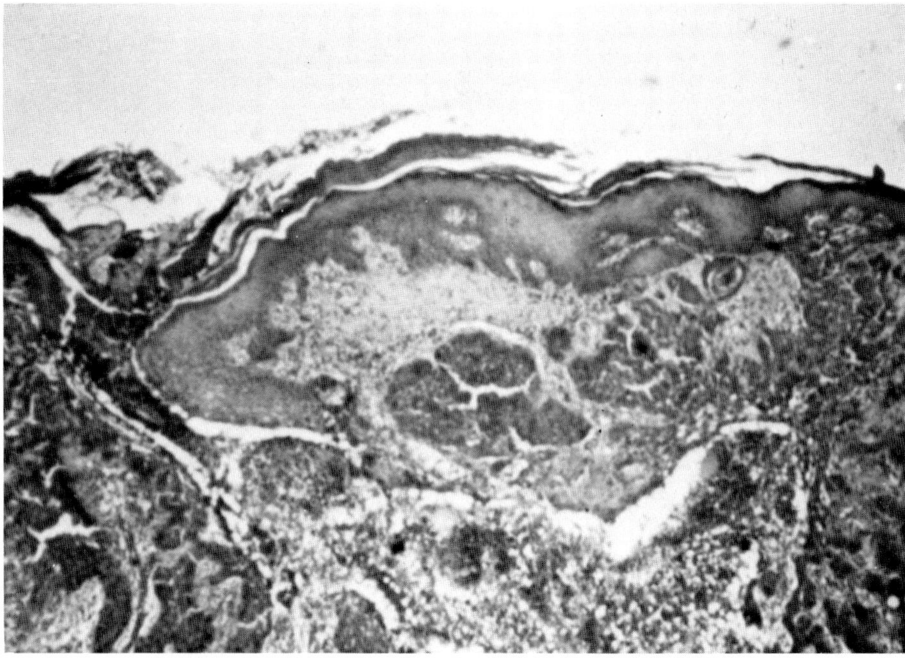

Figure 7.51. Photomicrograph of basal cell carcinoma. Tumor in dermis. Overlying epidermis is intact, which is responsible for the rolled edge around the ulceration.

tion can be the sequela. When untreated, the lesion may become malodorous and fungating. Berger et al. (42) state that "basal cell epitheliomas of the sole occur with extreme rarity."

Squamous cell carcinoma (epithelioma) lesions may or may not ulcerate and are more prevalent in males (Figs. 7.52 and 7.53). Metastasis is rare and is usually induced by trauma. The diagnosis is confirmed by histopathological examination. Squamous cell carcinomas are malignant, but have an activity similar to benign growths. They may, however, metastasize.

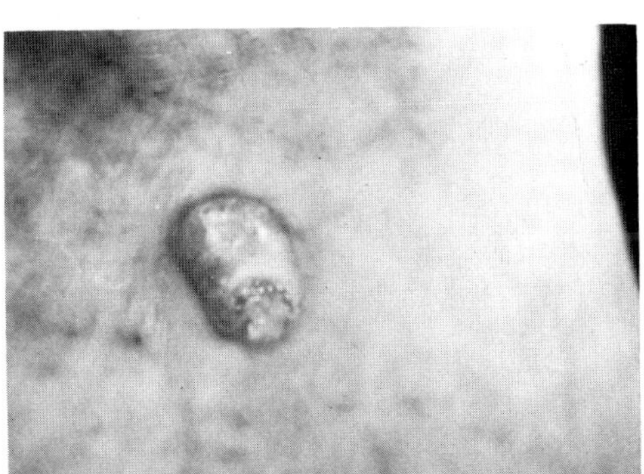

Figure 7.52. Epithelioma. Ulcerated skin nevus.

The squamous cell carcinoma usually occurs at sites exposed to sunlight or other actinic radiation. In contrast to basal cell lesions, they are opaque or present an ulceration with a large central fungating mass. Squamous cell carcinoma rarely occurs on the feet, but the astute diagnostician will evaluate suspicious lesions, their regional lymph node reactions and any evidence of pulmonary metastasis.

Hlavac (43) describes a rare calcifying epithelioma. Unlike other epitheliomas, this lesion does not metastasize. The etiology is unknown, and radiographic examination resembles calcinosis circumscripta. The pathology, however, is different, containing nests of poorly staining epithelial cells and lobules of eosinophilic invaded tissue separated by dense fibrous connective tissue. Occasional giant cell reactions with calcareous degeneration may be present.

Galinski et al. (44), in a study of the literature, report on two cases of squamous cell carcinoma of recent origin occurring on the feet. Many of these growths

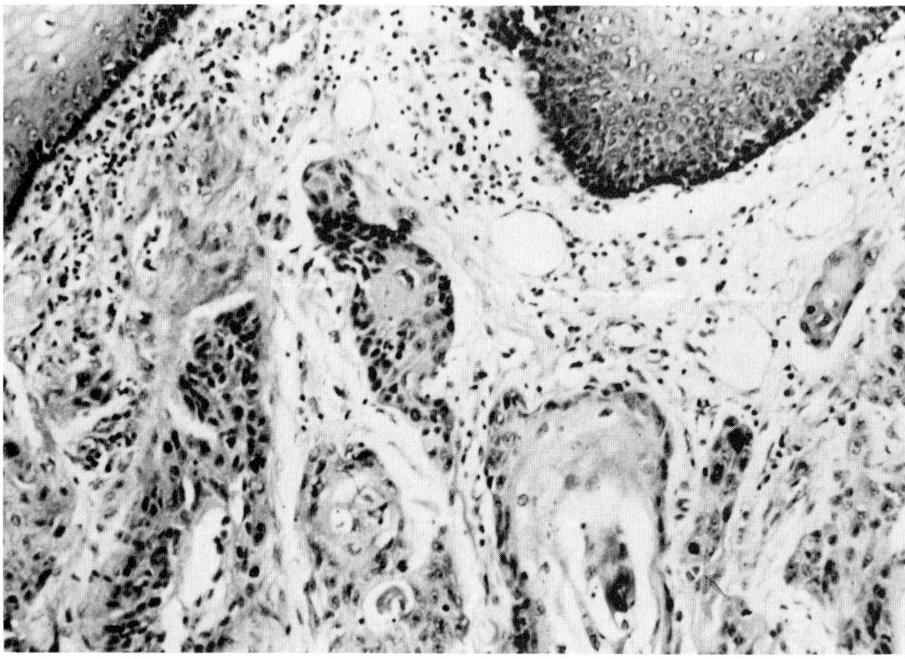

Figure 7.53. Photomicrograph of squamous cell carcinoma—epithelioma. Islands of tumor composed of abnormal squamous cells. Several pearls are noted. Abnormal mitotic figures are present.

have been reported in podiatric literature. Of significance is the location of these lesions beneath the hallux nail and the fourth toenail. The changes in the nail bed are characteristic and require differentiation from ulcers due to trauma, granulomas, basal cell carcinomas, malignant melanoma, verrucas and onychocryptosis, The nail plate is unusually elevated from its bed, a serosanguinous fluid may exude and the nail bed color will vary from a deep red to blue-black. According to Galinski et al., "the malignant character of the cancer is noted by the lack of a limiting layer of fibrous capsule, presence of a number of irregular mitotic figures and the invasion of lymphatic spaces by the neoplastic cells." Histologic studies are imperative, and early surgical excision and/or amputation is advised.

Three cases of biopsy-proven squamous cell carcinomas occurring on the plantar surface of the foot are reported by Snider and Demuth (45). Although this condition is uncommon, the authors caution the doctor to perform a biopsy of plantar lesions that are atypical or chronic. In each case reported, the patient had initially been treated for a plantar verruca. Treatment following laboratory studies consisted of excision and skin grafts.

Epithelial cancer of a toe originating locally from an inflamed heloma molle aggravated by "corn remedies" has been reported. The malignancy diagnosed upon biopsy and subsequent surgical removal as a squamous cell epithelioma was accompanied by an extreme cellulitis of the foot. The malignant growth measured 1½ × 2½ cm.

Squamous cell carcinomas on the foot have appeared clinically as ulcerations about 0.5 cm in diameter with surrounding induration and infiltration. The margins are elevated, hard and undercut. The base resembles poor granulating tissue and is gray in color.

Carcinoma may be caused by prolonged exposure to x-rays. The new growth has the microscopic characteristics of a squamous cell lesion. This lesion is accompanied by a numbness, roughening and fissuring of the skin. The fissures become painful, and the skin may become a mottled gray to dark brown. A general inflammatory infiltration and typical squamous cells are present on microscopic examination.

A personal case of a malignant fibrous histiocytoma and a review of the literature by Smith et al. (46) indicate the variety of this lesion. Podiatrists must consider this lesion in a differential diagnosis of a large, firm subcutaneous mass. At operation, the mass is usually well-encapsulated, white and freely movable. However, microscopic studies may reveal spindle-shaped histiocytes, large multinucleated giant cells and a well-developed capsular structure. Regional lymph glands must be carefully examined for metastasis. Wide excision of the lesion is recommended. Consultation is indicated to evaluate the need for chemotherapy, radiotherapy or amputation, because this lesion is not usually invasive despite its malignancy. An extranodal lymphoma (Fig. 7.54) is rarely found in the foot.

Treatment. Robins (47) reported a 98% cure rate in the chemosurgical treatment of basal cell carcinoma where electrodesiccation, surgery and irradiation had failed. The treatment consists of dichloroacetic acid applications to the mass to break down the keratin in preparation for further treatment. Zinc chloride is then applied to fix the tissues. After several hours, the lesion is removed. The tissue is fixed and mapped prior to examination, and the boundaries are checked for tumor tissue. The process is repeated until all boundary tissue is negative.

Wide excision of both basal and squamous cell carcinomas is recommended. Oncology consultation is mandatory.

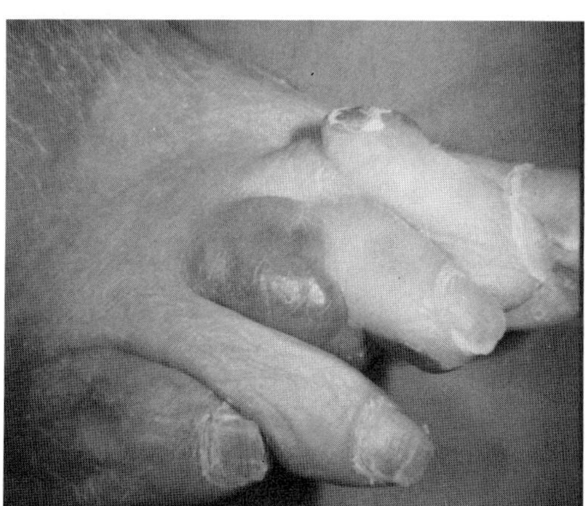

Figure 7.54. Extranodal lymphoma third toe.

Synovial Sarcoma. These rare tumors are malignant growths of connective tissue origin involving the tendon sheaths and synovial membranes. The duration of symptoms varies from several months to several years. Pain, swelling and abnormal function of the limb are the usual outstanding symptoms.

The tumor is attached to or invades the tendon, synovial membrane or joint capsule. It is usually soft, white and fleshy (depending on its vascularity), or it may have a velvety, purplish appearance.

Jaworek (48) describes a case of synovial sarcoma over the midportion of the shaft of the second metatarsal. On excision, this lesion measured 2.5 × 2.8 × 1 cm. Of significance to podiatrists is the need for early examination of any firm mass that is adherent and presents marked vascularity, rapid growth and histopathological mitotic cells. The presence of a pathology confirmation alone is not enough. A search for metastasis in this case revealed metastases to the tarsal and ankle joints resulting in the lifesaving surgical amputation of the limb above the knee within a week of complete body scanning.

Treatment. Extensive surgical removal of the growth and regional lymph glands followed by radiation therapy may be adequate treatment. Amputation is indicated where metastasis is in evidence.

Neuroma. Tumors of the nerves are not common. Traumatic neuromas (amputation neuromas) may be seen at the end of amputated stumps and are excruciatingly painful.

Hard, indurated tumors on the tendons or in subcutaneous tissues may be neurofibromas, as seen in Recklinghausen's disease. They occur in all parts of the body and are usually multiple. Occasionally a neurofibroma may prove malignant on histologic examination. The ankle joint is the usual site of a neurofibrosarcoma. Neurofibromas are often grayish-white in color.

Neurofibrosarcoma may arise from the tendon sheaths or joint capsules. Many of the sarcomas containing spindle cells originate from connective tissue cells in or around the nerve tissue. The round cell sarcomas grow rapidly and present an irregularly outlined tumor that is pink in color and prone to metastasis.

Treatment. Total excision of the mass is the treatment of choice.

Morton's Neuroma. McElvenny (49) and Betts (50) have expanded the earlier studies of Morton by surgically removing and performing gross and microscopic examinations of neurofibromas on the most lateral branch of the medial plantar nerve in the third intermetatarsal space. Grossly, the outside of the tumors is soft and contains connective tissue cells and fat cells; the central portion is dense, fibrous in texture and gray-white in color (Figs. 7.55–7.60).

Trauma or irritation of the nerve is thought to be etiologic. The neurofibromatous lesion is usually found between the bases of the proximal phalanges of the third and fourth toes. The nerve at this point is rather thickened due to its origin from the communicating branch of the lateral plantar nerve and the most lateral branch of the medial plantar nerve. This neurofibroma is sometimes enveloped by a bursal sac and also has tendencies toward development of an angioneurofibroma. Multilocular ganglionic cysts have also been anatomically associated. Some pathologists describe a neurinoma as the etiologic factor. This is generally the result of a thickening of the sheath of Schwann. Neurinomas can involve any of the distal nerves. Scotti (51) states that the affected nerve becomes demyelenized; nerve fibers are lost and fibrosis with localized swelling of the nerve occurs.

In a 15 year histopathological review of the author's records concerning excision of Morton's neuroma in the third intermetatarsal space, it was found that all lesions involving nerve revealed perineural fibrosis, intrafasicular edema, fibrosed V-P corpuscles and, in long-standing lesions, terminal hyalinization. Operative reports in over 200 cases reveal a predisposition to the medial digital nerve branch to the fourth toe in over 75% of the cases.

Bartolomei and Wertheimer (52), in a review of 97 hospital patients who had

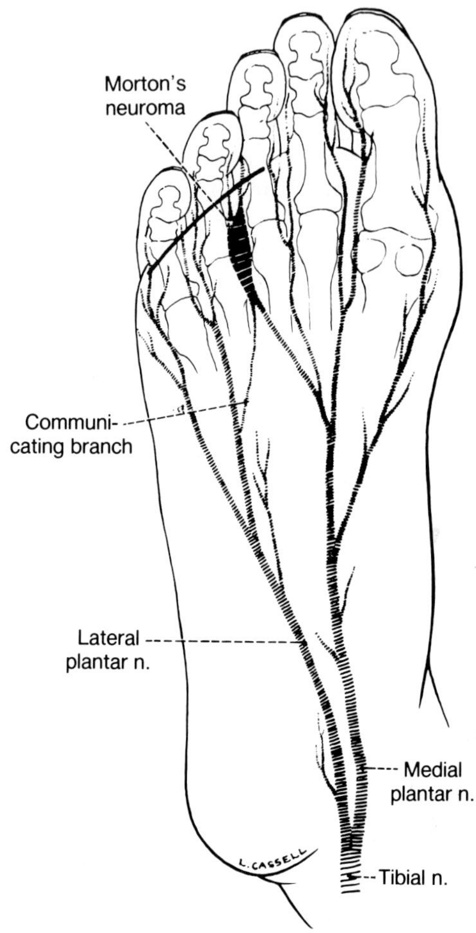

Figure 7.55. Morton's neuroma. (Courtesy RT McElvenney.)

interdigital neuroma excision, found that two-thirds of the lesions occurred in the third metatarsal interspace with the second interspace affected about one-half as often. Four-fifths of the patients were female, and 85% of the patients were overweight. Seventy-five percent of the unilateral neuroma patients presented with forefoot varus, and the majority of bilateral neuroma patients presented with a flexible forefoot valgus.

Pain in Morton's neuroma is dull at first, with a slight burning and stinging and a peculiar feeling of discomfort involving the fourth metatarsal and fourth toe. In the second stage of this illness, the patient has severe excruciating pains spasmodically. This discomfort is real and so severe that it often radiates to the second, third, fourth and fifth toes and frequently to the posterior calf muscles. The patient is compelled to remove the shoes, flex, extend and compress the toes in an effort to gain relief.

In the later stages the slightest provocation, such as alterations in the pavement, trying on shoes, a misstep or even atmospheric conditions or nervous strain, results in attacks of the characteristic pain, hysteria and nausea.

This lesion is most commonly found in women at any age and is characterized by a painful affliction of the foot that is often resistant to conservative treatment. The symptoms are produced by a tumor on the most lateral branch of the medial plantar nerve pinched between the third and fourth metatarsal heads or proximal phalanges.

Frost (53), in his series of 78 plantar neurectomies on 60 patients, calls attention to unilateral multiple neurofibromas. He proposes a diagnostic nerve block to rule out the possibility of more than one lesion. Unilateral multiple neurofibromas were observed in 7 of the 60 cases. Frost was the first to recognize this possibility, and he wisely advised a diagnostic test. He notes that the tumor can occur in more

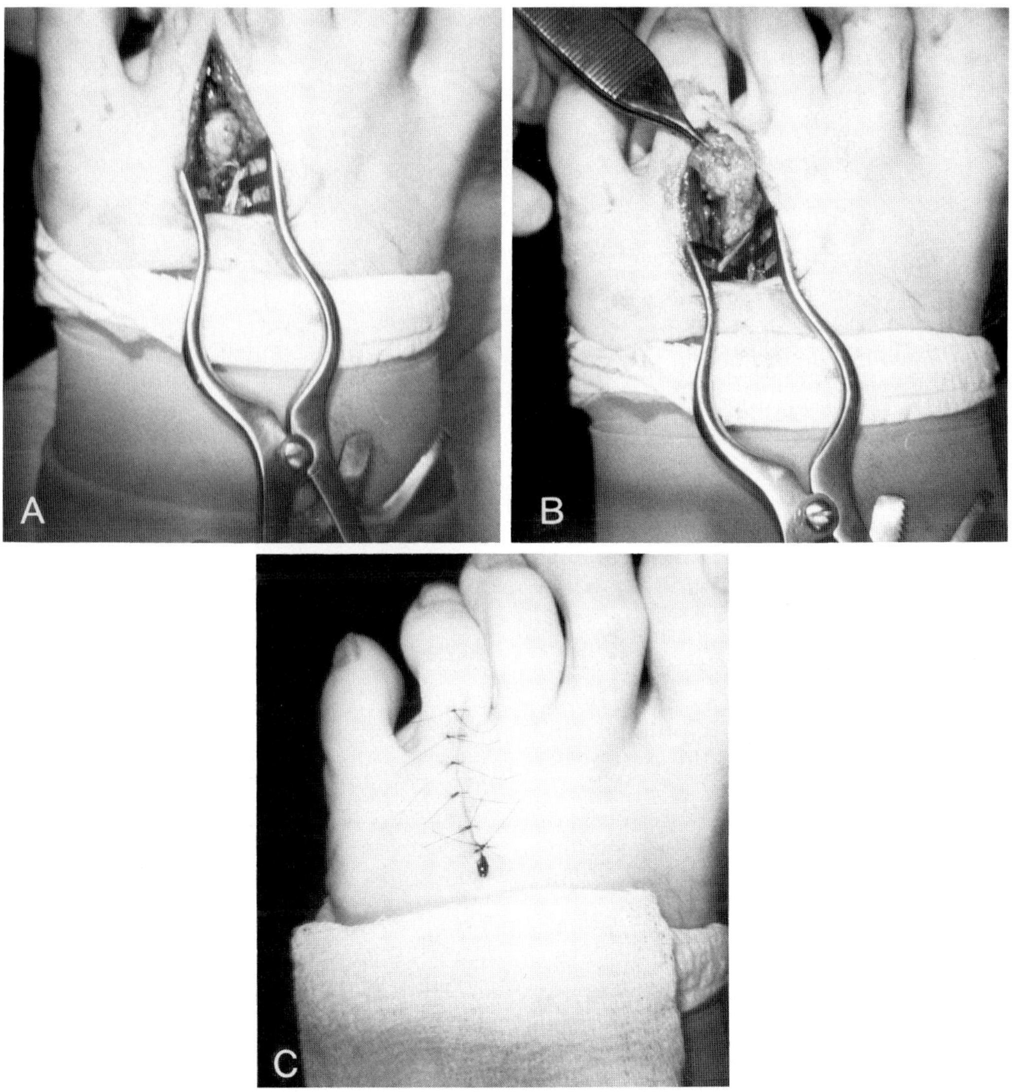

Figure 7.56. *A, B, C,* Typical presentation of Morton's neuroma.

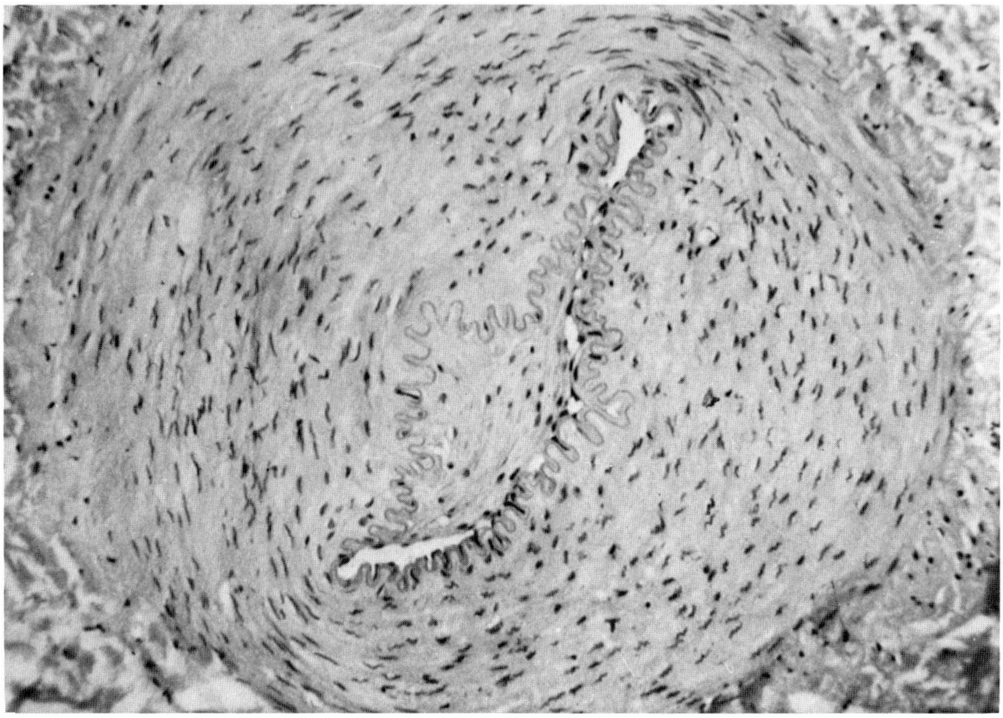

Figure 7.57. Photomicrograph of fibrosed artery (low power). Often seen in close proximity to Morton's neuroma. Note the fibrosis.

than one intermetatarsal space. An injection of a local anesthetic accompanied by a metatarsal raise may relieve pain.

Cozen (54) notes that a point of tenderness can be felt in the web between the toes, usually between the third and fourth but sometimes between the fourth and fifth or second and third toes. A diagnostic aid is a painful click elicited when the metatarsal heads are pressed together. It is significant only if pain accompanies the click. Cozen states that injection of 0.5 ml of hydrocortisone into the region of the neuroma affords relief and should be considered before subjecting the patient to surgery.

Davidson (55) presents a diagnostic approach to the differentiation of a heel neuroma from the commonly accepted impression of a plantar bursitis. He states, "A very firm pressure must be applied with the thumb from the plantar aspect of the heel. A cord-like structure will be felt called by Cohen the 'lamp cord' sign. The pain is excruciating at the site of the cord-like structure while 90% of the remainder of the heel is pain free." Other evidence of a nerve involvement is the presence of a Tinel's sign and the radiation of pain up-

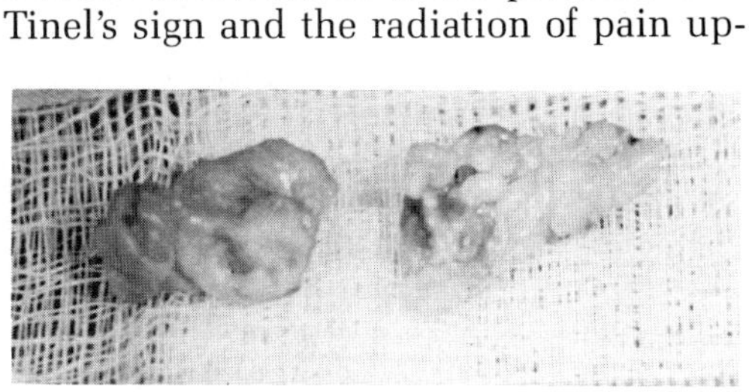

Figure 7.58. Gross specimen removed from third interspace—Morton's neuroma.

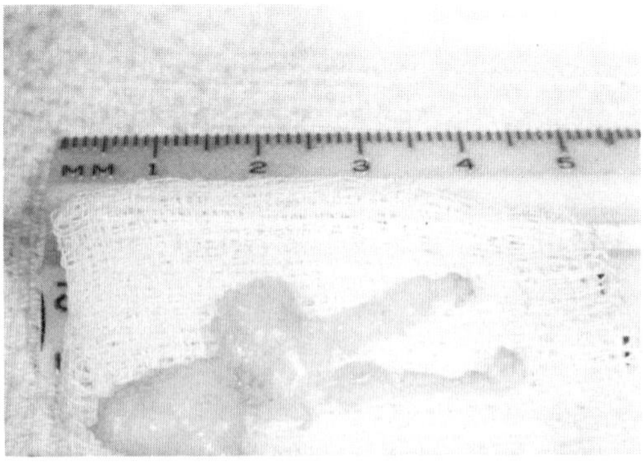

Figure 7.59. Morton's neuroma at bifurcation of digital nerves.

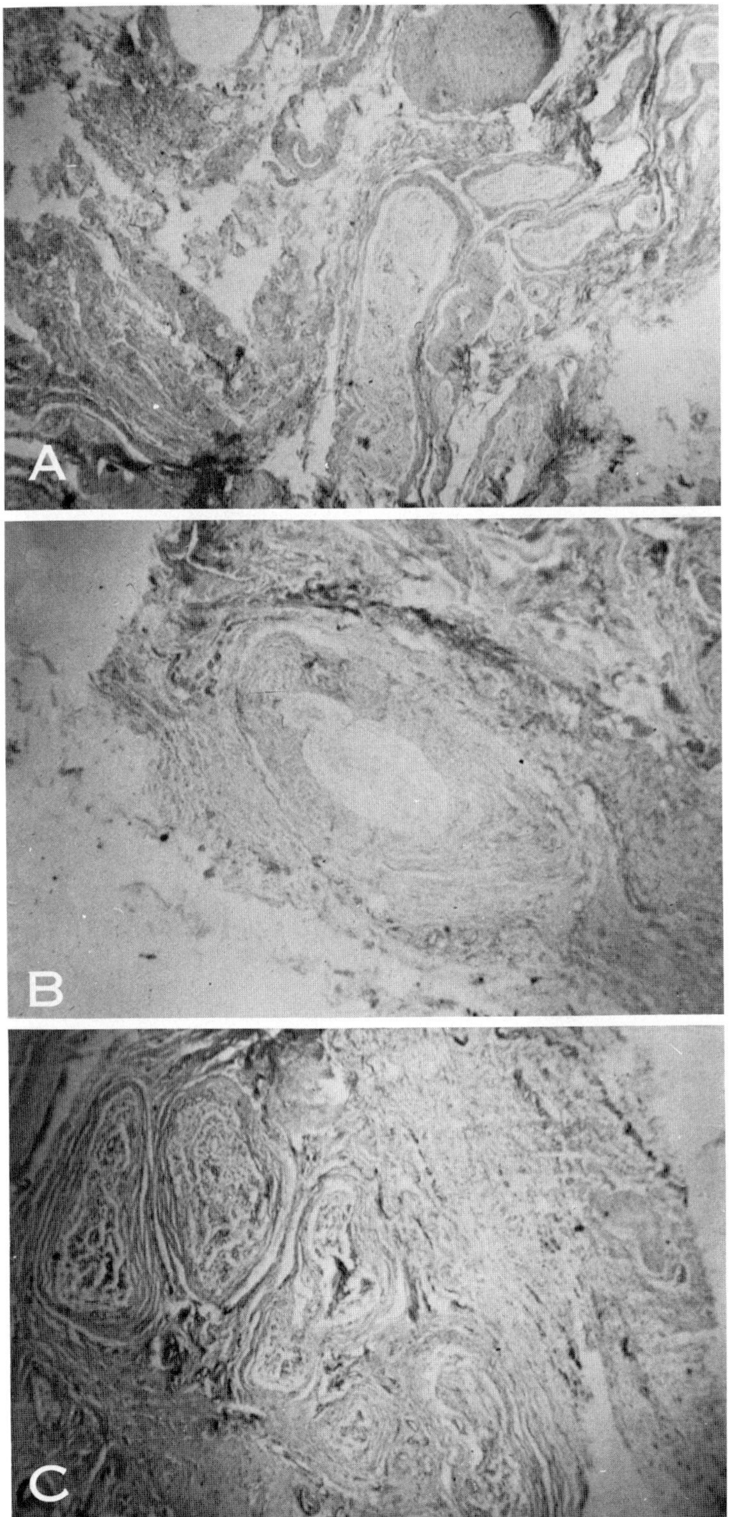

Figure 7.60. Major microscopic components of Morton's neuroma. *A,* Perineural fibrosis; *B,* fibrosed Vater-Pacini corpuscle; *C,* intrafasicular edema.

ward along the course of the medial calcaneal branch to its nerve trunk, the posterior tibial behind the medial malleolus. Both Cohen and Davidson recommend surgical excision of the mass.

Carrier et al. (56) describe the histologic appearance of Morton's neuroma as a perineural fibrosis manifest generally in hypermobile feet of middle-age women. Clinically, the patient may be of any sex or age. The authors, together with the expertise of Smith and Weil, describe the part that biomechanical dysfunction plays in the overall etiology. They note that hyperextended digits place tension on the digital plantar nerve distal to the heads of the metatarsals and the transverse metatarsal ligament. Tension and shearing forces play a part in trauma to the nerve caused by compression of the malfunctioning superstructure.

It has been the author's experience, over the past 20 years, that neurilemomas affecting the foot and ankle occur infrequently. Neurilemomas have characteristic pathological changes, according to Anderson (57). The capsule is generally thick, larger lesions are solid and highly cellular (Antoni A cells) or loosely arranged and less cellular (Antoni B cells); dense cells are spindle-shaped and nuclei present a fine granular chromatin and are long and narrow. Palisading of nuclei is not unusual, and a fasciculation pattern of the tumor cells can be expected. Antoni B cells are not as narrow and elongated as other neoplastic cells. Hyalinization, thickening of blood vessel walls, often results in hemorrhage, thrombosis and necrosis. Organized granulation tissue, together with cystic changes and macrophages undergoing fat and hemorrhagic degeneration, is common in benign neurilemoma.

Silverman (58) discussed the diagnosis and conservative treatment of 110 cases of Morton's neuroma. Silverman contends that weightbearing radiographs of the unshod foot and additional weightbearing views of the shod foot provide a basis for understanding the biomechanical alterations that exist in the metatarsus. Rotation and juxtaposition of the metatarsals are considered to be one of the etiologic factors. Silverman feels that the pathology is in a direct ratio with the extent of rotation. In the advanced stages, the metatarsal bones impinging on the nerve are spread apart to provide room for the enlarged nerve.

The treatment recommended consists of proper footgear and weekly injections of corticosteroids perineurally often accompanied by a posterior tibial nerve block. Faulty pathomechanics of the foot are corrected or maintained in a functionally normal position.

Treatment. There are several approaches to treatment for Morton's neuralgia or neuroma. Conservative methods are used first, followed by more radical measures when necessary. Relief of pain can be obtained in 40 to 60% of such cases by prescribing adequate footgear and constructing a foot orthotic device that lifts the fourth metatarsal bone into a different position. This is believed to relieve the compression on the digital branches of the lateral plantar nerve.

The second technique, which is sometimes used along with the first mechanical procedure, is to inject a local anesthetic-steroid mixture (0.75 ml .25% marcaine and 0.25 ml hexadrol) into the third intermetatarsal space, directing the needle downward and forward from the dorsum to between the heads of the metatarsals. Raise a wheal about ½ inch proximal to the third and fourth metatarsophalangeal joints, and then direct the needle point plantarwise through the intermetatarsal area to the plantar surface of the foot just superficial to the plantar skin. Withdraw the needle approximately ⅛ inch, and then inject the remainder of the solution. This approach may give the patient complete relief for periods of from 1 day to several months. Complete alleviation of the symptoms is common.

Additional injections may be necessary. The author recommends a maximum of three injections over a several week period before discarding this form of therapy.

Steinberg (59) prefers a therapeutic test with vitamin B_{12} and lidocaine solution. A 2% lidocaine hydrochloride solution, 1:100,000 epinephrine, is mixed with a standard vitamin B_{12} solution, 100 μg. of B_{12}/ml. Equal parts of each solution to make a mixture of 3 ml is used for injection. He suggests injecting 1½ ml into each of the third and fourth intermetatarsal spaces. Results have been gratifying in a high percentage of cases.

Polokoff (60) discusses a negative galvanism technique for treatment of Morton's neuralgia. using an aseptic procedure and local infiltration of anesthesia into the third intermetatarsal space, a negative galvanic needle is inserted into the site of the digital branches of the nerve to the third and fourth toes. The indifferent electrode is attached to the sole of the same foot or any other part of the body. The current is turned up to 5 mA. As the current volume is increased, the patient may feel heat, at which time the current is reduced 2 to 3 mA to tolerance. Pressure from the plantar pushes the nerve up between the metatarsals, allowing for easier contact with the needle electrode. When the tissue appears easy to penetrate with the negative current and when resistance has been removed in about 8 to 12 min of treatment, the machine is turned off and the needle electrode withdrawn. Warm foot soaks aid in resorption of the destroyed tissue. According to Polokoff, patients are relieved of discomfort without undue surgical risk.

In the author's opinion, Polokoff's technique may be too destructive to adjacent tissues not involved with the pathology.

In the resistant case, the following procedure is recommended. After administration of adequate anesthesia, a longitudinal proximal to distal incision is made over the third intermetatarsal space extending approximately 4 cm from the dorsal medial aspect of the fourth toe back into the space. This incision is deepened through the dermis and subcutaneous tissue. The tissues are retracted, exposing the transverse plantar metatarsal ligament. The ligament is incised longitudinally, and the metatarsal heads are separated. Pressure is exerted from the plantar surface between the heads, forcing the plantar nerve up into the operative site. The nerve is cleansed of adjacent clinging fascia and grabbed by an Allis forceps. Then the nerve is excised approximately 1.5 cm proximal to its bifurcation and forward from its bifurcation at its digital extensions to the third and fourth toes. The entire mass presents itself as a gray-white tissue and is delivered through the operative wound. Subcutaneous tissues are rejoined with interrupted 4-0 dexon sutures. Skin margins are approximated with interrupted 5-0 nylon sutures. Deep sutures are not used so as to avoid nerve entrapment and fibrosis. Care must be taken to incise the nerve proximal to the level of the transverse metatarsal ligament. There is a 5% incidence of amputation neuroma occurrence. The wound is carefully closed in layers. Very often one finds many small nerve fibers gathered around in a fine wire-like mass just distal and lateral to the bifurcation of the nerve. Microscopic examination is necessary for proper evaluation of the lesion.

Pincus (61) recommended the plantar approach as being less damaging to tissue and providing better visualization.

Ganglions. These lesions (ganglionic cysts) are not new growths, but are the result of herniation of a tendon sheath or joint capsule (Figs. 7.61–7.63). Very often

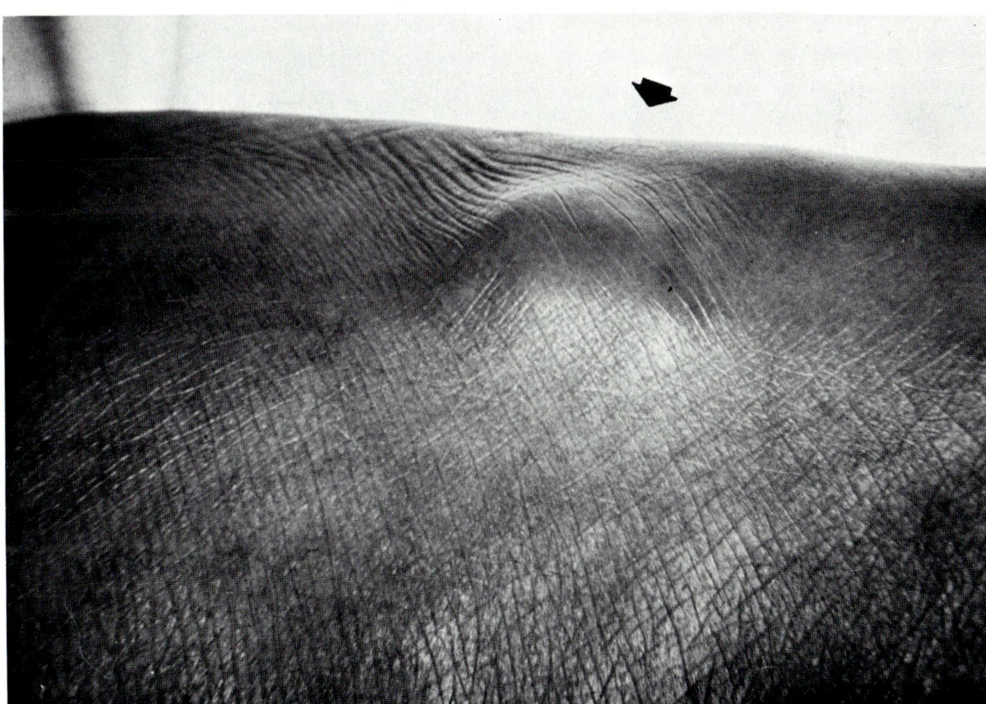

Figure 7.61. Ganglion on dorsal surface of the foot.

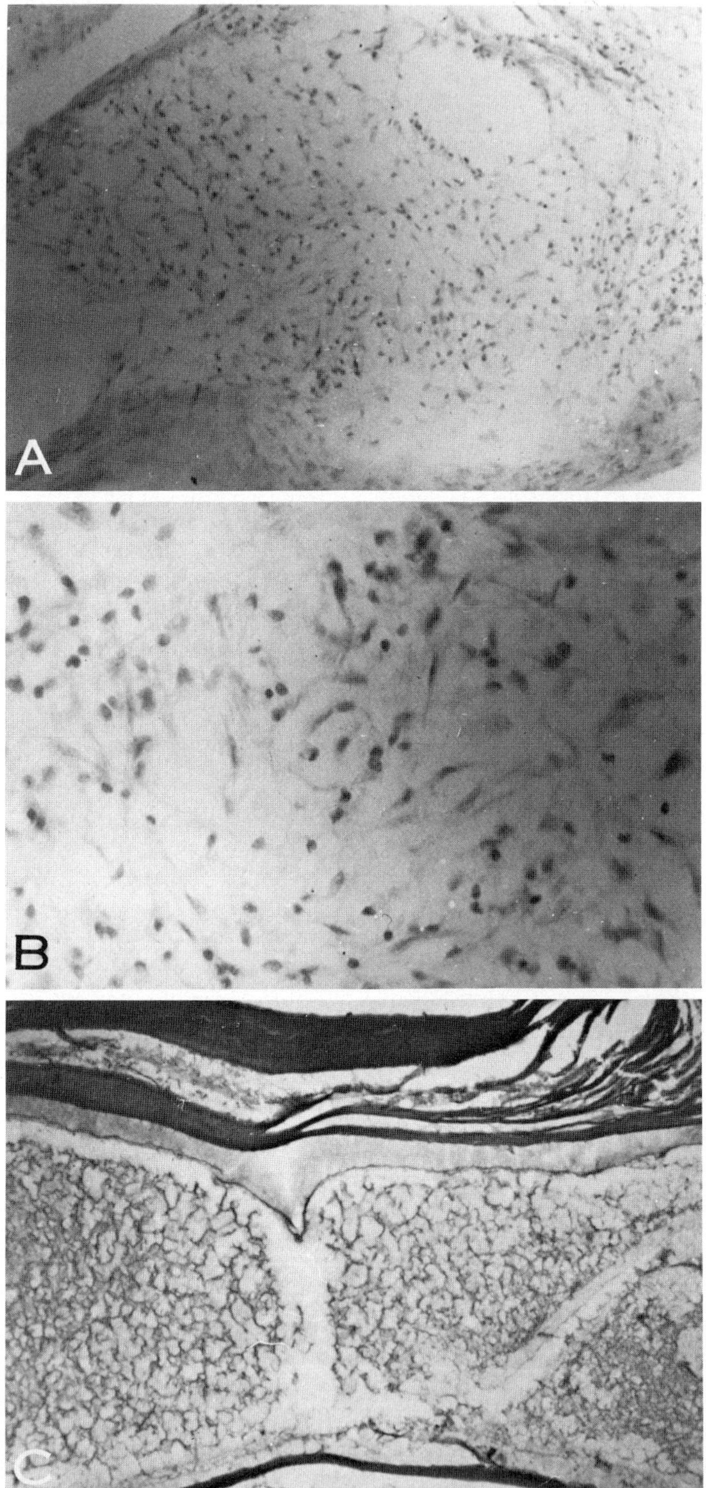

Figure 7.62. *A,* Photomicrograph of ganglion. *B,* Large spaces represent ganglion stroma. Myxomatous tissue between ganglion cyst spaces. Triangular-spaced myxomatous tissue. *C,* Ganglion (low power). Well encapsulated edematous myxomatous stroma.

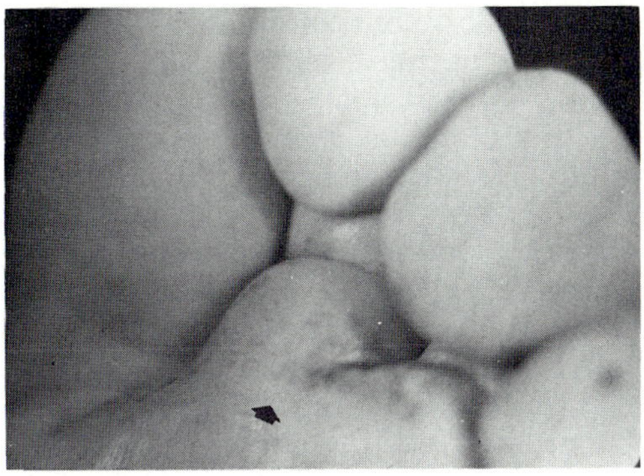

Figure 7.63. Ganglion, plantar surface of second toe.

crepitus on motion and movement of the "growth" with the function of the tendon allow for simple interpretation. Ganglions are common on the anterior of the ankle and dorsum of the foot. The extensor tendons are most often affected. Ganglions are circumscribed subcutaneous herniations of tendon sheaths or joint capsules and contain a clear viscid fluid that sometimes becomes jelly-like in character. The capsules are continuations of the tissue from which they develop and are firm and fibrous. The skin is smooth and freely movable over the ganglion, which commonly resembles a bursa. It has a fibrous outer coat and an inner synovial layer resembling the synovial membrane of a joint. A ganglion must be differentiated from a bursa, synovioma and xanthoma. This may be accomplished by aspiration and biopsy.

Treatment. The treatment of a ganglion can be frustrating. Surgical intervention often results in a collapse of the lesion unless great care is taken to dissect the mass in toto. The author advises making an incision to one side of the mass using blunt dissection to free the tissues around the ganglion. It is necessary to handle the lesion carefully while dissecting and to free the mass from its surrounding attachments. Should the ganglion be the result of a herniation of the joint capsule, it is necessary to free the mass from the surrounding tissue as it is grasped firmly with Allis forceps. Then it can be excised from its attachment. After removal of the ganglion it is essential to use adequate subcutaneous closure of the tissue layers, followed by compression bandaging to close the dead space created by removal of the mass.

Many techniques have been used other than surgical excision with various results. One method involves the use of field block anesthesia followed by aspiration of the fluid within the ganglion using a 10 ml syringe and 18 gauge needle. After irritation (needling) of the walls of the lesion, compression bandages are used to flatten the collapsed mass. The end result is often gratifying, with the irritated inner lining of the ganglion adhering to its opposite wall, resulting in obliteration of the lesion. The use of corticosteroids in 0.3 to 0.5 ml dosages injected directly into the cavity is helpful in relieving inflammatory changes. The author does not advise the use of sclerosing agents in ganglion treatment.

Bursitis. Trauma, infection and metabolic disorders are usually the cause of bursitis (Figs. 7.64–7.68). Traumatic bursitis is often found at those joints that are exposed to shoe pressure. The more common sites for bursitis are at the medial aspect of the first metatarsophalangeal joint, the fifth metatarsophalangeal joint at its lateral surface, the base of the fifth metatarsal laterally, the dorsum of the interphalangeal joints of the toes, the tuberosity of the navicular, the medial tubercle on the plantar surface of the calcaneus, the posterior bursa between the skin and the attachment of the Achilles tendon, and the anterior bursa between the

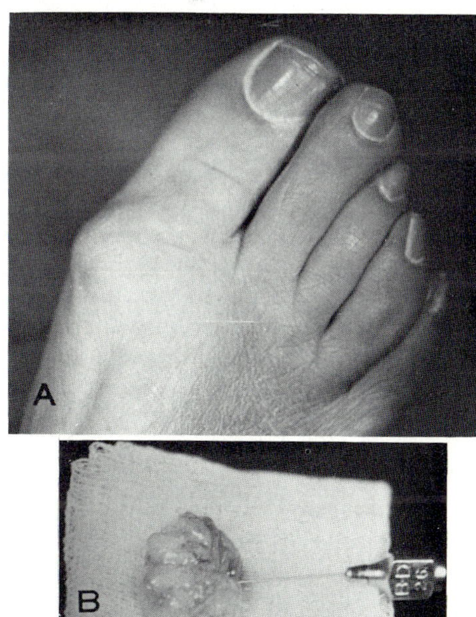

Figure 7.64. *A,* Chronic bursitis, first metatarsophalangeal joint, gross specimen, multilobulated mass. *B,* Gross specimen.

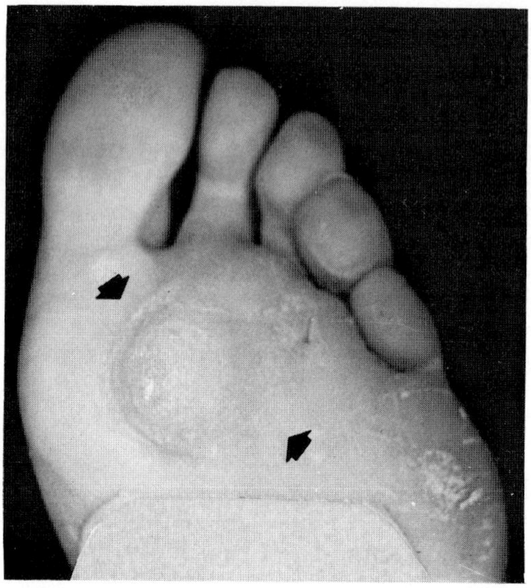

Figure 7.65. Bursitis with overlay of callus, plantar surface of second metatarsal.

Achilles tendon and the upper angle and posterior surface of the calcaneus. Intermetatarsal bursitis and bursitis secondary to rheumatoid arthritis and gout are not uncommon.

Occasionally inflamed bursae develop at the medial and lateral malleolus, as well as at the plantar surface of metatarsal heads from strain or trauma. The trauma may be acute or multiple and minimal in character. A sudden blow or kick or having the part stepped on may cause a bursitis. Exposure to extremes of temperature may be an exciting factor. Old frostbites or chilblains may predispose to bursitis.

Pathology. With trauma a local hyperemia may develop, followed by marked distention of the bursa. In swelling of the bursa the synovial fluid often breaks through the sac along the lines of least resistance.

Distended areolar tissue may occur in the intermetatarsal space or under any of the metatarsal heads from abnormal friction or pressure. The sesamoid region at the plantar surface of the first metatarsal head is often inflamed. Bursae may be acutely inflamed or subacute or chronic. A highly inflamed bursa must be differentiated from infectious lesions, periarticular arthritis, effusions or edema of inflammation.

Occasionally bursae are infected by invasion of bacteria from an abrasion or through a small opening in the skin. The infection of callus-covered bursa through injudicious cutting or contact dermatitis from "corn remedies" is common. A sinus infection, sometimes involving low-grade osteomyelitis, may develop. Cellulitis and lymphangitis are often sequelae to secondarily infected bursae.

Radiographic examination of bursae may disclose multiple loose bodies within the bursa or in the adjacent articular capsule. The capsule or articular ligaments undergo fibrosis, chondrification and later calcification. Very often the bone underlying the inflamed bursa decreases in density as a result of the local hyperemia. This superficial demineralization must not be interpreted as early osteomyelitis or infectious periostitis.

Patients with rheumatoid arthritis are prone to develop an inflamed bursa. In

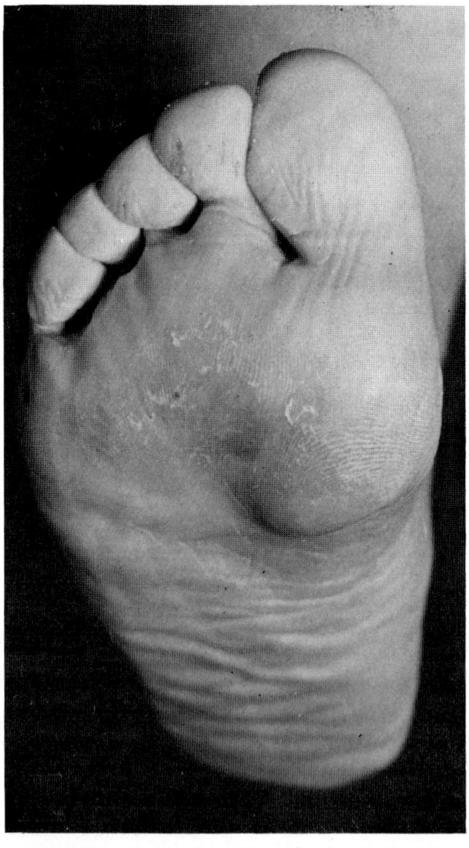

Figure 7.66. Acute bursitis, plantar first metatarsophalangeal joint.

gout the swelling is diffuse and acute, involving most of the soft tissues in the adjacent area.

Clinical Manifestations. Clinically the gross lesion is usually circumscribed, elevated and even in outline. Its surface is smooth, and the tissue's texture usually ranges from soft to fibrous and firm. It may range from a soft, normal-colored, chronically developed hypertrophied tissue to a deep red or blue, firm, nodular mass or a bright red, tense, hot, painful mass in acute inflammation.

Occasionally a bursa may develop between the metatarsal heads or shafts. It is manifest clinically by pain on weightbearing, especially while the patient is wearing a constricting shoe. Circumscribed swelling, tenderness on palpation, redness and heat are noted over the affected intermetatarsal space on the dorsum of the foot. Pressure exerted in opposing directions on the fifth and first metatarsals toward the midline of the foot usually elicits excruciating pain in intermetatarsal bursitis.

Bursa-like developments have been found in the third intermetatarsal space enveloping a Morton's neuroma that has developed on the most lateral branch of the medial plantar nerve.

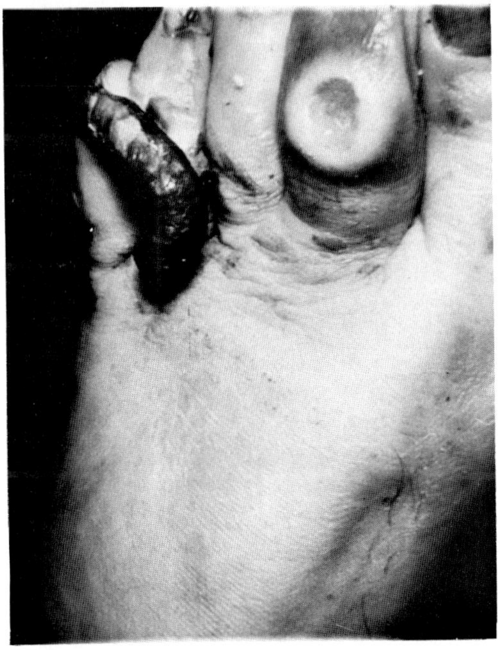

Figure 7.67. Breakdown of infected bursa in diabetic patient, onychogryphosis, ulcer.

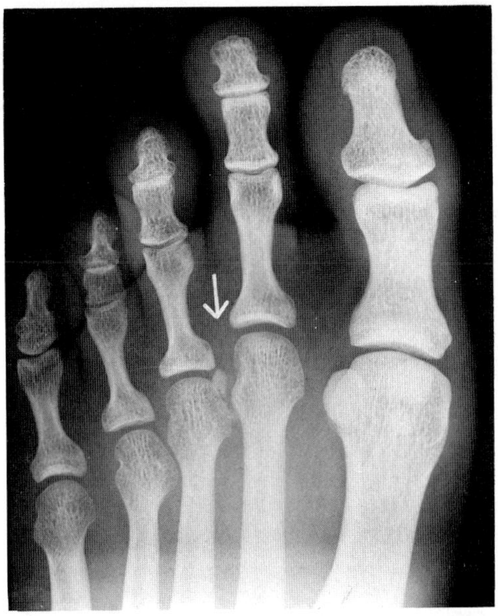

Figure 7.68. Bursitis, intermetatarsal calcification. (From FO Gamble, I Yale: *Clinical Foot Roentgenology.* Baltimore, Williams & Wilkins, 1966.)

Treatment depends on whether the bursitis is acute, subacute or chronic. In acute bursitis, eliminate trauma, treat any infection present and protect the affected part. Occasionally, heat aggravates and cold ameliorates acute symptoms. Burow's solution dressings generally reduce the swelling and inflammation.

Injections of minimal dosage of corticosteroid compounds or chymotrypsin, 0.1 ml to 1.0 ml, help relieve acute pain and generally reduce the size of the bursa. In independent studies, Locke (62) and Rosen (63) note a high percentage of good results in treating bursitis by injection of dexamethasone 21-phosphate and lidocaine in combination. White (64) described the highly effective betamethasone injection for acute and chronic inflammatory disorders. Intra-articular and intralesional injections are relatively free of postinjection flare.

Medical ionization with magnesium sulfate shrinks the mass. Galvanism with iodine often reduces the size of the bursa and decreases pain.

Antibiotics are used in the presence of infection.

In subacute bursitis, treatment is bascially the same as that for acute problems.

Aspiration and the use of ultrasound followed by protection of the affected part are helpful.

Following aspiration the intrabursal injection of 0.1 ml to 1.0 ml of chymotrypsin reduces the size of the bursa.

In chronic bursitis, excision of the growth en masse relieves pressure on underlying tissues. Provide for elimination of pressure by construction of a protective shield. Physical therapy may be needed.

Surgical excision of the mass and any degenerative calcification within the bursa by sharp and blunt dissection may be indicated.

If gout or rheumatoid arthritis is a suspected factor, diagnosis should be confirmed by laboratory studies.

Where bursae exist on the plantar surface of the weightbearing foot, relieve the acute symptoms and maintain relief through proper shielding. Various dynamic moldable materials may be used to construct an orthosis with cutouts at the site of bursal swelling.

The complications of bursitis, such as cellulitis, sinus tract formation, calcifications, ulceration, or underlying bone and joint involvement, can be treated according to the degree of pathology noted (Fig. 7.69).

Xanthoma. In examining 150 patients with elevated blood cholesterol levels, Bloomquist (65) noted that 22 were found to have xanthoma of the Achilles tendon (Figs. 7.70–7.72). In some instances the presence of xanthoma was an indication of hypercholesterolemia. Marcinko et al. (66) present a review of the literature, a case report of bilateral Achilles tendon xanthomatosis and a synopsis of types I through V lipoprotein phenotypes, including common signs, symptoms and risk factors. Characteristic fusiform swell-

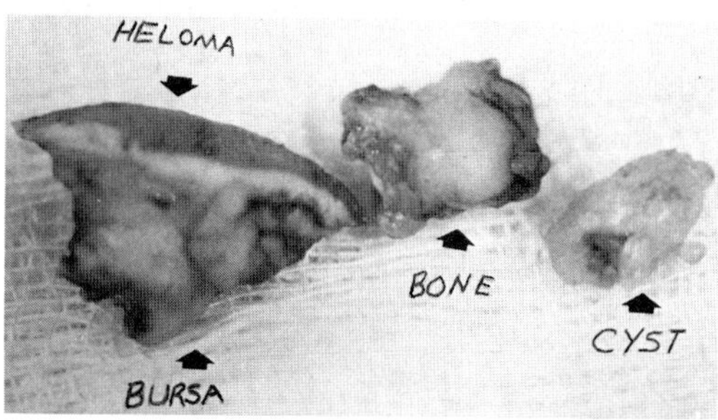

Figure 7.69. Arthroplasty, heloma, bursa, bone, inclusion cyst. Gross specimens.

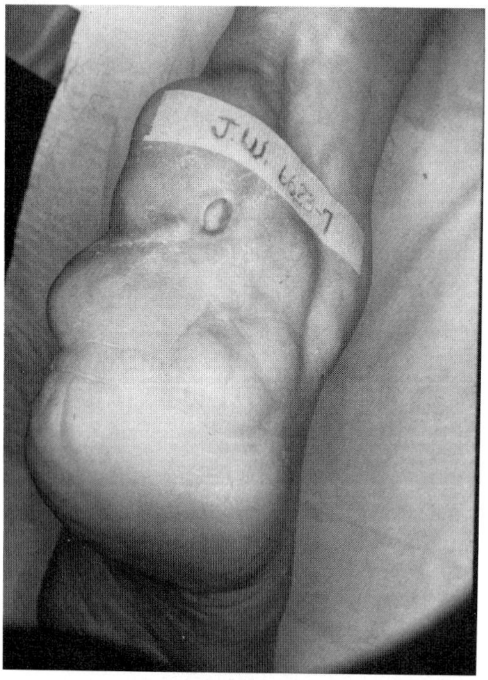

Figure 7.70. Xanthomatosis heel; ulcer. (Courtesy of M Shapiro.)

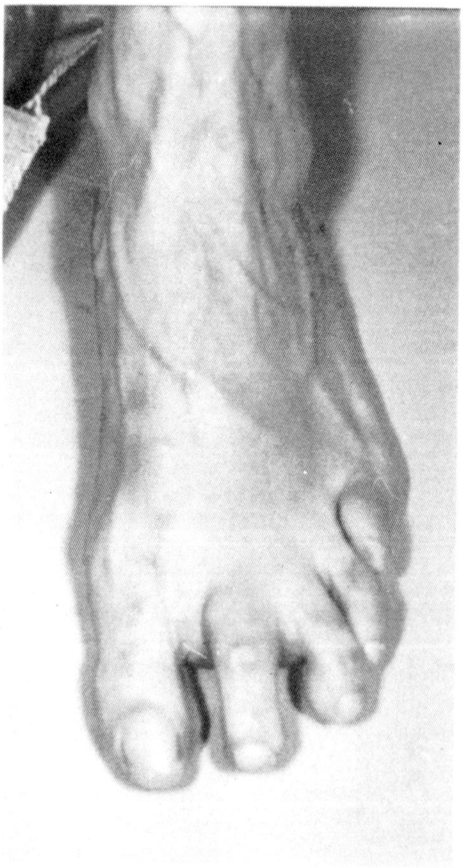

Figure 7.71. Xanthoma forcing the toes apart.

ings were noted, with some containing calcific deposits. The tendon was thickened and tender. Xanthoma cells, giant cells, cholesterol and connective tissue degeneration are noted histologically. X-ray examination shows evidence of rounded, clearly delineated masses of increased soft tissue density.

Xanthomas may occur around the ankle joint and toes and on the plantar surface of the foot. Small lesions around the toes may have to be differentiated from mucoid cysts.

Xanthoma tuberosum multiplex are well-defined neoplastic nodules or macules associated with jaundice and occur around the larger joints of the body. They involve the palms, soles and extensor surfaces of the extremities.

Treatment of xanthoma is based on the location and the extent of the lesion. Should these lesions affect the normal function of the foot and diminish the ability for adequate weightbearing, surgical removal is suggested. However, it is wise to limit surgical intervention because the patient with multiple lesions of this type is generally ill and requires treatment for the medical problems that exist.

Leiomyoma. These lesions are not common on the foot and, when they do occur, involve cutaneous or vascular tissue (67). In the last 45 years, less than 24 cases of cutaneous leiomyomas have been reported in the literature. Cases have been reported in the podiatric literature by McCain and Galinsky, Girelli, Rakow, Potter, Giese, Lobbato, Godfrey, Perles and Rota.

Berlin et al. (67) and Hosey (68) report three cases and one case, respectively, of vascular leiomyoma, and in each case the gross subcutaneous lesion was tinged a bluish-white color. The mass was generally oval and nodular. The lesions are generally freely movable and may resemble a ganglion. Pain may run the gamut of being negligible to severe and neuritic-like. The leiomyoma must be differentiated from a cord-like phlebitic process in a vein and a superficial neurofibroma upon gross surgical examination. Review of 11 cases excised by the author over the past 20 years

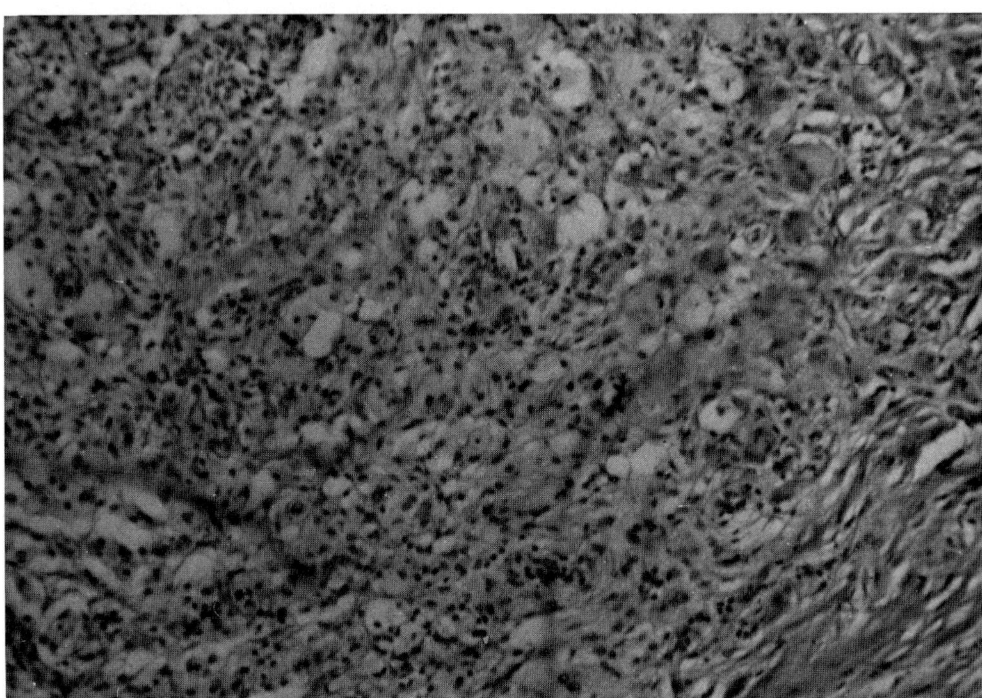

Figure 7.72. Photomicrograph of xanthoma (low power). Note large and small giant cells in a cellular stroma with hemosiderin deposits.

reveals a predisposition to plantar skin. It is obvious that a great variety of subcutaneous and exotic lesions have to be differentiated from leiomyoma. A clinical interpretation cannot be trusted. Gross and microscopic examination of the excised lesion by a qualified pathologist is mandatory. Stout (69) in a review of this lesion, classified leiomyoma lesions and estimated that 10% are capable of secondary malignant changes.

Treatment of painful leiomyoma lesions is excision.

Giant Cell Tumor of Tendon Sheath. Giant cell tumor of tendon sheath has been described by Coster (70) as a benign synovioma. Floyd et al. (71) report on two cases. However, a search of the literature does not show evidence of many reports of these lesions on the foot (Figs. 7.73 and 7.74). However, it is the author's opinion that podiatric surgeons are removing giant cell tumors of tendon sheaths regularly and should report them in the professional literature. Coster disagrees with prevalent literature concerning giant cell tumors being caused by alterations in lipoid metabolism. He has not been able to document such etiologic factors. He reports a giant cell tumor on the plantar medial aspect of the great toe.

Giant cell tumors appear more commonly about the fingers, wrists, metatarsals, ankles and knees. They are often referred to as tendon sheath tumors or myeloid tumors containing giant cells. They are to be differentiated from ganglions. Lipid-laden giant cells and the presence of hemorrhagic deposits containing variable amounts of lipids, hyperplastic synovial tissue and granulation tissue are characteristic of this benign inflammatory mass.

Galinski and Vlahos (72) discuss the proliferative and degenerative reactions in villonodular synovitis. The lesions are benign synoviomas and are often referred to as giant cell tumors or proliferative synovitis. Clinically, the distended synovial tissue creates pressure and pain in the adjacent tissues. The area is warm to touch

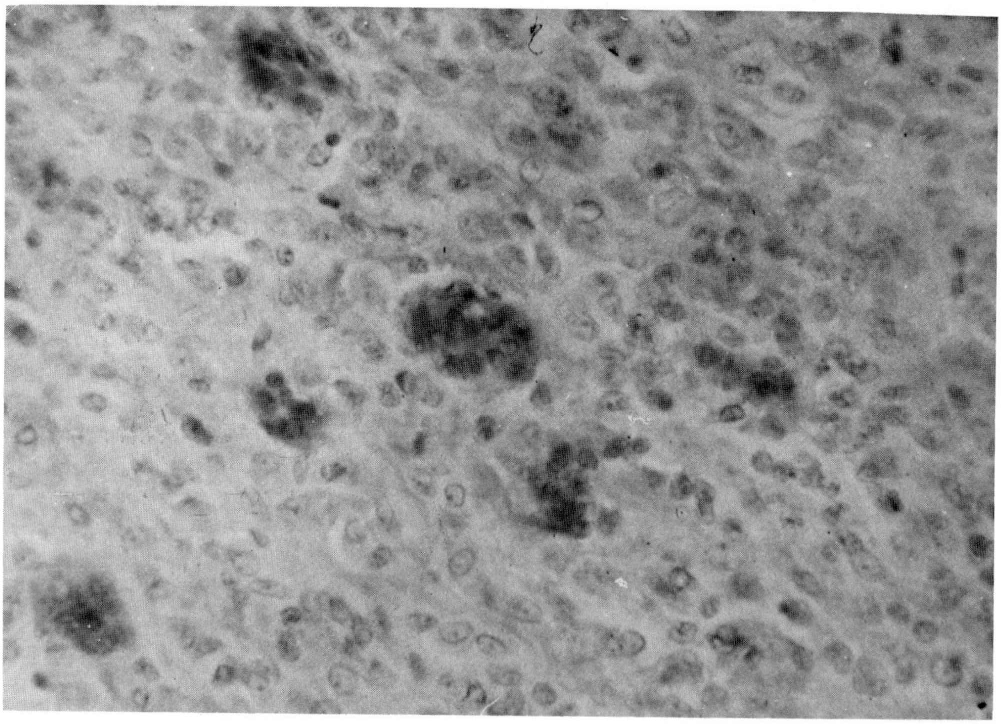

Figure 7.73. Photomicrograph of giant cell tumor. Note large and small giant cells. Typical findings in xanthoma, tenosynovitis, bursitis.

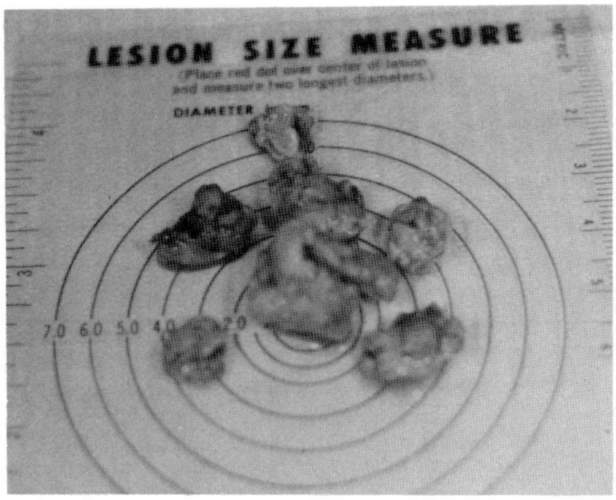

Figure 7.74. Giant cell tumor in the first intermetatarsal space. Gross specimen is multilocular.

and swollen. Trauma appears to be the etiologic factor, but is not always demonstrated. Pain is out of proportion to clinical findings. The lesion may be present for months or years before the patient seeks consultation. Villonodular synovitis may occur at any age, but is more prevalent in the second, third and fourth decades, during periods of greatest activity. Sex is not a factor. Radiotherapy or total synovectomy appears to be the treatment of choice. This proliferative synovitis appears differently on gross postsurgical excision depending on what synovial structures are involved and the age of the pathology. According to Galinski and Vlahos, pathology may vary from polyhedral cells with spindle-shaped nuclei to large histiocytes, foamy cytoplasm and focal areas of hemosiderin pigmentation and macrophages. Pathologists agree that degenerative changes occurring in late treatment do not result in degenerative hyperplasia, but are secondary to metaplastic alterations in embryonic mesenchyme in the synovial cavity. The tarsal joints and synovial sheaths are most commonly affected. Radiographic examinations are not productive unless a degenerative joint change is obvious (Fig. 7.75).

LaPorta et al. (30) describe the diagnosis and surgical treatment of a large yellow-pink, ovoid, firm "partially calcified nodule." Although the diagnosis was consistent with a "tumoral calcinosis," the significance of this presentation is in its appreciation of the theory of an inborn error of phosphorus metabolism. A hyperphosphatemia without significant changes in calcium, blood phosphatase, urea or nonprotein nitrogen is often part of the criteria necessary for a definitive diagnosis. Black and Sladek (73) review turmoral calcinosis in the foot and hand.

The gross description of this lesion is not unlike calcinosis of the nail sulcus as described by Frost (74).

Treatment. Excision of giant cell tumors of the tendon sheath, other synovial tissue lesions and calcifying lesions is the treatment of choice.

References

1. Gamble FO, Yale I: *Clinical Foot Roentgenology.* Baltimore, Williams & Wilkins Co, 1966.
2. DuVries HL: *Surgery of the Foot.* St. Louis, CV Mosby Co, 1978.
3. Nickel WR: Nevi: Clinical and pathological evaluation. *Plast Recon Surg* 22:123–138, 1958.
4. Levene M, et al.: Distribution of skin tumors on the sole of the foot. *The Chiropodist* 14:11, 1959.
5. Berlin SJ: A laboratory review of 67,000 foot tumors and lesions. *J Am Podiatry Assoc* 74:341, 1984.
6. Estersohn HS, Stanoch JF: Pyogenic granuloma: A literature review and two cases. *J Am Podiatry Assoc* 73:29, 1983.

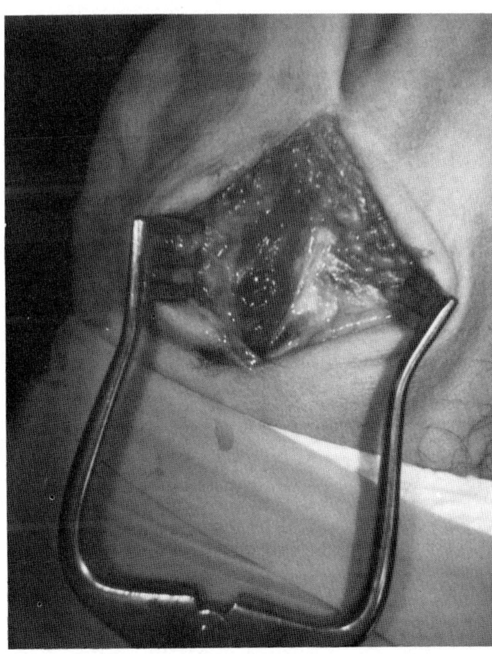

Figure 7.75. Atypical herniation of fourth dorsal interosseus muscle sheath simulating villonodular synovitis.

7. Steinberg MD: Benign, multiple acanthoma of the toes: A new concept entity. *J Natl Assoc Chirop* 40:50–54, 1950.
8. Politz MJ, Miller ML: Subcutaneous granuloma annulare of the foot. *J Am Podiatry Assoc* 73:147, 1983.
9. Silver SH, Glickman FS, Wanderer G: Granuloma annulare—A case report. *J Am Podiatry Assoc* 51:127, 1961.
10. Kamalam A, Yesudian P, Thambiah AS: Cutaneous infection by cryptococcus laurentii. *Br J Dermatol* 97:221–223, 1977.
11. Harris ED, Jr: Biology of the joints. In *Textbook of Rheumatology*. Philadelphia, WB Saunders Co, 1981.
12. Cohen J: Pseudorhematoid nodules in an adult. *J Foot Surg* 22:203–206, 1983.
13. Yale I, Yale J: *The Arthritic Foot and Related Connective Tissue Disorders*. Baltimore, Williams & Wilkins, 1984, pp. 237–239.
14. Beckett JH, Jacobs AH: Recurring digital fibrous tumors of childhood: A review. *Pediatrics* 59:401–406, 1977.
15. Lerman JS, Winarick SI: Acquired digital fibrokeratoma. *J Am Podiatry Assoc* 66:522–523, 1976.
16. Verallo VVM: Acquired digital fibrokeratoma. *Br J Dermatol* 80:730, 1968.
17. Toth S: Vater-Pacinian corpuscle, a case report. *J Am Podiatry Assoc* 247:48, 1975.
18. Burns AE, Harvey CK: Plantar fibromatosis. *J Am Podiatry Assoc* 73:141, 1983.
19. Daniels AE: Keloids: An enigma of surgeons. *J Foot Surg* 23:279–282, 1984.
20. Benhard L, et al.: Hypertrophic hemangioma vs hemangiopericytoma. *J Foot Surg* 22:308–313, 1983.
21. Oughterson WW, Tennant R: Angiomatous tumors of the hands and feet. *Surgery* 5:73–100, 1939.
22. Yale JF: Cutaneous mucous cysts of the toes. *J Am Podiatry Assoc* 57:457–463, 1967.
23. Politz MJ: Hemangioma of the digits. *J Am Podiatry Assoc* 66:515–518, 1976.
24. Cox K: Subcutaneous hemangioma of the foot. *J Am Podiatry Assoc* 70:318, 1980.
25. Berlin SJ: Hemangioma of the foot. *J Am Podiatry Assoc* 60:63, 1970.
26. Plotnick DL: Glomus tumor. *J Am Podiatry Assoc* 50:126, 1960.
27. Sandel RK: Unilateral multiple glomus tumors. *J Am Coll Foot Surg* 4:130, 1966.
28. Freed JB: Glomangioma: The physiologic effect of traumatized arteriovenous shunts. *J Am Podiatry Assoc* 55:198–200, 1965.
29. LaPorta GA, Pressman M, Novicki D, Marzzaco J, Davis WS: Tumoral calcinosis of the foot. *J Am Podiatry Assoc* 66:498–504, 1976.
30. LaPorta GA, Davis WS, Scarlet J: Glomus tumor of the foot. *J Am Podiatry Assoc* 66:568–529, 1976a.
31. Rubinstein SA, Jenkins WM, Conant MA, Volberding PA: Disseminated Kaposi's sarcoma in male homosexuals. *J Am Podiatry Assoc* 73:413–417, 1983.
32. Yale I, Yale JF: Kaposi cell sarcoma—report on two cases. *J Am Podiatry Assoc* 56:165–168, 1966.
33. Ferguson LK: *Surgery of the Ambulatory Patient*. Philadelphia, J B Lippincott, 1955, pp. 199–201.
34. Heller AG: A prophylactic surgical procedure. *J Am Podiatry Assoc* 48:258–259, 1958.
35. Davis MC, McLeod R, Beardmore GL, et al.: *Primary Cutaneous Melanoma: A Report From the Queensland Cancer Fund*. American Cancer Society, 1976.
36. Commack KV: Moles—Benign or potentially malignant? *J Mich State Med S* 55:1353–1354, 1956.
37. Pack GT: The pigmentated mole and malignant melanoma. *Va Med Monthly* 84:111–119, 1957.
38. Walker RD, Cunningham DJ: Malignant melanoma of the foot. *J Foot Surg* 22:230–233, 1983.
39. Mihm MC, Fitzpatrick TB, Lane Brown MM, Raker JW, Malt RA, Kaiser JS: Early detection of primary cutaneous melanoma. *N Engl J Med* 289:989–996, 1973.
40. Gumport SL, Harris MH, Kopf AW. Diagnosis and management of common skin cancers. *Amer Cancer Soc*, Prof Educat Publication no. 3373-P.E., 1975..
41. Jacobs EL, Block BR: Basal cell carcinoma of the foot. *J Am Podiatry Assoc* 66:554–556, 1976.
42. Berger RA, Auerbach R, Orentreich N: Basal cell epithelioma of the sole. *Arch Dermatol* 94:317–391, 1966.
43. Hlavac H: Calcifying epithelioma of Malherbe. *J Am Podiatry Assoc* 66:477–483, 1976.
44. Galinski AW, Shapiro LJ, Waldman M: Squamous cell carcinoma of the foot. *J Am Podiatry Assoc* 66:550–553, 1976.
45. Snider BL, Demuth R: Plantar squamous cell carcinoma. *Cutis* 18:195, 1976.
46. Smith LS, Lenet M, Sherman M: Malignant fibrous histiocytoma. *J Am Podiatry Assoc* 66:459–464, 1976.
47. Robins P: Chemosurgery for skin cancer patients. A report. *NY U Med Center*, 1970.
48. Jaworek TA: Synovial sarcoma (a case report of foot involvement). *J Am Podiatry Assoc* 66:544–546, 1976.
49. McElvenny RT: The etiology and surgical treatment of intractable pain about the fourth metatarsophalangeal joint. *J Bone Joint Surg* 25:675, 1943.
50. Betts LO: Morton's metatarsalgia: Neuritis of the fourth digital nerve. *Med J Aust* 1:514, 1940.
51. Scotti TM: The nature and pathogenesis of the lesion in Morton's metatarsalgia. *J Am Podiatry Assoc* 52:750–753, 1962.
52. Bartholomei FJ, Wertheimer SJ: Intermetatarsal neuromas: Distribution and etiologic factors. *J Foot Surg* 22:279–282, 1983.
53. Frost L: A treatment for paronchia with concomitant onychocryptosis. *J Am Podiatry Assoc* 49:197–201, 1959b.
54. Cozen L: Neuroma of the plantar digital nerve: A new method of treatment. *Clin Orthop* 11:224–226, 1958.
55. Davidson MR: Heel neuroma—Identification and removal. *J Am Podiatry Assoc* 67:431–435, 1977.
56. Carrier P, Janigan J, Smith S, Weil L: Morton's neuralgia: A possible contributing etiology. *J Am Podiatry Assoc* 65:315–321, 1975.

57. Anderson WAD: *Synopsis of pathology*, ed 2. St. Louis, C V Mosby Co, 1971.
58. Silverman LJ: Morton's toe or Morton's neuralgia (its recognition and treatment). *J Am Podiatry Assoc* 66:749–756, 1976.
59. Steinberg MD: The use of vitamin B_{12} in Morton neuralgia. *J Am Podiatry Assoc* 45:41–42, 1955.
60. Polokoff M: Negative galvanic procedure for Morton's neuralgia. *J Am Podiatry Assoc* 51:31–36, 1961a.
61. Pincus A: The syndrome of plantar metatarsal neuritis (Morton's toe). *J Am Podiatry Assoc* 52:746–749, 1962.
62. Locke RK: Local injection of combined dexamethasone 21-phosphate-lidocaine in non-articular foot disorders. *J Am Podiatry Assoc* 53:510–514, 1963.
63. Rosen MR: An injectable steroid anesthetic combination in disorders of the foot. *J Am Podiatry Assoc* 53:514–516, 1963.
64. White DD: Betamethasone in certain inflammatory states of the foot. *J Am Podiatry Assoc* 56:234–236, 1966.
65. Bloomquist G: Xanthoma of the tendo achilles. *Acta Radiol* 57:45–48, 1962..
66. Marcinko DE, et al.: Achilles tendon hypercholesteremic xanthoma. *J Foot Surg* 23:398–401, 1984.
67. Berlin SJ: *Soft Somatic Tumors of the Foot: Diagnosis and Surgical Management. Mt. Kisco, NY, Futura Publishing Co Inc, 1976.*
68. Hosey TC, et al.: Vascular leiomyoma. *J Am Podiatry Assoc* 74:93–95, 1984.
69. Stout AP: Solitary cutaneous and subcutaneous leiomyomas. *Am J Cancer* 29:435, 1937.
70. Coster AA: Giant cell tumor of tendon sheathe. *J Am Podiatry Assoc* 66:538–541, 1976.
71. Floyd EJ, et al.: Giant cell tumor of the tendon sheath: A report of two cases. *J Am Podiatry Assoc* 73:312, 1983.
72. Galinski AW, Vlahos M: Pigmented villonodular synovitis in podiatric medicine. *J Am Podiatry Assoc* 66:471–476, 1976.
73. Black JR, Sladek GD: Tumoral calcinosis in the foot and hand. *J Am Podiatry Assoc* 73:153, 1983.
74. Frost L: Digital calcinosis—A case report. *J Natl Assoc Chirop* 47:71–73, 1957.

Suggested Readings

Aho, CO: Case report: Plantar cystic tumor of first toe. *J Am Coll Foot Surg* 4:13–14, 1968.

Allen AC, Spitz S: Malignant melanoma: A clinicpathological analysis of criteria for diagnosis and prognosis. *Cancer* 6:1–45, 1953.

Asboe-Hansen G: Hypertrophic scars and keloids: Etiology, pathogenesis and dermatologic therapy. *Dermatologica* 120:178–184, 1960.

Bailey OT: The cutaneous glomus and its tumors-glomangioma. *Am J Pathol* 11:915, 1935.

Balkin SW: Villonodular tenosynovitis—A case report. *J Am Podiatry Assoc* 53:282–283, 1963.

Berman H: Some aspects of cutaneous malignancy. *Am J Med Sci* 233:456–472, 1957.

Berlin SJ, et al.: Leiomyoma of the foot, a review of the literature and report of cases. *J Am Podiatry Assoc* 66:450–458, 1976.

Berlin SJ, Donick II, Block LD, Costa A: Ganglion cysts and metatarsalgia. *J Am Podiatry Assoc* 66:491–495, 1976b.

Booher RJ: Lipoblastic tumors of the hands and feet. *J Bone Joint Surg* 47-A:727–740, 1965.

Bourns HK, Sanerkim NG: Mucoid lesions (mucoid cysts) of the fingers and toes: Clinical features and pathogenesis. *Br J Surg* 50:860–866, 1963.

Brohner MD: Morton's toe or Morton's neuralgia. *J Natl Assoc Chirop* 39:18–26, 1949.

Buneson EE: Neuroma of the first metatarsal interspace—A case history. *J Am Coll Foot Surg* 5:35, 1966.

Burwell EN: An unusual tumor of the foot. *Br J Surg* 52:708–711, 1965.

Campanelli M: Juvenile melanoma (a case report). *J Am Podiatry Assoc* 56:461–463, 1966.

Cangialosi CP, Schnall SJ: Kaposi sarcoma of the foot, a case report. *J Am Podiatry Assoc* 66:525–527, 1976.

Cedrone D: A short review of classification and etiology of tumors. *J Am Podiatry Assoc* 50:19–23, 1960.

Charache H: Squamous cell carcinoma of extremities. *Surg Gynecol Obstet* 68:1002–1006, 1939.

Citron J: Case report: Benign mummifying epithelioma. *J Am Coll Foot Surg* 4:42, 1965.

Colson GM, Wilcox A: Phalangeal metastases in bronchogenic carcinoma. *JAMA* 137:995, 1948.

Conway D: Postoperative development of an epidermal cyst. *J Am Coll Foot Surg* 4:7–8, 1965.

Cornell JA: Malignant growths of the feet. *Chirop Rec* 20:234–235, 1937.

Cortese CJ: Cavernous hemangioma of the foot. *J Foot Surg* 15:72–76, 1967.

Dueriling WM: Cutaneous neuroma. *Arch Dermatol Syph* 19:226, 1929.

DuVries HL, Cascino JP: Massive neurofibroma (neurinoma) *J Int Coll Surg* 18:5, 1952.

Feldman AC: Lipoma, a case report. *J Am Coll Foot Surg* 5:36, 1966.

Fielding MD (ed): *Skin Tumors of the Foot. Diagnosis and Treatment.* New York Futura Publishing Co, Inc, 1974.

Fields FS, Imanuel H, Marcus S: Elephantiasis nostras (case report and view of the subject). *J Am Podiatry Assoc* 66:28–31, 1976.

Fisher ER: Malignant blue nevus. *Arch Dermatol* 74:227, 1956.

Frank SC: Case report—Plantar fibromatosis. *J Am Coll Foot Surg* 4:9, 1965.

Freeman DW: Case history—Early squamous cell carcinoma. *J Am Coll Foot Surg* 51:142–143, 1966.

Freigenberg S: Fibromatosis of the plantar fascia. *J Am Coll Foot Surg* 5:30, 1966.

Frost L: Morton's metatarsalgia unilateral multiple neurofibromata. *J Am Podiatry Assoc* 49:62–66, 1959.

Frykberg R, Erben JK: The biochemistry and physiology of the surgical scar. *J Am Podiatry Assoc* 67:3–8, 1977.

Galinski AW: Moles and malignant melanomas. *J Am Podiatry Assoc* 63:35–45, 1973.

Gasser FJ: Report of two unusual neoplastic cases. *J Am Coll Foot Surg* 4:26–27, 1965.

Gelfarb M, Michaelides P: Plantar fibromatosis. *Arch Dermatol* 85:278–281, 1962.

Gemmett RA: Plexiform neuroma (a case report). *J Am Podiatry Assoc* 56:330–331, 1966.
Genovese VH: An unusual neuroma site. *J Am Coll Foot Surg* 4:33, 1965.
Gilman M: Excision of ganglionic cyst and exostosis. *J Am Coll Foot Surg* 5:41–42, 1966.
Godfrey CE: Case report—Vascular leiomyoma. *J Am Coll Foot Surg* 4:19, 1965.
Goldstein S: Office management of intermetatarsal neuralgias. *J Am Podiatry Assoc* 48:529, 1958.
Green AL: Case report of a typical Kaposi's hemorrhagic sarcoma. *J Am Coll Foot Surg* 4:21–22, 1965.
Hara B: Carvernous hemangioma. *J Am Coll Foot Surg* 5:30–31, 1966.
Hauser EDW: Neurofibroma of the foot. *J Am Podiatry Assoc* 121:1217, 1953.
Hennessee MT, et al.: Benign schwannoma—Clinical and histopathologic findings. *J Am Podiatric Med Assoc* 75:310–314, 1985.
Hoffner ML: Case report: Excision of plantar fibroma with secondary painful internal scar formation. *J Am Coll Foot Surg* 5:38–39, 1966.
Hunter GA, Hellier FF: Tumors of the palm and sole resembling basal cell epithelioma. *Br J Dermatol* 72:285–287, 1960.
Hyman AB, Michaelides P: Basal-cell epithelioma of the sole *Arch Dermatol* 87:481–485, 1963.
Janik A: Tumors of tendon sheathes. *Ann Surg* 85:897–911, 1927.
Job CK, Riedel RG, et al.: Squamous cell carcinoma arising in leprosy. *Int J Leprosy* 32:37–44, 1964.
Johnson EW, Ghormley RK, Dockerty MB: Hemangioma of extremities. *Surg Gynecol Obst* 102:531–538, 1956.
Kheng Khoo T, Ban Tze, K: A sweat gland tumor of the mixed salivary type of the right middle toe. *Med J Malaya* 2:128–133, 1964.
King ESJ: Malignant tumors of tendon sheathes. *Aust and NZJ Surg* 10:338–353, 1941.
Kleinberg S: Angioma of the foot. *J Bone Joint Surg* 24:367–371, 1942.
Kulchar GV: Benign and malignant tumors of the foot. *JAMA* 124:761–766, 1944.
Kwittken J, Negri L: Malignant blue nevus. *Arch Dermatol* 94:64–69, 1966.
Lanham RA: Plantar fibromatosis of the foot. *J Am Coll Foot Surg* 4:37–38, 1968.
Levin AS, Titchenal WO, Clark J: Tarsal tunnel syndrome secondary to neurilemoma. *J Am Podiatry Assoc* 67:429–431, 1977.
Lewis HM, Stensaas CO, Okun MR: Basal cell epithelioma of the sole. *Arch Dermatol* 91:623–624, 1965.
Liberman R, Ketai N: Plantar fibromatosis. *J Am Podiatry Assoc* 63:304–309, 1973.
Mason S: Case report of calcified bursa. *J Am Coll Foot Surg* 4:12, 1965.
McCain LR, Galinski AW: Pedal leiomyoma, a case report. *J Am Podiatry Assoc* 59:399, 1969.
McCarthy, DJ (ed), Montgomery, R (assoc ed): *Podiatric Dermatology*. Baltimore, Williams & Wilkins, 1986.
McClain J, Kanat IO: Plantar inclusion cyst: A review of the literature. *J Foot Surg* 23:454–456, 1984.
Meadow EN: Myxoma on the plantar surface (a case report). *J Am Podiatry Assoc* 56:463–464, 1966.
Michael BH: Juvenile melanoma. *J Am Coll Foot Surg* 5:135–136, 1966.
Mowbray DT: Angiofibroma involving the short saphenous vein and sural nerve. *Chirop Rec* 17:61, 1934.
Neufeld RI, et al.: Verrucous squamous cell carcinoma of the foot. *J Am Podiatry Assoc* 75:300–305, 1985.
Oloff-Solomon J, et al.: Rheumatoid nodulosis in the foot: A variant of rheumatoid disease. *J Foot Surg* 23:382–385. 1984.
Pack GT: *Tumors of the Hands and Feet*, ed 3. St. Louis, C V Mosby Co, 1939.
Packer A: Post traumatic neurofibroma: A case report. *J Am Podiatry Assoc* 53:756–757, 1963.
Parven HA: Excision of a fibroma of unusual size and location. *J Am Coll Foot Surg* 5:118–119, 1966.
Pascher F, Sims CF: Basal cell epithelioma of the sole. *Arch Dermatol* 69:475–481, 1954.
Paul GR, Leach, RE, Beetham WP: Pulmonary carcinoma metastasis to the great toe. *JAMA* 208:2163, 1969.
Perry GM: Villous synovitis, a case report. *J Am Podiatry Assoc* 53:757–758, 1963.
Rakow RB: Leiomyoma of the foot (a case report). *J Am Podiatry Assoc* 56:24–25, 1966.
Richter PA, Black JR: Recurring Kaposi's sarcoma of the foot (A case report). *J Am Podiatry Assoc* 75:162–165, 1985.
Sachs W, MacKee GM, Schwartz OD, Pierson HS: Junction nevus-nevocarcinoma. *JAMA* 135:216–218, 1947.
Schaffer B: A clinical appraisal of pigmented nevi in the light of present day histopathologic concepts. *Arch Dermatol* 72:120–132, 1955.
Scheimer OM: Case report—Massive intermetatarsal inclusion cyst. *J Am Coll Foot Surg* 4:10, 1965a.
Scheimer OM: Case report—invasive malignant melanoma. *J Am Coll Foot Surg* 4:18–19, 1965b.
Shaffer B: Pigmented nevi. *Arch Dermatol* 72:120, 1955.
Shaw RE: Xanthoma tuberosum. *J Am Coll Foot Surg* 4:14–15, 1965.
Solomon S: Excision of a typical nodular hydradenoma. *J Am Coll Foot Surg* 5:80–81, 1966.
Spinelli JA: Case report—Hemangiofibroma. *J Am Coll Foot Surg* 4:15–16, 1965.
Spinosa FA: Leiomyoma of the foot. *J Foot Surg* 24:68–70, 1985.
Steinberg RI, Harant W: Giant cell tumor of the foot. *J Am Podiatry Assoc* 66:534—537, 1976.
Steinhart AN: Squamous cell carcinoma of the foot: Case presentation and review of the literature. *J Am Podiatry Assoc* 70:330, 1980.
Stoler WA: Fibrolipoma with calcified organized thrombi. *J Am Coll Foot Surg* 5:35–36, 1966.
Stout AP: Liposarcoma—Malignant tumor of lipoblasts. *Ann Surg* 119:86–107, 1944.
Stout AP: *Tumors of Soft Tissues*. Washington, DC, Armed Forces Institute of Pathology, 1953.
Sutro CJ: Synovial sarcoma of the soft parts in the first toe: Recurrence after a 35-year interval. *Bull Hosp Joint Dis* 37:105–109, 1976.
Taylor, PC: Case report—Malignant melanoma of the great toe. *J Am Coll Foot Surg* 4:45–46, 1965.
Thompson SG: Epithelioma cuniculatum: An un-

usual tumor of the foot. *Br J Plast Surg* 18:214–217, 1965.
Toth AP: Xanthoma—A case report. *J Am Podiatry Assoc* 53:600–601, 1963.
Toth S: Perineural fibrosis—A case report. *J Am Podiatry Assoc* 53:755, 1963.
Weed JH: Nocardiosis of the foot—A case report. *J Am Podiatry Assoc* 53:561–563, 1954.
Wolf DS: Cavernous hemangioma. *J Am Podiatry Assoc* 59:446–447, 1969.
Yasuda T, Kawoda A, Yasuda J: Eccrine poroma. *Arch Dermatol* 90:428–431, 1964.
Zislin S: Intermetatarsal bursa producing a neuroma syndrome. *J Am Coll Foot Surg* 5:62–63, 1966.
Zugerman I: Basal cell epithelioma of the sole. *Arch Dermatol* 76:247–249, 1957.

8

Arthritic and Other Inflammatory Disorders

Arthritic disorders affecting the foot and ankle are many and varied (Table 8.1). It is beyond the scope of this text to discuss the total impact of the arthritic foot and ankle on the body complex. The reader is referred to Yale's *The Arthritic Foot and Related Connective Tissue Disorders* (1).

Acute painful arthritis of the feet often manifests as sudden spasms of the musculature involved with the biomechanics of the joint and is usually accompanied by redness, swelling, limited function and/or structural changes in the affected extremity (Figs. 8.1–8.5). Early interpretation of the etiology may be difficult (Table 8.2). Solicito et al. (2) discuss the use of radionuclide bone and joint imaging in arthritic and related diseases. The authors conclude that bone and joint scans are diagnostically helpful when bone and joint disease has not progressed far enough to be apparent on standard radiographs. The first stage, joint pool image, points out areas of hyperemia, making it easier to determine which joints are involved, and the second phase, bone scan, points out metabolic changes in calcium, as well as hyperemic areas. Differentiation of joint involvement from extra-articular lesions and septic arthritis from synovitis and osteomyelitis is enhanced. A positive gallium scan is a strong indication of the existence of an infective process. Radiographic findings include diminished joint space, periarticular bone destruction and bone formation, soft tissue swelling, joint subluxation and dislocation, periosteal reaction, soft tissue calcification and osteoporosis.

Pain may be relieved by ice packs, analgesics, nonsteroidal anti-inflammatories (NSAIDs), muscle relaxants, mild sinusoidal stimulation and passive exercises under ethyl chloride spray (see Chapter 3, The Painful Foot, and Chapter 13, Podiatric Treatment). When pain has been relieved, spasm subsides with improved function. A comprehensive examination may then be performed in order to establish a definitive diagnosis (1).

A good comprehensive case history is essential to establishing a diagnosis of chronic arthritis in the feet. Function and abnormal structural deformities provide additional information about the patient's limitations that should improve planning successful management.

The principles of kinesiology and physiological exercises must be followed with care. The osteoarthritic changes are slow and insidious. Even with the best intentions, treatment can be ineffectual due to conservative management, inadequate therapeutic management or the patient's failure to follow instructions. With limited function of joints, muscles become weak and atrophied. If physiotherapeutic measures, foot and ankle orthoses and biomechanical treatment measures fail, surgical correction may be necessary (1).

Arthritic and Inflammatory Disorders

Periarthritis of the Metatarsophalangeal Joints (Periarticular Fibrocitis).

Table 8.1.
Arthritic Manifestations in the Foot and Ankle

1. Polyarthritis of unknown etiology: rheumatoid arthritis, Reiter's syndrome, ankylosing spondylitis, Behcet's syndrome, polychondritis, polyfibrocytis, psychogenic arthralgia and palindromic recurrent rheumatism
2. Osteoarthritis: osteoarthrosis, degenerative joint disease, hypertrophic arthritis, senescent arthritis
3. Traumatic arthritis: from macrotrauma and multiple minimal cumulative microtrauma
4. Arthritis due to collagen disorders: scleroderma, dermatomyositis, systemic lupus erythematosus (SLE)
5. Arthritis due to vitamin deficiency: scurvy, rickets
6. Neurotrophic arthritis: diabetes, syphilis, syringomyelia, congenital pain insensitivity, myelopathy of pernicious anemia, paraplegia, hereditary sensory neuropathy, familial interstitial polyneuropathy of Déjérine and Sottas, peripheral nerve injury, leprosy, yaws
7. Arthritis due to known cause: amyloidosis; malignancy; hemochromatosis; frostbite; benign bone and soft tissue tumor; pregnancy; obesity; chondrocalcinosis; CPPD; gout; viral infection—rubella, mumps, chickenpox, polio, smallpox, hepatitis; bacterial infection—meningococcus, *Haemophilus infleunzae,* coliform, *Salmonella,* pneumonia, tuberculosis, gonorrhea, *Streptococcus, Staphylococcus, Proteus, Pseudomonas, Escherichia coli;* superficial fungus infections—maduromycosis, *Sporothrix, Candida;* deep fungus infections—coccidiodomycosis, histoplasmosis, blastomycosis, cryptomycosis, aspergillosis; parasitic infections—rickettsial, Lyme arthritis
8. Arthritic-associated diseases

Hyperthyroidism	Osteolysis
Ulcerative colitis	Erythema nodosum
Sarcoidosis	Cutaneous periarteritis nodosa
Sjögren's syndrome	Sickle cell disease
Whipple's disease	Leukemia
Psoriasis	Pseudohypertrophic osteoarthropathy
Pigmented villonodular synovitis	Hypertrophic osteoarthropathy
Hyperparathyroidism	Melorheostosis
Chronic active hepatitis	Hemophilia
Osteitis deformans	Periarticular osteoporosis
Osteochondromatosis	Sudeck's atrophy
Osteochondritis dissecans	Hyperlipoproteinemia II A
Regional enteritis	

This is a painful enlargement of the tissues of the plantar surface of the metatarsal heads. The condition may result from dancing excessively in high-heeled shoes and from wearing narrow and/or thin-soled shoes; it may be secondary to a compensated rearfoot or forefoot varus or a partially compensated or uncompensated equinus or be due to multiple minimal trauma. Periarticular fibrocitis of the second metatarophalangeal joint is often the first painful joint symptom associated with rheumatoid arthritis. The underlying structures are painful to palpation and weightbearing, and the patient complains of a throbbing pain and usually a dull ache. Swelling is present, and limitation of function typically occurs. An adventitious bursa or cyst may develop subcutaneously. Gout or rheumatoid arthritis may be an underlying factor. Marked soft tissue thickening and effusion are present. Calcifications may develop in degenerated tissue or a bursa. The joint space is widened or narrowed depending on the degree of effusion and extent of trauma. A stress fracture must be ruled out by radiographic examination.

Jacoby et al. (3), reporting on the examination of 200 consecutive inpatients with rheumatoid arthritis, note that some abnormality occurred in the great toe in particular in 196 feet.

Treatment. Oral analgesics, NSAIDs and muscle relaxants are helpful. Shortwave, ultrasound and other physical modalities may be necessary to relieve pain.

Felt raises skived to remove weightbearing from the affected part are placed in shoes or strapped to the foot. Use of a balanced foot orthosis to distribute weight from the affected part is generally successful.

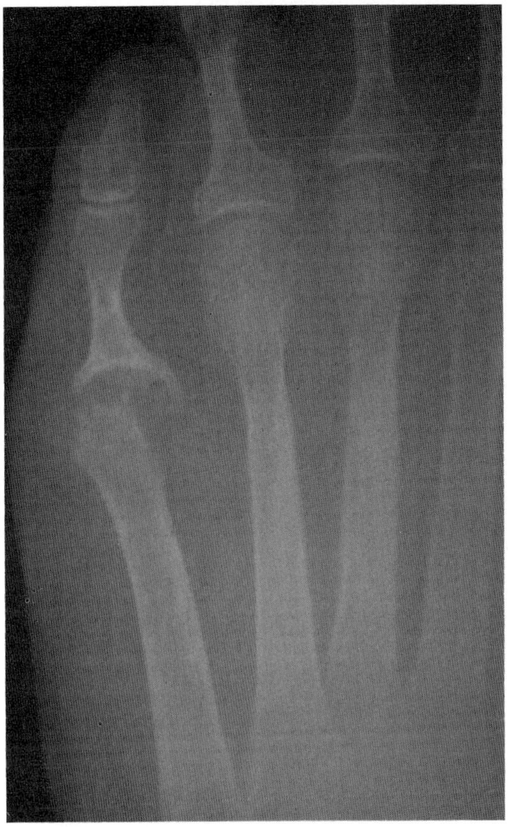

Figure 8.1. Rheumatoid arthritic destruction of fifth metatarsophalangeal joint.

The foot can be rehabilitated by low-voltage sinusoidal currents and active and passive exercises.

If pain persists, an injection of local anesthetic followed by injection of 0.4 ml of an effective corticosteroid into the acutely inflamed site relieves discomfort.

Epiphysitis of the Metatarsals. In examining children prior to complete union and ossification of their epiphyses, the examiner must be cautious in interpreting forefoot symptoms.

A history of injury to the forefoot from a misstep, a jump from a height in which the patient landed on the ball of the foot or direct trauma should lead the podiatrist to suspect epiphysitis of the metatarsals. This condition is characterized by swelling on the dorsum of the foot over the affected epiphysis. The second, third and fifth metatarsal epiphyses are usually involved. Often the styloid apophysis of the fifth metatarsal base may be displaced. This epiphysis is not constant. Pain on palpation is noted at the head of the affected metatarsal. Slight heat and bluish-red discolorations are present around the affected parts and involve the toes. The extensor tendons are usually contracted and very often inflamed with limitation of function accompanied by pain and swelling.

X-ray Examination. A soft tissue swelling follows the fascial planes. The

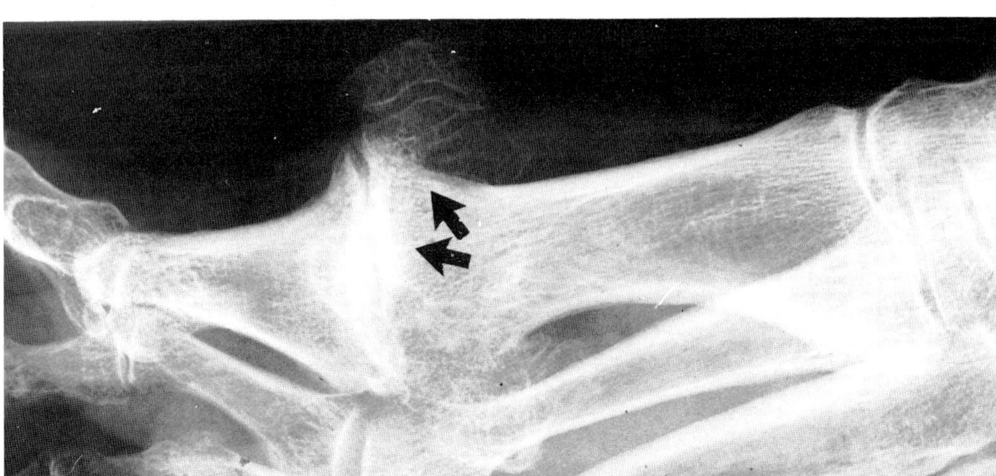

Figure 8.2. Osteochondroma. Severe deformity involving first metatarsophalangeal joint. There are marked soft tissue swelling, lipping, osteophytes, and destruction of articular cartilage.

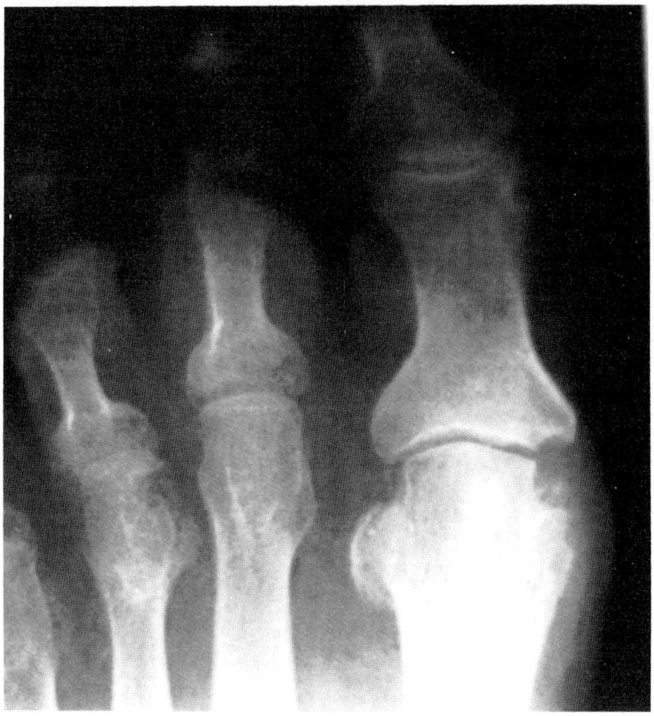

Figure 8.3. Severe gout. 58-year-old black male with severe loss of bone substance and tophaceous deposits. Deposits must be differential from calcium pyrophosphate dihydrate.

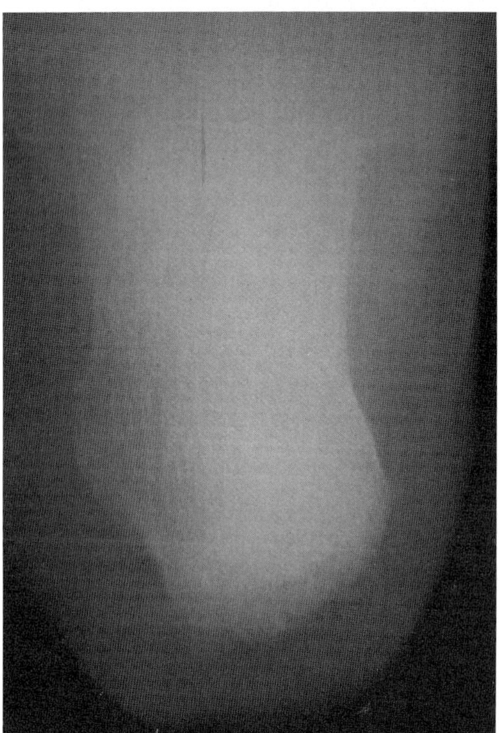

Figure 8.4. "Fluffy" periostitis of the calcaneus secondary to Reiter's syndrome.

joint may have an effusion presenting a symmetrical fusiform outline. The epiphysis may be subluxated at the metaphysis. In long-standing cases, a local demineralization may be evident anterior to the epiphyseal line. Very often a frac-

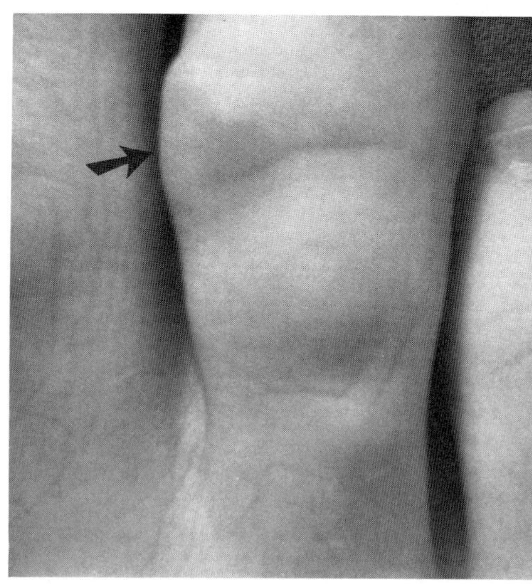

Figure 8.5. Heberden's Nodes: A thickening of the distal articulation of a toe or toes.

ture involves the metaphyseal end of the bone. Fibrocartilaginous tears at the epiphyseal line may be suggested but not visible. When the injury occurs in early childhood and is of sufficient severity, a failure in future normal longitudinal development of the bone may be possible. The epiphysis is very often displaced with trauma.

Treatment. Physical therapy, such as whirlpool, ultrasound, infrared, short wave and contrast foot baths, helps relieve pain. Immobilization by adhesive materials, plastic dressings, Celastic, plaster and orthoses are necessary to maintain a limitation of motion. Firm footgear and rigid foot orthoses coupled with shoe wedging to limit motion and protect the affected part are indicated in epiphysitis. A Jones bar on the sole of the shoe relieves excessive trauma.

Injection of corticosteroids prior to maturation and union of the epiphysis is not usually acceptable treatment because corticosteroids tend to stimulate maturation and thus inhibit normal bone growth.

Mild analgesics generally help bring about relief during the period of repair.

Sesamoiditis. Painful sesamoids suggest injury. Predisposing etiologic factors include: plantar flexed first metatarsal, forefoot valgus, spasm or contracture of the peroneus longus, limited dorsiflexion of the first metatarsal with subtalar pronation, and dorsal contracture of the hallux at the first metatarsophalangeal joint. Swelling, pain, discoloration and sometimes crepitus at the plantar surface of the head of the first metatarsal are the usual symptoms (Figs. 8.6 and 8.7).

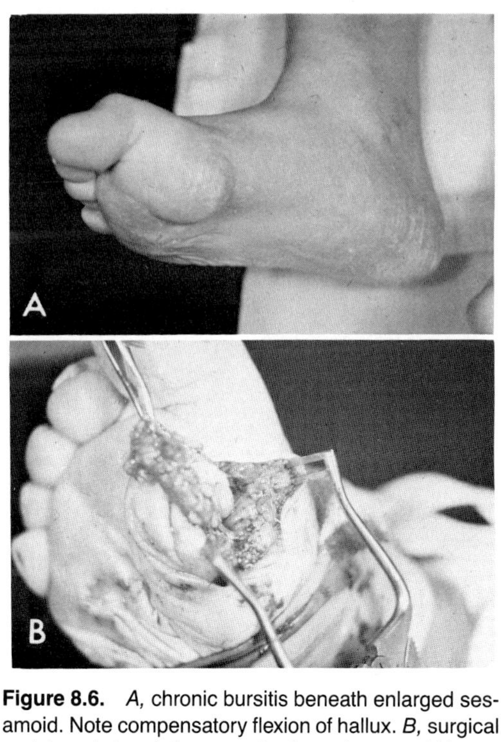

Figure 8.6. *A,* chronic bursitis beneath enlarged sesamoid. Note compensatory flexion of hallux. *B,* surgical excision of chronic bursa and enlarged sesamoid bone.

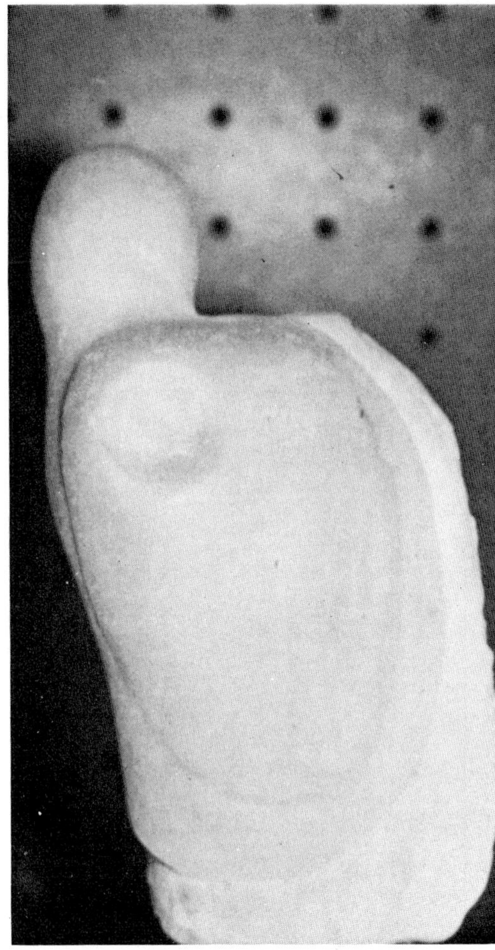

Figure 8.7. Latex shield may be modified to protect a bursa, intractable plantar keratosis or sesamoiditis in poor surgical risks. (Courtesy of Liquid Rubber Appliance Laboratory)

Ingersoll (4) described this problem as a "sesamoidalgia." He refers to enlarged sesamoids, displaced sesamoids, anomalous sesamoid bones, traumatically fragmented sesamoid bones and fusion or adhesion of one or both sesamoid bones. Clinical examination presents marked edema with

Table 8.2.
Differential Diagnosis of the More Common Foot Arthritides

	Male-female ratio	Fever	Involvement	Joint appearance	X-ray findings	Joints affected	Special considerations
Rheumatoid arthritis	1:2–3	Low grade	Multiple, migratory	Periarticular swelling and joint effusion	Narrowing of joint spaces with chondro-osseous lytic lesions, osteopororis (Fig. 8.1)	Prox IPJs, MPJs	Fusiform prox. IPJs, second MPJ periarticular fibrocitis is often first clinical sign, late periarticular nodules
Osteoarthritis	1:1	Absent	Multiple, nonmigratory	No periarticular swelling or redness	Narrowing of joint spaces with lipping (Fig. 8.2)	Distal IPJs, ankle	Heberden's nodes (Fig. 8.5)
Acute gout	15:1	High	Monoarticular	Marked periarticular swelling, redness and joint effusion	Normal, narrowing of joint space with cystic lesions in chronic cases (Fig. 8.3)	First MPJ, plantar fascial and Achilles tendon insertion	Tophaceous deposits, elevated blood uric acid
Chondrocalcinosis	2:1	Low grade	Monoarticular	Marked periarticular swelling, redness and joint effusion	Periarticular calcification	Knee	Calcium pyrophosphate crystals in synovial fluid
Rheumatic fever	1:1	High	Multiple, migratory	Marked periarticular swelling with occasional joint effusion	Negative	Ankle, knee	Rash, carditis, subcutaneous nodules, ASO titer +
Reiter's syndrome	2:1	Low grade	Oligoarticular, asymmetric	Sausage toe, no redness, enthesitis	Osteolysis with periosteal new bone formation (Fig. 8.4)	Fifth MPJ, plantar fascial and Achilles tendon insertion, hallux interphalangeal joint	Urethritis, conjunctivitis, keratoderma blenorrhagica, diarrhea, mucocutaneous lesions, HLA-B_{27} 65–80% +

redness that may involve the entire metatarsophalangeal articulation. Pain and often crepitus are felt on palpation over the affected bones. Bursitis is common.

One sesamoid may be grossly enlarged compared to the other. Occasionally a sesamoid is comminuted or presents a fracture. However, an interpretation of fracture must never be made unless a definite fracture line is present. Stippling or multiple hazy areas of demineralization may be visible in a sesamoid that has been painful for some time. This local demineralization usually occurs with marked hyperemia and resultant resorption of bone elements. Sesamoids may have spurs, osteophytes and lipping at their margins. Frequently a tear of the fibrocartilaginous attachment of one part of a multipartite sesamoid from the other may be noted on x-ray examination. Subluxation or dislocation of the sesamoids is a common cause of sesamoiditis.

Treatment. Debride overlying tylomas and shield or disperse pressure from the affected parts by using conventional shielding, either parallel stress pads as described by Sansone (5) or the well-known dancer's pad used for many years by podiatrists.

Inject a local corticosteroid into a bursa beneath the sesamoids if necessary.

Short wave and ultrasound therapy twice weekly help relieve pain. Analgesics should be prescribed if pain persists.

Firm-soled, well-fitting footgear with anterior heels or Jones bars are helpful in relieving multiple minimal trauma.

Construction of semirigid foot orthoses with a cutout under the sesamoids may be necessary.

Properly posted Rohadur orthoses may correct the subtalar valgus and compensate for a first metatarsal equinus that often predisposes a patient to sesamoiditis.

Partial or total surgical removal of a chronically painful, dislocated or subluxed tibial sesamoid may be necessary. This is accomplished by an incision at the medial plantar aspect of the metatarsal head.

Hypertrophy of the First Metatarsocuneiform Articulation. Thickening of the first metatarsocuneiform joint is not uncommon. Frequently only one aspect of the articulating surface of the affected part presents osteophytic changes at the anterior surface of the medial cuneiform or the posterior articulating surface of the first metatarsal base. Usually the dorsal and medial aspect of the articulation are involved.

On gross examination the enlargement on the dorsum of the foot looks like a tumorous mass. Careful examination may reveal an inflamed superficial tissue with overlying helomas of 1 to 3 mm. A bursal sac may overlie the enlarged bone. Very often this lesion is found alone without bone pathology. X-ray examination should substantiate these findings.

The pathology in the affected part suggests enlargement and thickening of the joint capsule due to chronic irritation.

The involved bone is hypertrophied, and an overlying adventitious bursa may be noted. Often the bursa is hypertrophied, inflamed and fibrotic. The sac fluctuates in size depending upon the degree of friction and irritation. The overlying skin is thickened and commonly develops helomas. Occasionally the tendon of the extensor hallucis longus becomes inflamed, resulting in a tenosynovitis over the hypertrophied bone. Pressure on the medial branch of the medial dorsal cutaneous nerve may cause paresthesias along the inner side of the great toe. The medial marginal veins and an anastomotic branch overlying the hypertrophied joint may become inflamed by pressure, causing a local phlebitis. Local infection may occur at the site of pressure.

X-ray examination may reveal hypertrophy of the margins of the first metatarsocuneiform joint. The joint space narrows, and the margins of the articulating surface show evidence of lipping, osteophytes, spurs or exostoses. Occasionally an accessory bone may develop over the body of the cuneiform. This must be differentiated from a calcification in the soft tissues or a degenerative calcareous tendonitis. Bursae may degenerate, become fibrous and eventually calcify, leaving flaky amorphous, calcareous deposits.

Treatment. Excise the dorsal heloma. If a bursal sac is acutely inflamed, a corticosteroid of choice may be injected.

Remove eyelets on shoes overlying the enlarged bone, and shield the affected part with felt. A soothing ointment should be used.

Construct a permanent shield of latex, felt latex, plastic or silicone gel. A foot orthosis to control pronation relieves the stress from the first metatarsocuneiform joint.

If pain persists, local applications of ultrasound or injections of corticosteroid medications into the painful articulation are helpful.

Surgical excision of a chronic bursa and its underlying bony prominence will relieve pain and eliminate the cause.

Shortened Metatarsal Segments. With the advent of Dudley Morton's theories on the shortened first metatarsal segment, there has been much concern about the shortening or dystrophic involvements of one or more of the lesser metatarsal bones.

Morton felt that many of the existing foot complaints of a biomechanical nature were related, either singly or in combination, to a shortened first segment, hypermobility of the first segment or posteriorly placed pivotal sesamoids.

Podiatric observers have noted that shortening and hypermobility of the fifth metatarsal segment occur with the same frequency as the shortened first. Relief of symptoms has been accomplished through treatment of short metatarsals by affording better weight distribution.

Frequently the fourth metatarsal is short but well-developed. Faulty weight distribution results in subsequent tyloma formation under the pivotal heads of the longer metatarsals. The toes are usually dorsiflexed, the extensor tendons are contracted and a concavity is present over the fourth head on the dorsum of the foot (Fig. 8.8). Occasionally two or more metatarsals may be shortened. It is conceivable that a neurotrophic disorder or an injury to the distal epiphysis of a metatarsal could result in early union and a cessation of growth. The danger of shoe-fitting fluorscopic devices producing cumulative x-ray injuries to the epiphyses is great. Reports of early union of the epiphyses from accumulation of exposures to x-rays are not uncommon. Shortening of any of the long metatarsal bones may result.

With shortening of the fifth metatarsal, the fifth toe usually falls medially against the fourth toe and very often causes a heloma molle.

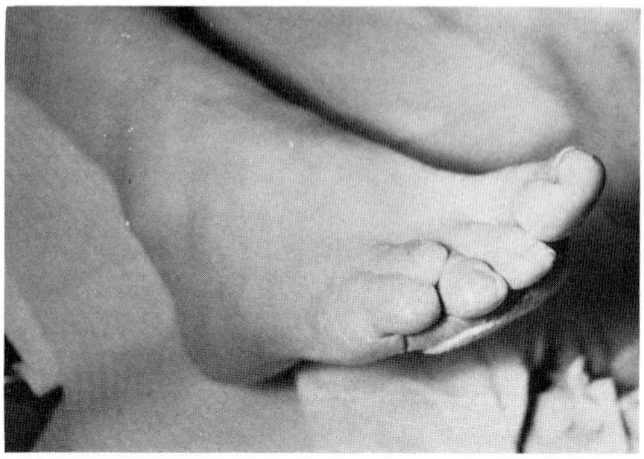

Figure 8.8. Brachymetapodia, fourth metatarsal bone. Note short dorsiflexed fourth toe with underlapping third toe.

X-ray studies of the foot on weightbearing give the necessary information in suspected cases of shortening and variations in the metatarsal parabola.

Sansone (6) describes the metatarsal parabola as representing the area of weight transmission in the forefoot. It varies according to the width and length of the foot. Sansone suggested a "Rule of Forefoot Weight Distribution. The arc of the metatarsal parabola deviates directly with any inconsistence in the metatarsal lengths and the regular weight distribution pattern varies accordingly." He discussed variations in metatarsal length and the pathology they caused. Compensating pads are prescribed to provide proper forefoot balance.

Treatment. X-ray examination establishes the presence of short or elongated metatarsal segments.

Deep excrescences occurring under longer metatarsals are debrided and shielded. The site of excrescences is marked off with skin pencil, and impressions are taken for construction of an accommodative orthotic device. Felt latex orthoses are constructed to accommodate the shortened bones and the deep excrescences commonly found on fulcrum-serving long bones.

If feet are hypermobile, a rigid orthosis is constructed for the rearfoot with a flexible accommodating forefoot extension.

Weiner (7) recommended a felt pad for metatarsalgia that covered a wide area of the metatarsus. It is longer and wider than the conventional metatarsal pad, extending from the interdigital spaces backward to the bases of the metatarsals. It covers all the metatarsal heads with a long forward bevel to the interphalangeal joints.

Sansone (6) described balancing of the forefoot parabola. For short metatarsal bones, extensions beyond the metatarsal heads of ⅛- to 3/16-inch pieces of felt are used to balance the foot. Cutouts are made under longer metatarsal heads while other covered metatarsals accept more of the body weight. Pads are devised to balance the forefoot when there is a long second metatarsal, Morton's syndrome, a pseudoshort metatarsal, a short first and second metatarsal, a metatarsus proximus or when the second and third metatarsals are long, the first and fifth are short, the first or the first and second are long and the fourth and/or the fifth are short.

Rigid orthoses are necessary to control rear foot subtalar valgus and forefoot varus or valgus incidental to this problem.

Strain at the Attachment of the Plantar Fascia and Flexor Digitorum Brevis. The plantar fascia and short plantar flexors of the toes originate at or near the medial tubercle of the plantar surface of the calcaneus. The onset of pain is very often acute, yet many instances are reported in which a dull pain, persisting for several weeks or months, had become progressively worse. Pain is noted in the region of the plantar fascial attachment and also anterior to this along the course of the painful structure. Weightbearing and digital pressure under the medial tubercle of the calcaneus elicit pain. Swelling, when present, is usually slight. The condition is unilateral when caused by trauma, but if it has an infectious origin a bilateral affliction is not uncommon.

Pathological changes or organic bone disturbances may be the result of constitutional defects, such as syphilis or tuberculosis, or may follow gonorrheal and rheumatic diseases, Reiter's syndrome or ankylosing spondylitis.

An increase in body weight, long working hours on the feet and a vocation of standing or walking on hard inelastic surfaces cause strain. A strained plantar fascia may be caused by jumping from a height, the use of a foot pedal or a sudden change from a high to low flat-heeled shoe, which causes an excessive pull on the musculature. When high heels are worn for a prolonged period of time, the musculature contracts. The change on weightbearing without shoes or wearing flat-heeled shoes causes strain. Prolonged rest in bed weakens the musculature. Strain of plantar connective tissue is usually accompanied by pain on arising after a period of rest.

Treatment. Pain is relieved by oral NSAIDs. Whirlpool, ultrasound, paraffin baths, short wave and infrared treatments are helpful. Contrast foot baths at home bid for several days are helpful.

Adhesive immobilization by low Dye strapping shortens the distance between the origin and insertion of the plantar musculature and fascia and thus relieves strain.

In an acutely inflamed plantar fascia, injections of corticosteroids at trigger points help relieve symptoms.

Changing shoes from flexible shanks to firm rigid shanks is mandatory. Flexible shanks allow for stretching of already inflamed plantar structures.

If a structural deformity exists the problem should be corrected. Foot orthotic devices are helpful.

Plantar Calcaneal Exostosis. The calcaneal spur that causes pain on the plantar surface of the heel is defined as a bony projection extending from the tuberosity of the calcaneus, forward and downward in the direction of the plantar fascia (Fig. 8.9). It may appear sharp, sclerosed, condensed or neatly demarcated with central reticulation.

The patient complains of a painful heel on arising in the morning or following periods of rest. The pain is acute with each step and in the early stages disappears after a few steps, only to return after prolonged weightbearing or stress. It feels

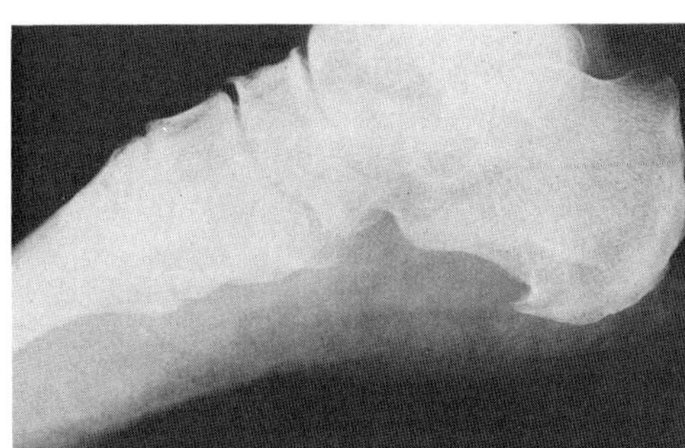

Figure 8.9. Plantar calcaneal exostosis. Note the degenerative lipping and osteophytes at the dorsal posterior and anterior articulations of the navicular.

like a nail sticking into the foot or as a bruise localized to a definite area in the heel. The medial tubercle at the plantar surface of the calcaneus is painful, and an inflamed plantar fascia or an acute bursitis may coexist. The x-ray examination is essential for diagnosis.

The podiatrist must be aware that the heel is often the site for acute pain of gout accompanied by a high blood uric acid. Secondary gout—precipitated by thiazide diuretics, trauma, salicylates, alcohol, penicillin, insulin and/or thiamine or riboflavin ingestion—may be manifested as acute pain at the insertion of the plantar fascia. Reiter's syndrome, hyperlipidemia and ankylosing spondylitis must be differentiated from it (Table 8.3).

Treatment. Short wave and ultrasound treatments every 2 or 3 days and contrast foot baths at home tid are recommended. Analgesics by inunction and oral pain-relieving medication are helpful.

Adhesive immobilization by low Dye strapping with a ¼ inch felt raise may be used. The posterior skive is abrupt to raise the body of the calcaneus off the medial tubercle. Occasionally a donut-shaped felt or sponge pad around the painful area is helpful.

Injections of lidocaine and/or corticosteroids into the soft tissues adjacent to the spur are indicated when pain persists. They relieve an acute bursitis that often accompanies the spur.

Construction of a foot orthotic device designed to cradle the heel with a high longitudinal raise is desirable to alter weight distribution and relieve pain. A rigid foot orthosis is desirable if it is well-fitted.

Table 8.3.
Lipoprotein Phenotypes[a]

Phenotype	Elevated lipoprotein(s)	Predominantly elevated lipid(s)	Serum appearance	Comment
Type I	Chylomicrons	Triglycerides	Cream layer; clear	Low risk of ASCVD[b] Pancreatitis Eruptive xanthomas
Type IIa	Low-density lipoprotein (LDL)	Cholesterol	Clear	Highly atherogenic Tendon xanthomas Xanthelasmas
Type IIb	LDL Very low-density lipoprotein (VLDL)	Cholesterol Triglycerides	Turbid	Atherogenic
Type III	Intermediate-density lipoprotein (IDL)	Cholesterol Triglycerides	Turbid	Atherogenic (PVD)[c] Palmar xanthomas
Type IV	VLDL	Triglycerides	Turbid	Atherogenic Glucose intolerance
Type V	Chylomicrons VLDL	Triglycerides	Cream layer; turbid	Low risk of ASCVD Pancreatitis Insulin deficiency Eruptive xanthomas

[a] From R Sloan. Hyperlipedemia. *Am Fam Physician,* 174, 1983.
[b] ASCVD = atherosclerotic cardiovascular disease.
[c] PVD = peripheral vascular disease.

Carleton (8) described a leather Shaffer shell designed to distribute weightbearing to the structures anterior to the calcaneus and just posterior to the metatarsal heads. The heel area is cut out, and a ¼-inch thick sponge skived at its margins is placed on top of the shell. Both top and bottom are covered.

A metal, Prenyl, Rodan or Rohadur or other firm, rigid or semirigid foot orthotic device may be constructed to realign the weightbearing foot and remove pressure from the site of pain. The success of treatment depends on the skill of the foot specialist, rather than the material used.

Analgesics with muscle relaxants or NSAIDs may be prescribed for relief of pain and secondary spasm, e.g., methacarbamol, 500 mg (Robaxin); chlorzoxazone (Paraflex, Parafon), 250 mg two tablets qid; Paraflex, 250 mg and acetaminophen, 300 mg, two tablets qid; and methacarbamol, 400 mg, with aspirin, 325 mg (Robaxisal).

Posterior tibial nerve blocks may be necessary in the acutely painful heel. Injections of 0.5 ml of corticosteroid directly into the painful site are also helpful in relieving acute pain. Michael (9) reported excellent results using injections of triamcinolone acetonide, 10 mg/ml. (Decadron, Kenalog, Aristocort, Aristospan and Depo-Medrol are all useful injectible corticosteroids.)

Sinus Tarsi Syndrome. This condition is often misdiagnosed. This post-traumatic arthritis of the subtalar joint may be caused by a sudden eversion foot injury or the multiple minimal microtrauma of adverse subtalar joint function. An aching-type pain associated with the dorsalateral aspect of the foot just anterior and distal to the lateral malleolus is experienced. The discomfort is worse upon arising.

Treatment. Must be first directed toward efficient functioning of the subtalar joint through the use of foot orthoses. Symptomatic treatment consists of steroid-local anesthetic injections into the sinus tarsi and oral NSAIDs. On rare occasions, the soft tissue contents of the sinus tarsi must be excised. Subtalar synchondrosis, syndesmosis and synostosis must be differentiated. Tomograms may be useful (10).

Calcaneal Bursitis. Calcaneal bursitis occurs on the plantar surface of the heel, usually at the origin of the plantar aponeurosis at the medial calcaneal tubercle (plantar calcaneal bursitis), just anterior to the Achilles tendon between it and the posterior superior surface of the calcaneus (anterior calcaneal or retrocalcaneal bursitis) or just posterior to the Achilles tendon between it and the skin (posterior calcaneal bursitis). It manifests as a soreness of the affected area of the heel that soon becomes moderately swollen, red and painful to touch. Plantar calcaneal bursitis commonly develops in the presence of a plantar calcaneal exostosis and excessive subtalar pronation. Anterior and/or posterior calcaneal bursitis commonly develop in the presence of a posterior superior calcaneal exostosis and/or excessive subtalar pronation.

Treatment. In extremely painful plantar calcaneal bursitis, bed rest is indicated along with analgesics, corticosteroid local injections and other anti-inflammatory oral medication.

Ritchie (11) recommends phenylbutazone (Butazolidin) or Butazolidin Alka for short-term treatment of bursitis; 100 mg qid for 7 consecutive days taken after meals is an acceptable dose. Oxyphenbutazone (Tenderil), one tablet 3 to 4 times daily for 3 to 5 days, is anti-inflammatory. Phenylbutazone and oxyphenbutazone are currently not recommended for treatment of bursitis. Other NSAIDs such as sulindac, ibuprofen, or naproxen are recommended.

Plantar intrabursal injection of anti-inflammatory medication is made easier when a posterior tibial nerve block is instituted first. Using aseptic techniques, aspiration may be instituted following local anesthesia. Leaving the 18 gauge needle in the plantar bursa, a second syringe with 0.2 to 0.5 ml of the corticosteroid of choice is attached to the needle and injected intrabursally.

A donut pad ¼ inch thick may be cemented to the heel or bound down with adhesive tape. A low Dye and ¼ inch thick felt longitudinal and metatarsal pad dressing may be applied.

Insufficient Adipose Covering. Often one sees asthenic individuals with insufficient adipose tissue around the heel. This condition may develop following prolonged bed rest and inactivity in the elderly and the young.

Treatment. Rubber heels on shoes and a sponge in the heel seat are helpful. If the tissue is acutely inflamed, bed rest and elevation removes inflammatory exudates.

Closely fitting plastic or rubber heel cups or foot orthoses high enough to accept weight on the medial longitudinal arch remove pressure from the heel. Moldable insole material serves to break the shock of weightbearing. A high medial longitudinal felt shoe pad lifts pressure from the heel.

Calcaneal Periostitis. Periostitis of the calcaneus manifests as a soreness of the heel with severe pain on weightbearing and palpation. Evidence of a soft tissue mass or subperiosteal calcific deposits may be found on x-ray examination. The most common site of tenderness is palpated at the sides of the calcaneal body. Soft tissue swelling is common.

The author has seen several cases of calcaneal periostits following infections of the teeth, nose or throat. There is generally a slight elevation in skin temperature overlying the area of inflammation. Tenderness and swelling of the heel have been observed following the use of penicillin for an infection far removed from the foot. Stress fractures of the calcaneus must be ruled out.

Treatment. If stress is caused by the patient being overweight, weight reduction is indicated.

Plastic or rubber heel cups protect the heel from trauma. Fiberglass, metal, Rohadur or leather orthoses to relieve weightbearing from the affected heel may be necessary. A plaster cast, flexible casting or Celastic immobilization of the heel may be used in acute states.

Isolation of an infecting organism is necessary to establish the etiology and prescribe the proper antibiotics. Arthritic disorders should be differentiated.

Osteochondrosis of the Calcaneus. (Synonyms include apophysitis of the calcaneus, avascular necrosis of the calcaneal apophysis, osteochondritis of the calcaneus, calcaneal osteosis, and Sever's disease.) Gamble and Yale (12) define an apophysis as any outgrowth, swelling or process, especially a bony process that had never been entirely separated from the bone of which it forms a part, that does not enter into the formation of a joint and that is not covered by cartilage. An apophysis is a traction epiphysis. Apophysitis, an inflammation of the posterior epiphysis of the calcaneus, is most common in boys between the ages of 8 and 12 (Fig. 8.10). Direct trauma or multiple minimum injury to the apophysis may be etiologic (13). Muscular stress on the Achilles tendon may cause a tenderness along the cartilage line. Infections and circulatory changes in the epiphyseal cartilage may cause discomfort in the apophysis. This condition is usually unilateral. Krantz (personal communication) felt that calcaneal apophysitis is probably caused by microtrauma.

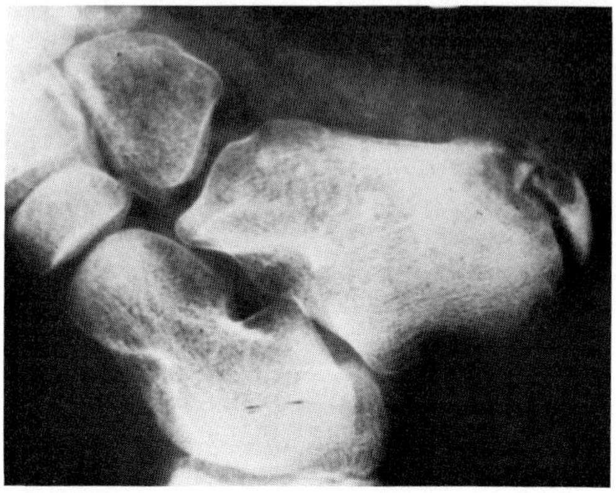

Figure 8.10. Traumatic calcaneal apophysitis with fracture of the apophysis. (From FO Gamble and I Yale: *Clinical Foot Roentgenology.* Baltimore, Williams & Wilkins, 1966)

The apophysis is placed at a distinct disadvantage by virtue of the attachment on its posterior surface of the Achilles tendon. When the osteochondrotic changes become severe, osteitis and destructive lesions may occur, and in some cases, periostitis may be evident. The apophysis may fail to develop properly if untreated, possibly resulting in a faulty ossification. Krantz found that children with medium to high arches and soft tissue equinus seem to be subject to this problem. Excessively pronated feet may also be etiologic.

At first the pain is described as a dull ache over the midportion of the posteror surface of the apophysis. The pain may then become more severe, extending to either side of the posterior of the heel. The slight pain in the back of the heel becomes severe when climbing stairs, jumping or running. Pain and difficulty in walking are most severe after a period of rest. This is called poststatic dyskinesia. Pain on palpation is noted at the posterior plantar angle of the heel. A thickening of the tissues may be felt laterally and on the plantar of the apophysis. Dorsiflexion of the foot may cause pain at the apophysis. Pain is less marked when a ¼ inch felt pad is placed in the heel seat to relieve the pull of the Achilles tendon. Pressure of the shoe counter causes pain. Swelling may be present, and very often the patient walks with a limp, as in an equinus gait. This is especially true in the morning with the first steps. The pain disappears with motion, only to return when the patient gets tired.

Treatment. Prescribe oxford tie shoes with rigid shanks, extended counter, rubber heels, leather soles and a snug fit in heel and arch. The patient should refrain from wearing soft soles, flexible shanked shoes or sneakers.

It is wise to limit the use of short wave and ultrasound currents to the developing apophysis, as they cause alterations in the cartilage growth.

Rheumatic fever should be ruled out. A CBC, sedimentation rate, heterophile and latex fixation examination are also necessary for diagnosis.

Relieve strain on the Achilles tendon and plantar musculature by strapping and padding the affected foot in a supinated position. Use heel cups and foot orthoses to control associated biomechanical problems. Protection from repeated trauma can be ensured by decreasing physical activities and using a sponge heel seat.

In severe cases, a plaster cast to limit a child's activity may be necessary for a few weeks to relieve inflammation.

Use of corticosteroids in young patients is discouraged. Analgesics are helpful in relieving pain. Salicylates, 10 grains q 4 to 6 h prn, are usually adequate.

Anterior Achillobursitis (Synonyms include Albert's disease, achillodynia and anterior calcaneal or retrocalcaneal bursitis.) Anterior Achillobursitis is an inflammation occurring in the bursal sac lying between the Achilles tendon and the upper portion of the posterior surface of the calcaneus.

This inflammation may result from excessively pronated feet with a positive Helbing's sign, trauma or, more rarely, gout, rheumatoid arthritis, Reiter's syndrome, tuberculosis, ankylosing spondylitis, and gonorrhea. When inflammation is the result of disease, the onset is slow, but in trauma the symptoms appear rapidly. A severe twist of the foot, especially in a high-heeled pump, may produce this condition. Sudden jumps, constant strain on the Achilles tendon, stiff shoe counters or a kick or blow to the heel may cause this inflammation. Haglund's deformity may be etiologic.

Pain is localized over and around the sides of the tendon just proximal to its insertion. Use of the foot and digital pressure may cause pain. Swelling and inflammatory changes may be evident on either side of the Achilles tendon.

Treatment. Sources of trauma should be eliminated. The heel should be elevated with a ¼-inch raise in the heel seat. Salicylates, indomethacin (Indocin), propoxyphene hydrochloride (Darvon) and acetaminophen (Tylenol, Valodol), 325 mg tablets, are helpful in controlling pain. Injection of corticosteroids or other anti-inflammatory agents in less than 0.4 ml amounts directly into the bursa affords relief. Ultrasound every other day is also helpful.

In severe cases, the heel should be immobilized by adhesive tape or a plaster cast, and oral analgesics may be prescribed.

If systemic disease is the underlying cause of the condition, consultation may be indicated.

Posterior Achillobursitis. This is an inflammation of an adventitious bursa (posterior calcaneal bursitis) occurring between the skin and the Achilles tendon just above its insertion into the calcaneus (Figs. 8.11 and 8.12). It may be caused by friction and pressure from shoes that do not fit properly, such as those with stiff counters, tight shoes, high-heeled pumps, sling backs and poorly shaped shoes. Rheumatoid arthritis, chilblains and frostbite affecting the heel often cause this condition, which is more common in females. Prominence of the posterior superior aspect of the calcaneus and excessive pronation are predisposing factors.

Pain is caused by friction and pressure from the shoes. Bullae may develop. The bursal sac forms at the margin of the counter, often becoming red, hot and swollen. Sometimes fissures develop in the skin. The bursa may become chronic and cause pain at the slightest provocation. The skin over the bursa may ulcerate.

X-ray findings show a large, soft tissue mass of increased density just above the attachment of the Achilles tendon. Occasionally, the bursal sac degenerates and calcification takes place. An exostosis may be present at the attachment of the tendon. The posterior superior angle of

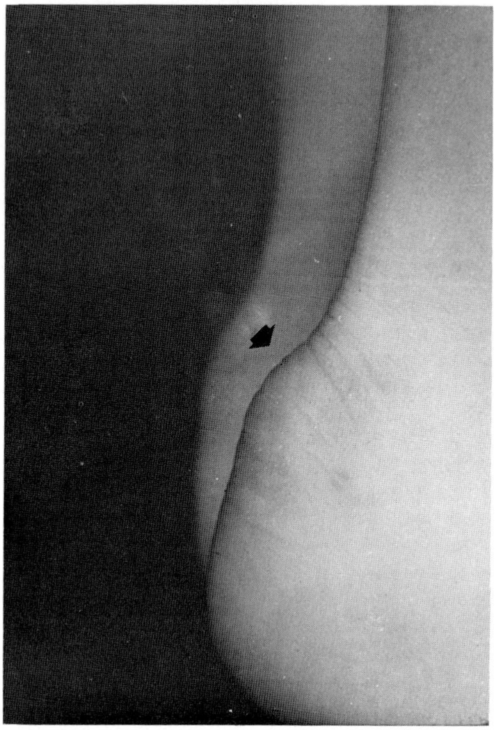

Figure 8.11. Posterior achillobursitis. X-ray examination may reveal an underlying bony prominence requiring surgical correction.

the heel may protrude as in Haglund's deformity.

Treatment. Frostbite and chilblains should be treated. Vasodilators are helpful, and protection from the cold is necessary. Remove pressure of the shoe by elevating the heel seat. A felt or foam donut pad over the inflamed part to relieve pressure is helpful. Injections of an acetylated corticosteroid into the bursa relieves pain. Oral NSAIDs may be helpful. Ultrasound, hot packs and topical analgesic ointments are also used.

Construct a permanent shield from a cast or directly over the part. Latex or liquid plastic are materials of choice. Silicone gel has simplified the technique of pad construction.

Surgical excision of a chronic bursa or underlying bony prominence is indicated in intractable cases.

Haglund's Deformity. In Haglund's deformity, the posterosuperior angle of the calcaneus extends upward and backward (Figs. 8.13 and 8.14). The pressure of the Achilles tendon against this bony prominence results in severe pain. An x-ray of the part establishes the diagnosis of a bony prominence of the posterior superior aspect of the calcaneus. It is the author's opinion that this prominence is a normal anatomic varient.

Over a period of years, the prominent bone may undergo degenerative changes. Irregularity of the cortex with loss of substance and subcortical demineralization are often found with this disorder. Subacute or chronic bursitis is often associated. Arthritic disorders must be differentiated.

Treatment. Permanent shields may relieve pressure from the bony prominence. Raising the heel seat ¼ inch lifts the bone away from the pressure of the counter.

Local physical therapy and oral analgesics or NSAIDs are indicated for relief of pain in acute inflammations.

Surgical excision of the bony prominence is necessary for complete relief. A chronic bursa may be excised.

Traumatic Tenosynovitis. This is an inflammation of the tendon sheath due to excessive use (Fig. 8.15). The inflammatory symptoms may result from slow, prolonged friction over a tendon, such as may occur from ice skating, long hikes, multiple twists of the ankle, strap shoes and pressure on the extensor hallucis longus tendon from pumps. Sudden direct

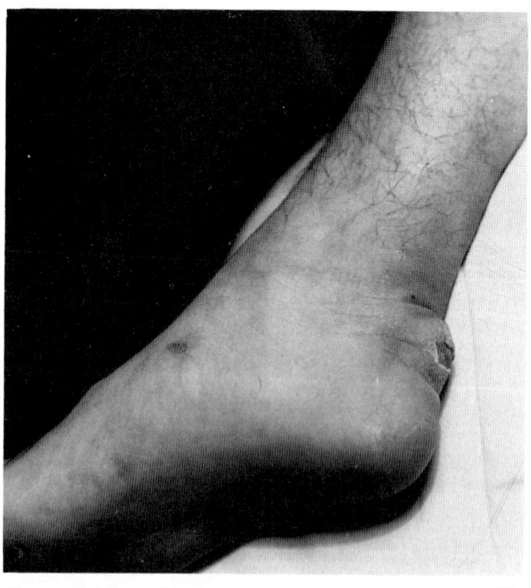

Figure 8.12. Ulceration over posterior achillobursitis. (Courtesy of D Mowbray)

injury, such as dropping an article on the foot, may cause tenosynovitis. A tenogram analysis, after injecting contrast media into individual tendon sheaths, is helpful in diagnosing stenosing tenosynovitis.

Tenosynovitis is most common around the ankles. As the tendons pull at an angle, they are subjected to a great amount of friction. Usually there is pain on motion and crepitus within the inflamed sheath, but on direct pressure pain is slight. The tendon sheath becomes hot, swollen, painful and tender, and in the slow, prolonged cases, marked fibrosis takes place. Over the Achilles tendon the multiple minimal frictions from the counter of a woman's shoe may cause fibrosis of the tendon. The overlying tissues may or may not show evidence of inflammatory changes. The extensor hallucis longus and the tibialis anterior and posterior tendons are frequently affected.

Treatment. Rest and removal of the causative agent are necessary. Ultrasound and immobilization help relieve pain and inflammation. Local injections of corticosteroids (no more than three injections during a 6 month period) may be used in conjunction with aspirin, 10 grains q 4 to 6 h prn for pain. NSAIDs reduce swelling and relieve pain.

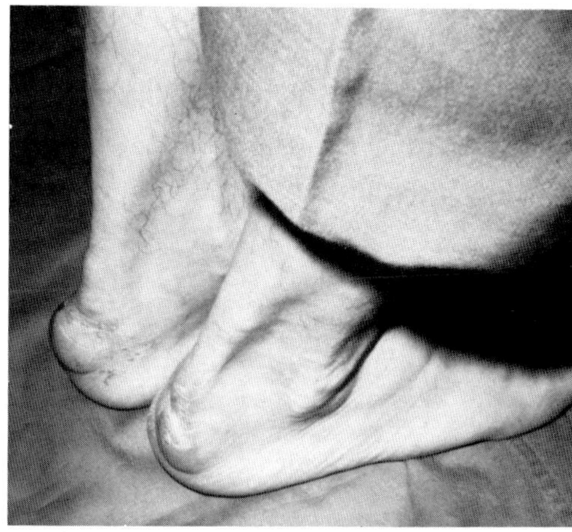

Figure 8.14. Haglund's deformity with overlying chronic bursitis.

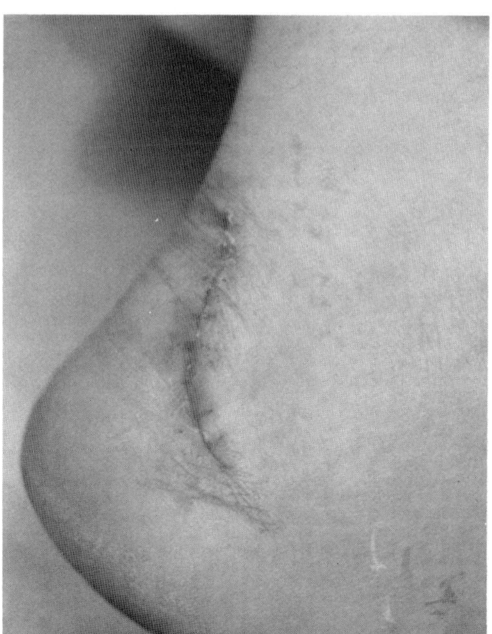

Figure 8.13. Surgical approach to anterior and posterior achillobursitis, as well as Haglund's deformity of the heel.

Pyogenic Tenosynovitis. This condition is usually caused by the introduction of bacteria through a wound over a tendon sheath or by the extension of infection from the surrounding area through a puncture wound or laceration.

Objectively, the lesion presents all signs of acute inflammation accompanied by a marked degree of impaired function. Fluctuation is noted after organization of the pus. The severity of the condition is manifested by increased temperature and leukocytosis. Lymphangitis and adenopathy may be present.

Treatment. Culture and sensitivity tests performed after incision and drainage identify the infecting organism and the antibiotic(s) of choice.

A hot magnesium sulfate poultice over the acutely infected tendon is helpful. Remove all pressure and apply moist heat with rest and elevation of the afflicted part.

Rupture of the Plantaris Tendon. This traumatic condition characteristically affects tennis players and is known as "tennis leg." The patient feels a sudden, sharp pain in the calf of the leg when landing on the foot after a high jump. The pain is described as a snap or "whiplash" type of trauma. Discomfort is great on dorsiflexion of the foot. The pa-

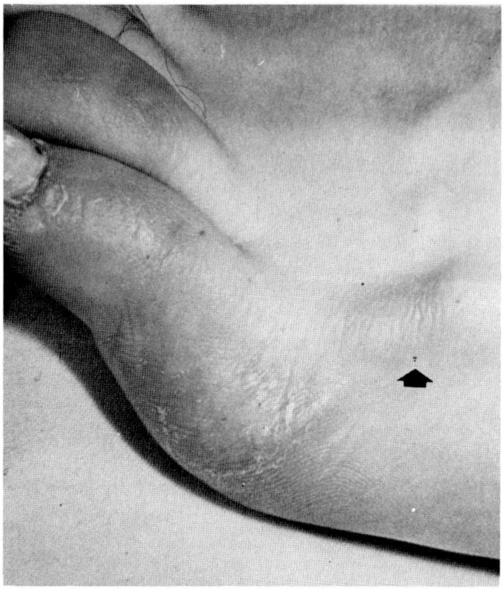

Figure 8.15. Tenosynovitis. Note discoloration and distention of extensor tendon sheath.

tient walks on the toes and is relieved by elevation of the heel by mechanical means.

This condition may be seen in people of all ages, especially middle-aged females. Direct or indirect trauma may be etiologic. After a marked, sudden pull of the calf muscles, symptoms may become evident. Objectively, the middle of the calf may become discolored as if contused, and slight edema may be seen. Pain on palpation is evident. Predisposing factors are overuse, senility, pathological changes, physiological predisposition, occupations requiring stair climbing or sudden movement, fatigue or trauma. The podiatrist must rule out rupture of the fibers of the Achilles tendon or specific damage to the gastrocnemius and soleus muscles.

Treatment. Early treatment consists of rest and application of ice bags to the painful site.

Oral enzymes should be used to reduce swelling and to dissipate hemorrhage. Muscle relaxants relieve spasms. Oral NSAIDs provide relief.

Elevate the heel with a ¼ inch heel pad in the shoe and immobilize it by strapping the foot in the extended position or by applying a plaster cast to immobilize calf muscles. A gelatin cast is helpful in mild cases. The patient may have to use a cane or crutches in walking because the foot is placed in an extended position.

Analgesics to relieve pain and facilitate early function will help bring about a rapid recovery in 3 to 5 weeks.

Plantar Fasciitis. The plantar aponeurosis is easily strained when severe stress is placed on excessively pronating feet. The attachment to the medial tubercle of the plantar surface of the calcaneus is very often inflamed from continued pull or microtrauma.

Symptoms have been described that resemble strain of the plantar fascia, but present few of the predisposing causes.

Although the onset is acute and pain is localized in the ankles, subtalar joints, plantar surfaces of the heels and the origin of the plantar fascia, the symptoms present a definite entity. They must be differentiated from infectious, rheumatoid and other anthritides.

The symptoms are severe with acute onset affecting the parts mentioned above. Increased temperature and swelling of the affected area are noted. Sedimentation rate is always high. Both males and females, usually between the ages of 3 and 30, may be affected.

Careful history taking discloses a recent febrile disease about 3 to 6 weeks before onset. The disease runs its course in from 10 days to 3 weeks. Penicillin reactions have resulted in a similar acute plantar fasciitis.

X-ray findings are reported to be indefinite and of little diagnostic value.

Plantar fibromatosis may develop following acute inflammation.

Nodular fasciitis or infiltrative fasciitis is a tumor-like fibroblastic proliferation that resembles a sarcoma, but is clinically benign. Rosenberg (14) describes the lesion as usually occurring in adults, possibly as a virus-induced inflammatory process. The overlying skin may be raised with slight brownish discoloration. It appears suddenly and is characterized by rapid growth. It may be a single lesion measuring 4 mm to about 4 cm in diameter. Total excision of the mass is indicated. It is comparatively rare on the foot.

Galinski (15), having repaired 20 cases of herniation of the plantar fascia, describes the common sites and reports on three cases. He states that strapping and padding serve as a truss and often relieve discomfort. Use of an orthotic device may be indicated to reduce the hernia and limit stress. If pain persists, surgical correction is indicated. The medial and lateral plantar nerves must be carefully preserved during the blunt and sharp dissection required to expose and repair the herniation.

Miller and Bodman (16) review the literature on the differential diagnosis of nodular fasciitis. It appears that the literature is confusing about the potential for metastasis of these lesions due to their variable pathology. The onset is usually abrupt, and experience indicates that the lesion generally subsides with rest and removal of any etiologic irritants. Radical surgery should be approached with caution.

Treatment. Heat, rest and elevation of the part and use of antiinflammatories are the usual treatment. Carisoprodol (Soma) and methocarbamol (Robaxin) may be used successfully in the treatment of pain and spasm. NSAIDs are often helpful.

Adhesive immobilization by means of a low Dye and ¼ inch felt longitudinal metatarsal dressing to reduce strain is indicated.

Blood studies are often necessary to differentiate infections and rheumatic disorders of systemic origin.

Myalgia. This is a symptom affecting single muscles or groups of muscles and is characterized by varying degrees of pain, stiffness and disability. Because the pain of myalgia is increased with movement of the muscle, the affected muscle is held in a certain position of immobilization in order to avoid motion. The pain is in some cases caused by a slight neuritis affecting the intramuscular sensory nerve ending and may also be due to inflammations and abnormal movement of the muscles themselves.

Strains or overuse of the muscles may cause myalgia. Acute infections often result in acute myalgic states.

In addition, the cause of chronic myalgia may be chronic intoxication with alcohol, lead poisoning, diabetes or gout. Chronic infections, such as syphilis, tuberculosis and septic infections, and unusual strain from lack of proper muscular balance and postural instability may cause chronic myalgia. It may also be caused by lesions involving joints or bones.

Acute cases may last from a few days to a week, whereas chronic cases continue with remissions and exacerbations for months or years.

The plantar flexors and plantar fascia are very often affected by this involvement. Although the central portion of the plantar fascia is most tender and painful, usually the localization of pain is at the medial tubercle of the calcaneus at the origin of the short flexors of the toes. The peroneal and anterior tibial muscles are readily affected. The calf muscles, when painful, should be thoroughly checked in order to differentiate myalgia from other lesions. Myalgias must be differentiated from myositis, dermatomyositis, myositis ossificans and fibrocitis.

Treatment. Analgesics, NSAIDs and oral muscle relaxants help relieve pain. Pentazocine hydrochloride (Talwin), 50 mg q 3 to 4 h, may relieve the pain when the usual analgesics have failed.

Chronic intoxications must be corrected. Disease and infections should be controlled by proper medication.

Muscle and joint disorders are corrected to relieve strain. Physical medicine using hot packs, ultrasound, short wave and other heat-producing modalities are good adjunctive treatment.

Steinberg (17) discusses treatment for the short muscles of the foot. He uses a spot injection of a solution of local anesthetic, chlorobutanol and saline. Results were good with reduction of pain and restoration of functions. Rarely were more than two or three injections given into the myalgic "spot."

Arthritis Treatment Based on Etiology and Judgment

A thorough interrogation, history and examination, including radiographs and laboratory interpretations, are essential before establishing a tentative or positive diagnosis of joint disease (Table 8.4). Relief of pain by prescribing analgesics and anti-inflammatory agents may serve to mask the symptoms in an undiagnosed case of arthritis. Most adverse drug reactions can be minimized when one knows the patient's history of drug habits and

Table 8.4.
Differential Diagnosis: Most Types of Arthritis

Disease	ASO	Latex agglutination	Sheep cell agglutination	CRP	ANA	BFP VDRL	LE prep	Special considerations
Osteoarthritis	–	–	–	–	–	–	–	Heberden's nodes
Rheumatoid arthritis (Fig. 8.16)	–	+ 68%	+ 50–60%	+	20% +	May be +	10% +	Periarticular fibrocitis 2nd MPJ
Rheumatic arthritis	↑	Usually negative	Usually negative	+	Usually negative	Often +	–	Carditis usually
Systemic lupus erythematosus (SLE)	–	+ in 34%	Sometimes +	+	+ 99%	Often +	60–75% +	
Gouty arthritis	–	–	–	±	–	–	–	Uric acid ↑
Pseudogout	–	–	–	±	–	–	–	Normal blood chemistry
Tuberculous arthritis (Fig. 8.17)	–	–	–	+	–	–	–	TBC skin test +
Septic arthritis (Fig. 8.18)	–	–	–	Usually negative	–	–	–	Blood cultures may be +
Traumatic arthritis (Figs. 8.19–8.21)	–	–	–	Usually negative	–	–	–	History of micro or macro trauma
Reiter's syndrome (Fig. 8.22)	–	–	–	±	–	–	–	65–80% HLA-B_{27} +

Normal values: ASO titer 166 Todd units ↓; Latex agglutination 1:40 ↓; Sheep cell agglutination 1:32 ↓

CRP — negative; ANA — negative

current medications being used and their doses, precautions, reactions and interactions. The extent of joint disease and its etiology, pain tolerance of the patient and the dosage necessary to relieve pain should govern the type of medication chosen. X-ray examinations should be evaluated carefully during the acute and chronic phase of arthritis. Laboratory results should be studied and used in establishing therapy (Table 8.5). In any event, a conservative approach to treatment is mandated.

I. ACUTE PHASE
   A. Reduce pain
      1. Nonnarcotic analgesics (anti-inflammatory, nonsteroidal) can be useful
      2. Anti-inflammatory medication alone
      3. Analgesics alone, intrasynovial injections of single joints
      4. Rest of the affected part (adhesive, splint, plaster cast, or bed rest)
   B. Reduce swelling
      1. Ice packs (acute phase)
      2. Enzymes (early or late)
      3. Aspiration of fluid in joint or bursa under field block or nerve block anesthesia
      4. Elevation of affected part
   C. Reduce stiffness
      1. Muscle relaxants (nonnarcotic)
      2. Contrast foot baths
      3. NSAIDs or analgesics
      4. Passive and active range of motion exercises
   D. "Genetic engineering" may be beneficial in the near future
II. CHRONIC PHASE
   A. Establish presence or absence of painful nonreversible bone or joint pathology
      1. Injection techniques (local anesthetics, and peri- and intra-articular steroids)
      2. Oral NSAIDs or analgesics
      3. Injections or oral intake of gold compounds prescribed by internist or rheumatologist where indicated for rheumatoid arthritis
      4. Immunosuppressive medication techniques where indicated
      5. Physical therapeutic measures, including stretching, active and passive movements, exercise, traction, etc, to relieve residual joint stiffness and pain
      6. Hypnosis, autosuggestion, medical relaxation
   B. Correct deformity and relieve pain
      1. Orthotic devices to accommodate deformity, improve function and reduce pain
      2. Surgical excision of hypertrophic bone to correct deformity, improve function and reduce pain

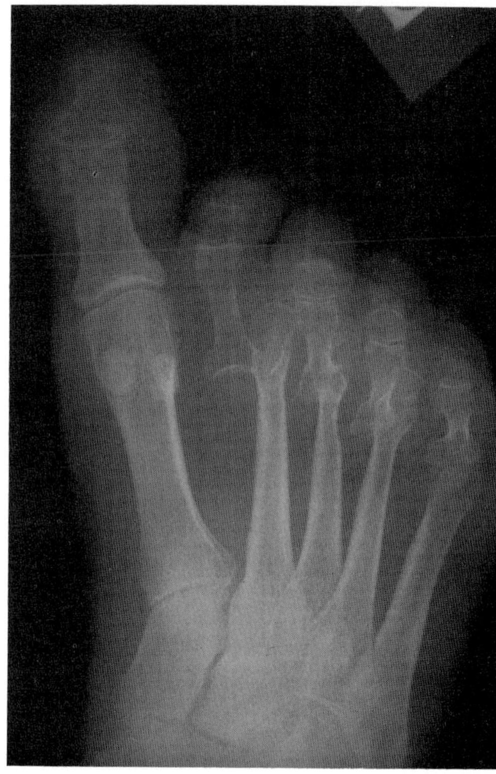

Figure 8.16. Rheumatoid arthritic lesser toe dislocations.

Table 8.5.
Synovial Fluid Analysis[a]

	Gross appearance	Mucin clot	Synovial cells	Crystals	Cartilage Debris	Serum-joint Glucose dif. (mg/100ml)
Normal	Straw/clear	Good	10–600 25% polys	0	0	0–10
Osteoarthritis	Yellow/clear	Good	1000 ± 50% lymphs	0	Frequent fibrillar fragmentation	0–10
Rheumatoid arthritis	Yellow/green, cloudy	Poor	8,000–40,000 70% polys	Cholest. crystals late	0	Average 30
Rheumatic arthritis	Yellow, slightly cloudy	Fair	10,000 ± 50% polys	0	0	0–20, average 10
Systemic lupus erythematosus	Yellow, slightly cloudy	Good	3000 ± 10% polys	0	0	10–20
Gouty arthritis	Yellow/white, milky	Poor	10,000 ± 75% polys	Many urate	0	Average 20
Pseudogout	Slightly yellow, cloudy	Good	6000 ± 75% polys	Few to many $CAPO_4$	0 to many	Average 20
Tuberculous arthritis	Yellow, cloudy	Poor	25,000 ± 40–50% polys	0	0	Average 60
Septic arthritis	Gray-red, turbid	Poor	80,000 ± 90% polys	0	0	Average 60
Traumatic arthritis	Cloudy, bloody	Good	2000 ± many RBC's	0	1 ±	Average 10

[a] From Sisson AJ: *Handbook of Clinical Pathology.* Philadelphia, JB Lippincott Co, 1976, p. 226.

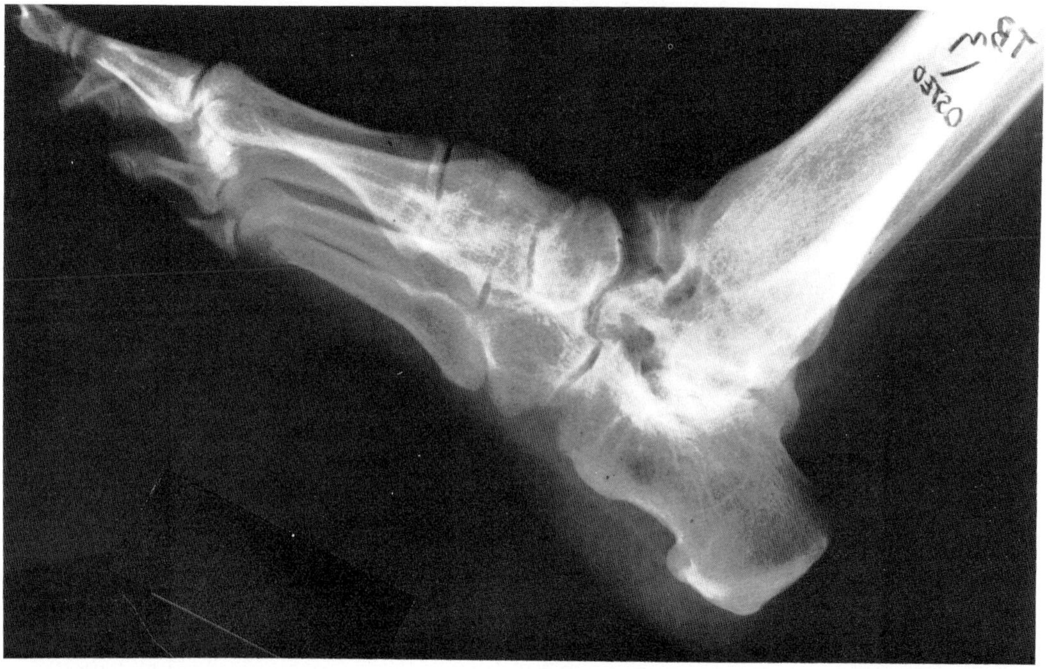

Figure 8.17. Tuberculous arthritis, secondary to tuberculosis osteomyelitis. Note destruction of subtalar, midtarsal and talonavicular joints. Note the talocrural fusion. Destruction is transverse to the long axis of bone.

3. Osteotomy, ostectomy and other corrective procedures to reestablish as near normal joint congruency as possible
4. Surgical implants of bone or synthetic substances to create partial or substitute joints where feasible
5. Physical therapeutic treatment

Regional Nerve Blocks

The author has found nerve block techniques to be beneficial in providing a physiological response to inflammation. The relief is especially effective when the anesthetic of choice is combined with 1:200,000 epinephrine in selected cases. Podiatrists have demonstrated safe and excellent results in hundreds of thousands of cases when epinephrine is used in this dilution, despite the concern expressed previously in some of the medical literature. Obviously, the patient's circulatory status must be assessed, and good judgment is expected and mandatory.

Injections of local anesthetics for regional anesthesia may involve posterior tibial, sural, saphenous, superficial and deep peroneal and digital nerve blocks. In many instances, long-lasting local anesthetics without epinephrine can be the anesthesia of choice.

Techniques described by Steinberg and Block (18), Kaplan and Kashuk (19) and Locke and Locke (20) are of great importance in a review of the proper type of local anesthetic techniques used by podiatrists.

Corticosteroids

The injection or ingestion of corticosteroids must be performed with a general appreciation of their physiological function and pathological complications. It has been hypothesized that, if the blood level of cortisone drops, the hypothalmus is stimulated by the CNS to supply more cortisone. This action is further accom-

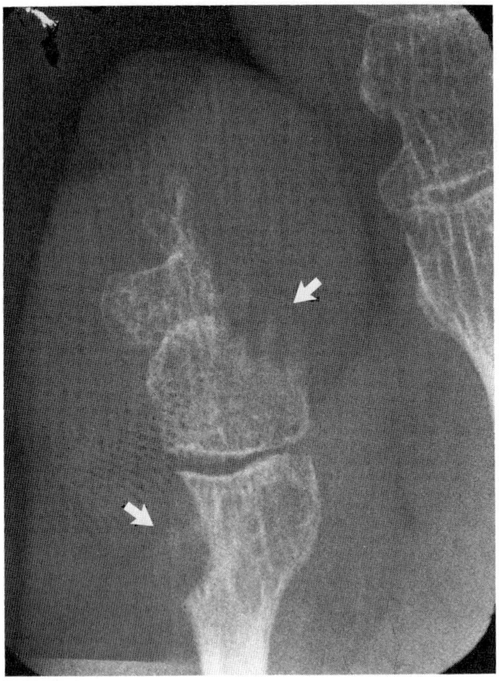

Figure 8.18. Pyogenic arthritis and osteomyelitis of the phalanges. Infection of fifth toenail extended back to the middle, and distal phalanx prior to incision and drainage. The head of the proximal phalanx is saucerized with loss of bone substance that is hazy and indistinct.

plished by the anterior pituitary serving as an intermediary stimulus to the elaboration of ACTH and outpouring of cortisone from the adrenal cortex. The bloodstream level of cortisone is satisfied, and the tissues become nourished, resulting in a physiological dependence on the hypothalamus and the anterior pituitary to maintain a proper level.

The long-term injection of corticosteroids can result in atrophy of the adrenal cortex. Corticosteroids are catabolic and can result in subcutaneous atrophy. They decrease the necessary build-up of essential proteins in the tissue and lead to hyperglycemia and glycosuria. Cortisone affects the body electrolytes by causing a retention of sodium, water, and fluorides while stimulating excretion of potassium.

Cortisone alters physiology in the diabetic patient, resulting in the development of an intolerance to insulin. However, steroid-induced diabetes is fortunately reversible if the diabetic patient is not brittle. Due to the body's inability to metabolize protein, one can expect to see radiographic evidence of systemic demineralization of bone.

Cortisone is a nonspecific anti-inflammatory agent that is capable of limiting connective tissue repair. Skin incisions or wounds may repair at the normal level; however, subcutaneous connective tissue repair is diminished. The sedimentation rate and C-reactive protein levels are usually reduced during cortisone therapy.

Dexamethasone sodium phosphate is a water-soluble inorganic ester of dexamethasone. It can be used by injection for short-term therapy for acute episodes of rheumatic disorders and exacerbations of joint and collagen disorders. It may serve as short-term replacement for adrenocorticoid insufficiency.

The intra-articular injection of corticosteroids is useful in the relief of painful joints. However, the joint spaces in the foot are rarely wide enough to allow for entry of the needle without damage to the articular cartilage. Talocrural joints are approached with care so the steroid can be deposited intrasynovially, not intracartilaginously. The smaller joints can be placed in traction while injecting a cor-

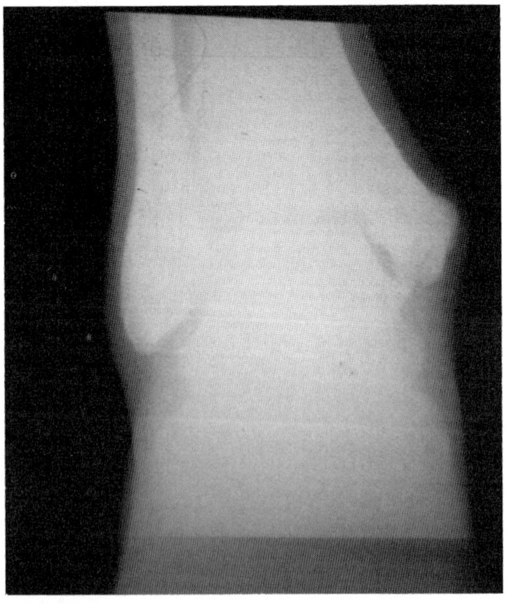

Figure 8.19. Traumatic arthritis secondary to medial malleolar fracture.

ticosteroid anti-inflammatory agent into the synovial spaces. A field block of a local anesthetic may precede the intrasynovial injection, but is usually not necessary. The doctor ensures that he or she has entered the joint space by aspirating synovial fluid.

The volume of injected solutions must be determined by the judgment of the therapist. Consideration is given to the recommended mg/ml dosage of the injectable corticosteroid. If the part is not helped by a single injection, additional injections are usually doomed to failure.

Because the intra-articular injection of a corticosteroid does not correct, reverse or allay the disease process, it should be used sparingly. Where joints are severely deformed, the addition of a foreign substance by injection can only serve as a source of irritation. Care must be exercised not to demineralize bones by frequent injections of steroids. Avoiding injections into blood vessels and nerves is mandatory. Many joints have been destroyed by frequent deposition of steroids, resulting in instability of the articulation.

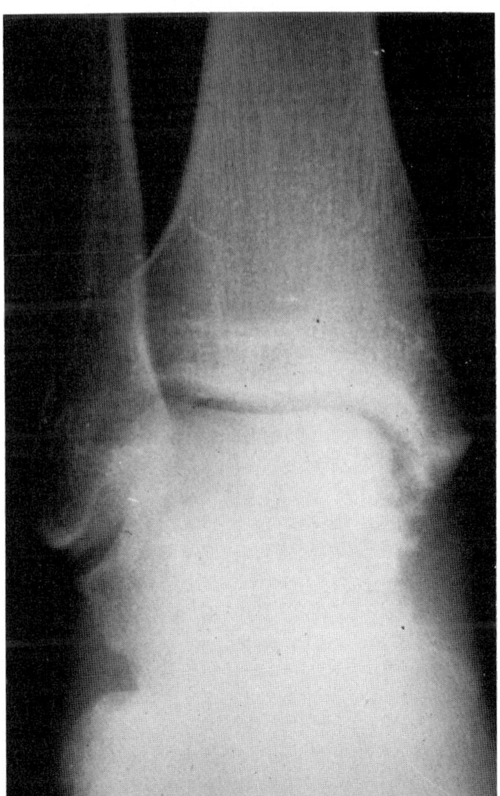

Figure 8.20. Traumatic arthritis talotibial articulation.

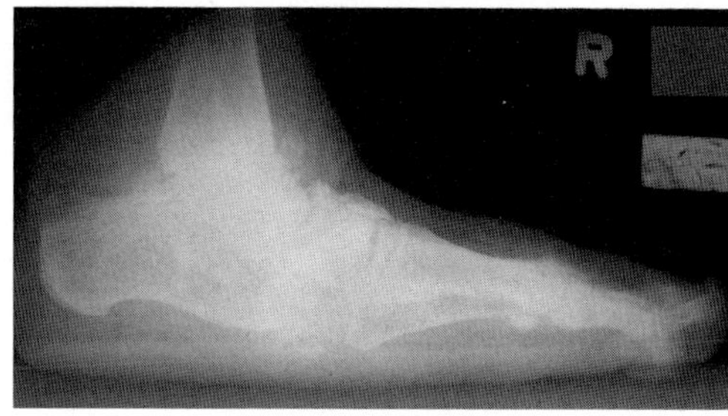

Figure 8.21. Traumatic arthritis secondary to congenital abscence of tarsal bones.

The parenteral steroids are generally similar to oral glucocorticoids in their potency. The use of steroids systemically is fraught with adverse reactions and complications. The clinician must be selective in using intra-articular injections of steroids in local foot joints.

The systemic therapy of glucocorticoids should be the choice of the internist and rheumatologist. Their use for local foot joint disease in the absence of systemic arthritis is rarely indicated. The author prefers the prescription of a nonsteroidal anti-inflammatory analgesic drug of choice and local judicious intra-articular injections of steroids or local anesthetics.

A few of the steroids for intra-articular foot injections are briefly mentioned below. The technique is to inject the steroid into the synovial space under sterile aseptic conditions. A small amount of synovial fluid is aspirated to indicate penetration of the synovium. The needle remains intact as the syringe is replaced with the steroid to be injected. Care must be exercised not to penetrate the articular cartilage.

Dexamethasone sodium phosphate is a synthetic adrenal cortical steroid, supplied for intra-articular injection as 4 mg/ml, with rapid onset and short duration for acute disorders. It is available in 5 or 10 ml multidose vials as a sterile aqueous solution that can be injected intra-articularly or in soft tissue as adjunctive short-term therapy following an acute inflammation or exacerbation of a chronic or subacute problem. Systemic fungal infections may be exacerbated following the

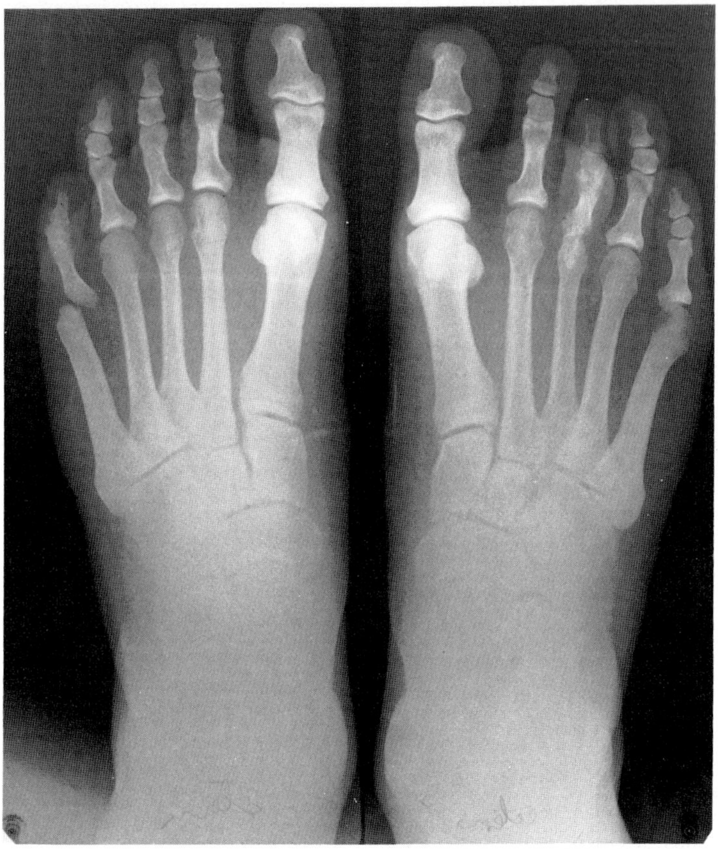

Figure 8.22. Reiter's syndrome. Migratory olygoarthritis. Note third toe right foot, fifth toe left. Patient also has plantar fasciitis.

injection of betamethasone sodium phosphate. Care must be exercised not to inject intravenously. Injections are best used 1–2 weeks apart, not to exceed three injections into the same joint every 6 months; 0.25–0.5 mg is the dosage of choice for most joints in the foot.

Triamcinolone diacetate (Forte) is useful for intra-articular or soft tissue injection at 40 mg/ml. The clinician must be fully aware of the indications, contraindications and adverse reactions of all corticosteroid medications.

Methylprednisolone acetate, as an aqueous suspension, reacts similarly to other anti-inflammatory steroids. Among the several adverse reactions is the possibility of a postinjection flare. This may be caused by many intra-articular or soft tissue acetylated steroid injectables.

Arthritic Medication (see Chapter 3, The Painful Foot)

Although aspirin has been of proven benefit for the relief of pain, swelling and stiffness of joint diseases, it is universally accepted that combinations of acetylsalicylic acid with other chemicals may ameliorate some of its toxic and physiopathological effects. New antiarthritic drugs that are of nonsteroidal anti-inflammatory organic acid origin are appearing regularly and enjoying the respect of the medical and arthritic community.

Gastric mucosa may be irritated by the ingestion of acetylsalicylic acid as it is absorbed in the stomach, hydrolyzed and reacts with esters in the liver. The anti-inflammatory activity is basically produced by salicylates binding with serum albumin. When combined with magnesium and choline (Trilisate tablets), the salicylate is effective as a single daily dose, permitting a sustained therapeutic level. The choline is metabolized readily, and the magnesium is excreted without difficulty when normal renal function exists. The delivery of 500 mg of salicylate compares favorably with an aspirin that delivers only 244 mg of salicylate in a single-dose form.

Salicylates have an antiblood clotting effect and, like most drugs, can be the source of sensitivity, as well as pathology. Aspirin may cause a microbleeding problem, demonstrated by an assay of fecal blood, when used for prolonged therapy. Bleeding time is increased as platelet aggregation is decreased, and a decrease in blood prothrombin becomes a secondary liability to the ingestion of aspirin. With bleeding problems secondary to aspirin, a chronic deficiency anemia is also possible.

The very young and the aged treated with salicylates should be carefully monitored for CNS and auricular complications. Patients receiving salicylates for treatment of arthritis must be subjected to frequent renal and liver profiles to ensure that problems are not developing on the biochemical and cellular level. This testing is done before clinical symptoms of physiological dysfunction occur.

A generalized distribution of erythematous skin lesions, breathing difficulties and shock are not uncommon with high dosages of acetylsalicylic acid. If one is allergic to the drug, abdominal upset, vomiting and often an acute allergic reaction occur.

Aspirin in high doses is said to decrease hyperuricemia. As with all other drugs in the formulary, the doctor should be aware of the problems that accrue when multiple medications create interaction complications. This is an especially frequent concern with the arthritic patient who is usually being treated for multiple health problems by more than one physician.

In recent studies of clinical patients by surgeons treating transient ischemic attacks (TIA), Carson et al. (21) suggest that aspirin may not be helpful against stroke. In fact, Carson states, "It may only mask cerebrovascular symptoms." He continues with his report by noting, "aspirin does more than inhibit platelet aggregation at sites of plaque build-up, it hinders formation of thromboxane A_2 from arachidonic acid metabolites." Of further interest are the higher dosages that arthritic patients usually require to relieve pain and stiffness. Aspirin inhibits prostacyclin synthesis at arterial walls. This process of prostacyclin synthesis is also reduced by atherosclerosis that may very well be a coexisting complication in arthritis affecting the lower extremities.

Despite the concern about aspirin one must recognize the great value of the drug and the important part it plays in relief of painful arthritis in the foot and other anatomical sites. Combinations of salicylates with an antacid, with magnesium and choline, or in other combinations may provide relief of pain, stiffness, swelling, and limit gastrointestinal complications.

Sulindac (Clinoril) claims to be effective when prescribed 200–400 mg daily when compared to 2400–4800 mg daily of aspirin in osteoarthritis and rheumatoid arthritis. In acute gouty arthritis, 400 mg daily of sulindac are as effective as 600 mg of phenylbutazone. Similar dosages appear to be helpful in the acute tenosynovitis and bursitis so often associated with rheumatoid or traumatic arthritis. Clinoril does inhibit platelet function and is best prescribed in starting doses of 150 mg bid. The use of this drug must be monitored closely so as to avoid bleeding tendencies and liver or renal dysfunction.

NSAIDs are ulcerogenic, may aggravate high blood pressure, cause frontal headaches and/or aggravate hepatic or renal disease. Those medications containing sodium (Naprosyn, Anaprox, Tolectin) and Butazolidin may lead to fluid retention. NSAIDs should not be prescribed for patients with active peptic or gastric ulcer, malignant hypertension, a history of angioneurotic edema, nasal or rectal polyps or allergic reaction to acetylsalicylic acid. NSAIDs are also known to cause blurred vision. They should be prescribed with caution, and consultation with an ophthalmologist is indicated if symptoms persist. Withdrawal of the medication should promptly relieve symptoms. If the patient is retaining fluid and is hypertensive, allergic or has a history of cardiopulmonary disorders, the doctor must use good judgment and skill in prescribing any anti-inflammatory drug. Prothrombin times, SGPT, serum creatinine and urine protein should be monitored regularly when patients are receiving NSAIDs.

The anti-inflammatory action of aspirin and the NSAIDs has proven to be effective in inhibition of prostaglandin biosynthesis. Joint swelling, redness, heat and pain produced by prostaglandins are the result of physiochemical mediators at the cellular level. Prostaglandin is one of the excitants of acute and chronic inflammation, along with histamine, kinins, and other substances known and those not yet discovered.

Naproxen (Naprosyn), in 250, 375 or 500 mg tablets bid, is prescribed for mild to moderately severe, acute or chronic arthritic pain. Periarticular inflammations are often helped by naproxen when bone- and cartilage-degenerative changes are minimal. It is essential to recognize that potential gastrointestinal bleeding is a factor to be dealt with when prescribing naproxen. It is capable of decreasing platelet aggregation and increasing bleeding time. The doctor must be fully aware of the involvement, however minimal, of all body systems. Careful selection of dosage based on a thorough history and physical examination is vital. A dose of 500 mg bid. has proven to be useful in severe cases of rheumatoid or osteoarthritis.

Tolmetin sodium (Tolectin DS, 400 mg), like aspirin and all other NSAIDs, seems to cause similar problems with gastrointestinal bleeding and a variety of reactions.

In severe rheumatoid arthritis, remission-inducing agents, such as gold salts, levamisole and penicillamine; immunosuppressive drugs, such as azathioprine and cyclophosphamide; and potentially toxic drugs, such as methotrexate and hydroxychloroquine (Plaquenil) have been used recently for relief of symptoms not otherwise relieved by other medications. Long-term controlled studies about the use and toxicity of low-dose methotrexate therapy are needed before the use of this drug is increased.

There are many analgesics available for the treatment of acute and chronic pain, some more effective than others. Indomethacin (Indocin), phenylbutazone (Butazolidin), oxyphenbutazone (Tandearil), gold compounds, ibuprofen (Motrin), allopurinol (Zyloprim), and steroids all have their indications and contraindications for use in the treatment of arthritis in the foot.

Choline magnesium trisalicylate (Trilisate) 1000–1500 mg bid has proven to be as effective as ibuprofen (Motrin) 600 mg tid for relief of the pain, inflammation and morning stiffness of rheumatoid arthritis in double-blind controlled clinical evaluations by 11 investigators. It appears to be better tolerated than aspirin, with no evidence of fecal occult blood loss. Endoscopic examination suggests less gastric bleeding and peptic ulceration when using choline magnesium trisalicylate in the rheumatoid patient. This drug was as effective as indomethacin (Indocin) in reducing morning stiffness and nocturnal joint pain and in extending time to the onset of fatigue. The long-term use of any of these NSAID medications, regardless of the published reports, must proceed with the utmost of caution. They are not without a capability to create both subjective complaints and objective pathology.

Ibuprofen (Motrin) has proven useful for relief of severe pain when prescribed qid 300–800 mg, or every 4–6 hours for an acute arthritic flare. Long-term use at a reduced dose may be the treatment of choice if one is to avoid gastrointestinal upset or other complications.

Ketoprofen (Orudis) taken 75 mg tid or 50 mg qid, not to exceed 300 mg a day, and suprofen (Suprol) taken 200 mg 4–6 times a day, not to exceed 1600 mg a day, have relieved the chronic arthritic patient where ibuprofen (Motrin) has not.

Meclofenamate sodium (Meclomen) equals indomethacin for the relief of osteoarthritis. It can prove helpful in both osteoarthritis and rheumatoid joint discomfort. Indomethacin (Indocin) has been the analgesic anti-inflammatory agent of choice by many when used for rheumatoid arthritis, one 25 mg or 50 mg capsule after meals and at bedtime. The dosage is later reduced to the lowest dose providing the desired clinical response.

Piroxicam (Feldene) in 20 mg capsules provides an antipyretic, analgesic and anti-inflammatory effect in a once-daily dose. The action of Feldene does not provide greater relief than aspirin in large doses. However, the incidence of fecal blood loss is less with Feldene. This nonsteroidal analgesic is useful in treating adult rheumatoid arthritis and osteoarthritis.

Beaver (22) makes a note in his review of the methods for clinically measuring analgesic efficacy that "the need to put repeat-dose studies of analgesics on a quantitative footing as firm as currently exists for single-dose studies constitutes the most important challenge for clinical analgesimetry."

Balagot et al. (23) contend that the mode of action of D-phenylalamine is due to its ability to block enkephalinase. Relief of chronic pain by this amino acid is accomplished by the oral route to a total dose of 750–1000 mg. Pain in osteoarthritis was successfully relieved in 3–4 weeks. D-Phenylalamine, it is postulated, acts as an analgesic due to its ability to block some enzymes, such as enkephalinases, in the CNS. According to the researchers, enkephalinases destroy enkephalins, which are naturally occurring opiate-like substances produced in the brain and spinal cord that diminish sensitivity to pain.

The key to positive treatment is prescribing the minimal effective dose of a medication and using good judgment. Consultation is always valuable and should be pursued when indicated.

The doctor should be guided by clinical and laboratory research when treating the acute or chronic arthritic. Although the symptomatology of an arthritic disorder may be controllable, the disease process is relentlessly progressive. This is an important concept for the arthritic patient to understand. There is no place for poor judgment that extends the symptomatology of the arthritis to vital organs. Doing so can result in irreversible pathology. The family practitioner, internist, orthopaedic surgeon, allergist, immunologist, hematologist, dermatologist, dentist, podiatrist and a variety of subspecialists have a stake in the well-being of the arthritic patient. However, only skilled, experienced and well-trained personnel should make up the therapy team with the rheumatologist as the pivotal specialist.

References

1. Yale I, Yale JF: *The Arthritic Foot and Related Connective Tissue Disorders*. Baltimore, Williams & Wilkins, 1984.
2. Solicito V, Jacobs AM, Oloff LM, et al.: The use of radionuclide bone and joint imaging in arthritic and related diseases. *J Foot Surg*, 23:173–182, 1984.
3. Jacoby RK, Vidigal L, Kirkup J, Dixon AJ: The great toe as a clinical problem in rheumatoid arthritis. *Rheumatol Rehabil* 15:143–147, 1976.
4. Ingersoll TE: Sesamoidalgia. *J Am Podiatry Assoc* 45:15–24, 1955.
5. Sansone RE: Parallel strip padding for weight stress distribution and redirection. *J Am Podiatry Assoc* 60:193–198, 1970.
6. Sansone RE: Forefoot imbalance due to alteration of metatarus parabola. *J Natl Assoc Chirop* 47:219–227, 1957.
7. Weiner H: Some comments on metatarsalgia. *J Natl Assoc Chirop* 47:460–462, 1957.
8. Carleton FJ: An effective appliance for calcaneal spur. *J Natl Assoc Chirop* 44:35–36, 1954.
9. Michael B: Management of calcaneal spur inflammation with triamcinolone acteonide. *J Am Podiatry Assoc* 51:801–803, 1961.
10. Schlefman BS, Katz FN: Tomographic interpretation of the subtalar joint. *J Am Podiatry Assoc* 73:65–69, 1983.
11. Ritchie J: Phenylbutazone for non-specific inflammation. *J Am Podiatry Assoc* 56:124–125, 1966.
12. Gamble FO, Yale I: *Clinical Foot Roentgenology*. Baltimore, Williams & Wilkins, 1966.
13. Yale JF: Growth center injuries of the foot. *Arch Pod Med Foot Surg* 1:129–140, 1973.
14. Rosenberg A: Nodular fasciitis—A case report. *J Am Podiatry Assoc* 59:400–402, 1969.
15. Galinski AW: Calcaneodynia-herniation. *J Am Podiatry Assoc* 67:646–650, 1977.
16. Miller TJ, Bodman MA: Nodular fasciitis; A podiatric review and report of a case. *J Am Podiatry Assoc* 66:465–470, 1976.
17. Steinberg HH: Myalgia of the foot. *J Wis Soc Chirop* 5:7–10, 1957.
18. Steinberg MD, Block P: The use and abuse of epinephrine in local anesthetics. *J Am Podiatry Assoc* 61:341–343, 1971.
19. Kaplan EG, Kashuk K: Disclaiming the myth of use of epinephrine in local anesthetics. *J Am Podiatry Assoc* 61:335–339, 1971.
20. Locke RK, Locke SE: Nerve blocks of the foot. JACEP, 5:698–702, 1976.

21. Carson SN, Demling RH, Esquivet CO: Aspirin failure in symptomatic atherosclerotic carotid artery disease. *Surgery* 90:1084–1092, 1981.
22. Beaver WT: Measurement of analgesic efficacy in man. Paper delivered at the Third World Congress on Pain, Edinburgh, Scotland, September, 1981.
23. Balagot RC, Ehrenpreis S, Kubato K, Greenberg J: Analgesia in mice and humans by D-phenylalamine: Relation to inhibition of enkephalinase. Paper delivered at the Third World Congress on Pain, Edinburgh, Scotland, September, 1981.
24. Sisson JA: *Handbook of Clinical Pathology*. Philadelphia, JB Lippincott Co, 1976, p. 226.

Suggested Readings

Annunziato EJ, Pressman MM, Gorecki GA: Frostbite arthritis of the foot. *J Foot Surg* 23:116–120, 1984.

Banninga HS: Musculoskeletal disorders: Treatment of pain and spasm. *Med Times* 8:1440–1443, 1960.

Black JR, Cahalin C, Germain BF: Pedal morbidity in rheumatic diseases (a clinical study). *J Am Podiatry Assoc* 72:360, 1982.

Canter KG: Rheumatoid nodules in the foot. *J Foot Surg* 17:35–37, 1978.

Cinzio JR: Myofascial syndromes in the lower extremity and their diagnosis. *J Am Podiatry Assoc* 53:195–198, 1963.

Cooper CT, Jr: Hansen's disease: A podiatrist's experience. *J Am Podiatry Assoc* 65:300–309, 1975.

DeLorimer AA: *The Arthropathies, A Handbook of Roentgen Diagnosis*. Chicago, Year Book Publishers, 1946.

Golding DN: Polyarteritis presenting with leg pains. *Br Med J* 1:277–278, 1970.

Harrington DB, Chen TA: The anatomy of joints (gross, histologic, and fine structures). *J Am Podiatry Assoc* 72:222–227, 1982.

Haverhill fever (erythema arthriticum epidemieum), Editorial. *JAMA* 113:941–942, 1939.

Helfand AE: Arthritis in older patients as seen in podiatric practice. *J Am Podiatry Assoc* 57:85, 1967.

Kelly WN, et al: *Textbook of Rheumatology*, vols. 1 and 2, ed 2. Philadelphia, WB Saunders Co, 1985.

Locke RK: Local steroid injection therapy. *Podiatry Q* Summer: 19–26, 1961.

Locke RK: Steroids in podiatric management of arthritis. *J Am Podiatry Assoc* 57:164–167, 1967.

Marcinko DE, Dollard MD: Physical and mechanical properties of joints (the pathomechanics of articular cartilage degeneration) *J Foot Surg* 25:3–13, 1986.

Mennell J: Spray: Stretch for the relief of pain from muscle spasm and myofascial trigger points. *J Am Podiatry Assoc* 66:873–876, 1976.

Newman AW: Case report: Juxta articular rheumatoid nodule. *J Am Coll Foot Surg* 4:10, 1965.

Roth A, Trosko P, Boxer MD: Osteoarthritis of the tarsal bones of the foot. *J Am Podiatry Assoc* 72:244–247, 1982.

Subotnick SI: The practical value and research potential of synovia analysis of joints within the human foot. *Proc Res Alumni Assoc Calif Podiatric Med Center* 1:1–16, 1972.

Talbot JH (ed.): *Seminars in Arthritis and Rheumatism*, vol. 14, no. 3. Orlando, FL, Grune and Stratton, Inc, 1985.

9

Biomechanical Disorders

Podiatric medicine considers the deformities of the foot in light of their relationship to function, discomfort and pain. Because time and space do not permit a thorough study of biomechanical relationships and treatment of foot deformities this chapter considers the biomechanical implications of congenital and acquired abnormalities in the foot and discusses a variety of painful pathological entities, most of them related to a malfunctioning foot. No attempt is made to elaborate on the biomechanical mechanisms involved. However, a study of these conditions provides an adequate background for their diagnosis and treatment.

Additional information about the x-ray findings is described in *Clinical Foot Roentgenology* (1). Ross (2) reviews the literature and discusses the use of computed tomography (CT) in the diagnosis of foot disorders. Floyd et al. (3) feel a CT scan is the diagnostic modality of choice for subtalar joint evaluation. Because of the CT scanner's ability to distinguish subtle densities, syndesmosis, synchondrosis and synostosis involvement of the subtalar joint are readily appreciated. Nuclear magnetic resonance (NMR) may have even greater application to podiatric medical practice than CT. Future studies will help to clarify the use of NMR and its applicability to the diagnosis of foot pathology.

In discussions of the biomechanical problems affecting the foot, the author has been impressed by the ability of foot specialists to relate faulty foot structure and function to the complaint of pain. The science of biomechanics is undergoing revolutionary changes. A strong effort by a small group of scientists is fueling a steady flow of working propositions and definitions. Texts are standardizing diagnoses and treatment of structural and functional disorders.

On the basis of its internal structures, the ball of the foot can be divided into three transverse areas, each with a different mechanical function: (1) an area proximal to the heads of the metatarsals in which the retinacula cutis are developed into a series of transverse bands and in which the deep fibers of the plantar aponeurosis form ten sagittal septa connected to the deep transverse metatarsal ligament and through this the proximal phalanges of the toes; (2) an area below the heads of the metatarsals in which vertical fibers from the joint capsules and the sides of the fibrous flexor sheaths form a cushion below each metatarsal head and in which fat bodies cover the digital nerves and vessels in their passage between the cushions; and (3) a distal area that comprises the interdigital web. The superficial fibers of the plantar aponeurosis are inserted into the skin of this distal area, and below the superficial fibers of the plantar aponeurosis, the plantar interdigital ligament forms a series of transverse lamellae connected to the proximal phalanges by a mooring ligament that arches from one fibrous flexor sheath to the next. When the metatarsophalangeal joints are extended, the fibers of the three areas are tensed, and the skin is anchored firmly to the skeleton. The direction of the fibers in the distal and proximal area promotes the transfer of forces exerted on the skin during pushoff and braking respectively, whereas the intermediate area is adapted to bear the weight of the body (Fig. 9.1). A concentration of Pacinian corpuscles is found along the digital nerves in the weightbearing area below the transverse metatarsal ligament. The nerves for the second, and especially for the third, interspace are close to or in contact with the sharp proximal edges of the sagittal septa.

The feet are subject to many anomalies of congenital and hereditary origin. These may vary from mild genetically predetermined deformities to severe deforming states requiring surgical correction to enable the pedal extremities to perform useful biomechanical functions.

Abnormal Motions of the Foot

According to Root et al. (4), abnormal motions of the foot include abnormal pronation, abnormal supination and restricted motion (Table 9.1). **Abnormal pronation** may be a result of compensation for a bony or soft tissue abnormality of a part of the lower extremity, a response to any condition that prematurely loads the medial aspect of the foot, a result of a neuromuscular disorder causing muscle imbalance, or may be due to pain in the articular or periarticular tissues causing tonic muscle spasm.

Planal dominances of the subtalar, ankle and midtarsal joints determine the primary plane of compensation of the foot as a unit (5). Common foot deformities compensated for by abnormal foot pronation include forefoot varus, a plantar flexed fifth ray, forefoot valgus, rearfoot varus, a plantar flexed first ray and minimal ankle equinus (Fig. 9.2). Extrinsic deformities compensated for by abnormal pronation include internal tibial torsion, internal femoral torsion, tibial varum, a short gastrocnemius muscle, short hamstrings, limb length inequality, a short ileopsoas muscle and any condition causing the femur to remain internally rotated during gait. Common causes of premature medial loading of the foot resulting in abnormal

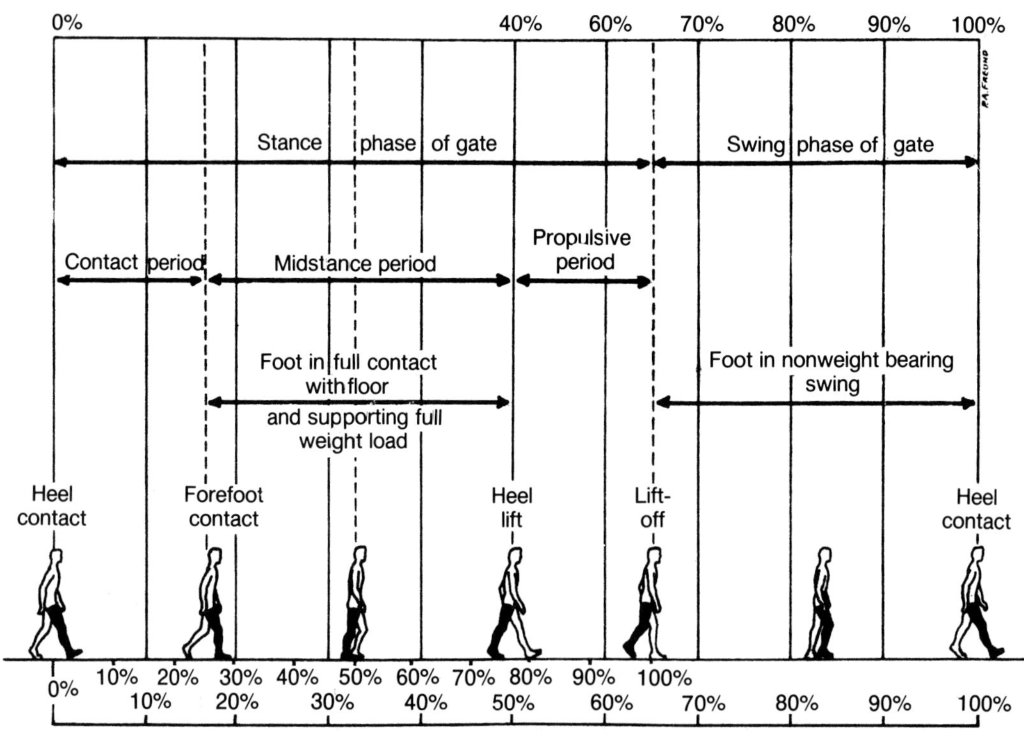

Figure 9.1. One complete gait cycle of the right limb. (Reprinted with permission from HF Hlavac, *The Foot Book—Advice for Athletes,* Mountain View, CA, World Publication, 1977, p. 89.)

Table 9.1.
Review of Foot Types and Biomechanical Disorders (Fig. 9.3)

Foot Types	Nonweightbearing description	With weightbearing the foot may compensate by:	Plantar lesions usually develop under metatarsal heads	Descriptive synonyms
Sagittal plane				
Ankle joint:				
Uncompensated equinus	Measurement shows limited dorsiflexion	None (uncomp.)	Diffuse lesions 2–4	"Toe walker" (part of clubfoot)
Compensated equinus	Foot is plantarflexed	STJ & MTJ pronation (comp.)[a] or MTJ subluxation (comp.)	2, 2–4[b,c] Varies	Pes planus, P. valgoplanus[d] "Rocker bottom," "vertical" Talus (Fig. 9.4)
Uncompensated calcaneus	Limited plantarflexion	None (uncomp.)	Around heel	"Heel walker"
Compensated calcaneus	Foot is dorsiflexed	STJ & MTJ supination (comp.)[a]	5th–1st	Pes cavus
Frontal plane				
Subtalar joint (STJ):				
Uncomp. subtalar varus	Neutral position of the STJ is inverted from the tibia	None (uncomp.)	5th[c]	Calcaneal varus, (part of clubfoot) heel varus
Comp. subtalar varus		Subtalar pronation (comp.)[a]	Nucleated 2nd 2–5[b,c]	Pes planus, "weak foot"
Subtalar valgus	Neutral position of the STJ is everted from the tibia	Foot is "flat." No force on talus to compensate	Varies	Pes valgoplanus[d]
Midtarsal joint (MTJ):				
Uncomp. forefoot varus	Forefoot (plane of the metatarsal heads is inverted from the rearfoot bisection of the calcaneus)	None (uncomp.)	5th[c]	Medial imbalance
Comp. forefoot varus		Subtalar and midtarsal pronation (comp.)[a]	Nucleated 2nd 2 & 5[b,c]	Pes valgoplanus[d]

Table 9.1.—continued
Review of Foot Types and Biomechanical Disorders (Fig. 9.3)

Foot Types	Nonweightbearing description	With weightbearing the foot may compensate by:	Plantar lesions usually develop under metatarsal heads	Descriptive synonyms
Uncomp. forefoot valgus	Forefoot is everted from the rearfoot (as above)	None (uncomp.)	Nucleated 1st (tibial sesamoid)	Pes cavus
Comp. forefoot valgus		Subtalar supination (comp.)[a]	Nucleated 1st Diffuse 5th	Pes cavus Posterolateral imbalance
Transverse Plane				
Midtarsal joint (MTJ):				
Forefoot adductus	Forefoot (anterior to MTJ) is adducted on the rearfoot	No need to compensate because both the heel and the forefoot are on the supporting surface	None, but tend to aggravate other problems by making foot rigid	Often grouped under metatarsus varus, met. adductovarus, met. adductus (part of clubfoot)
Tarsometatarsal joint:				
Metatarsus adductus	Differentiated by x-ray Metatarsus is adducted on the lesser tarsus			

a Compensation is an abnormal but not necessarily pathological attempt by the body to neutralize an abnormal force from another part. Compensation produces abnormal secondary muscle pulls, affecting joint positions and forefoot abnormalities; in treatment, we attempt to prevent compensation by supporting the abnormality.

b Hypermobility is defined as either excessive motion or motion at a time when there should be none. Hypermobility of the first ray develops whenever the foot is pronated from its neutral position; therefore lesions develop under the second metatarsal head. Whenever hypermobility is present, hallux abductovalgus will tend to develop.

c Pinch callus develops under the medial plantar aspect of the hallux where the upper meets the lower of the shoe.

d Shows "positive" Helbing's sign.

(Reprinted with permission from Hlavac HF: *The Foot Book: Advice for Athletes.* Mountain View, CA, World Publications, 1977, p. 89.)

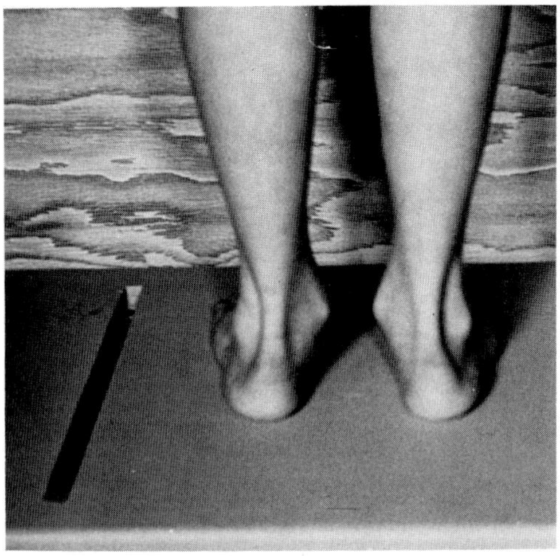

Figure 9.2. A compensating intoeing gait may develop in this pronated foot problem.

pronation include external femoral torsion, obesity, external tibial torsion, rearfoot valgus, tibial valgum, an abnormally pronated foot at the end of the swing phase of gait and any condition causing the femur to remain externally rotated during gait. The following types of muscle imbalance and tonic muscle spasm may cause abnormal pronation: chronic muscle spasm of the peroneus brevis or gastrocnemius and tonic muscle spasm of the peroneus brevis (peroneal spastic flatfoot), peroneus longus, gastrocnemius or tibialis anterior.

Abnormal supination of the foot may be caused by CNS disease, lower motor neuron disease, compensation for an everted forefoot position or a soft tissue or bony ankle equinus preventing heel contact to the floor (5). Yale and Hugar (6) classify the supinatory deformity of pes cavus (talipes arcuatus, talipes plantaris, hollow foot, clawfoot, nondeforming clubfoot) into anterior, posterior, and combined cavus. Anterior cavus, in which the forefoot is in plantar flexion in relation to the rearfoot, is further classified into global and local cavus. Global cavus is defined as total forefoot equinus, and local cavus is described as having the first ray in equi-

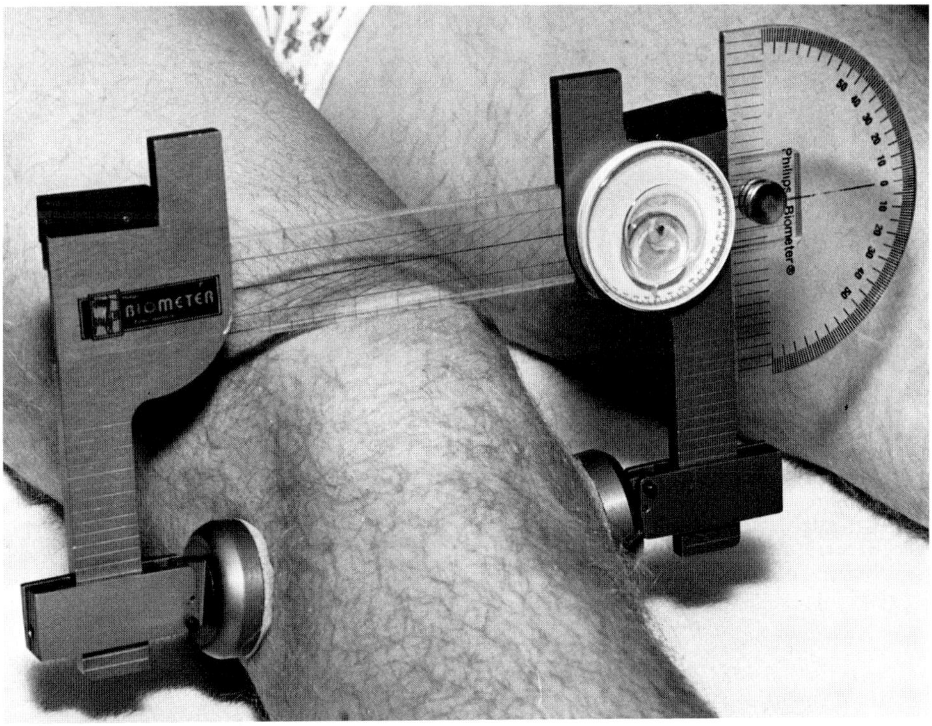

Figure 9.3. The Phillips Biometer shown being applied to the epicondyles of the femur to measure external and internal rotation of the leg. The instrument can measure 15 to 17 pathomechanical problems of the lower extremities with accuracy and reliability. (Courtesy of Robert Phillips, DPM.)

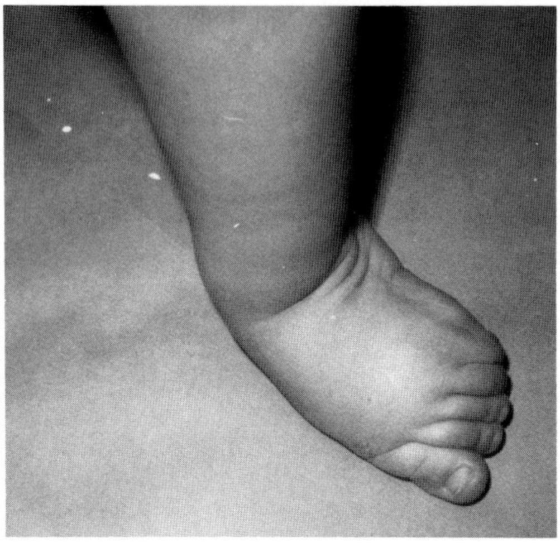

Figure 9.4. Severe pes valgoplanus.

nus. Posterior cavus occurs when the calcaneus approaches the vertical, and in combined cavus there is both a forefoot equinus and rearfoot calcaneus (Fig. 9.5). Etiologic factors include muscle paralysis, congenital bone and soft tissue deformity, muscle overactivity, underlying metabolic disorder and improper footgear.

Pes cavus is almost always associated with a neurological disorder. Often the underlying disorder cannot be identified, resulting in a diagnosis of idiopathic pes cavus. The following neuromuscular diseases have been implicated: muscular dystrophy, Déjèrine-Sotta's interstitial hypertrophic neuritis, Charcot-Marie-Tooth disease, polyneuritis, traumatic lesions of the sciatic nerve, poliomyelitis, myelomeningocele, diastenalomyelia, spinal cord tumors, Freidreich's ataxia, Roussy-Levy syndrome, cerebral palsy, dystonia musculorum deformans, Marie's cerebellar ataxia, olivopontocerebellar atrophy, heredopathia atactica polyneuritiformis, spinal dysraphism, infections, trauma and hysteria (6–9) (see Chapter 5, Neurological Disorders).

The author has found a gastrocnemius or gastrocnemius-soleus equinus associated with an uncompensated or compensated cavus deformity. Because the knees must prematurely flex during the gait cycle, more body weight is borne by the low back musculature at the $L_{4,5}S_1$ level, resulting in low back muscle spasm. Concomitant stress at the insertion of the plantar fascia and Achilles tendon predisposes to plantar fasciitis (heel spur syndrome) and Achilles tendonitis, respectively, as well as triceps surae muscle spasm. Soft tissue foot equinus is a common finding associated with a sharp growth spurt of the long bones during the teenage years. The posterior leg muscle groups do not elongate as quickly as their osseous counterparts, resulting in triceps surae and hamstring muscle pain ("growing pains") and spasm. Control of adverse foot function through a foot orthotic device, combined with stretching-flexibility exercises for the posterior leg muscle groups, is effective (see Chapter 12, Sports Medicine).

Common forefoot deformities caused partially or wholly by abnormal subtalar joint pronation include hallux abductus or abductovalgus, hallux limitus or rigidus, hammertoe, digiti quinti varus, and tailor's bunion (10–14). McCarthy et al. (15, 16) review the processes of chondrogenesis and osteogenesis employing light microscopy, scanning electron microscopy, cryomicrotomy, and transmission electron microscopy relative to common osseous foot deformities.

Disorders

Metatarsus Adductus (Varus). Flexible metatarsus adductus generally escapes detection until the infant starts to walk, but associated problems may be noted at birth. The common clinical presentation involves a hypermobile musculature, especially at the hip, resulting in inward rotation at the acetabulum in gait. Examination of all the body joints may reveal lax articular ligaments with hyperextensibility of the muscles with active or pas-

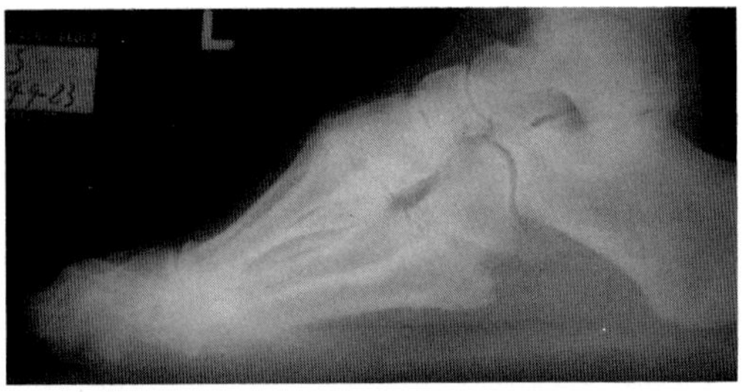

Figure 9.5. Combined cavus deformity.

sive function. The joints are flaccid in the hip, knee, ankle and foot. A true metatarsus adductus however, is a fixed adductus located in the forefoot only, with a normal or somewhat everted rearfoot (Fig. 9.6). Metatarsus adductus is usually apparent at birth or by the third or fourth month. The fixed type of metatarsus adductus is observed early enough for serial cast correction.

Frequently, the patient with an intoe gait presents a severely pronated foot with inward rotation of the calcaneus on its long axis, a prominent tuberosity of the navicular or subluxated talar head and poor muscular function. Careful examination may disclose that the intoe gait is often a compensatory reaction to the great strain on the leg muscles from improper foot function and faulty weight distribution. The external rotators of the hip are often weak. Contractures of the internal rotators may be a factor. Intoe gait may result as a compensatory change from myositis or dystrophic and neurogenic factors.

Where structural deformity exists in a marked adductus or varus, the patient generally has equinus, and the condition must then be considered a clubfoot (talipes equinovarus).

Treatment is based on the appearance of the foot at rest and its ability to perform in stance and in gait. An evaluation of the relative strength of the various muscle groups is most important in deciding on proper therapy. The extremities should be placed through various passive ranges of motion, and the podiatrist must decide whether there are restrictions in both active and passive motion at the hip or knee or in the foot. A limitation of active or passive external rotation of the limb at the acetabular articulation may be the result of a tightness of the ligaments and internal rotators at the hip. Normally, the gluteal and inguinal folds should be equal and bilaterally symmetrical. The knee joint flexes and extends both actively and passively. The ankle joint should perform its function within a normal range. Abduction, inversion, eversion and adduction must be tested both actively and passively to detect restrictions that could create the intoe gait. The gross appearance of the foot in gait and stance must be properly appreciated at this time. Deep and superficial reflexes should be evaluated and measurements in limb length and girth considered to rule out neurological disorders and deformities of the extremities.

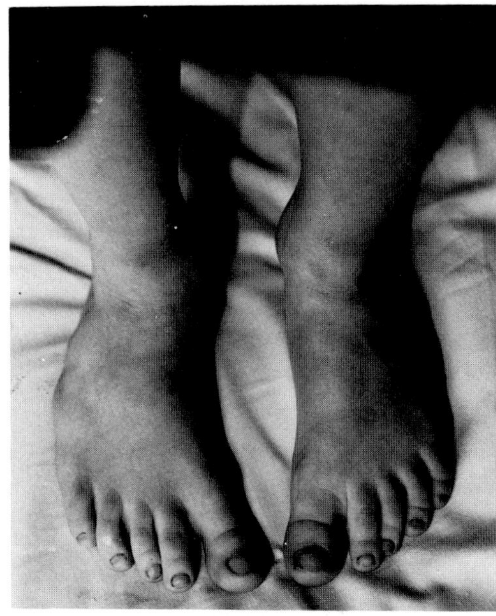

Figure 9.6. Metatarsus adductus (varus).

If, following propulsion, the patient brings the leg and foot into internal rotation and adduction prior to heel strike, one can assume that the problem is not a foot deformity but a compensatory change due to muscular contraction. This performance may be necessary for the relief of some discomfort or restriction elsewhere in the extremities. Conversely, if, on complete weightbearing of the foot, the knees appear knocked, the intoe may be a compensatory change due to severe subtalar valgus and compensatory forefoot varus.

Clinical findings must be evaluated by proper radiographs as outlined by Gamble and Yale (1).

Treatment. Early treatment in infancy is accomplished by plaster casting the fixed forefoot adductus (varus) in an overcorrected position. Periodic cast changes may correct the problem. The use of the Brachman Skate, Irving Yale Club Foot Splint, Ganley Splint, Fillaur Bar, Dennis Brown Bar, Friedman Shoe and Equinovarus Shoe may assist in reversing the deformity.

Scheimer (17) states that the use of plaster of paris casts is by far the best treatment for metatarsus varus.

Care must be taken to hold the rearfoot in as close a neutral subtalar position as possible when splinting or casting so as to avoid an iatrogenic flatfoot.

It has been the author's experience that most torsional abnormalities of the upper and lower legs rectify themselves with time and good functional foot control. Plaster casting and/or forced external rotation night splints used in the treatment of internal tibial torsion often lead to knee instability and subtalar pronatory collapse. Although the treatment of asymptomatic pronatory foot conditions in children remains controversial, the author has found great value in early functional control of adverse subtalar pronation for the prevention of adult symptoms and/or deformity.

Active and passive exercises, stretching of the forefoot and internal hip ligaments, physical therapeutic massage and manipulation are indicated. Gait training is imperative.

When the patient starts walking, straight last shoes will help. Care should be taken to ensure that the corrective procedures do not permanently deform the foot in a valgus state. Such shoe corrections as lateral wedges to force the feet out should never be used without compensatory medial longitudinal support and a Thomas heel.

In most cases of flexible intoeing the author prescribes a straight last shoe, external rotation gait exercises and a Celastic Whitman build-up in the shoes with a lateral extension under the fifth segment. Various metals, Rohadur or fiberglass, Whitman or Roberts foot orthoses, may be necessary. The patient wears a toe cutout shoe at night with a strap extending from one shoe to the other to rotate the limbs externally. This is the treatment of choice except when contractures require the use of a Brachman Skate, Dennis Brown or other bar splint. Surgical correction is rarely necessary. Active and passive stretching helps. Less damage to the structure of the foot is noted when tendoachilles lengthening is performed where indicated.

Counter correctors or similar straps attached to the shoes may be used as night and sleep retainers.

Hip and knee pathology should be treated by an orthopaedic surgeon.

Hallux Adductus (Varus). The classical clinical appearance presents the great toe widely separated from the second toe. The abductor of the great toe exerts considerable pull causing this deformity. Congenital hallux adductus (varus) is rare. When it is found early before the bony transformations take place, the joint may be corrected by orthodigital treatment.

Joseph et al. (18) classify hallux varus according to etiology. The congenital type is divided into primary, secondary (associated with clubfoot) and teratogenic (Fig. 9.7) The acquired type of hallux varus is divided into posttraumatic, following burns, due to chronic arthritis and idiopathic acquired hallux varus of middle age. Iatrogenic hallux adductus (varus) subsequent to hallux abductus (valgus) surgery is another acquired type. The authors present a study of 30 cases and note a progressive tendency toward hallux varus in an unshod population.

Regardless of the therapy selected, the end result will depend on judicious use of orthoses, exercises and corrective forces of an active and passive nature. One word of caution at this point should be made about the overtreatment of infants and children: The podiatrist must be constantly aware not only of the need for corrective forces and their application but also of the damage that may accrue in epiphyseal cartilage from their injudicious use.

Treatment. Treatment of congenital hallux adductus (varus) depends on whether the deformity is localized to the hallux or a part of a varus of the first metatarsal segment. In the event treatment is started early, it is wise to have the child wear a varus shoe or the opposite shoe on the affected foot. A plaster cast may be necessary to correct this deformity.

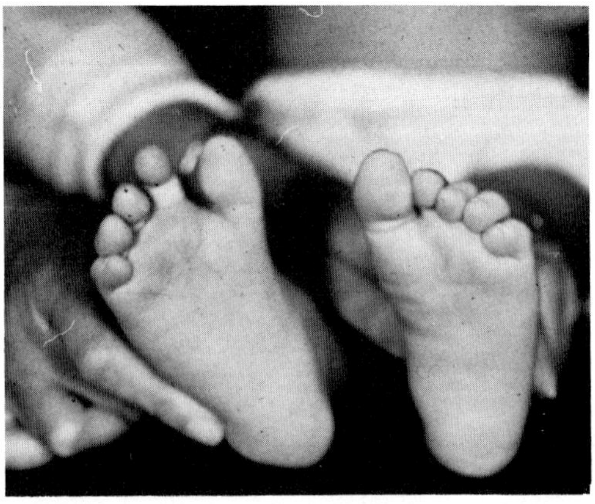

Figure 9.7. Congenital hallux varus—short first metatarsal. Note cleft in first interdigital space.

If therapy is instituted rather late, it may be necessary to construct an orthodigital device to bring about correction. Such a device can be constructed out of felt and latex or latex and other materials, such as tubegauze or plain bandage impregnated with latex or silicone gel. The application of a ring around the hallux coming over the dorsum of the foot connected to one or more of the lesser toes or encompassing the entire forefoot may produce an adequate force to bring about correction. This device pulls the hallux closer to the foot in line with the lesser toes. More sophisticated treatment may involve surgical syndactyly of the hallux to the second toe. Occasionally the treatment of choice is a surgical shortening of the adductor hallucis oblique and transverse tendon at its attachment. Lengthening the abductor tendon and incision of the medial joint capsule are also helpful. Syndactylizing the hallux to the second toe may be necessary to realign the hallux.

X-ray examination may suggest the need for surgical intervention.

Overlapping and Underriding Toes. These deformities commonly involve the lesser toes (Figs. 9.8–9.10). The author has seen many cases of underriding hallux; usually a hallux valgus coexists with the deformity. The great toe may extend under the second toe and sometimes under the third toe. The hallux nail, receiving the brunt of weightbearing by the dorsiflexed second toe, becomes atrophic, grayish, yellow or brown in color. The hallux may also override the second toe with severe contractures of the adductor hallucis, joint capsule and articular ligaments. Very often the extensor hallucis longus appears as a bow string due to its great longitudinal pull.

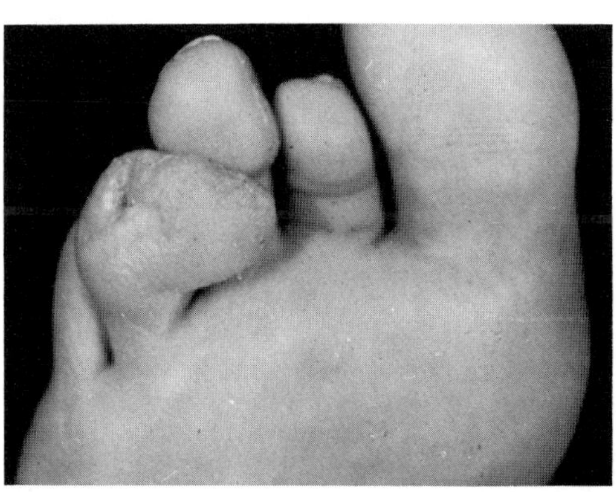

Figure 9.8. Underlapping fourth toe. Ulceration and sinus tract.

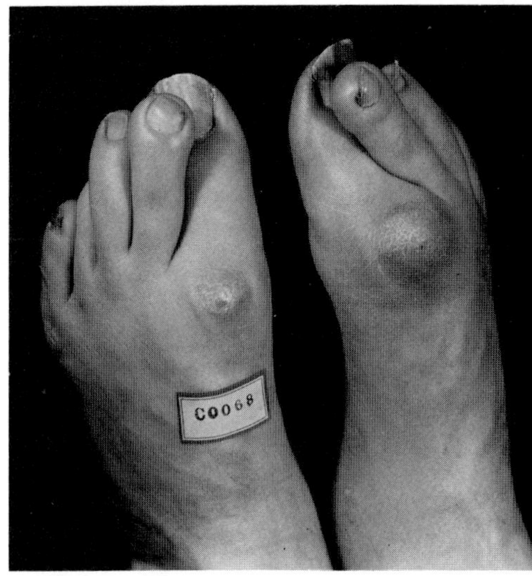

Figure 9.9. Overlapping second toes. Hallux limitus, dorsal bunion.

Observation of the feet of many children and adults reveals a characteristic hypermobile deformity of the lesser toes. The second toes of many individuals—often of Italian extraction—are contracted through pull by extensor muscles and articular ligaments to the point of dislocation. In addition to this contracture, there are flexions of the distal phalanges on their long axis either medially or laterally, resulting in severe deformity. The third toe is similarly involved, but more often presents an underlapping to the second toe that is contracted. The fourth toe is usually rotated on its long axis and underlapping the third. Many of the deformities occur at the interphalangeal joints with normal metatarsophalangeal joints. The fifth toe may overlap the fourth with contractures of the skin and joint capsule, as well as the extensor tendon.

These patients develop helomas from abnormal friction, and many patients develop hypertrophied nails from trauma. They also have difficulty in buying shoes that fit well.

Treatment. Treatment depends on the degree of deformity, the age of the patient and the extent of deformity as it relates to disturbances of the biomechanics of the foot. The usual physiological functions of the foot may not be affected by the minor deformities of the toes. However, the presence of underlapping or overlapping toes

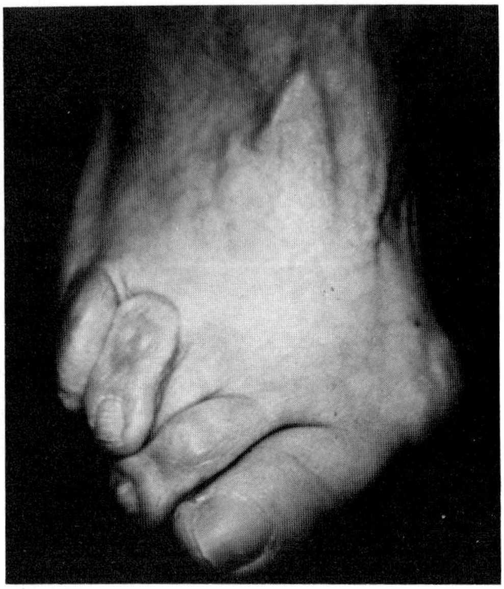

Figure 9.10. Overlapping toes. Second and fourth toes over third.

may alter foot function, creating postural disturbances at a distance from the site of a local deformity. Conversely, tight long flexor muscles may pull toes down to a deformed state when the flexor digitorum brevis muscles become atrophied.

Treatment may be conservative or surgical. Conservative treatment of these deformities depends on the use of adequate footgear to provide sufficient room for function of the deformed toes. Also, it is essential that the toes be placed on a plane that allows for maximum function within the limitations of the deformity. This can be done by judicious use of orthodigital corrective forces as prescribed by Budin, Polokoff, Whitney, McGlamry, Rosoff, and others. Roven (19) demonstrates a simple rubber sling for correction of overlapping fifth toe. This was a modification of Budin's (20) elastic traction loop sling. The use of orthodigital corrective or accommodative devices to increase the efficiency of the affected parts is indicated when surgical intervention is a risk. These devices include functional splints, removable crests and crests located on functional or accommodative foot orthoses (Fig. 9.11).

The surgical treatment of these disturbances may consist of a combination of surgical intervention and splinting in order to maintain the correction. The podiatrist may use the techniques of "Z" plasty, tenectomy, tenotomy, tendon lengthening, capsulotomy, syndactyly, arthroplasty, removal of an exostosis and resecting portions of capsular tissues to tighten up the articulation with suturing. Often it is essential to use two or more of the above techniques for correction. The author corrects these deformities with a middle phalangectomy to bring about a more even balance between the flexors and extensors of the toes. A surgical approach, described by Roven as "phalangeal set," which necessitates transverse incision of digital tendons and joint capsules without bone removal, has proved beneficial in correcting minor digital deformities (Figs. 9.12 and 9.13).

Polokoff (21) using his ingenious techniques, describes a single ring traction appliance to pull down a contracted third toe. This device may be used in inoperable contractions of a toe or following tenotomy or tenectomy. The clinician should spend time developing some expertise in the Polokoff techniques to ensure a broad scope of therapeuatic methods in the relief of minor toe deformities.

Fusion Deformities (Figs. 9.14–9.18). Cases are reported of congenital synostosis in several articulating bones. With congenital absence of articular cartilage,

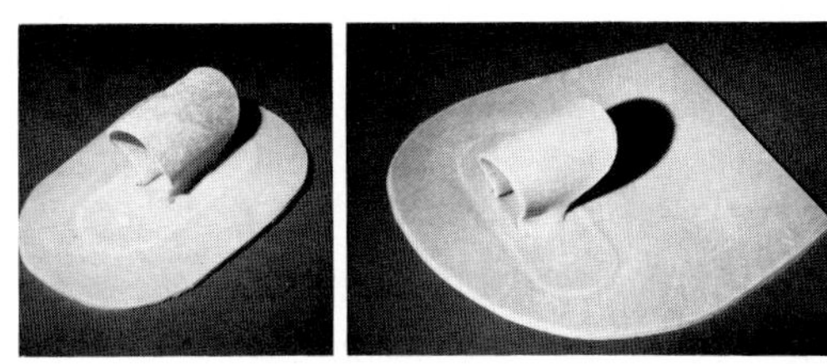

Figure 9.11. (*Left*) Budin splint. Transverse for overlapping toe. (*Right*) Budin splint. Longitudinal for hammertoes.

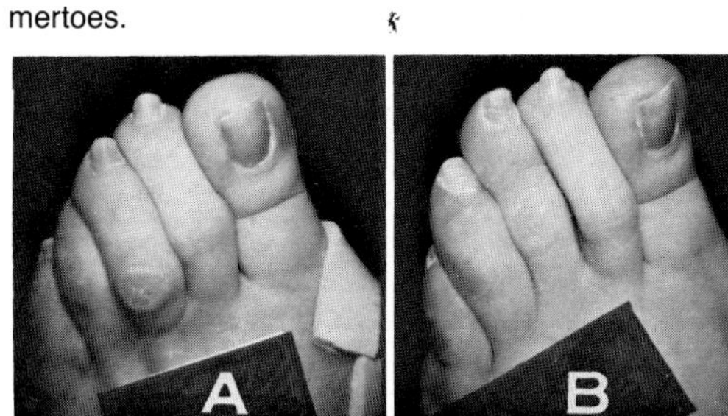

Figure 9.12. Correction of hallux and lesser toes.

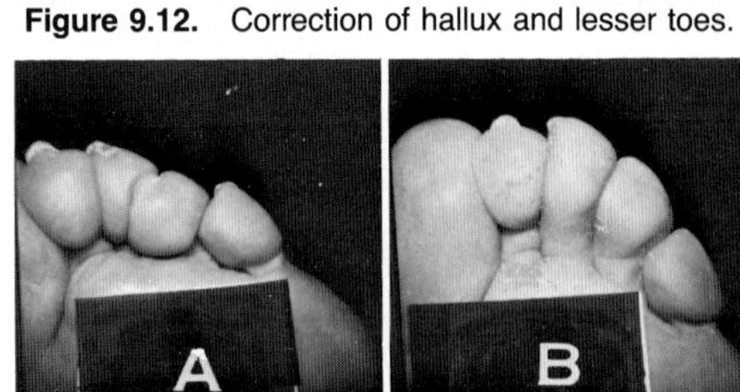

Figure 9.13. Phalangeal set. (Courtesy of M Roven.)

the apposing bone surfaces may unite and form a complete fusion. Bilateral fusion of the calcaneocuboid articulations has been reported. The tarsometatarsal articulations are often fused without pathological findings, and therefore the fusion must be construed to be of genetic origin. Syndactylism is a fusion deformity involving the soft tissue of the toes. The most common syndactyly is between the second and third toes followed by a syndactyly between the hallux and second toe. Occasionally, the phalanges are fused, resulting in claw foot. Rarely is treatment necessary for soft tissue syndactyly. If function is compromised or there is great psychological distress concerning the deformity, surgical desyndactylization may be performed. Weinstock et al. (22) describe a new surgical approach to desyndactylization utilizing two full thickness grafts.

Fusion deformities may also cause the various bars to develop between two or more tarsal and metatarsal bones. In this classification is found the talocalcaneal-cuboid or the talonavicular-calcaneal synostosis. The treatment for these fusion deformities depends upon the extent of the deformity and the patient's ability to pursue normal activities with the affected foot. The proper application of a rigid orthotic device often alleviates the discomfort that commonly develops when a mechanical dysfunction exists due to synostosis. The orthosis is constructed to a cast of the foot. Under no circumstance should the patient with fusion deformities wear flexible-soled or shanked shoes. The motion produced by gravitational pressure against a flexible weightbearing surface increases the stress on the bony bars. Fracture of the bar is capable of causing a disabling deformity of a foot.

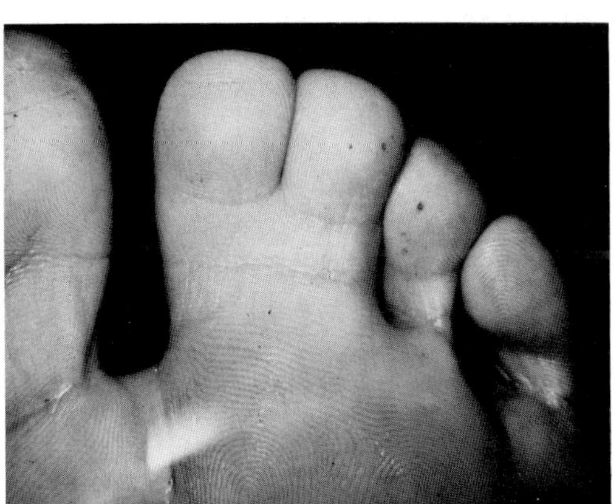

Figure 9.14. Syndactylism.

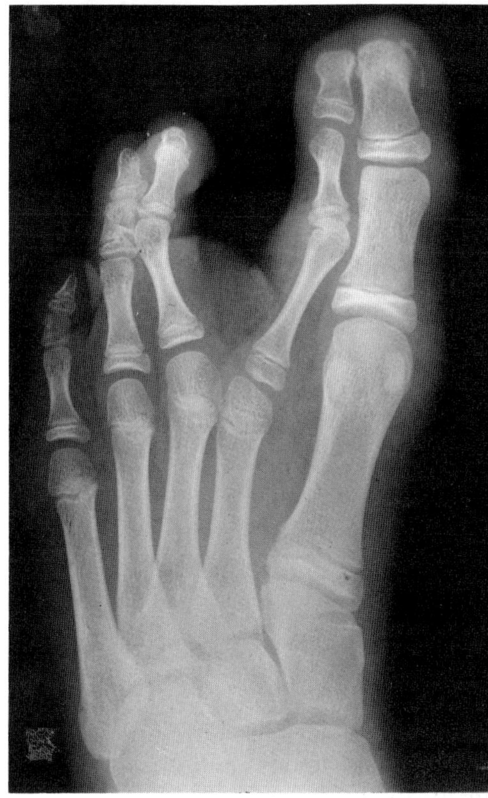

Figure 9.15. Syndactylism.

Polydactyly (polyphalangia, supernumerary toes). The fifth toe, as well as all other toes, may have a rudimentary center for development of an extra toe. Often the toe may have its own corresponding metatarsal, or it may arise from the base of the proximal or distal phalanges or the heads of the metatarsals or form an accessory metatarsal shaft.

The treatment of polydactyly is based on the physiological factors entering into the case and the ability of a patient to wear conventional footgear. The proper approach to treatment is surgical intervention as early as possible to eliminate the extra toe. Where additional metatarsals exist, surgery to remove the extra toes and their articulating metatarsal bones is necessary. Another important reason for surgical intervention in this deformity is to remove emotional stress in patients who are often overly sensitive about the condition. Christensen et al. (23) present three cases of polydactyly and review the classification, genetics and surgical correction of this congenital deformity (Table 9.2).

Agenesis. This condition should be differentiated from intrauterine amputations of skeletal parts. In agenesis there is sudden cessation of further bony growth, and the skin and subcutaneous tissue extend beyond the abruptly completed skeletal parts. The soft tissues may look like the absent skeletal part through their shape, although bony support is absent. The defect is in the skeleton, and the parts show no evidence of ever having been present.

True skeletal intrauterine amputations occur where there is involvement of more than one extremity. There may be clinical and radiographic evidence of sloughing off. The soft tissues have multiple creases to differentiate them from true agenesis as previously described.

Treatment. Treatment of this involvement is cosmetic unless the extent of agenesis results in faulty function and gait. The author advises the early use of cosmetic devices to maintain emotional stability, as well as to maintain adequate foot function and good foot posture.

Agenesis of a toe or entire forefoot may be accommodated in a shoe by a prosthetic device with shaped fillers. The prosthesis can be molded over a cast to fit the foot. An impression of the forepart of the shoe can be constructed with the foot in the shoe by stuffing wet papier mâché into the toe section. Other materials, such as rubber butter, silicone gel or felt impregnated

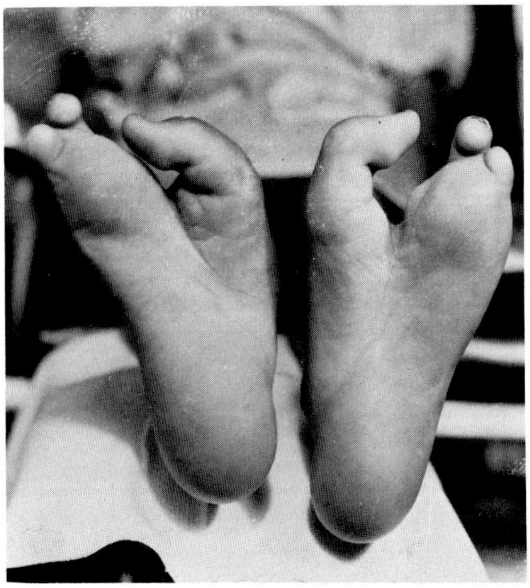

Figure 9.16. Claw foot.

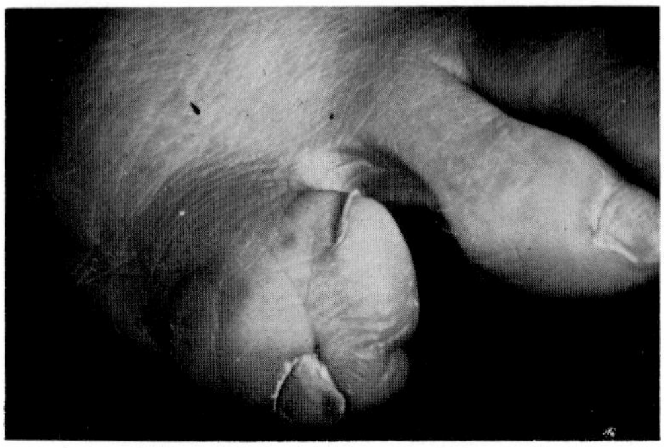

Figure 9.17. Synpolydactylism.

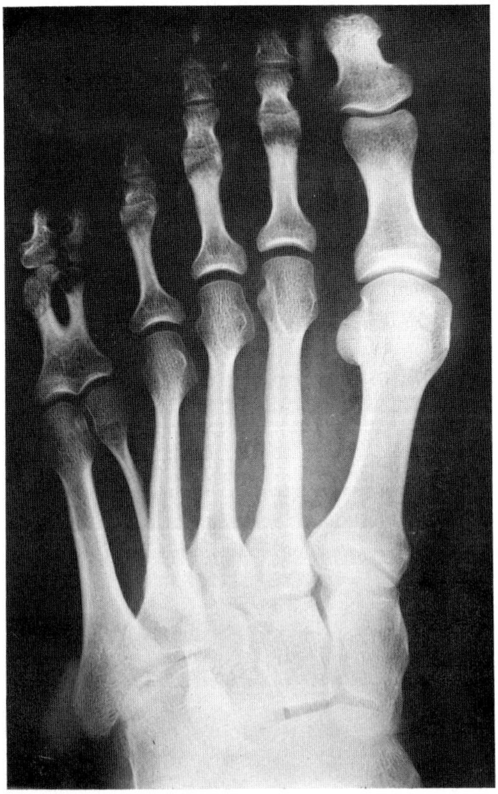

Figure 9.18. Synpolydactylism.

Table 9.2.
Syndromes Associated With Polydactyly[a]

Postaxial polydactyly	Preaxial polydactyly
Ellis-van Creveld syndrome	Acrocephalopolysyndactyly (Carpenter's syndrome)
Infantile thoracic dystrophy (Jeune's disease)	Acrocephalopolysyndactyly with leg hypoplasia
Hydrometrocolpos-postaxial polydactyly syndrome	Greig cephalopolysyndactyly syndrome
Trisomy 13-15 with polydactyly	Mohr-Claussen syndrome
Median cleft of upper lip with polydactyly	Majewski syndrome
Saldino-Noonan syndrome	Townes syndrome
Orofaciodigital syndrome III	Polydactyly-imperforate anus, vertebral abnormalities
Laurence-Moon-Bardet-Biedl syndrome	Bilateral aplasia of tibia
Biemond's syndrome	Holt-Oram syndrome
Opitz C syndrome	Hand brachydactyly with foot polydactyly
Weyers acrofacial syndrome	
Meckel syndrome	

[a] From Christensen JC, et al: Congenital polydactyly and polymetatarsia: Classification, genetics, and surgical connection. *J Foot Surg* 20:151–158, 1981.

with latex, may be used for molding. The podiatric device is ideally a well-fitting, comfortable prosthesis. Ground smooth, covered with soft leather and fit into a shoe, the prosthesis enables the patient with agenesis to be a normally functioning individual with a minimum of physical or emotional instability.

A prosthetic device with simulated toes can be fit over the stump. In many instances it may serve necessary cosmetic purposes. The device can accommodate certain pressure points that exist with agenesis. Cutouts, buildups, wedging and depressions allow for accommodation and relief of pressure pain. Engelmeir (24) describes an excellent technique for fabrication of a prosthetic replacement for missing toes.

Brachymetatarsia. This condition is generally seen in hypoplastic malformation of the metatarsal bones. The author has seen several cases of unilateral shortening of the fourth metatarsal bone. This bone is usually well formed but prematurely developed and ossified at the epiphyses. Cases of unilateral shortening have been observed associated with neurological disorders unnoticed in childhood. Cases of bilateral shortening of the fourth metatarsal bones and bilaterally shortened third and fourth bones are also in the author's files. This development is considered to be either congenital or acquired. Trauma to an epiphysis may result in premature closure and cessation of bony growth.

Scheimer and Chamas (25) present a review of the literature and a case study of brachymetatarsia. Possible etiologic factors predisposing to one or more short lesser metatarsals include trauma, congenital abnormality, Down's syndrome, Turner's syndrome, pseudohypoparathyroidism, malignancy, Albright's hereditary osteodystrophy, diastrophic dwarfism, multiple epiphyseal dysplasia and myositis ossificans.

Treatment. Treatment for brachymetatarsia is based upon maintenance of good foot function. The construction of a prosthetic device to maintain proper foot balance is indicated. This device is chosen based on the extent and degree of deformity and the ability of the part to function without pain.

Shortened metatarsal bones create faulty weight distribution as adjacent longer metatarsal bones must accept a greater share of weight-bearing. Construction of a prosthesis is aimed at developing a broad distribution of body weight. Extensions of weight-distributing material beneath the short bone allow it to assume its responsibility in maintaining good stance and gait.

Some foot surgeons have used a lengthening sliding osteotomy followed by several weeks of traction with a modicum of success. Lengthening procedures are performed for biomechanical and cosmetic reasons. Cylindrical bone grafts from adjacent metatarsals, autogenous calcaneal bone grafts and fifth metatarsal head transfers have been reported.

Absence of Toes (Fig. 9.19). The fifth toe often develops with two phalanges. The proximal phalanx appears unusually long with a normal-sized distal phalanx. Absence of toes is common and is often seen with absence of other bones in the extremities. Cases of congenital absence of one or both sesamoids have been reported. Very often the distal phalanx appears fused to the middle, giving a double phalanx appearance where only a single phalanx exists. This condition is rarely of clinical significance. However, a prominent base of the distal phalanx may be the underlying etiology for a heloma.

Treatment. Correction of foot deformities and faulty foot function due to absence of toes or bones of the feet must be considered early. Artificial toes may be constructed using silicone rubber. These may be incorporated into a latex forefoot prosthesis. Surgical excision of deformed bones may be indicated. Accommodative orthotic devices may be necessary.

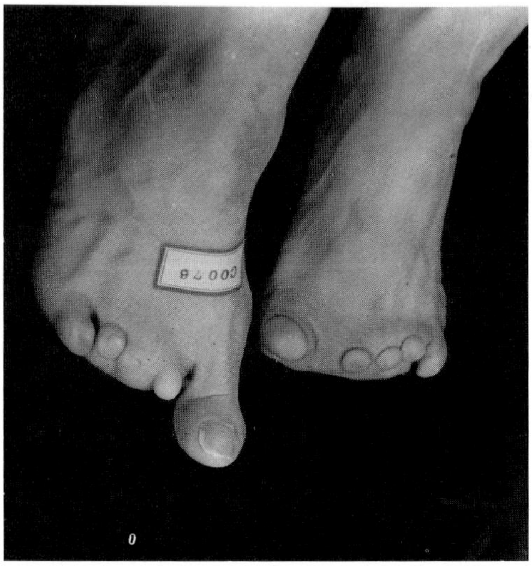

Figure 9.19. Congenital absence toes. (Courtesy of D Mowbray.)

Deformities of the Accessory Bones of the Foot (Fig. 9.20). The accessory bones of the foot are often referred to as sesamoid bones. The only constant sesamoid bones are those that occur beneath the first metatarsal head. They develop by separate centers of ossification within the tendons of the flexor hallucis brevis. These bones may commonly be seen on the radiograph as multipartite. The tibial or medial sesamoid is often seen as a bipartite bone. However, it is not unusual to find the tibial sesamoid in many parts. Each part is attached to its adjacent member by fibrocartilaginous tissue and is developed from a separate center of ossification.

All accessory bones may show evidence of trauma or pathology. The sesamoid bones beneath the first metatarsal head are subject to fracture and dislocation.

Sesamoids beneath lesser metatarsals are not uncommon. They are often multiple when present under the metatarsal heads and present a complete cortex and central ossific pattern. These sesamoids or ossicles are also commonly seen at the plantar surface of the interphalangeal joint of the great toe and must not be confused with calcium deposits.

The os trigonum, located at the lateral portion of the posterior surface of the talus, often is attached to and forms a part of the talus. Plantar flexion of the ankle or a sudden severe trauma may result in a fracture of this posterior process or a tear of its fibrocartilaginous attachment.

The os tibiale externum is posterior medial and slightly plantar to the tuberosity of the navicular. It is not necessarily bilateral as many observers have stated. This accessory ossicle may be attached by cartilage to the tuberosity of the navicular and become a part of it, or it may become displaced from its articulation with the body of the bone and develop degenerative arthritis. Often it is inflamed from the pressure of excessive pronation when prominent on the medial aspect. A prominent tuberosity of the navicular may fracture with severe trauma, resulting in a simulated os tibiale externum with a pseudoarticulation from nonunion. An acute adventitious bursitis may develop over the prominent bone.

The os vesalianum, os cambelli, os intermetatarseum, os cuneiforme intermedium, secondary calcaneus, accessory os cuboideum, Pirie's bone, os fibulare and os tibiale are shown in Figure 9.20. These bones must be differentiated from fracture fragments or calcifications of the soft tissues; when overlapped by bone they are often mistaken for nonreticulated areas, compact islands or innocuous bone nodules.

The presence of an os vesalianum sometimes results in a prominence at the fifth metatarsal base with an overlying callus.

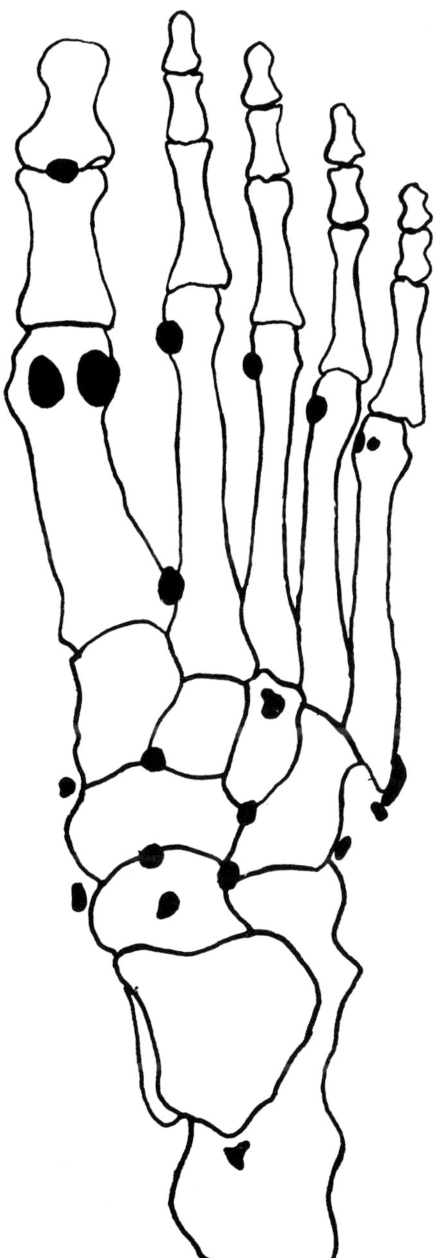

Figure 9.20. Accessory bones of the foot.

Acute bursitis may develop between the callused skin and the prominence of bone.

The os fibulare at the distal end of the fibular malleolus must be differentiated from fractures of the lateral malleolus or displacement of the distal epiphysis. A cortical tear may result from an inversion injury of the ankle and rupture of ligaments. The torn cortex may simulate an accessory ossicle.

The os tibiale at the distal end of the medial malleolus must also be differentiated from fracture or epiphysis. Often a tear of the accessory bone from its fibrocartilaginous attachment simulates a fracture. Remember that the accessory ossicle has a complete smooth cortical outline.

There is a 2-year lag between ossification of the sesamoids in males and ossification of the sesamoids in females, but there is negligible difference in the sex distribution of accessory bones.

Calcifications are amorphous with no evidence of cortex or internal architecture on the radiograph. They must not be confused with ossifications as seen in accessory bones.

Treatment. Treatment of the accessory bones of the foot depends upon the status of the bone in function and structure. A sesamoid bone beneath the lesser metatarsals may be innocuous unless it has been crushed, subluxated or torn from its adjacent tissues. Resting the part with the use of felt and adhesive tape for a period of time is necessary to allow for complete repair and relief of pain. An orthotic device properly constructed to take pressure off the affected part may be indicated. Subluxation of sesamoids beneath the interphalangeal joints of the toes—most frequently the great toe—may be treated by immobilization, traction or both.

Damage done to the os trigonum is easily relieved with local injection of an anesthetic and steroid, followed by adhesive tape immobilization. A fracture of the posterior process of the talus is treated by immobilization with rigid or flexible castings to allow for repair of the fractured part. After the fracture has healed, physiotherapeutic measures may be used to hasten relief of pain and increase mobility. Rarely a symptomatic nonunion develops and must be excised.

Treatment of a painful os tibiale externum may be either conservative or surgical. When constructing an orthotic device for an abnormally pronating foot with an associated os tibiale externum, it is essential that the podiatrist consider that a very high medial flange may result in great pressure over the os tibiale externum. It is not uncommon for a bursitis to develop over an os tibiale externum where a rigid orthotic device with a high flange presses on the bony prominence. The author suggests that the flange be kept low and below the prominence of bone or that a pocket for the bony prominence be provided in the orthosis. Where traumatic arthritis has developed between the tuberosity of the navicular and the os tibiale externum, it may be necessary to excise the os tibiale externum if it is too large and interferes with the functioning of the foot. A semielliptical incision is made over the affected part, the attachment of the tibialis posterior is exposed, the os tibiale externum is dissected free from its attachments and closure is instituted in such a way as to maintain the integrity of the tibialis posterior tendon.

Hammertoe (Figs. 9.21 and 9.22). The common digiti flexus or hammertoe deformity causes untold misery. This deformity usually affects the second and fifth toe, but may occur in any toe. The proximal phalanx is dorsiflexed on the metatarsal head, the middle phalanx is plantar flexed, and the distal phalanx is flexed or extended.

Hammertoes may be congenital, hereditary or acquired by trauma or disease; they are usually bilateral. The second toe, because it is the longest toe, is easily traumatized by short stockings or by short or extremely pointed shoes. Hallux abductovalgus deformities are common with extreme deformities of the second toes (Fig. 9.23) Rheumatoid arthritis and osteoarthritis may be etiologic (Fig. 9.24).

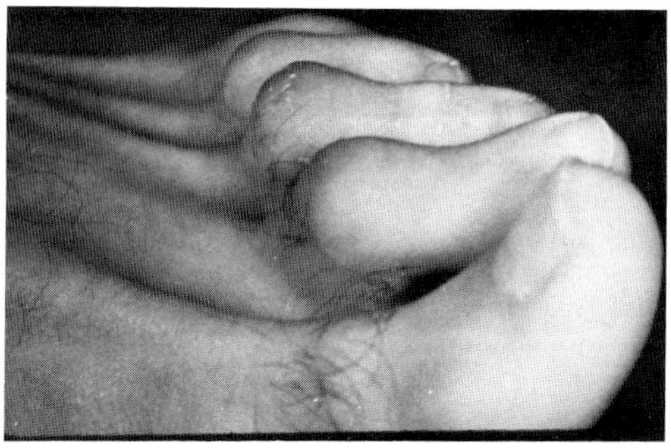

Figure 9.21. Multiple hammertoes with contraction of extensor tendons.

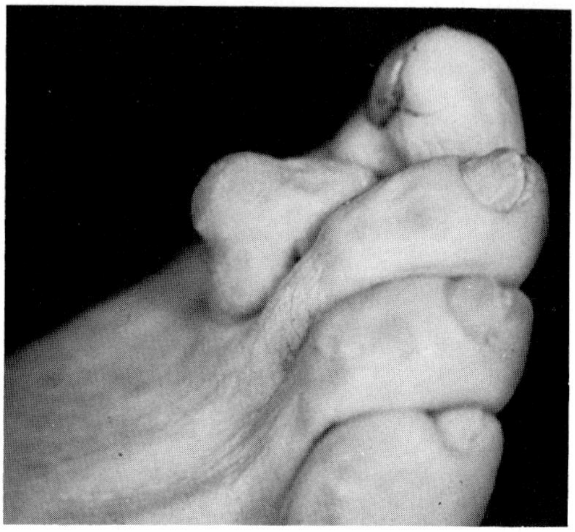

Figure 9.22. Hammertoe.

The proximal interphalangeal joint is the highest point dorsally and is readily traumatized by shoes. Helomas, tylomas and bursae result from friction and pressure. The tip of the distal phalanx is very often flattened out, broadened and covered by a heloma or tyloma. The above excrescences break down in circulatory or trophic disease, creating an excellent focus for infection and subsequent sinus or trophic ulcer. The great toe may overlap or underlap the second toe. Callus tissue develops at such points of pressure as the plantar surface of the second metatarsophalangeal joint, the dorsum of the proximal interphalangeal joint and the distal end of the toe. Contractures of the extensor and flexor tendons, fascia and glenoid and collateral ligaments are noted. The skin on the plantar surface is contracted and very often fissured. The joints are enlarged and deformed. Ankylosis, usually of a fibrous nature, may result.

X-ray examination may disclose a calcified sinus or calcification of the bursa in long-standing lesions. Sequestration and a focal necrosis of bone may be in evidence. Lipping, osteophytes and loss of substance at the chondro-osseous margins are common (Fig. 9.25).

Polokoff (26) describes and illustrates an orthotic device fabricated in the podiatrist's office on the patient's foot. This device made of a dental cotton roll, surgitube, liquid latex, rubber cement, moleskin, 1/16 and 1/8 inch adhesive felt has a

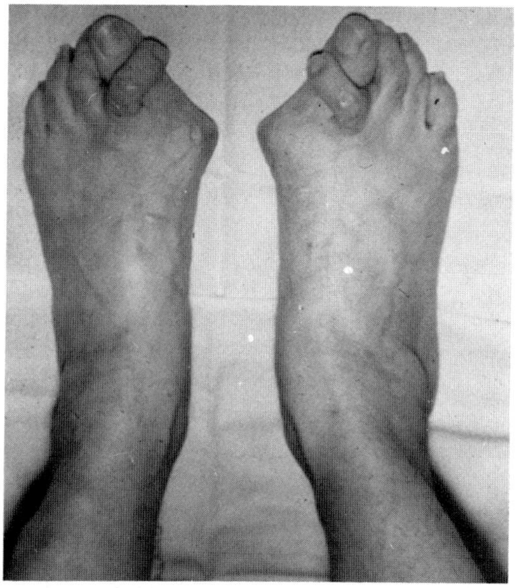

Figure 9.23. Hallux valgus—overlapping second toes.

four-fold purpose. "It encourages weight-bearing by the lesser toes, relieves weight load from 2nd, 3rd and 4th metatarsal heads, forces soft tissue back under the metatarsal heads and extends contracted toes to remove pressure from distal and dorsal helomas." The simplicity of construction of these pads is illustrated by Polokoff.

Treatment. The treatment of hammertoe may be conservative or surgical. Conservative treatment may include wearing of different footgear to eliminate pressure on the affected part or use of accommodative orthodigital devices to relieve compression on the deformed toe. Conservative treatment is desirable in those cases that present poor surgical risks, as only surgical intervention can correct an established hammertoe. In the early states and especially in children, the use of adhesive materials to straighten deformed toes is often sufficient. Polokoff (personal communication) developed an original double-ring hammertoe device constructed from 1/16 inch Polokoff felt. Budin splints help keep the toe in alignment.

Plaster impressions and latex, plastic or silicone shields constructed over the cast have been used by podiatrists for many years. Moldable plastic materials and silicone products are currently being used along with tubegauze to create accommodative devices for hammertoes. Inlay depth shoes allow freedom in the forefoot and relief of pressure. These shoes have a removable insole about 1/4 inch thick that can be ground down to accommodate dorsiflexed toes.

Surgical treatment of hammertoe is described in the treatment of chronic helomas (see Chapters 6 and 11). The initial incision may be longitudinal, elliptical, or curvilinear depending on the pathology. A transverse incision is made through the dorsal capsule, and incision of the collateral ligaments is then made close to the bone. Upon making the dorsal and lateral incisions of the articular capsule and ligaments, the head of the proximal phalanx is delivered into the surgical wound. The joint is resected through the neck of the proximal phalanx using a bone forceps, Stryker reciprocal saw or ultrahigh-speed airdrills. Very small bites are made into the bone through the neck in order to preserve the integrity of the shaft of the bone and to reduce the possibility of splintering. The head and its articular cartilage are delivered into the wound and removed. The cut surface through the neck of the proximal phalanx is then rasped smooth, and closure of the skin is effected by the use of interrupted 5–0 nylon skin sutures that also include the capsule. The capsule may be repaired prior to skin closure with interrupted 4–0 dexon sutures.

Another technique used by the author is making a transverse semielliptical incision around the painful excrescence overlying the joint and excis-

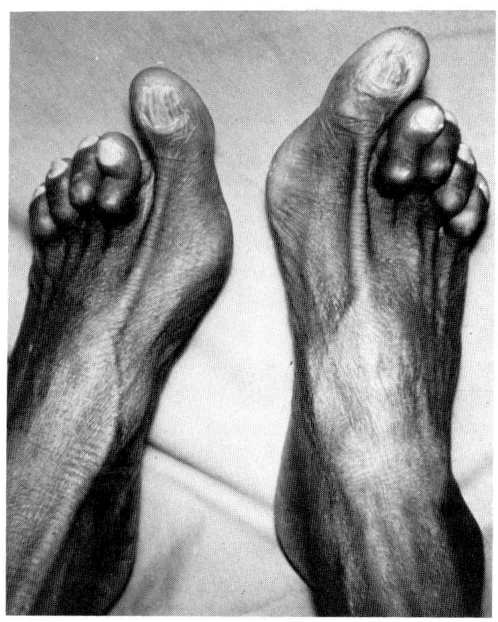

Figure 9.24. Severe rheumatoid arthritis. Hammertoes. Note contraction of extensor tendons, prominent proximal interphalangeal joints with flexion of middle phalanx and extension of distal phalanx.

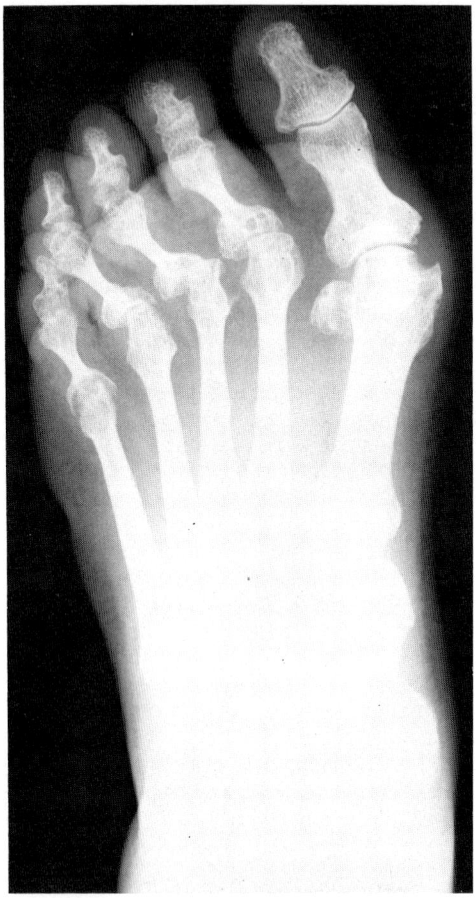

Figure 9.25. X-ray, rheumatoid arthritis. Note lateral deflection of toes. Atrophic loss of substance chondro-osseous margins of bone.

ing the excrescence and its underlying bursa. The joint is exposed, and the same procedure described above is followed (Fig. 9.26).

In some cases it is necessary to perform a tenectomy, tenotomy or lengthening on the extensor tendon to the affected toe. In severe cases where there is a subluxation or dislocation at the metatarsophalangeal articulation, it is helpful to do a capsulotomy at the metatarsophalangeal joint. A "V" extension-shortening osteotomy performed at the surgical neck of the affected metatarsal is effective in reducing the dorsally subluxed hammertoe. Another technique used when there is a dislocation at the metatarsophalangeal joint is to make an incision at the medial or lateral aspect of the toe exposing the entire proximal phalanx and then dissecting out the proximal phalanx or removing the base of the proximal phalanx in order to realign the toe. The author finds it is best to remove the entire proximal phalanx in order to correct both the metatarsophalangeal deformity and the deformity at the proximal interphalangeal joint. Surgical syndactyly must be accomplished if this technique is to be successful.

When the deformity exists without enlargement of the joint margin, removal of the middle phalanx may be in order. The middle phalangectomy has been most successful when the middle phalanx is short, resulting in good closure and little evidence of postoperative flaccidity. The treatment of choice with involvement at the distal interphalangeal joint is middle phalangectomy or middle phalangeal head resection (Figs. 9.27 and 9.28). In this procedure, two transverse semielliptical incisions are made over the middle phalanx, and the entire phalanx is dissected from its attachments. Closure is made in the usual manner.

It is essential in some instances to create a bony ankylosis in order to straighten the affected toe. To do this, the head of the proximal phalanx is dissected out, and the base of the middle phalanx is resected. The parts are apposed either by subcutaneous suturing to effect good apposition of the part or by pinning the bones with a Kirschner wire or Steinman pin. The author's experience indicates that pinning is unnecessary for interphalangeal joints and creates unnecessary trauma. A bony ankylosis results if the part is splinted and maintained in close apposition following removal of the base of middle phalanx and the head of the proximal phalanx.

When only soft tissue is involved in hammertoe deformity, cutting the plantar capsules and flexor tendons may correct the condition. This has been called "phalangeal set" by Roven (27) (Fig. 9.29).

Polokoff (28) describes a double-ring toe traction device to restore a rotated toe to its normal position, to force phalanges of a toe into extension, to relieve excessive pressure on metatarsal heads by providing the toes a share of the weightbearing, to reduce maceration and to protect dorsal

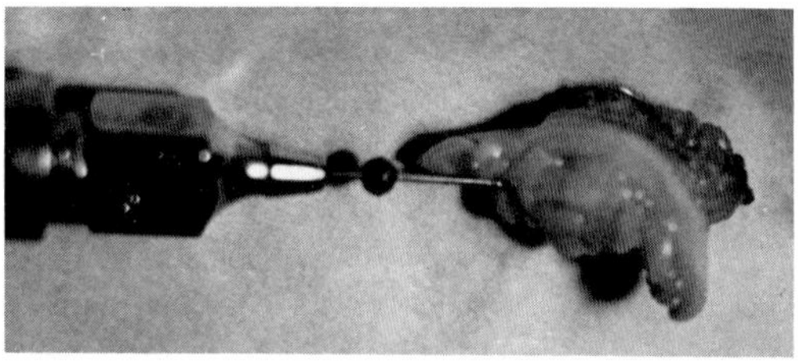

Figure 9.26. Distended subhelomal bursa beneath elliptical section removed during surgical correction of hammertoe.

prominences. Polokoff uses a ⅛-inch special felt bearing his name. (The reader should study the details of fabrication of these pads as provided in the January 1976 issue of the *Journal of the American Podiatry Association*.)

Coates, in personal communications (29), and in a well-written paper described the construction of silicone devices moldable in a brief minute. Coates is able to control the "softness, hardness, shape, shade and processing time" of these washable devices. Part II of his paper (30) illustrates each step in the construction of a silicone orthodigital device.

Sharrard and Smith (31) claim good results in 15 out of 17 patients following tenodesis of the flexor hallucis longus for

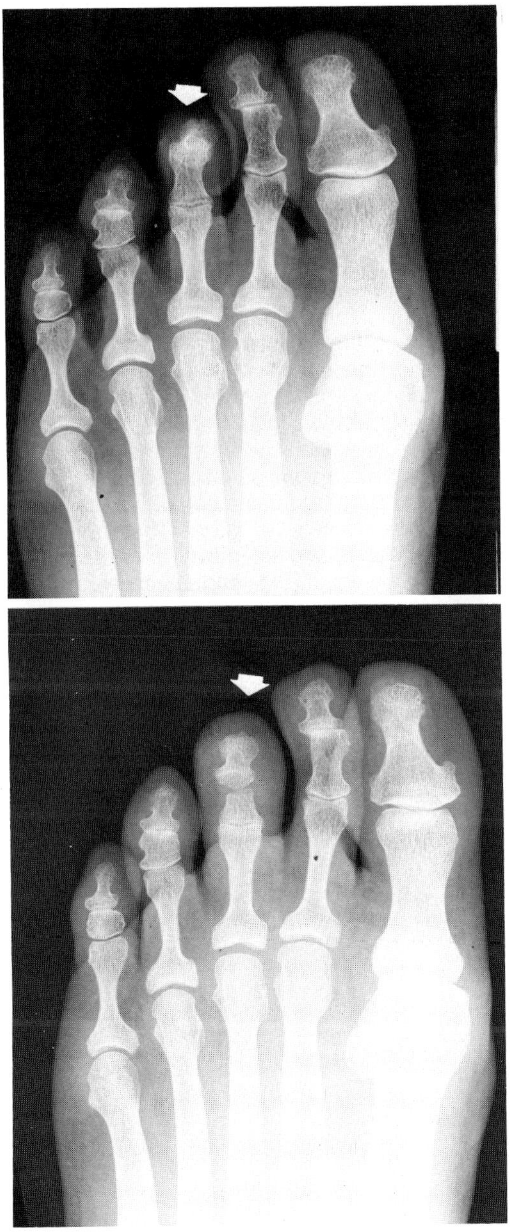

Figure 9.27. *Top,* preoperative mallet toe. *Bottom,* correction of mallet toe, distal interphalangeal joint.

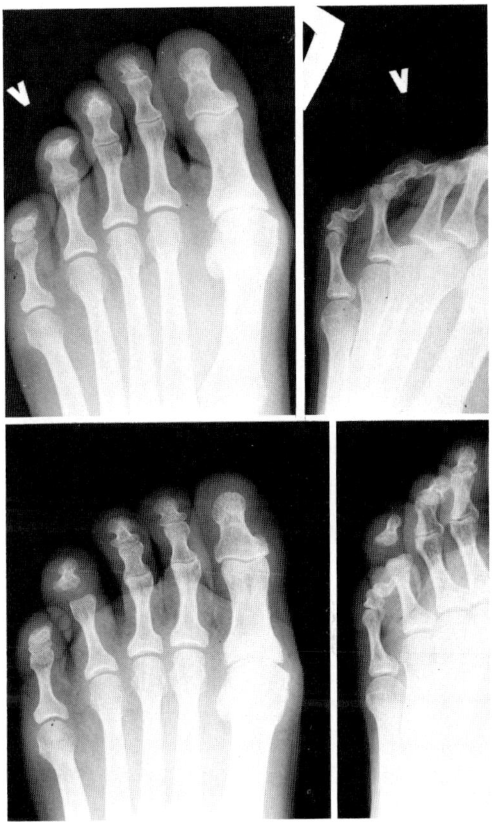

Figure 9.28. Middle phalangectomy for correction of hammertoe.

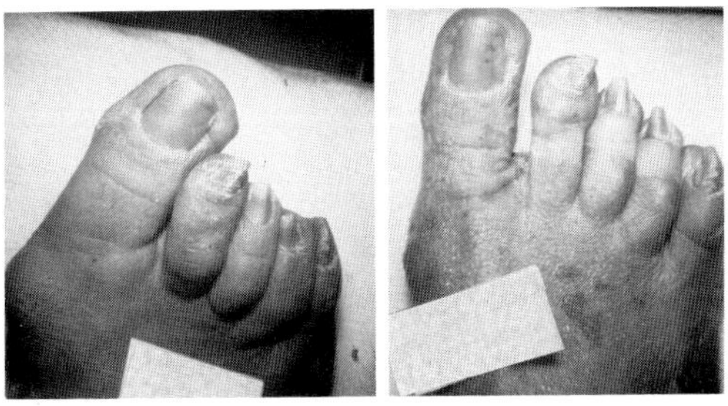

Figure 9.29. Correction of hallux and lesser toes by osteotripsy and phalangeal set.

paralytic clawing of the hallux in childhood.

Haber et al. (32), in a random study of 18 patients who had undergone surgery for correction of contracted fifth toes, conclude that biomechanical problems, especially affecting the flexor digitorum longus and quadratus plantae, dictate the need for postoperative orthotic control. They cite the pull being exerted by the imbalance produced by structural faults in the forefoot and rearfoot as exciting factors in the development and postoperative reoccurence of fifth toe contractures.

Hallux Flexus (Hallux Malleus). This deformity is a hammertoe of the great toe (hallux hammertoe) characterized by a dorsiflexed proximal phalanx on the first metatarsal head with plantar flexion of the distal phalanx (Fig. 9.30). This often is spoken of as a trigger toe. Lewin (33) feels that this condition is usually due to a stenosing tenosynovitis, a synovioma or sesamoiditis.

Hallux flexus has been observed in adolescents when the young adult develops rapidly before shoes are changed to compensate for increased foot size. In conditions of foot strain, the compensatory contracture of the extensor hallucis longus tendon makes an attempt to support the medial longitudinal arch by dorsiflexing the great toe. The flexor hallucis longus tendon is the antagonist in this case, resulting in the deformity of hallux flexus.

Drop foot deformities from poliomyelitis or spastic paralysis exert a great pull on the extensor muscles, leading to hallux flexus deformity.

Pes cavus, forefoot valgus, or plantar flexed first metatarsal may produce clawing of the lesser toes and hallux flexus.

A heloma, tyloma, or bursa may develop on the dorsum of the hallux with degenerative changes in the interphalangeal joint.

The author has noted hallux flexus in children who present an improperly developed interphalangeal joint. The articulating surfaces are not transverse but angulated, leaving an imbalanced joint and causing the toe to rotate in a slightly medial direction on its long axis.

Treatment. The treatment of hallux flexus may be conservative and palliative or surgical and corrective. The congenital or hereditary deformities that result in a strong pull on the extensor hallucis longus tendon should be treated. The podiatrist must decide whether simply lengthening the extensor hallucis longus tendon would correct the deformity or if a surgical procedure involving the interphalangeal joint as well is necessary. If a lengthening of the tendon is indicated, a longitudinal incision is made to one side of the extensor tendon. The incision is deepened to expose the tendon, and a Z-shaped lengthening of the tendon is performed. DuVries (34) has developed a technique in which he makes a small longitudinal incision at the medial plantar aspect of the interphalangeal joint, passes a small blade into the soft tissues adjacent to the bone and makes a transverse incision through the plantar capsular ligamentous tissues. The contracted tissues are released, and the toe straightens out from its flexed position. However, when bony changes have taken place on the dorsal aspect of the interphalangeal joint it is necessary to remove the head of the proximal phalanx or fuse the interphalangeal joint.

Treatment requires correction of stresses and strains that create a pull on the extensor hallucis longus tendon. This is followed by lengthening of the extensor tendon, incision of the plantar capsule at the interphalangeal joint and often a resection of the head of the proximal phalanx. Traction is of little help in treatment of this deformity.

Hallux flexus can be accommodated by an extradepth shoe, or the affected digit may be protected on its dorsal surface by a molded shield. Although this is a conservative approach, it may also be beneficial after surgery in some cases.

Digiti Quinti Flexus (Fig. 9.31). This is a flexion or hammertoe deformity of the fifth toe. The changes and symptoms are the same as those in digiti flexus. The digital branch of the extensor digitorum longus tendon appears as a bow string on the dorsum. The author has observed several cases of tenosynovitis affecting the extensor tendons in severe cases of digiti quinti flexus. A painful heloma with underlying bursitis is common. A sinus infection may be present, with periostitis of a phalanx visible on the radiograph. The sinus tract may be calcified if chronic. The margins of the articulating surfaces of the underlying joint present lipping and osteophytes.

Treatment (see Chapters 6 and 11). The treatment of digiti quinti flexus is the same as that of hammertoe on other toes as described above.

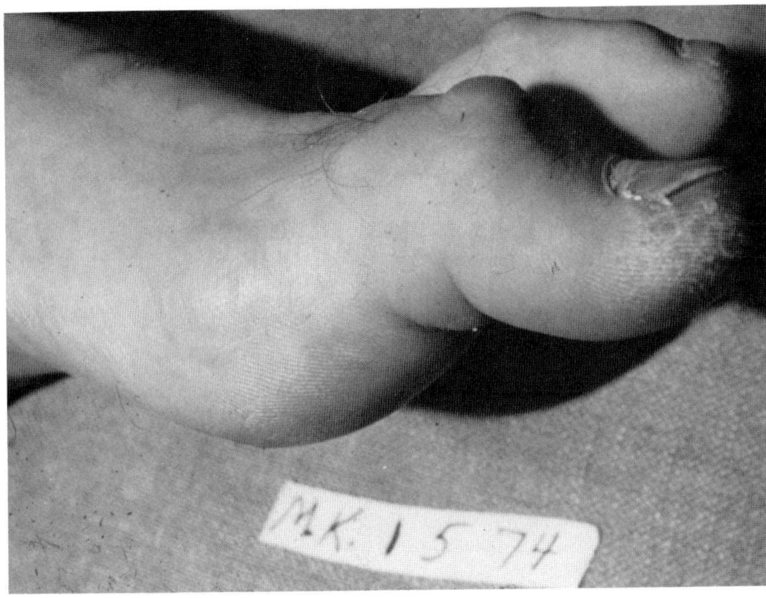

Figure 9.30. Hallux flexus. Subluxated hallux interphalangeal joint. Surgical reduction necessary.

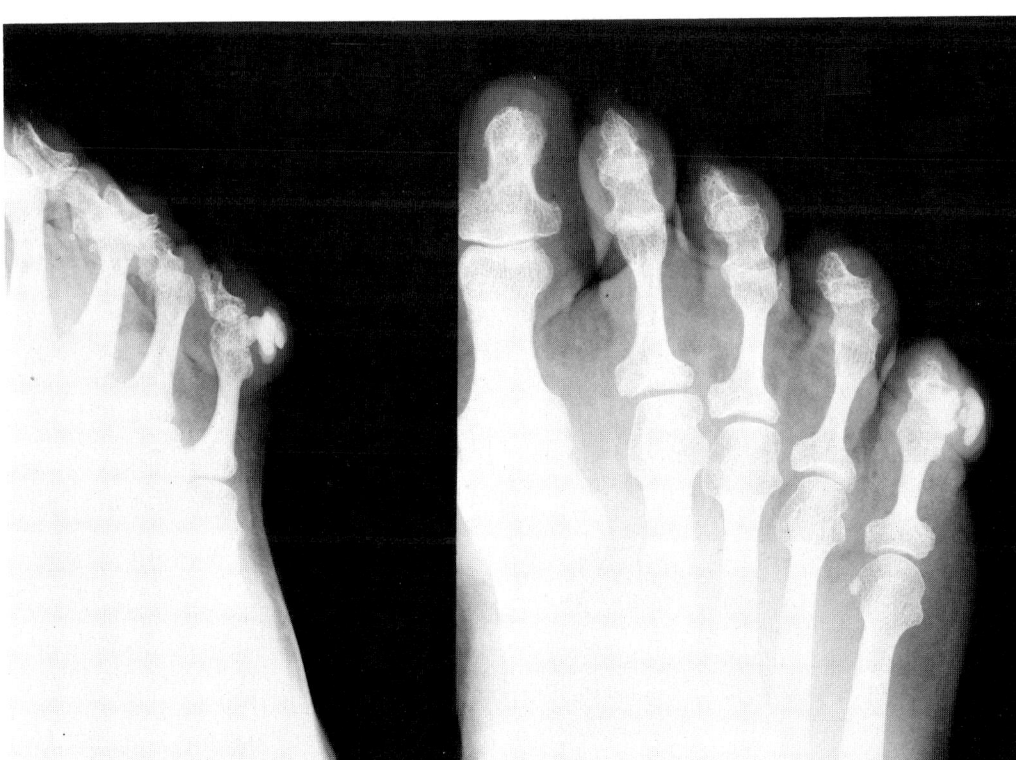

Figure 9.31. Digiti quinti flexus complicated by subhelomal calcification.

Lengthening of the extensor tendon or incision of the dorsal capsule at the metatarsophalangeal joint and the plantar flexors may be indicated.

Excision of a bursa or protection of the prominence of bone by temporary or permanent shields often relieves pain. Treatment of sinus tracts depends upon the extent of inflammation.

Goldhirsch (35) describes the following technique for correction of digital deformities. The dorsal skin and subcutaneous tissue around the extensor tendon is anesthetized. A no. 15 blade is used to puncture the skin. The blade is turned to contact the extensor tendon, and the tendon is cut. On occasion, the dorsal capsule is incised.

Digiti quinti flexus, as well as other flexion deformities of the phalanges, are easily corrected when soft tissue contractures are etiologic.

Roven (27) developed a semiclosed surgical technique for reduction of malaligned digits. He coined the term "phalangeal set" to describe the realignment of phalanges (Fig. 9.29). Under local anesthesia a stab incision is made at the level of interphalangeal joints to release contracted structures. Manipulation of the digits into a corrected position follows, resulting in correction of the deformity. This technique is especially useful where bony deformity is minimal in a digiti quinti flexus or other flexion deformities of the lesser toes.

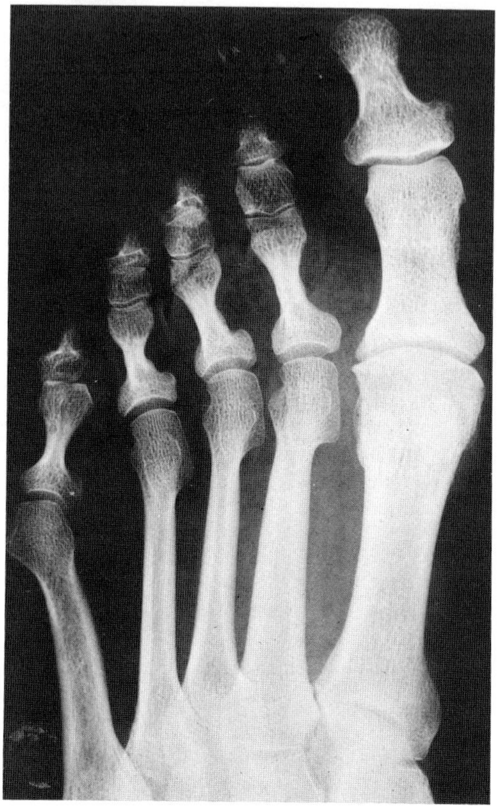

Figure 9.39. Digiti quinti varus. Note prominent lateral aspect head of fifth metatarsal.

Digiti Quinti Varus (Overlapping or Overriding Fifth Toe or Tailor's Bunion). This is a deformity of the fifth toe, similar to hallux valgus, in which the fifth metatarsal is abducted and the fifth toe is adducted and usually inverted (Figs. 9.38–9.40). The deformity may be caused by forefoot varus or pointed, narrow, inflared shoes and is usually associated with hallux valgus as a result of increased lateral pressure. Trauma and occupational stress are principal causes of tailor's bunion. Genetic factors are to be considered when deformities show up early in life in the absence of trauma.

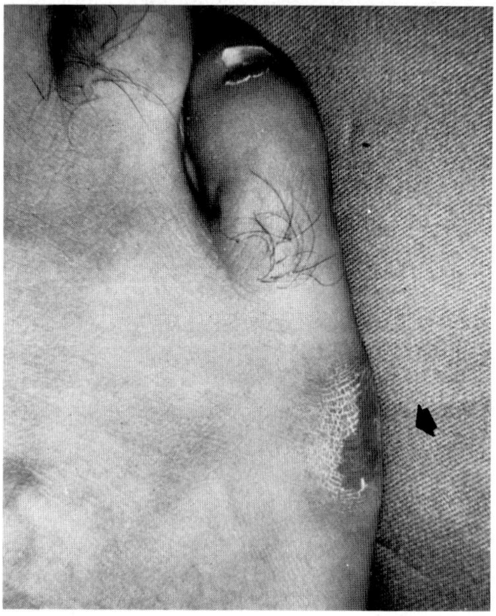

Figure 9.38. Digiti quinti varus. Note overlying tyloma.

Pathology. Friction on the lateral side of the head of the fifth metatarsal gives rise to helomas, tylomas, bursitis and bony prominences on the fifth metatarsal head. Contraction of the soft tissue structures on the inner side of the joint—the third plantar interosseous muscle, medial joint ligament, fourth lumbricale muscle, fascia and skin—results in adduction and rotation of the fifth toe.

Symptoms. Pain is evident from irritation of the shoe on the fifth metatarsal

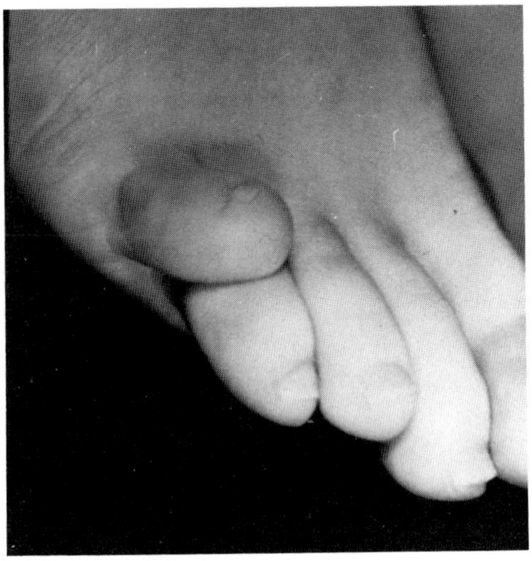

Figure 9.40. Digiti quinti varus with overlapping fifth toe.

head. The fifth toe may lie over or under the fourth toe. The lateral aspect of the fifth toe adjacent to the nail may be callused and painful, and a sinus tract infection or bursitis may be present beneath the painful heloma.

Roentgen Features. A hypertrophied fifth metatarsal head and an overlying soft tissue mass arc apparent. Superficial demineralization of bone with marked inflammation is noted. Effusion and soft tissue swelling may be present. Very often an infection may be evident to obscure the usual soft tissue response. A soft tissue calcification may be present in a chronic bursa or sinus tract over the enlarged joint.

Treatment (see Chapters 6 and 11). Digiti quinti varus does not necessarily present an overriding or overlapping fifth toe. However, the overlapping fifth toe may occur alone or with a digiti quinti varus. The treatment of choice in those cases that are poor surgical risks is accommodation of the lesion. This may require an alteration in footgear or the use of a shield to fit over the fifth toe and the prominence at the lateral aspect of the fifth metatarsophalangeal joint to protect it from shoe pressure. A shield can be constructed of felt, latex or plastic compounds. A plaster cast of the part is necessary, and a latex or plastic shield is created over the cast by the dip method.

It is often a simpler procedure to construct the shield on the toe in dynamic fashion. A shield may be constructed with a toe ring around the fifth toe overlapping the fifth metatarsophalangeal joint laterally with a cutout for the prominence. This can be coated with latex or silicone gel to give it firmness and memory. The patient is provided with a covering, such as Saran Wrap for the latex shield and is allowed to walk. The pad is dynamically shaped to the affected part.

Surgical correction of the digiti quinti varus should be conservative because of the importance of the digit in weightbearing (Fig. 9.41). If surgical intervention is necessary, the following procedure is used. A semielliptical incision is made above the fifth metatarsophalangeal joint and is deepened to expose the articulation. A lateral transverse incision is made through the joint capsule exposing the prominent head of the fifth metatarsal. The joint capsule is reflected back and preserved. This prominence of the head of the fifth metatarsal is removed by a Stryker bone saw, bone rongeur, bone forceps or ostetome. Bone resection follows the surface of the neck of the metatarsal forward to the articular cartilage. The rough bone surface is rounded off with a fine bone rasp.

Exostoses on the base of the proximal phalanx are rasped off without damaging the articular cartilage. Subcutaneous sutures are used to close the articular capsule; closure by layers is followed by skin closure. When there is a contraction of the tendon of the extensor digitorum longus to the fifth toe, it is necessary to do a tenectomy on this tendon followed by a cap-

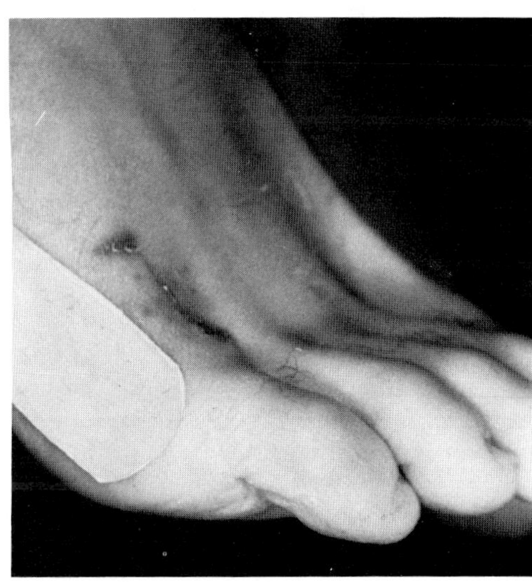

Figure 9.41. Corrective surgery for overlapping fifth toe. The extensor tendon and dorsal capsule of the fifth metatarsophalangeal joint are incised. A "Z" plasty incision allows for stretching of the contracted skin. Skin repair is by third intention. Same patient as in Figure 9.40.

sulotomy. A "Z" plasty to correct the contracted skin may also be in order if the toe is extremely contracted. When calcification of a sinus tract leading into a chronic bursa is present, it is advisable to remove the sinus tract by a circumscribed excision around the tract down to the bursal area. Dissection of the bursa is often necessary, and closure is accomplished in the usual manner.

Many cases are improved following a corrective adductory wedge osteotomy of the fifth metatarsal.

Hallux Valgus (Hallux Abductovalgus). This is a term given to the deformity in which the great toe is everted (valgus) or abducted and everted (abductovalgus) to an exaggerated degree and is kept in this position by accommodative changes in the cartilage, articular ligaments, joint capsule, sesamoids and tendons forming the first metatarsophalangeal joint (Figs. 9.32 and 9.33). Hallux valgus is most often caused by any condition leading to excessive subtalar pronation during the propulsive phase of gait and its development is aided by short, narrow shoes with pointed toes. Ill-fitting socks or stockings may create abnormal stress while the deformity is increased by a shortening of the extensor and flexor hallucis longus muscles that, in their backward pull, evert the hallux commensurate with the obliquity of the first metatarsocuneiform joint.

Any inflammation of the joint may be a predisposing cause. Metatarsus primus adductus may predispose to hallux valgus. The deformity is induced by changes following gout, rheumatism, infectious arthritis, traumatic arthritis and neurological lesions.

As a rule, both feet are affected although the deformity and symptoms are usually more marked on one side. About 30% of hallux valgus deformities are of congenital origin or of hereditary predisposition. The author has seen several cases in which members of three generations in the same family exhibited hallux abductovalgus.

Pathology. The first metatarsal adducts and the great toe abducts; the second and third metatarsals usually adduct slightly, whereas the fourth and fifth metatarsals abduct. The first metatarsal bone and the proximal phalanx may articulate on their lateral side by 50% or less. The cartilage on the exposed condyles of the metatarsal and phalanx usually becomes atrophied. Sesamoids are displaced laterally, with the lateral bone lying between the first and second metatarsal heads in the first intermetatarsal space. The tissues on the lateral side of the hallux joint undergo accommodative shortening, and the tissues on the inner side are stretched and lengthened. Metatarsus primus adductus with compensatory pronation is noted.

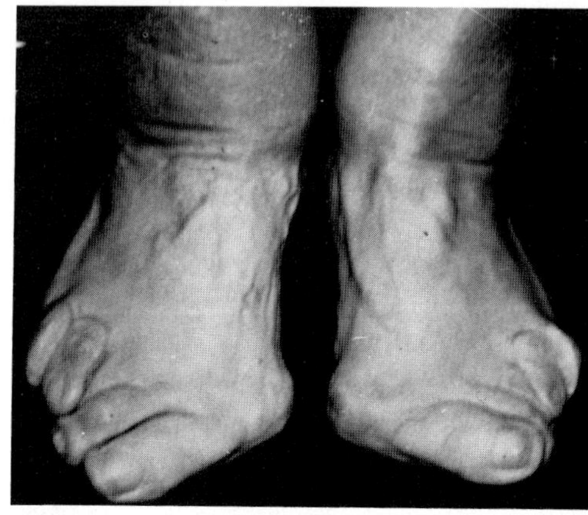

Figure 9.32. Severe hallux valgus bilateral.

The surface of the bone beneath the irritated periosteum becomes roughened and irregular; exostoses due to irritation and pressure develop at the medial and sometimes dorsal aspects of the first metatarsal head, thus aggravating the effects of lateral pressure by the shoe. The muscles around the great toe maintain and increase the deformity of hallux valgus. Once the deforming process has begun the muscles complete the deformity. Muscles are continually contracting, and when the resistance of bones is partially removed, as in the case of hallux valgus, the deformity progresses. The extensor and flexor hallucis longus tendons lie in the first intermetatarsal space, rather than above and below the first metatarsal.

The flexor hallucis longus lying between the heads of the flexor hallucis brevis holds the flexor hallucis brevis muscle from under the first metatarsal head along with the sesamoid developed in each of its tendons. The adductor hallucis holds the proximal phalanx laterally, being unresisted by the abductor hallucis that has slipped under the head of the first metatarsal bone or has been stretched by the shoe and pronation.

Symptoms. The complications of hallux valgus are more significant than the structural deformity itself. When the deformity is more pronounced the pressure of wearing shoes causes pain, tenderness and swelling, which eventually lead to the development of helomas, tylomas, bunions, septic bursitis and, when it penetrates the joint, septic arthritis. Infected sinuses are common over the deformed joint. Dorsal subluxation of the second toe and pain beneath the second metatarsal head are not uncommon.

The forefoot is hypermobile and spreads to allow for imbalance of the anterior metatarsal segments. Acute or chronic sesamoiditis may develop. Neuralgia caused by pressure on sesamoids and the periarticular structures may be present. Correction by the podiatric surgeon minimizes the complications of this deformity.

Roentgen Features. Marked lateral luxation of the hallux on the first metatarsal head with either an imbalanced joint space or narrowing of the articulation is visible on x-rays. The lateral aspect of the articulating surface of the metatarsal head is being impinged upon by the lateral aspect of the base of the proximal phalanx, which is rotated on its long axis.

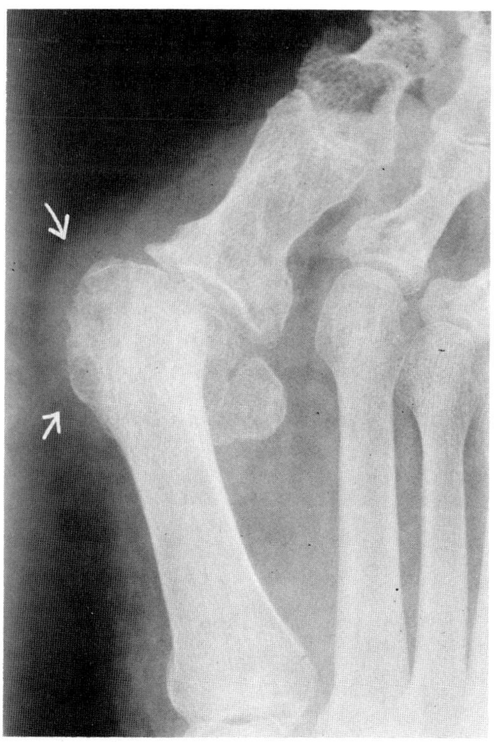

Figure 9.33. Severe hallux abductovalgus.

A subarticular sclerosis is noted just distal to the base of the proximal phalanx. This consists of a dense, sclerotic, irregular line extending completely across the base underneath the articulating cartilage. The sclerotic trabeculae mingle with the rest of the bone. Effusion may be evident within the articular capsule, whereas soft tissue swelling is present around the joint. A bursa is seen as a soft tissue mass or increase in soft tissue density overlying the deformed joint.

The head of the metatarsal may be altered in shape. A broad, flat, irregular, articulating surface is present, instead of the smooth, rounded surface normally seen. The margins of the joint may present osteophytes, such as lippings and sometimes spurs. Hypertrophy of the trabeculae may be noted at sites of great stress. In the acute stages superficial demineralization from hyperemia or cellulitis often develops at the metatarsal head. Occasionally the overlying bursa may degenerate and become calcified, presenting amorphous calcareous density overlying the joint on its medial aspect.

The sesamoids present degenerative changes, such as degenerative periositis, spurs and osteophytes. In severe deformity they are displaced into the first intermetatarsal space.

Care must be taken to rule out gout and rheumatoid or gonococcal arthritis.

Treatment (see Chapter 11, Podiatric Surgery). Correction of hallux valgus deformities depends on the degree of deformity, the extent of pathology and the presence of complicating factors. It is essential to appreciate all the pathology that exists in hallux valgus while attempting correction. In the early stages, conservative treatment can be moderately effective with the use of hallux valgus active and passive exercises and splinting of the joint by use of night splints as prescribed. Special low-voltage stimulation, stretching and traction devices, latex shields and splints, together with accommodative orthoses or footgear, may be helpful in the early stages (Figs. 9.34 and 9.35).

Where marked deformity exists and bony proliferation and pathology involving the joint are noted, surgical intervention is indicated. The various surgical techniques for correction of hallux valgus have been described extensively in surgical texts. Modifications by podiatrists have resulted in a high percentage of good to excellent results.

Surgery must be sophisticated enough to attempt correction of most of the gross pathology. Simple corrective surgical procedures are often suitable for relief of pain and elimination of obvious minor deforming states.

Melillo (36) discusses the criteria for selection of a particular corrective hallux abductovalgus technique over others. he establishes his choice by considering the metatarsus primus adductus angle, the presence or absence of motion at the first metatarsophalangeal joint, mild or severe axial rotation of the hallux and the degree of forefoot valgus.

The Silver-type technique is performed when the metatarsus primus adductus angle is small, hallux valgus is minimal and the bones appear to be well aligned.

The McBride bunionectomy may be indicated when the metatarsus primus adductus angle is less than 14° and the hallux valgus angle less than 35° (Figs. 9.36 and 9.37).

Melillo notes that the Akin procedure is desirable when there is less than 14° of metatarsus primus adductus angle, a great degree of hallux valgus angle, a congruous first metatarsophalangeal joint and closure of the epiphysis of the proximal phalanx of the hallux.

The Keller-type bunionectomy is most successful when the metatarsophalangeal joint is painful and rigid and presents with degenerative joint disease, an extreme hallux valgus angle, a metatarsus primus adductus angle of less than 15° and an elongated first metatarsal. Melillo has

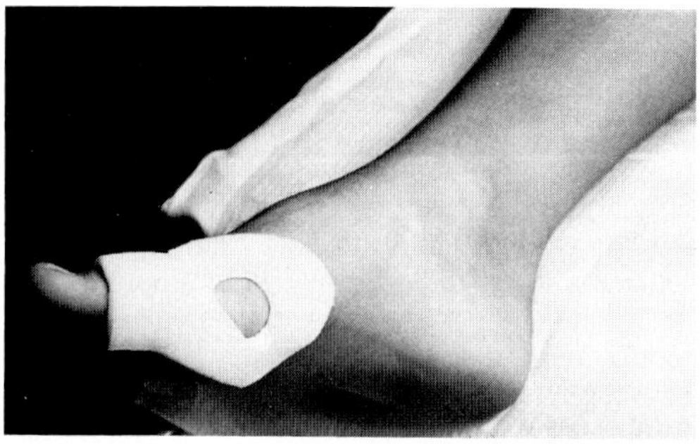

Figure 9.34. Bunion shield—tube foam. May be impregnated with liquid latex or silicone gel for construction of a permanent shield.

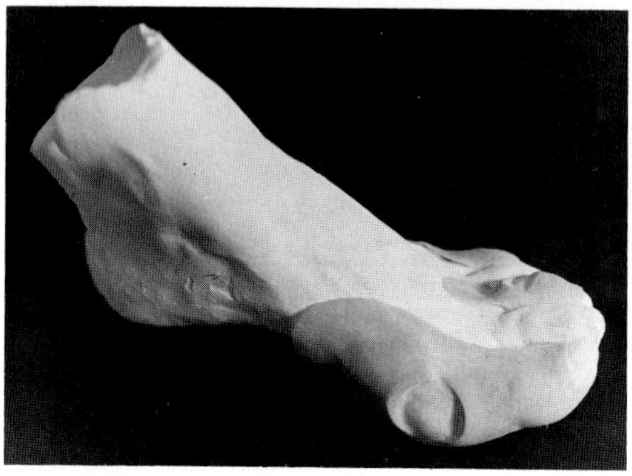

Figure 9.35. Latex shield for protection of bunion over hallux valgus. Note shields on third and fifth toes. (Courtesy of Liquid Rubber Appliance Laboratory.)

outlined preoperative, surgical and postoperative management for the above techniques, as well as for the Stone and Mayo bunionectomies, Mitchell osteotomy and the closed and open wedge first metatarsal osteotomies of choice.

Corrective procedures for hallux abductovalgus may include lengthening of the extensor hallucis longus, a lateral capsulotomy, excision of the lateral sesamoid, incision of the transverse and oblique adductor hallucis tendon at its attachment and reattachment to the lateral aspect of the metatarsal head, excision of prominent bone, insertion of Silastic (Dow) implant or Sil-

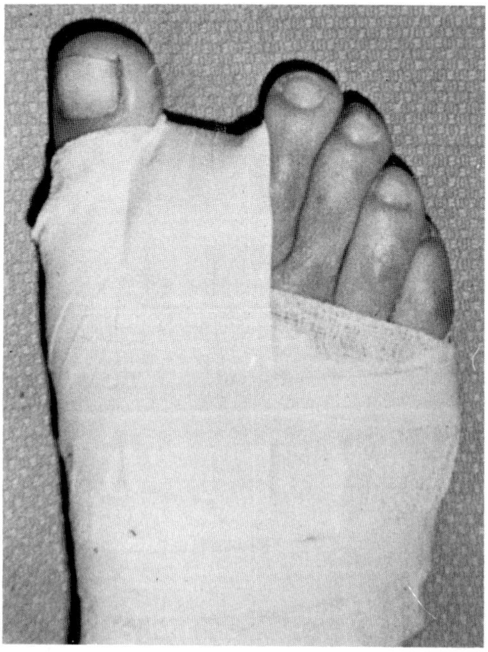

Figure 9.36. Postoperative bandage—hallux abductovalgus.

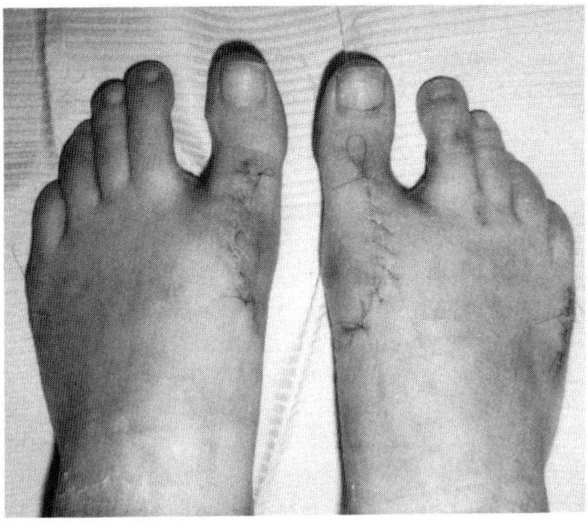

Figure 9.37. Modified McBride bunionectomy 2 weeks postoperative.

astic flexible hinged toe implant, an osteotomy at the neck or base of the metatarsal or a wedge osteotomy at the proximal or distal one-third of the proximal phalanx. The use of any one of the above procedures or a combination of several is available to the skilled podiatric surgeon. The reader is referred to the many excellent texts in podiatric surgery for detailed techniques.

Hallux Limitus (Rigidus). This is a painful affliction of the great toe characterized by a restriction of motion (limitus) or no motion (rigidus), particularly of dorsiflexion at the first metatarsophalangeal joint (Figs. 9.42 and 9.43). It may occur in young adults or at any age and is caused by excessive subtalar pronation at the propulsive phase of gait, overt trauma, such as stubbing the toe, a fall from a height, kicking a hard object or a low-cut shoe producing impingement and limitation of function.

Infection, osteoarthritis, rheumatoid arthritis and posttraumatic arthritis may result in the limitation of function. An acute flareup of first metatarsophalangeal joint pain and swelling may be due to primary gout or a hyperuricemia caused by thiazide diuretics.

Pathology. The affliction appears to be a form of periarticular fibrositis. The restriction of motion is caused by muscular spasm and accommodative changes of bone, ligaments and tendons. Protective spasms of soft tissues in recently traumatized joints may limit the motion of the hallux.

Symptoms. There is pain on motion and tenderness to touch, usually at the dorsolateral aspect of the joint. Swelling and redness are seen on the dorsum of the joint ("dorsal bunion"), and there is limited motion and pain on flexion and extension of the joint.

An enlarged metatarsal head or bony growths about the articulate margins may be palpated. Very often the distal phalanx is dorsiflexed from accommodative use as the fulcrum in walking.

Roentgen Features. There is a diminution of articular cartilage; osteophytes and lippings may be present at the articular margins, and a dorsal spur on the first metatarsal head extending upward and backward from the dorsal aspect of the head is common. The osteophytes are commonly seen at the external aspects of the articulating margins of the first metatarsophalangeal joint. Complete ankylosis of this articulation with loss of function is not unusual. Osteochondromas and osteochondritis have also been observed to produce this clinical picture of a rigid hallux joint. Calcareous deposits in the adjacent soft tissues, infection or tumor may

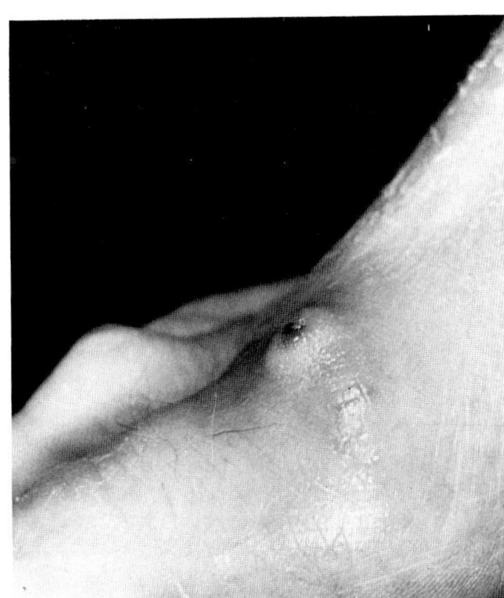

Figure 9.42. Dorsal bunion—sinus tract, bursitis, dorsal exostosis. Hallux joint limited in dorsiflexion, often associated with tyloma, plantar surface of the hallux interphalangeal joint and plantar surface of the fifth metatarsal head.

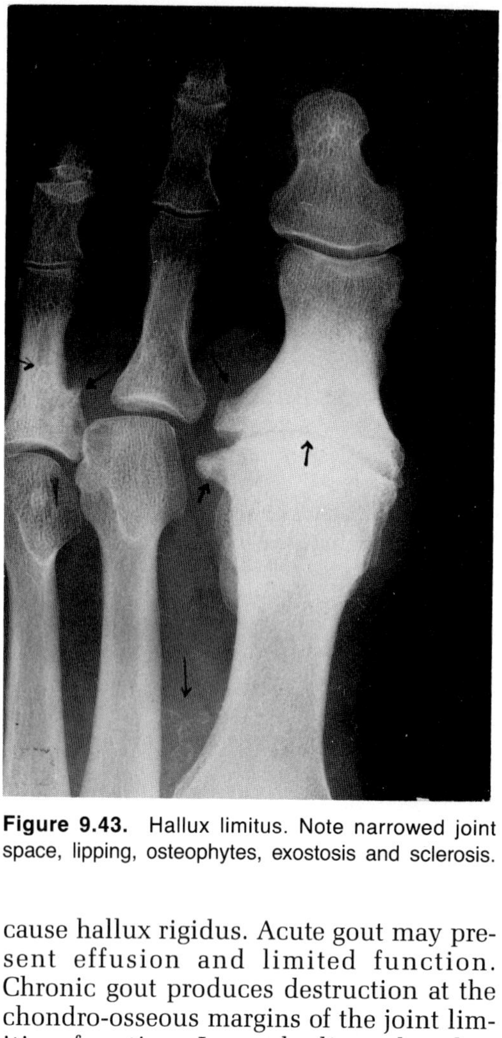

Figure 9.43. Hallux limitus. Note narrowed joint space, lipping, osteophytes, exostosis and sclerosis.

cause hallux rigidus. Acute gout may present effusion and limited function. Chronic gout produces destruction at the chondro-osseous margins of the joint limiting function. Loose bodies, chondromatosis or giant cell tumors may restrict normal function of the hallux joint. Gamble and Yale give definitive descriptions of the roentgen features.

Treatment (see Chapter 11). Limitation of function of the hallux may be due to fibrous ankylosis, complete bony ankylosis or contractures of the periarticular tissues. The purpose of therapy in most cases is to improve the functions of the foot, as well as the affected part. In most cases in which there is slight motion in the joint, greater motion can be achieved with proper treatment. Improvement of function can be initiated by using a local anesthetic to relax the periarticular tissues. This is followed by traction and plantar flexion of the first metatarsophalangeal joint.

In addition to traction, foot orthoses are used to relieve undue weightbearing on the affected part. A steel plate may be placed between the inner sole and the outer sole to splint and relieve function of the joint, thereby giving it an opportunity to relax. In acute pain and swelling, Grovit and Block (37) have shown that pain secondary to hyperuricemia due to thiazide diuretics can be relieved by injection of betamethasone acetate and betamethasone disodium phosphate into the affected monoarticular lesion.

Another technique is to use an orthotic device with a high medial longitudinal raise extending to just behind the sesamoids to transfer the weight from the affected joint to the lateral aspect of the foot. A properly posted rigid orthosis can relieve pain. The use of various bars on the sole of the shoe, such as a Jones bar and Denver heel, is helpful. The author has found that, where a hallux limitus exists, relief can be obtained with a Thomas heel, rigid shank and extended counter, which shift the weight laterally.

Joints that are completely ankylosed require entirely different care and treatment. Complete splinting of the joint by the use of a steel insole to keep the part from functioning is of great benefit in the relief of pain. However, if it is necessary to improve function where no function exists, surgical intervention may be necessary. This may involve the removal of any unusual exostoses, lipping or osteophytic changes around the margins of the joint. Resection of the base of the proximal phalanx is justified in extensive ankylosis. A Silastic (Dow) implant may be necessary to provide mobility in the severely damaged joint.

If infections are present, they must be properly treated with antibiotics and drainage. Tumors and exostotic overgrowths require surgical excision to improve function. Total resection of the head of the first metatarsal to increase mobility of the hallux joint is not recommended.

References

1. Gamble F, Yale I: *Clinical Foot Roentgenology, ed. 2.* Huntington, NY, RE Krieger, 1975
2. Ross, A: The use of computerized tomography in the foot. *J Foot Surg* 21:111–113, 1982.
3. Floyd EJ, et al.: Computed tomography scanning of the subtalar joint. *J Am Podiatry Assoc* 74:533–537, 1984.
4. Root ML, Orien WP, Weed JH: *Clinical Biomechanics—Volume II, Normal and Abnormal Function of the Foot.* Los Angeles, Clinical Biomechanics Corp, 1977, pp. 295–296.
5. Green DR, Carol A: Planal dominance. *J Am Podiatry Assoc* 74:98–103, 1984.
6. Yale AC, Hugar DW: Pes cavus: The deformity and its etiology. *J Foot Surg* 20:159–162, 1981.
7. Tachdjian MO: *Pediatric Orthopedics,* vol. II. Philadelphia, WB Saunders Co 1972, p. 1378.
8. Brachman PR: *Podiatric Orthopedics—Principles and Practices.* Park Ridge, IL, Podiatry Books Co, 1984.

9. Tax, HR: *Podopediatrics*. Baltimore, Williams & Wilkins, 1980.
10. Marcus, SA (ed), Block BH (assoc ed): *Complications in Foot Surgery—Prevention and Management*, ed 2. Baltimore, Williams & Wilkins, 1984.
11. Lemont H, Gibley CW, Jr: Prevalence of osteoarthritis of the foot. *J Am Podiatry Assoc*, 72:214–216, 1982.
12. Yale JF: Firm footings for the athlete (a preventive injury and self-help guide for those athletes involved in the running sports). Ansonia, CT, 1981.
13. Sgarlato TE: *A Compendium of Podiatric Biomechanics*. San Francisco, California College of Podiatric Medicine, 1970.
14. Clough JG, Marshall HJ: The etiology of hallux abducto valgus (A review of the literature). *J Am Podiatric Med Assoc* 75:238–244, 1985.
15. McCarthy J, et al: The morphogenesis of common osseous pedal lesions. Part I. Scanning electron microscopic analysis. *J Am Podiatry Assoc* 73:497–509, 1983.
16. McCarthy DJ, et al: The morphogenesis of common osseous pedal lesions. Part II. Transmission electron microscopy considerations. *J Am Podiatry Assoc* 73:549–560, 1983.
17. Scheimer OM: Chiropodical management of infantile metatarsus varus. *J Natl Assoc Chirop*, 47:435–443, 1957.
18. Joseph B, Jacob T, Chacko V: Hallux varus—A study of 30 cases. *J Foot Surg* 23:392–396, 1984.
19. Roven MD: A traction sling to affect an overlapping fifth toe. *J Am Podiatry Assoc* 49:376, 1959.
20. Budin H: Pain in the great toe joint. *J Exp Podiatry* 1:21–32, 1940.
21. Polokoff MM: Traction appliance for third toe. *J Am Podiatry Assoc* 65:1011–1012, 1975.
22. Weinstock RE, et al: Desyndactylization—A new modification. *J Am Podiatry Assoc* 74:458–461, 1984.
23. Christensen JC, et al: Congenital polydactyly and polymetatarsia: Classification, genetics, and surgical correction. *J Foot Surg* 20:151–158, 1981.
24. Engelmeir RL: Technique for prosthetic replacement of missing toes. *J Am Podiatry Assoc* 73:36–38, 1983.
25. Scheiner DE, Chamas CE: Brachymetatarsia: A review and case study. *J Foot Surg* 22:257–262, 1983.
26. Polokoff MM: Buttress appliance. *J Am Podiatry Assoc* 66:261–263, 1976b.
27. Roven MD: Phalangeal set. Paper delivered at the annual American Podiatry Association Meeting, Chicago, August, 1968.
28. Polokoff MM: Double ring toe traction device. *J Am Podiatry Assoc* 66:35–37, 1976a.
29. Coates IS: Silicone orthodigita and shielding. Part I. *J Am Podiatry Assoc* 66:648–651, 1976.
30. Coates IS: Silicone orthodigita and shielding. Part II. *J Am Podiatry Assoc* 66:706–711, 1976.
31. Sharrard WJ, Smith TW: Tenodesis of flexor hallucis longus for paralytic clawing of the hallux in childhood. *J Bone Joint Surg* 58:224–226, 1976.
32. Haber L, Winthrop L, Weiner S: Biomechanical findings in a random survey of fifth toe abnormalities. *J Am Podiatry Assoc* 65:206–211, 1975.
33. Lewin P: *The Foot and Ankle*. Philadelphia, Lea & Febiger, 1940.
34. DuVries HL: Lectures in surgery. Chicago, Illinois College of Chiropody and Foot Surgery, 1936–37.
35. Goldhirsch S: Tenotomy as an aid in orthodigita. *J Natl Assoc Chirop* 47:463, 1957.
36. Melillo TV: Gastrocnemius equinus—Its diagnosis and treatment. *Proc Res Alumni Assoc Calif Podiatric Med Center* 1:37–54, 1972.
37. Grovit M, Block P: Pedal manifestations of hyperuricemia due to thiazide diuresis. *J Am Podiatry Assoc* 58:176–177, 1968.

Suggested Readings

Bleck EE: Congenital clubfoot: Pathomechanics, radiographic analysis, and results of surgical treatment. *Clin Orthop* 125:119–130, 1977.

Bojsen-Moller F, Flagstad KE: Plantar aponeurosis and internal architecture of the ball of the foot. *J Anat* 121:599–611, 1976.

Bruno J: Gross muscle evaluation by the podiatrist. *J Am Podiatry Assoc* 57:309–315, 1967.

D'Amico JD: The postural complex I. *J Am Podiatry Assoc* 66:568–574, 1976.

DiPiero H: A device for measuring foot deviations. *J Am Podiatry Assoc* 51:203–205, 1961.

Gamble FO: Attitudes of subjects' feet in foot roentgenology. *Chirop Rec* 22:149–150, 1939.

Gamble F: *Applied Foot Roentgenology*. Baltimore, Williams & Wilkins, 1957.

Goff C: Gait and posture: A symposium. *Clin Orthop* 25:7–109, 1962.

Henenfeld M: Balance and imbalance. *J Natl Assoc Chirop* 46:817–825, 1956.

Hensinger RN: Rotational problems of the lower extremity. *Postgrad Med J* 60:161–167, 1976.

Hlavac H, Schoenhaus H: The plantar fat pad and some related problems. *J Am Podiatry Assoc* 60:151–155, 1970.

Hoffmeister FH: Dynamic balance therapy. *J Am Podiatry Assoc* 48:19–20, 1958.

Langenski OA, Ritsil AV: Supination deformity of the forefoot. *Acta Orthop Scand* 48:325–333, 1977.

Lapidus PW: Dorsal bunion. *J Natl Assoc Chirop* 29:9–13, 1939.

LaPorta G, Melillo T, Olenski D: X-ray evaluation of hallux abducto valgus deformity. *J Am Podiatry Assoc* 64:544, 1974.

Lewis LL: Pedal propulsive hinge as a key to normal foot function. *J Am Podiatry Assoc* 56:103–109, 1966.

McGlamry ED, Kitting RW: Equinus foot. *J Am Podiatry Assoc* 63:165–183, 1953.

McGlamry ED, McGlamry R (eds): Doctors Hospital Podiatric Education and Research Institute, Fourteenth Annual Surgical Seminar, Stamford, CT, April 18–21, 1985.

McCrea JD: *Pediatric Orthopedics of the Lower Extremity*. Mt. Kisco, NY, Futura Publishing Co, 1985.

Morton DJ: *The Human Foot*. New York, Columbia University Press, 1935.

Palmer R, Martz CD: Recovery of power in leg muscles following poliomyelitis. *Phys Ther Rev* 36:466–473, 1956.

Pepin W: Measurements of hip rotation and foot pronation and supination in school children. *J Am Podiatry Assoc* 53:181–186, 1963.

Phelps WM, Kiphuth RJH: *The Diagnosis and Treatment of Postural Defects*. Springfield, IL, Charles C Thomas Co, 1932.

Phillips RD, Phillips RL: Quantitative analysis of the locking position of the midtarsal joint. *J Am Podiatry Assoc* 73:518–522, 1983.

Phillips RD, Christeck R, Phillips RL: Clinical measurement of the axis of the subtalar joint. *J Am Podiatric Med Assoc* 75:119–131, 1985.

Roven MD: Accommodating the overlapping second toes. *J Am Podiatry Assoc* 57:425–426, 1967.

Russinoff RM: Pathogenesis of depressed metatarsal heads. *J Natl Assoc Chirop* 20:5, 1940.

Sgarlato TE: A Compendium of Podiatric Biomechanics. San Francisco, California College of Podiatric Medicine, 1971.

Sharp JT: Juvenile flat foot. *J Natl Assoc Chirop* 39:9–17, 1949.

Silverman LJ: Forefoot problems of the nondeforming clubfoot. *J Am Podiatry Assoc* 56:110–113, 1966.

Steindler A: *Mechanics of Normal and Pathological Locomotion in Man*. Springfield, IL, Charles C Thomas Co, 1935.

Sutton EH: Equal balancing of body weight. *Clin J Chirop Pedic Items* 12:159–161, 1942.

Tintocalis CA: A measuring device for orthopedic evaluation. *J Am Podiatry Assoc* 12:8–15, 1968.

Varzos PN: Hesperdin and ascorbic acid in conjunction with mechanotherapy for static foot problems. *J Am Podiatry Assoc* 51:861–865, 1961.

Whitney AK: Podokinetics *J Natl Assoc Chirop* 47:383–387, 1957.

Yale I: Nondeforming club foot. *Chirop Rec* 1939.

Yale I: Idiopathic osteochondrosis of the tarsal navicular. *J Natl Assoc Chirop* 41:41–44, 1951.

Yale I: Imbalanced forefoot. *Conn Chiropodist* 2:3–5, 1955.

Zitzlsperger S: The mechanics of the foot based on the concept of the skeleton as a statically indeterminate space framework. *Clin Orthop* 16:47, 1960.

10

Foot and Ankle Trauma

Trauma Axioms

The following principles should be followed when treating cases of foot and ankle trauma (1).

1. Protect and immobilize all injuries until a diagnosis is made.
2. Avoid unnecessary handling of injured parts. Gentleness and care in handling a broken limb are to be commended.
3. Absence of deformity and disability does not rule out fracture.
4. In the presence of an obvious fracture be suspicious that there are other fractures or dislocations.
5. Examine for vascular or nerve injury.
6. Persistent pain suggests improper splinting.
7. Date and time your findings and record them with care and accuracy.

Roentgen findings of trauma include interruption of the continuity of bone, dislocation of a joint, soft tissue swelling, altered vascular response and the presence of a foreign body. Comparative x-ray examination of the injured foot and/or ankle and the opposite foot and/or ankle is almost always helpful in making a definitive diagnosis.

Fractures

Phalangeal Fractures (Fig. 10.1)

The most common type of phalangeal fracture is the incomplete or complete, transverse or oblique so-called bedpost fracture of the proximal phalanx of the fifth toe. Phalangeal dislocations usually result from forced dorsiflexion injuries after falling from a height (Fig. 10.2). Tape immobilization for a period of 3 weeks is usually sufficient treatment for them (Fig. 10.3). Proximal and distal phalangeal fractures of the hallux are treated, depending on their severity and degree of displacement, with tape immobilization, metal, Celastic, or tongue depressor splint (Fig. 10.4). If caused by a direct blow over the toenail, the resulting subungual hematoma must be evacuated. An uncommon sequela to comminuted fractures of the great toe is vascular impairment requiring amputation.

Sesamoidal Fractures

Sesamoidal fractures involving the two constant sesamoids in the flexor hallucis brevis tendon occur (1) as a result of direct trauma after jumping from a height or (2) after multiple minimal trauma over a short period of time as occurs in a dancer. The medial sesamoid is injured more frequently than the lateral (Fig. 10.5). Sesamoidal fractures must be differentiated from bipartite and tripartite sesamoids. Sesamoidal x-ray views are indicated. Treatment consists of protection with accommodative padding and limited weightbearing. If pain persists the affected sesamoid can be excised. Fractures of the os tibiale externum, os peroneum, os vesalianum and os trigonum have been reported.

Metatarsal Fractures

Metatarsal fractures usually result from direct injury or in the case of the base of the fifth metatarsal, an inversion force (Fig. 10.6). Fractures of the base of the fifth

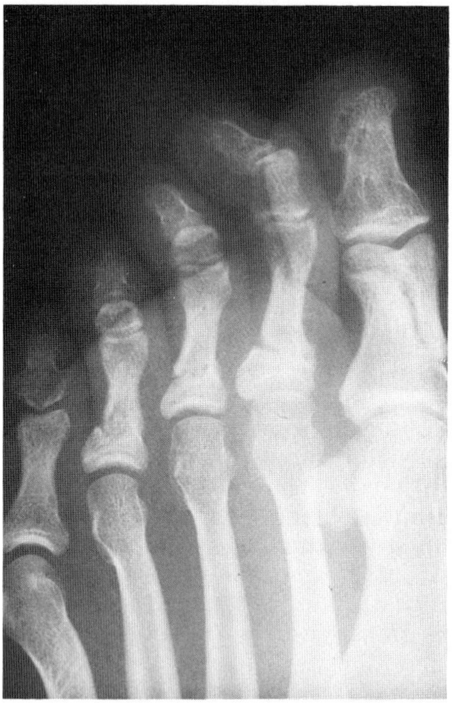

Figure 10.1. Healing first, second, third, and fourth toe phalangeal fractures.

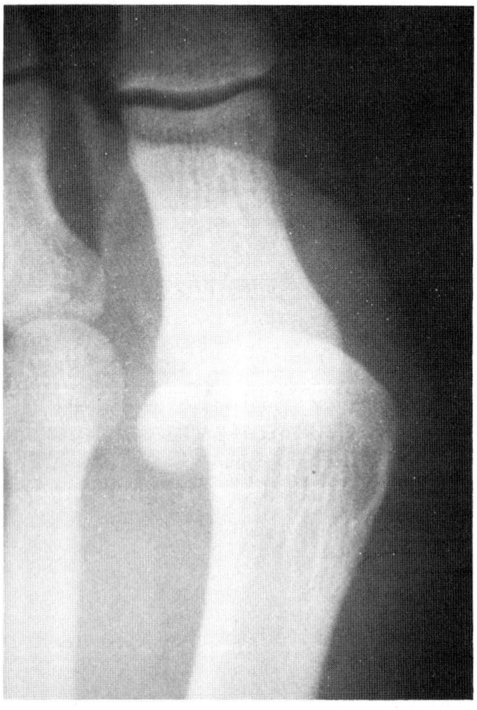

Figure 10.2. Hallux dislocation reduced by traction under local anesthesia.

metatarsal in children (ages 9–14) must be differentiated from fracture of the apophysis or the apophysis itself and the os vesalianum. Laurich et al. (2) present a rational treatment approach to fifth metatarsal fractures based on classification of injury mechanism and the injury itself. Fracture type, general health, age and activity level of the patient are all areas to be considered (Fig. 10.7). Fractures of the lesser metatarsals are more common than the fracture of the first metatarsal. Tape immobilization with or without a ¼-inch felt longitudinal metatarsal pad, Celastic

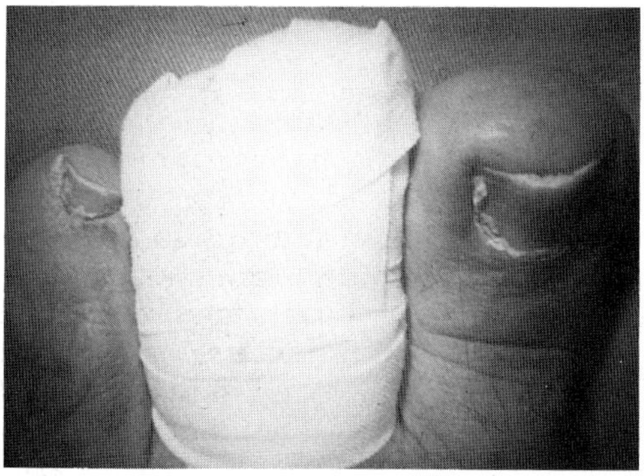

Figure 10.3. Tape immobilization for transverse fracture of proximal phalanx second toe.

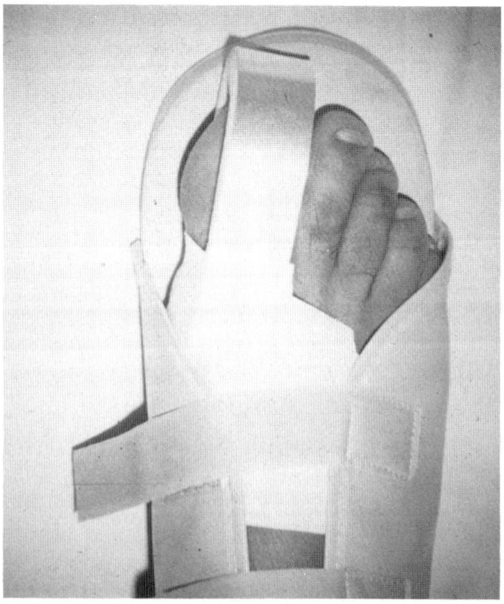

Figure 10.4. Hallux fracture splint.

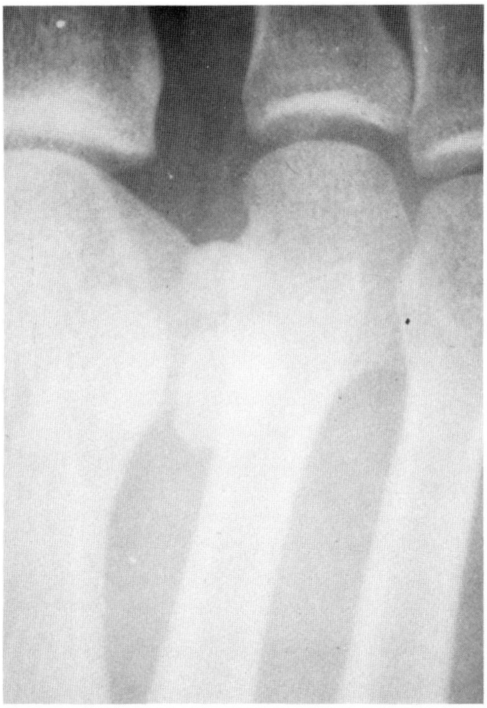

Figure 10.5. Lateral sesamoidal fracture.

or prenyl splint with a Reese shoe for 3–6 weeks is the treatment of choice. If there are no opposing surfaces at the fracture site, open reduction with insertion of a Kirschner wire for stabilization may be performed (3). Spector et al. (4) review 12 cases of lesser metatarsal fractures. Anatomical reduction, early mobilization and return to normal activity are stressed (Fig. 10.8). Maxwell (5) presents a thorough discussion of open and closed treatment for metatarsal fractures. Surgical treatment principles and Association of Osteosynthesis (AO) techniques are emphasized. The author has found transverse, oblique or spiral fractures involving the proximal one-third of the fifth metatarsal to heal by fibrous union initially and to proceed to osseous union 1 to 2 years later. Internal fixation is usually not needed. Healing of the great toe proximal phalangeal metaphysis following an Akin wedge osteotomy often is closely similar to the healing time and appearance of fifth metatarsal base fractures.

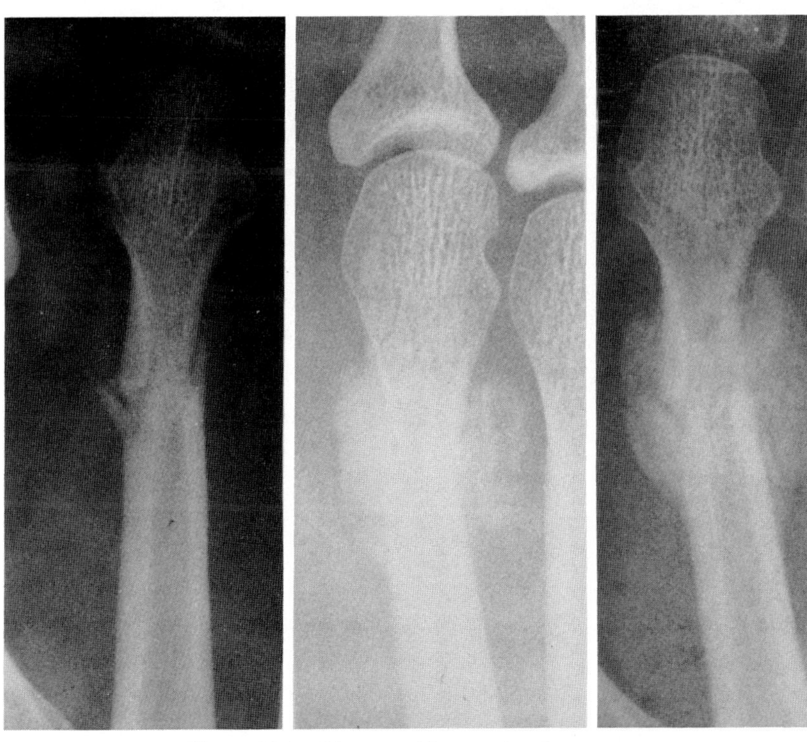

Figure 10.6. Metatarsal fracture healing response.

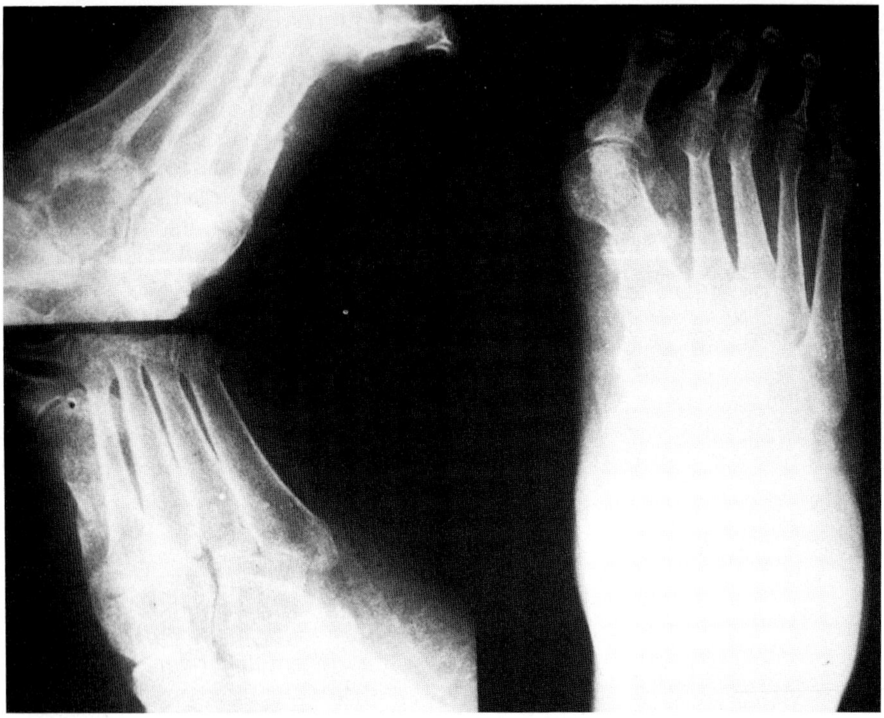

Figure 10.7. Healing first metatarsal fracture.

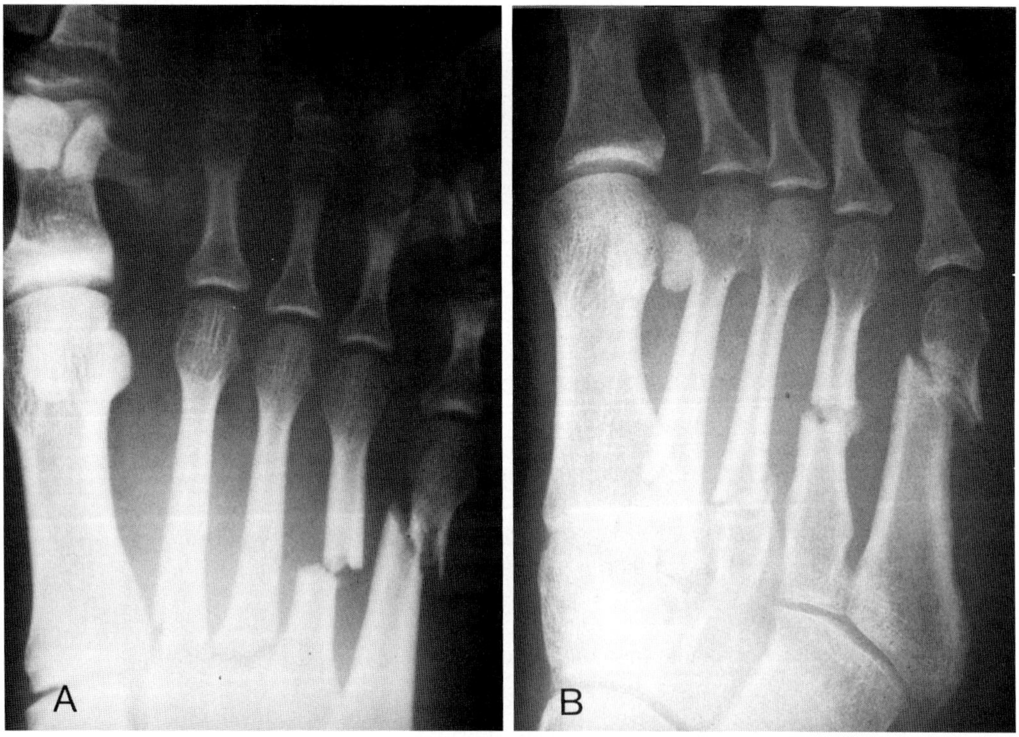

Figure 10.8. *A.* Second, third, fourth, and fifth metatarsal fractures at time of injury. *B.* Three weeks after closed reduction and immobilization.

Tarsometatarsal fracture/dislocation or Lisfranc's fracture dislocation is infrequent. The most common dislocation force is lateral and dorsal, with separation at the first and second metatarsal bases.

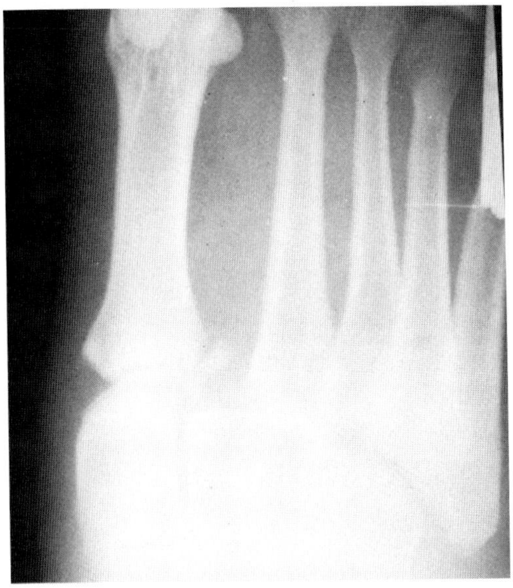

Figure 10.9. Tarsometatarsal fracture dislocation at time of injury.

The injury is usually not confined to the tarsometatarsal joints only. Fractures of metatarsals and ligamentous injuries are associated and must be reduced as soon as possible. This usually can be done with manual traction and manipulation. Internal fixation is sometimes necessary (Fig. 10.9).

Cuneiform Fractures

Isolated fractures of the cuneiforms are uncommon. The injury is usually a result of compression. The medial cuneiform is most likely to be affected (Fig. 10.10). An associated dislocation at the tarsometatarsal joint is the rule, rather than the exception. A resultant posttraumatic arthritis occurs frequently. Smith et al. (6) describe an uncommon case of fracture dislocation of the middle cuneiform.

Navicular Fractures

Fractures of the navicular can be divided into three types: avulsion, body and tuberosity. Medical tuberosity fractures result from an avulsion injury and must be differentiated from an accessory navicular,

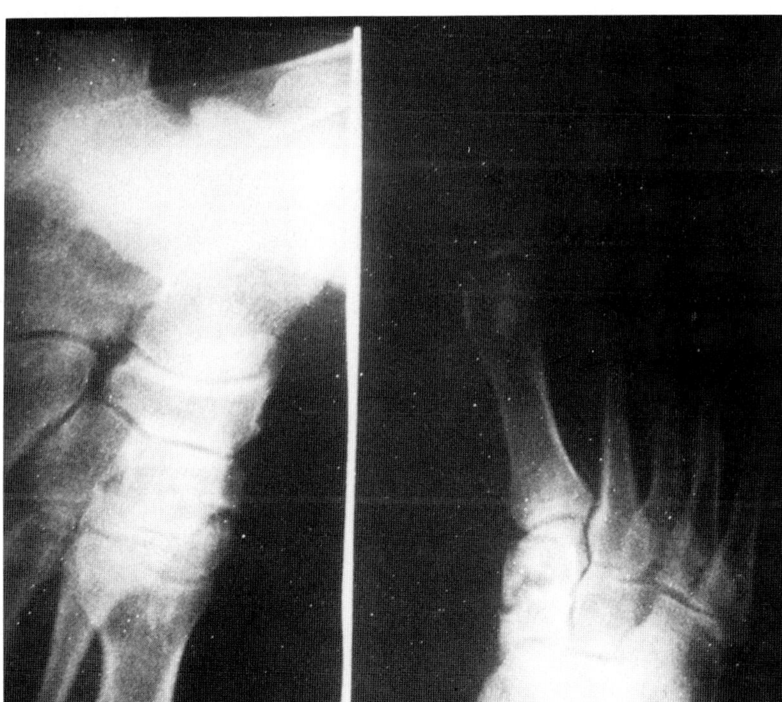

Figure 10.10. Medial cuneiform compression fracture.

os tibiale externum or prehallux (Fig. 10.11).

Chip fractures occur from glancing blows on the dorsum of this bone. Crushing fractures of the navicular usually result in posttraumatic arthritis. Tibialis posterior tendon rupture, plantar calcaneonavicular ligament rupture and medial collateral ankle ligament rupture must be ruled out. Depending on the fracture's severity, treatment in a well-molded splint or cast, for 4–6 weeks is indicated. Open reduction and internal fixation should be considered in cases where the fracture fragments cannot be reduced by closed reduction methods. Resultant talonavicular osteophytes, if they become symptomatic, must be excised. Maintenance of the medial longitudinal arch utilizing foot orthoses is essential after termination of the immobilization.

Cuboid Fractures

Isolated fracture of the cuboid is also quite uncommon (Fig. 10.12). It is usually a result of a compression force and is associated with concomitant dislocation. A

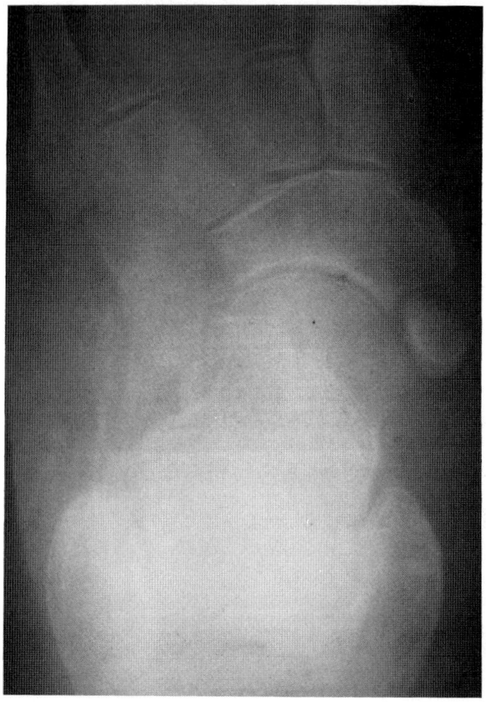

Figure 10.11. Avulsion fracture of the navicular.

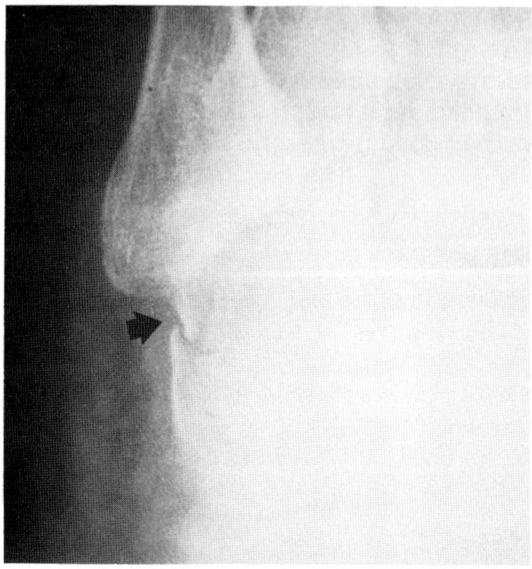

Figure 10.12. Cuboid fracture.

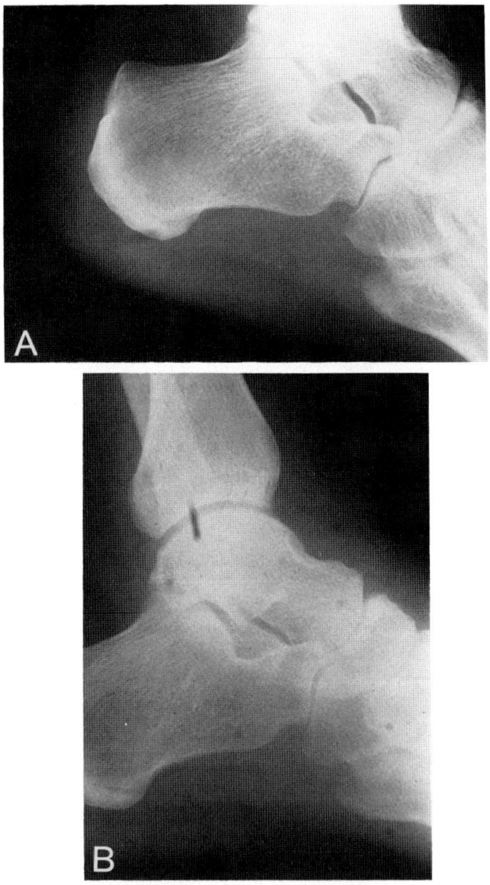

Figure 10.13. *A.* Painful loose body of bone between talus and navicular secondary to trauma. *B.* Loose body of bone excision.

chronic peroneus longus tenosynovitis may result if fracture displacement interferes with the gliding action of this tendon. Conservative treatment consisting of immobilization for 4–6 weeks is indicated.

Talar Fractures

Fractures of the talus result in prolonged and often permanent disability. The most common talar fractures are the talar neck fracture, fracture dislocation and fracture of the body of the talus. Associated ankle injuries are frequent.

Talar neck fractures usually occur as a result of forced dorsiflexion at the ankle joint. Reduction, which must be performed accurately and early, sometimes must be accomplished under a general anesthetic after which the foot is casted in equinus and eversion. Resultant aseptic necrosis is a prevalent finding. Ochwat and Hugar (7) discuss the classification, management and complications of talar neck fractures; present two cases; and review the literature. They emphasize immediate reduction of the displaced fracture in order to lessen the incidence of avascular necrosis and traumatic arthritis. A chip fracture of the anterior superior aspect of the talus or the posterior superior aspect of the navicular may also occur (Fig. 10.13).

Talar body fractures do not occur as frequently as do talar neck fractures, and their prognosis is not as good. If the joint surfaces are disturbed or if there is comminution, posttraumatic arthritis results. Anatomical reduction should be accomplished. Resultant incongruity of the subtalar joint may require future subtalar fusion (Fig. 10.14). Ganel et al. (8) report on three cases of severe plantar flexion of the foot associated with adduction and supination, which resulted in medial subtalar dislocation. Closed reduction in two patients and open reduction in one, with a 1- to 2-year follow-up, produced excellent results with no complications. Immediate closed reduction is recommended. If this does not reduce the dislocation, open re-

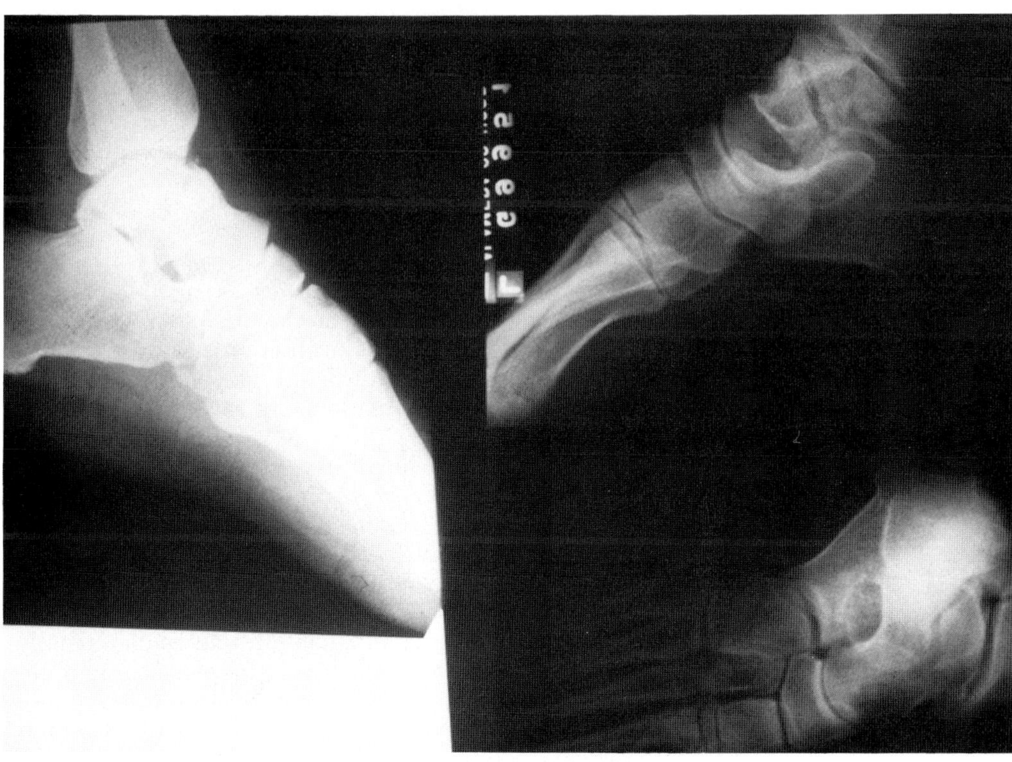

Figure 10.14. Talar body fracture.

duction is indicated. The practitioner must be alert to associated fractures of the medial malleolus, talus, proximal and distal fibula and base of the fifth metatarsal (Fig. 10.15). Complications include aceptic necrosis of the talus, ankle and subtalar arthrosis and ankle instability. A fracture of the lateral posterior process of the talus, as a result of forced plantar flexion at the ankle, must be differentiated from an os trigonum (9).

Osteochondritis Dissecans

Osteochondral fractures simulating osteochondritis dissecans of the talus should be immobilized until adequate healing takes place. If still symptomatic, these areas must be curetted. If the medial trochlear surface of the talus is involved an osteotomy of the tibia is sometimes necessary to gain adequate exposure. (Fig. 10.16). Portillo (10) reviews the diagnosis and treatment of osteochondritis dissecans of the talus. Although these lesions are of a traumatic nature, other etiologic factors include a hereditary tendency to exert shearing forces on either side of the talar trochlea over a prolonged period and the presence of localized ischemia. Xeroradiography and technetium bone scan may augment other radiologic diagnostic methods.

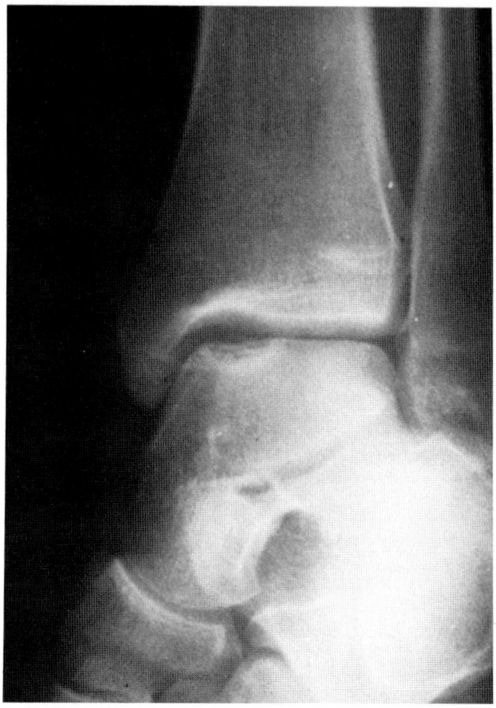

Figure 10.16. Painful progressive osteochondritis dissecans of the medial talar trochlea requiring curettage.

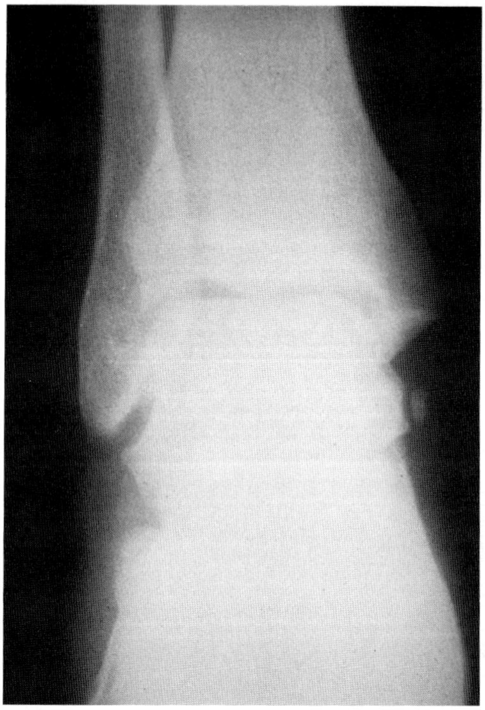

Figure 10.15. Unusual chip fracture of the talus.

Calcaneal Fractures

Calcaneal fractures are usually the result of falling from a height (Fig. 10.17). Careful x-ray evaluation should be made, including studies of the spine, as there is a 10–20% incidence of associated vertebral fractures. There are several classifications of calcaneal fractures and a variety of opinions regarding their type and treatment. The most common types are the tuberosity fracture, beak fracture, fractures not involving the subtalar joint and fractures involving the subtalar joint with depression. Tuberosity fractures can usually be treated effectively by plaster immobilization. In combination beak fracture and oblique fracture involving the subtalar joint, treatment varies from open reduction and fixation to early mobilization.

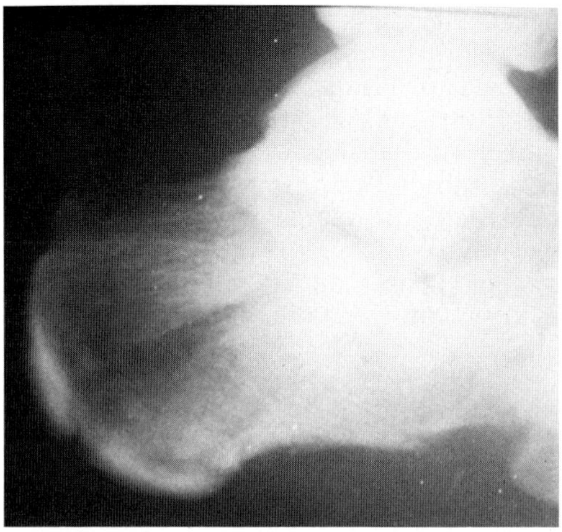

Figure 10.17. Calcaneal compression fracture.

The mechanism of injury of an undisplaced fracture of the anterior superior aspect of the calcaneus is obscure, although a twisting force is usually the cause. One's index of suspicion has to be high to search for this fracture (11) (Fig. 10.18).

Stress Fractures

In the early stage of a metatarsal stress fracture there is a feeling of weakness and possibly some pain on walking that disappears when the foot is rested. Excruciating pain may occur after 5 to 10 days with no treatment. The pain remains localized, and with continued weightbearing the color may progress from marked rubor to a deep cyanotic edema of congestion. Pain is increased by pressure on the head of the affected metatarsal and at the site of the fracture. When the head of the bone is grasped and gently manipulated, the pain is increased. Callus becomes profuse as a result of failure of early immobilization (Fig. 10.19). When the clinical findings are typical and the x-ray is negative, the lesion should be considered a fracture until proven otherwise.

Moss and Modad (12) describe a study in which 35 consecutive patients with stress fracture symptoms and 17 healthy control subjects were subjected to therapeutic ultrasound over the area thought to be involved with a stress fracture on one extremity, followed by ultrasound over the same area on the opposite extremity. The majority of patients with radiographically positive stress fractures experienced pain over the fracture site with ultrasound application.

Treatment consists of a ¼-inch felt metatarsal pad applied to the foot, an anterior heel applied to the shoe and/or the use of a wooden-soled shoe for 3–5 weeks. A plaster cast is not necessary for a patient who does not have to ambulate for prolonged periods of time. In over 3000 cases of documented x-ray-positive calcaneal and metatarsal stress fractures the most common site was both calcanei followed by one calcaneus. Contrary to what has been reported in the literature, the third metatarsal is by far the most common metatarsal affected, and not the second. No correlation with foot type could be found in 500 consecutive cases (13).

In the early stages of a calcaneal stress fracture there is soreness that seems to be in the ankle joint that disappears when the foot is rested. After 3 to 5 days the areas just below the malleolae become swollen. If the heel is grasped and pressure is applied, severe pain ensues. X-rays are negative at first. After 5 to 10 days callus formation is noted on x-ray as a linear line of increased density or sometimes simulating a cancellous bone island (Fig. 10.20). Here again, as with metatarsal stress fractures, when the clinical findings are typical and the x-rays are negative, the lesion should be considered a fracture until proven otherwise. Treatment consists of a 1-inch thick heel sponge and an MF heel

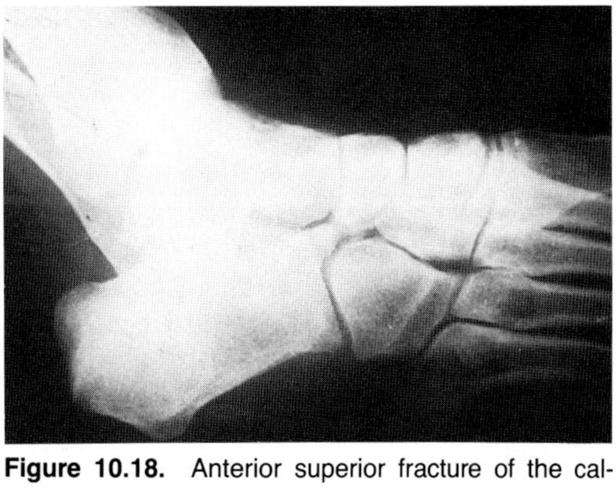

Figure 10.18. Anterior superior fracture of the calcaneus.

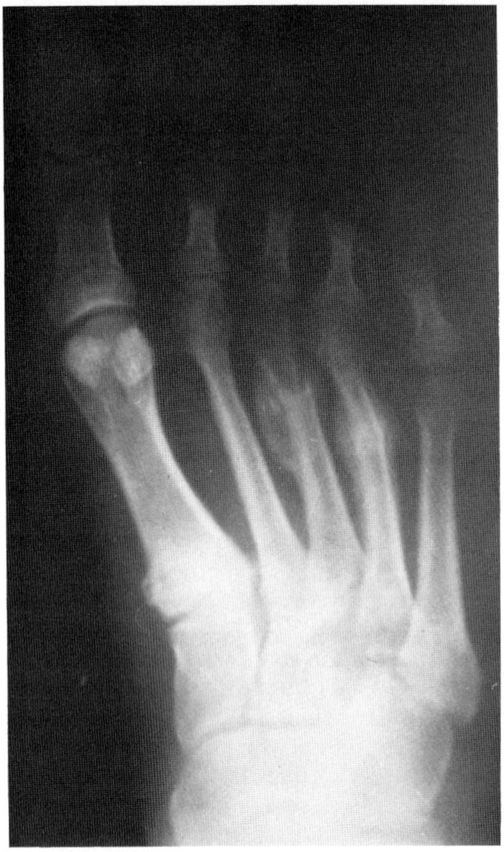

Figure 10.19. Healing third and fourth metatarsal stress fractures; 3 weeks with no immobilization and continued prolonged daily weightbearing.

cup or Tuli. The patient is instructed to use ice applications initially and not to engage in prolonged ambulation for 10 days. Distal, midshaft, and proximal tibial and fibilar stress fractures are not uncommon (Figs. 10.21 and 10.22). Limited ambulation and Gelocast immobilization for 3 to 4 weeks are sufficient treatment for distal lesions.

Ankle Injuries

One should keep three general considerations in mind when handling ankle injuries. When the foot is plantar flexed, the posterior portion of the talar trochlea advances in the mortise, resulting in an added space between the posterior portion of the talus and the malleolae. This creates lateral instability. Medial collateral ankle ligaments are stronger and longer than the lateral ligaments. The anterior aspect of the ankle joint is capsular, and the posterior aspect ligaments are thin.

The Lauge-Hansen classification of ankle injuries is a rational step-wise approach to the diagnosis of ankle injuries (14). Injuries, according to mechanism, are classified into clockwork and nonclockwork types. The clockwork classification system is based on the relationship of the ankle anatomy as compared to the face of a clock. Clockwork injuries are further divided into four stages. Clockwork injuries include supination eversion, pronation eversion and pronation dorsiflexion. Nonclockwork injuries include pronation abduction and supination adduction (15). Freer (16) presents a 2½-year experience involving 900 ankle injuries. Definition, classification and accurate diagnosis of injury are stressed. Heller and Vogler (17) review the use of diagnostic arthroscopy in ankle joint trauma.

The most common injury to the ankle is an inversion sprain involving the anterior talofibular ligament and often the calcaneofibular and the posterior talofibular ligament. The calcaneofibular ligament is

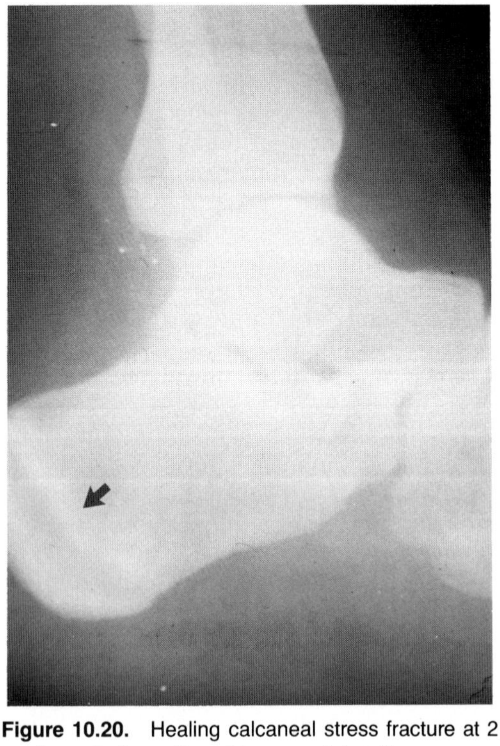

Figure 10.20. Healing calcaneal stress fracture at 2 weeks; note linear line of increased density.

the only component of the lateral collateral ligaments that is extracapsular. It is stronger than the anterior talofibular ligament. X-rays should be taken. If ankle instability is suspected clinically, x-rays are taken with the foot forcibly inverted. Ankle arthrogram may be diagnosticly helpful if performed within 48 hrs after injury.

Dowling et al. (18) present an excellent review of the radiologic diagnosis and assessment of lateral ankle ligamentous injuries. If there are no objective inflammatory symptoms to correlate with the patient's subjective complaint and the ankle has full range of motion and is stable with negative x-rays, an Ace bandage is applied to the ankle. If there are mild objective inflammatory symptoms with negative x-rays, a Gelocast is applied, and the patient is given crutches for 1 week. A tape strapping or Air-Stirrup Ankle Brace can be used instead of a Gelocast. If the objective inflammatory symptoms are moderate to severe with moderate to severe swelling and heat and/or discoloration and x-rays are within normal limits, the ankle is elevated 3 to 4 days to reduce the swelling after a compression dressing of webril and Ace bandage is applied. The ankle is then put into a well-molded short leg walking case for 3 weeks followed by a Gelocast for 1 to 2 weeks. Hice et al. (19) describe a plaster-synthetic cast with its many variations of use dependent on treatment requirements. In cases of chronic recuring lateral ankle sprains, conservative therapy consisting of application of a lateral heel flair and ankle support is prescribed. Surgical procedures include using the peroneus brevis tendon for stabilization and direct repair of the divided ligaments.

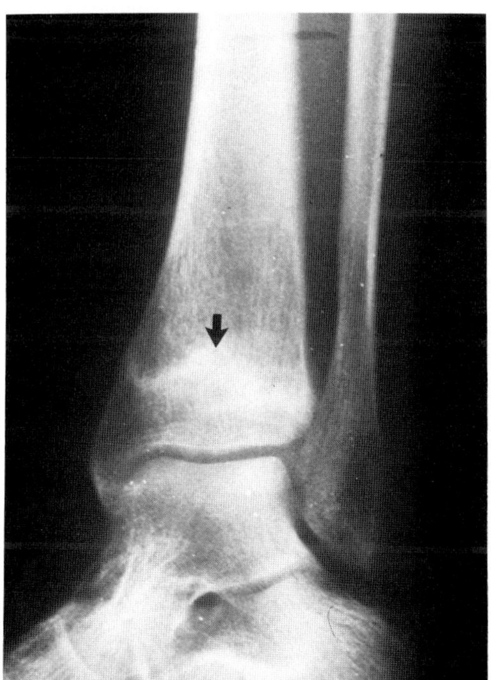

Figure 10.21. Healing distal tibial stress fracture at 4 weeks; note the irregular transverse line of increased density.

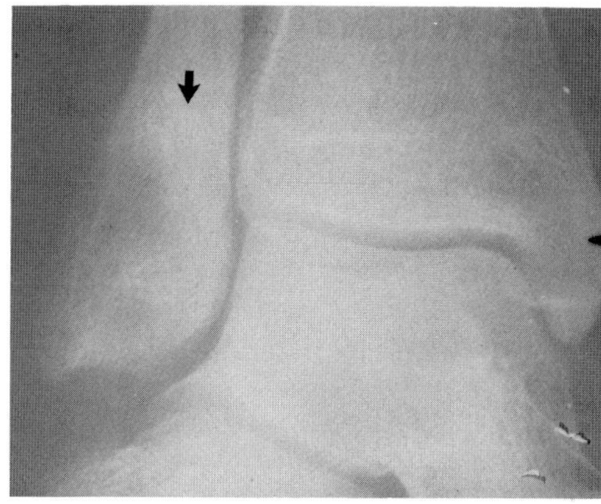

Figure 10.22. Healing distal fibular stress fracture at 4 weeks; note cloud-like area of increased density.

Cangialosi (20) reports on 20 surgical repairs of the anterior talofibular ligaments operated on between 10 and 30 months after injury. A lateral retinacular homograft was utilized with 11 to 36 months follow-up. Results in 14 repairs were excellent. Two cases resulted in restricted inversion. In three cases edema persisted for 4 months, and in one case the patient remained symptomatic due to rupture of the graft. Postoperative biomechanical treatment was stressed.

Ransom and Dailey (21) describe a technique for lateral ankle stabilization using the plantaris tendon instead of the peroneus brevis tendon. Sacrifice of the plantaris tendon, which has a medial insertion, has a positive effect on limiting calcaneal inversion whereas sacrifice of the peroneus brevis tendon results in more muscular inversion stress on the foot. Kaplan et al. (22) discuss chronic ankle instability and present seven cases involving the modified Chrisman-Snook ankle stabilization procedure with a 2–8 year follow-up. Interference with sural nerve function was described as a complicating factor. Other ankle stabilization procedures include the Evans, Watson-Jones and Lee tendon stabilization procedures; the use of unwoven carbon fibers as a scaffold in ligamentous repair (23); and the Campbell, Charnley, and Gallie fusion stabilization procedures. There is a high incidence of complications associated with lateral ankle stabilization procedures, including loss of tendon function, loss of motion, delayed healing, posttraumatic arthritis and extended postoperative rehabilitation (24, 25).

Foot orthotic devices with a lateral rearfoot extension to minimize inversion at heel strike have been very effective in preventing lateral ankle inversion injury and in the extended treatment of the recurring lateral ankle sprain. Ankle sprain is commonly seen in the presence of uncompensated rearfoot varus, forefoot valgus and rigid plantar flexed first ray. In the uncompensated cavorarus foot it is sometimes necessary to apply a full lateral extension to the orthotic device. Care must be taken to support the medial longitudinal arch so as to minimize abnormal subtalar pronation through midstance into propulsion. A lateral heel flair may be used on a walking shoe or applied to an athletic shoe to minimize the effect of ankle inversion forces at heel contact. Fractures of the lateral malleolus and base of the fifth metatarsal must be ruled out by x-ray before a diagnosis of lateral ankle sprain can be made.

The intensity of the abnormal force governs the type of injury produced. In most instances of inversion injury, there is an element of internal rotation and plantar flexion of the foot. Young people tend to tear ligaments and injure epiphyses. Older people tend to fracture the lateral malleolus. In inversion ankle injuries, lateral ankle ligaments tear, the lateral malleolus is fractured, a separation (diastasis) occurs at the distal tibiofibular syndesmosis, the medial malleolus is fractured and occa-

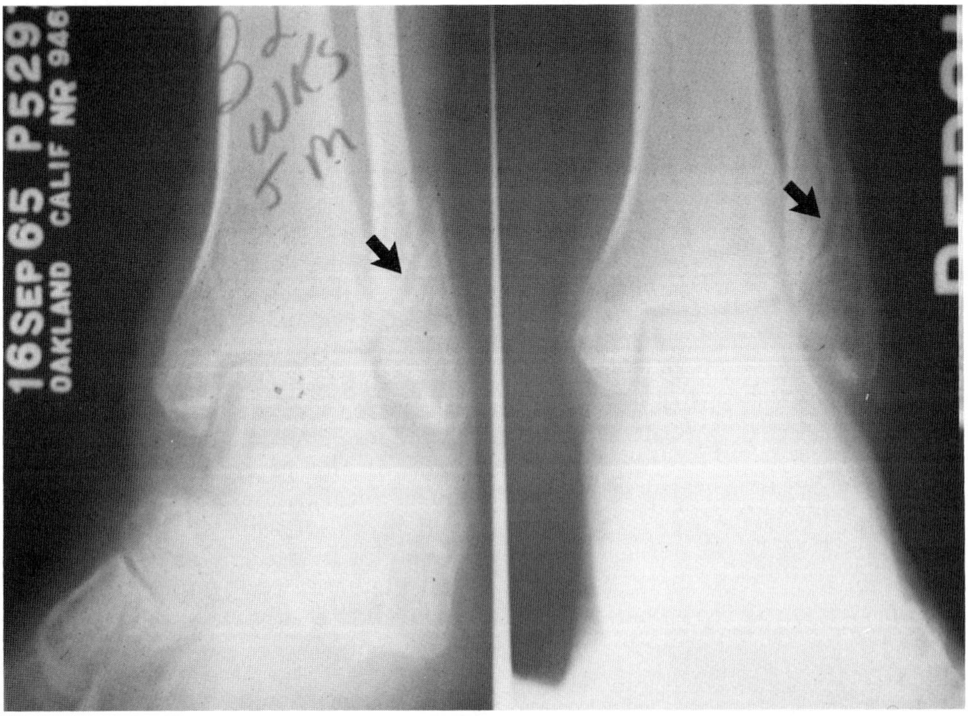

Figure 10.23. Healing slightly displaced oblique distal fibular fracture.

sionally the posterior lip of the tibia is fractured. Anterior ankle instability, occurring with rupture of the anterior tibofibular ligament results in abnormal anterior displacement of the talus in the ankle mortise. The eliciting of an "anterior drawer sign" is the primary diagnostic feature.

The most common type of ankle fracture that one sees is the incomplete or complete oblique nondisplaced distal fibular fracture without a tibiofibular diastasis (Fig. 10.23). These fractures are treated with well-molded short leg walking casts for 4 to 6 weeks followed by a Gelocast for 2 to 3 weeks.

Knudsen et al. (26) describe the Danis and Weber classification for diagnosis and treatment of ankle fractures. It is based on lateral ankle fracture fragment position and proper compression techniques for reduction. Prolonged fixation of the distal tibiofibular syndesmosis should be avoided. The normal movement in this area in the propulsive phase of gait should be maintained.

In eversion injuries of the ankle, the foot is everted, externally rotated and dorsiflexed. The medial collateral ankle ligaments are torn, the medial malleolus may be avulsed, the tibiofibular interosseous ligament may be torn and the lateral malleolus may be fractured below the level of the articular surface of the tibia. The deltoid ligament, consisting of the anterior talotibial, tibionavicular, tibiocalcaneal and posterior talotibial ligaments, is involved. Bimalleolar or trimalleolar fractures with or without distasis can occur from forced eversion or inversion (Fig. 10.24 and 10.25).

Dorsiflexion injuries are usually accompanied by some external rotation of the foot. If rotation is forced, a tear of the distal tibiofibular ligament may ensue. This is a difficult diagnosis to make. A forced dorsiflexion injury may result in a chip fracture of the anterior distal aspect of the tibia.

Epiphyseal Injuries

Terminology

Common usage has created two terms for the secondary growth centers in the bones of the foot; namely, epiphysis and apophysis. The word "apophysis" has come to be synonymous with the secondary growth center of the calcaneus. "The term was used by Galen and Oribuseus in the sense of a growth from a bone. It returned to popular usage in the 16th century. Gorraeus (1601) notes that it is a growth from a bone (tubercle or hump) and differs from an epiphysis. In the early 19th century the term was used for an epiphysis after the epiphysis had fused to the shaft of the bone" (1). Actually, an apophysis is an epiphysis that does not enter into the development of a joint (28). Apophyses may be found in several locations in the foot: at the posterior aspect of the calcaneus, the base of the fifth metatarsal and often at the medial tuberosity of the navicular.

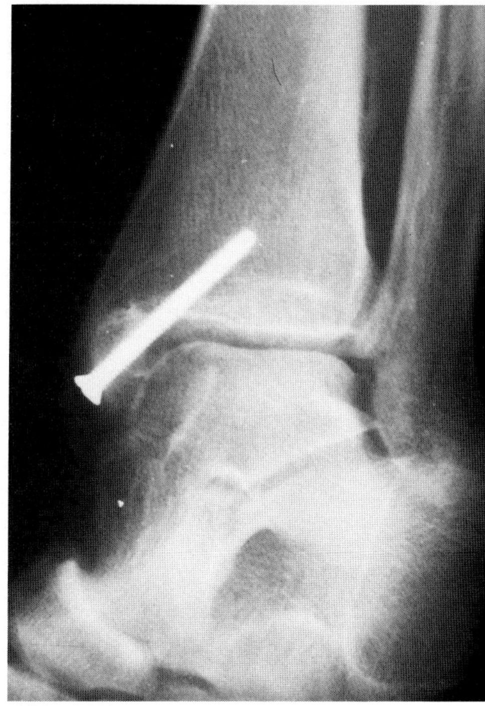

Figure 10.24. Reduced bimalleolar fracture with internal fixation.

The term "epiphysis" is used in this discussion for the secondary growth centers of the metatarsals and phalanges. The term "apophysis" designates the secondary growth centers of the calcaneus, fifth metatarsal base and navicular tuberosity (29).

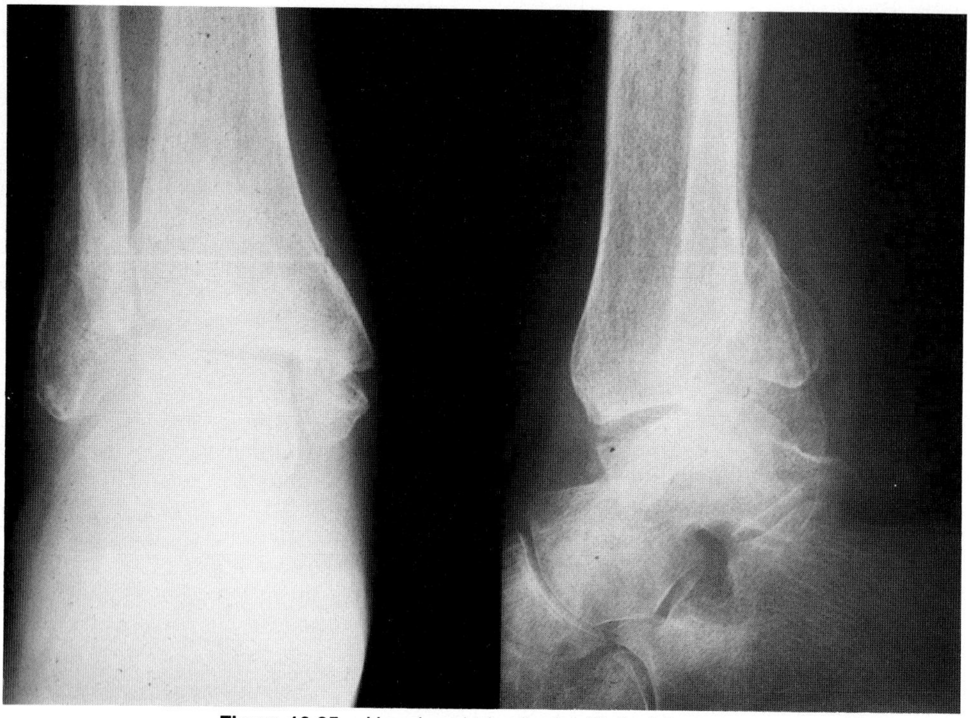

Figure 10.25. Unreduced trimalleolar (Cotton) fracture.

Anatomy

The epiphysis consists of three components: the ossification center of the epiphysis, cartilagenous growth plate or epiphyseal line, and the metaphysis or distal end of the diaphysis (30). Ossification centers appear in chronological sequence depending on age, sex and endocrine and nutritional factors. Unless deprived of blood supply, the growth plates in the normal foot mature and close, by about age 20 in males and 17 in females. The actual size and shape of the ossification centers in the bones of the foot vary with age and sex. Any bone of the foot may develop from several nuclei in a primary ossification center or secondary ossification centers. It is necessary to know the approximate age these centers appear, what they look like at different stages of development and when they close to appreciate "normal" development. It is quite difficult to differentiate centers of ossification of the small tarsal bones from fractures. Several ossifying cartilagenous nuclei may eventually unite into a primary ossification center. The same histologic process may form secondary ossification centers. If there are two or more fully formed ossification centers at a site of trauma, it is generally difficult to rule out an epiphyseal or cartilage ossification center injury (29).

Many studies have determined the chronological appearance of normal primary ossification centers and their time of complete ossification (31, 32, 33.) One must become familiar with the approximate time an epiphysis or an apophysis appears in order to differentiate it from a traumatic lesion. A familiarity with the approximate time of closure for secondary ossification centers is essential to avoid errors in interpreting symptoms following trauma.

Epiphyseal Injuries

Epiphyseal injuries may be present in 6 to 15% of children's fractures. Significant disturbances in development occur in only 10% of the epiphyseal injuries. These disturbances occur when the relationship of the fracture line interferes with the blood supply to the growth plate or epiphysis. Because the epiphyseal cartilage derives most of its blood supply from the capsular structures, its development may be affected subsequent to capsular injury. Ligamentous injuries commonly affect the epiphysis (30). Forces that would produce ligamentous injury in an adult could produce epiphyseal injury in a child. Joint capsule and ligamentous structures are 2–5 times stronger than the epiphyseal plate (34).

The classifications of epiphyseal injuries by Aitken (36) and Salter and Harris (37) are most useful for the purposes of this textbook. Five injury types may be differentiated. In the first type, the epiphysis is separated from the epiphyseal plate, which occurs most often in children under age 5 from a shearing force (Fig. 10.26). The majority of epiphyseal injuries found in the foot and ankle are of the second type. The fracture line extends into the metaphysis, fragmenting a part of the metaphysis. There is usually a separation of the epiphysis with a metaphyseal fracture. This metaphyseal fragment, found at the opposite side of the shearing and compression force, has been called the "corner sign" by Holland (37). In the third type of injury there is no separation of the epiphysis. This type is most commonly found at the distal tibia. The fragment must be reduced properly to obviate circulatory impairment resulting in growth disturbance. Types four and five are reportedly rarely found in the foot and occasionally at the distal tibia and/or fibula. In type four the fracture line traverses the epiphysis, epiphyseal plate and metaphysis. Growth arrest is common even with proper reduction. Nordentaft (38) reproduced injury to the cartilagenous growth plate of the distal tibial epiphysis of 40 animals. Permanent bony bridging occurred in 75.6% of those cases where epiphyseolysis combined with drilling through the basement plate was performed. Type five is reported to be quite rare. The contributing force is compression with no fracture element. The injury is very difficult to determine and often impossible to detect by radiographic studies. It may manifest at a future time with evidence of growth irregularity. The distal tibial epiphysis has been reported to be one of the most common sites affected by this type of injury.

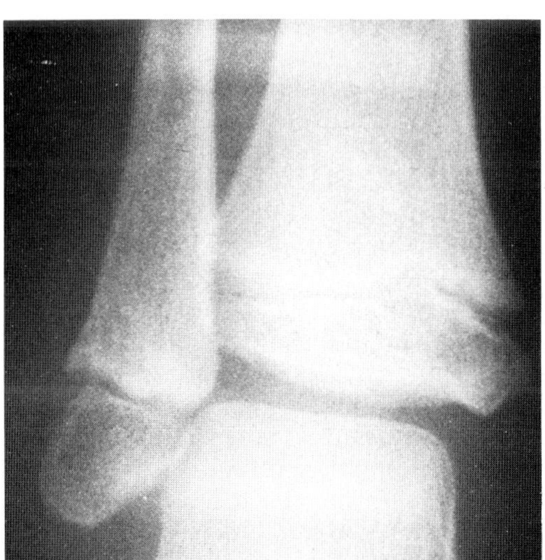

Figure 10.26. Subluxed distal fibular epiphysis with wide ankle mortise.

Apophyseal Injuries

It is entirely possible and even probable that many of the irregular calcaneal apophyseal growth centers result from a type five injury (29). Active children in the 8–12 year age group, particularly active boys, have a great deal of difficulty with heel apophysis discomfort. Many podiatrists have thought of these injuries in terms of aseptic necrosis, osteochondritis or osteochondrosis. In effect, however, they may be an unrecognized type one or type five epiphyseal injury. In many instances there may be several centers of ossification or a posttraumatic periostitis as well (Fig. 10.27). Although treatment objectives are often quite similar, it is important from a diagnostic standpoint to differentiate these types of injury. Many of these injuries may lead to some forms of posterior superior calcaneal prominence. These prominences predispose to shoe-related foot problems, including the common posterior achilles bursitis and retrocalcaneal bursitis. It is important to recognize and control a contributing pathomechanical foot problem.

When dealing with a pronated foot in a child, one often sees several nuclei of os-

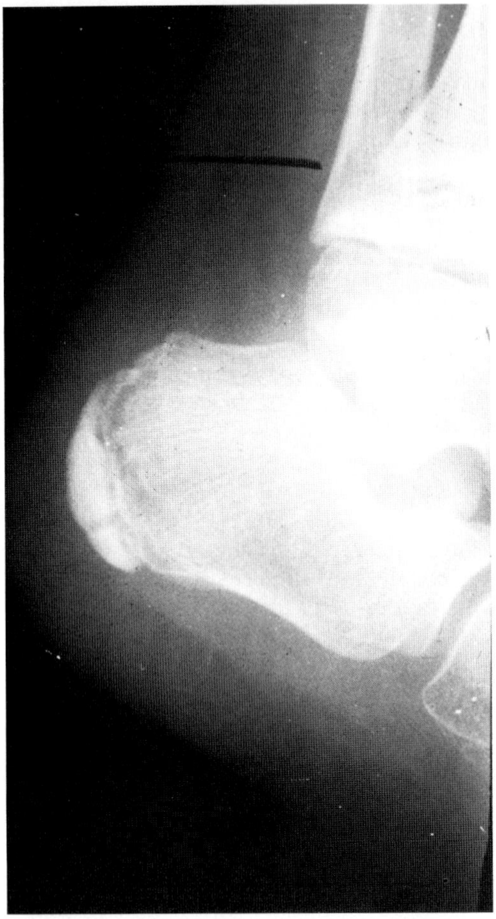

Figure 10.27. Irregular calcaneal apophysis.

sification or separate ossification centers presented in a number of tarsal bones. If a history of direct trauma is elicited and upon physical examination objective inflammatory syptoms are found, it is almost impossible to differentiate between normal growth center variations and growth center injuries. These variations must be recognized, traumatic lesions treated, and pathomechanical conditions controlled (29).

Treatment. The treatment of epiphyseal, apophyseal and growth center injuries varies with the type of injury presented. Comparison x-ray views should be taken in three planes to help differentiate an anomaly from an injury. Comparison x-ray examinations at 6-month intervals is often necessary when growth interference is suspected. Only in very exceptional cases must open reduction or open reduction with internal fixation be utilized. Because open injuries can be complicated by infection, prognosis is not as favorable. Closed reduction may be accomplished fairly easily in most epiphyseal injuries affecting the foot. Distal tibia and fibula epiphyseal injuries types two, three, and four are sometimes difficult to reduce. Tape may be utilized for digital epiphyseal injuries with or without Celastic or metal splints. Celastic or prenyl splints may be used effectively for injuries involving first and fifth metatarsal epiphyseal injuries. Heel cups and/or a sponge heel seat initially, followed by foot orthotic devices to control abnormal pronation, may be used for calcaneal apophyseal injuries. Plaster slipper casts may be utilized as needed in more involved cases. A firm shoe with a rigid and extended medial counter and steel shank or a Reese postoperative shoe should be used in combination with the indicated splint or slipper cast. Rarely is a below-the-knee walking cast indicated. A below-the-knee non weightbearing or walking cast, is indicated in distal tibia or fibula epiphyseal injuries, depending on the extent of injury.

Tendon Injuries

Tendon injuries affecting the foot and ankle include tendon and sheath inflammation as seen in Achilles tendonitis and extensor hallucis longus tenosynovitis, tendon dislocation as seen behind the malleolae and tendon rupture commonly found related to the Achilles tendon (see Chapters 11 and 12).

Tendons tend to rupture when stressed at the time that the attached muscle is contracting. Rupture may occur at the insertion of the tendon to bone or at the musculotendinous junction. Muscle tear usually precedes tendon rupture in children. Wicks et al. (39) report on 64 children with tendon injuries about the foot and ankle. Immediate tendon repair, except for the extensor hallucis longus (EHL), flexor hallucis longus (FHL) extensor digitorum longus (EDL) and flexor digitorum longus (FDL), was recommended. The authors found that repair of the long extensors and flexors may cause limitation in metatarsophalangeal range of motion, whereas not repairing these tendon ruptures did not lead to permanent deformity. Reinherz (40) recommends primary surgical repair of the FHL tendon within the first 8 hours of laceration using a lateral trap technique. A below-the-knee cast with nonweightbearing for at least 3 weeks, followed by passive mobilization or partial weightbearing for an additional 2–3 weeks, is advised. A tenogram may be helpful in differentiating a partial from a complete tendon rupture.

Acute dorsiflexion injuries of the foot may cause complete or incomplete tear of the Achilles tendon. Other etiologic factors include the presence of coronary artery disease, calcific deposits at the tendon insertion, Reiter's syndrome and other collagen disorders, long-term oral steroid therapy or steroid injection around the Achilles tendon, hyperlipidemia, gastrocnemius equinus and gastrocnemius-soleus equinus. Diagnosis is made by observing an indentation at the site of rupture, testing for active foot plantar flexion and squeezing the triceps surae group in order to note plantar flexion of the foot (Thompson's Test) (41). Ultrasonography has been utilized as a diagnostic tool (42).

Treatment approaches range from nonsurgical to immediate surgical intervention. The nonsurgical treatment involves 2 months casting of the foot in equinus, with gradual dorsiflexion as the casts are changed, followed by a heel lift and gradual stretching of the Achilles tendon (43). Surgical treatment may involve reapproximation of the torn tendon ends, the use of an autogenous Achilles tendon graft or the use of the plantaris tendon for repair (44, 45). Several conservative and surgical procedures have been performed for recurring subluxation and/or complete dislocation of the peroneus longus tendon at the level of the lateral malleolus. Recommended conservative treatment involves manipulative replacement of the tendon behind the lateral malleolus, placing the foot in a slightly everted position, followed by 6 to 8 weeks immobilization in a short leg walking cast.

Surgical indications are determined by the degree of tendon luxation, incidence of luxation, symptomatology, and their deleterious effect on the lateral ankle joint ligaments. Soft tissue procedures consist of tightening of the peroneal retinaculum and performing a fascia lata graft. An osteoperiosteal flap and wedge bone graft osteotomy of the lateral malleolus have been recommended for chronic dislocation of the peroneus longus tendon (Fig. 10.28) (46).

Goldman (47) describes a case of snapping tibialis anterior tendon. Differentiation from tibialis anterior tenosynovitis, bursitis and ganglion is stressed.

Kuwada et al. (48) believe patients with Achilles tendon rupture who are casted or treated by surgical repair with their foot in equinus predispose to rerupture.

Hosey and Werthheimer (49), in a retrospective study of eight Achilles tendon rupture repairs, find recreational activities requiring repeated rapid acceleration to be the primary cause of Achilles tendon rupture.

Nerve Injuries

Peripheral nerve injuries may be caused by traction, friction, compression or traumatic division. After a nerve is divided axons branch out in all direction in an attempt to find pathways for growth. If the

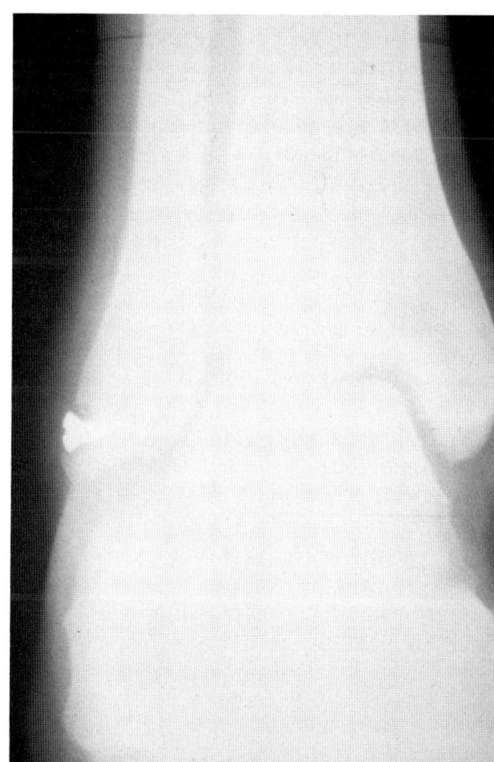

Figure 10.28. Postoperative view of Kelly bone wedge procedure for reduction of chronic dislocation of the peroneus longus tendon.

new fibers can find the sheath of the distal portion of cut nerve, they will grow along the nerve sheath and sensation will return. Usually the cut ends of the nerve will be fairly far apart, and the axons branch in all directions. If they mass together, an amputation (traumatic) neuroma results. This is seen at times after Morton's neuroma excision or amputation of a toe, foot or limb. If nerve fibers do cross the gap in the sectioned nerve and grow down the nerve sheath, the axons grow at rates averaging about 1 mm/day. Growth does not begin until approximately 10 days after nerve division, which is the time it takes for the motor or sensory neuron to overcome the original trauma. Nerve growth at the ankle level continues for 6 months. A peripheral nerve continues to conduct for up to 19 hours after it is cut. This is followed by a reaction of degeneration (Wallerian degeneration) for a period of 3 weeks. A record of sensory nerve regeneration may be kept by performing the starch-iodine test at regular intervals. Electromyographic (EMG) and nerve conduction velocity studies may be utilized to detect denervation and reinnervation, to follow the progress of the degeneration or recovery of a nerve, to detect nerve compression or to locate a lesion at the neuromuscular junction, peripheral axon, anterior horn or muscle itself. A decrease in nerve conduction and velocity helps locate the point of nerve pressure or injury and the lesion site of peripheral neuropathy.

Nerve injuries may be classified, according to degree, into three groups:

1. Neurotmesis: complete cut of the nerve (no recovery)
2. Axonotmesis: axonal damage with Wallerian degeneration with no loss of nerve continuity (recovery expected in 2–3 months)
3. Neuropraxia: nerve contusion with no actual damage (recovery expected in a few hours to as long as a week)

Nerve damage may be detected by means of the Tinel's sign–percussion-elicited tingling paresthesias coursing along the nerve from the site of damage or at the end of an advancing axon.

Treatment of a severed nerve—neurotmesis—involves primary repair through the epineurium with fine suture (50). If the nerve is torn it is attached to the soft tissues for a month until surrounding inflammation diminishes and it is then repaired. In an axonotmesis injury, when there is no sensory return after 6 months, the nerve is explored under local anesthesia and tested for conduction subsequent to repair by the use of external neurolysis and/or neurorrhaphy (51).

Injury of the medial cutaneous branch of the superficial peroneal nerve is commonly seen in cavus feet and in the presence of a first metatarsocuneiform exostosis from shoe pressure. This compression-type injury is also seen in athletes who lace their shoes snugly, who wear shoes with metal eyelets or who have a wrinkle in their sock or tongue of the shoe. Sural nerve injury and/or entrapment is seen as a sequela to lateral ankle injury. The first medial plantar digital nerve is often traumatized by ill-fitting footgear or inappropriate function leading to a diminished sensation or complete loss of sensation along the medial plantar aspect of the great toe.

Missile Wounds

The effect of a missile on tissue depends upon several factors: (a) the energy that the missile imparts to the surrounding tissue, (b) the surface area of the missile upon contact with the tissue, and (c) the nature of the tissue that comes into contact with the missile.

Low-velocity missiles with velocities less than 1,000 ft/sec as seen in civilian practice, injure only the tissue they contact; therefore, only the structures directly in the path of the missile are damaged. High-velocity missiles of a velocity greater than 1,000 ft/sec and usually around 3,000 ft/sec do not ordinarily pass clearly through tissue, except when fired at a very close range. High-velocity missiles "tumble" either in flight or when meeting the resistance of tissue, thereby increasing the surface area presented to the tissues.

During combat 75% of all missile injuries are produced by fragments and 25% by bullets. Fragment wounds in Vietnam resulted from the extensive use of mines, mortars and grenades by hostile forces (Figs. 10.29–10.32).

All wounds are debrided according to established principles. All nonviable fat and muscle are excised and easily accessible foreign bodies removed. As much bone as possible is saved to enhance stability of the structure. The debrided wound is covered with a single layer of fine-mesh gauze. The injured part is immobilized in a position of function using either a bulky dressing, splint or bivalved plaster cast. Delayed primary closure of clean wounds is performed.

Binson et al. (52) reports on primary and delayed primary closure in the treatment of noncombat-incurred open fractures. Seventy-eight patients with 82 open fractures comprised the study group. At the time of admission 14 wounds were classified as clean, 42 as slightly dirty, 15 as moderately dirty, and 11 as grossly dirty. Forty initial wound cultures were positive, and 42 were negative. Primary closure or delayed primary closure, the use of prophylactic and therapeutic cefazolin or clindamycin and internal fixation were not found to be significant in the development of clinical infection.

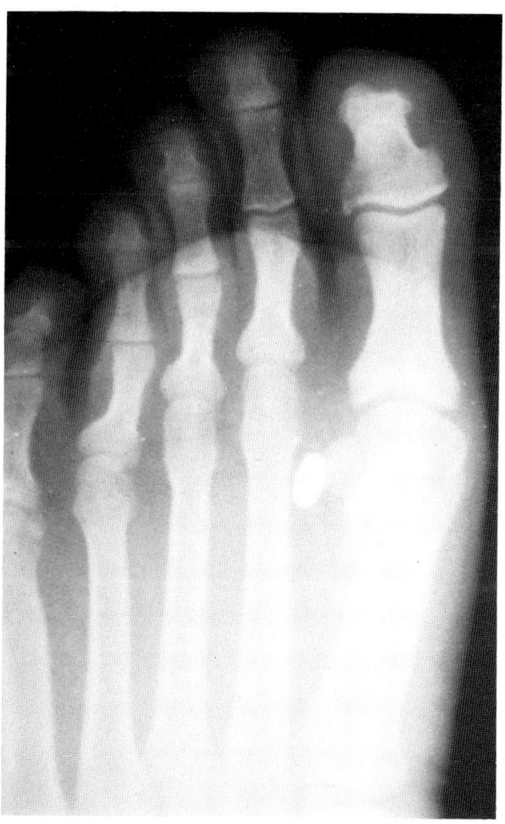

Figure 10.29. Low-velocity gunshot wound.

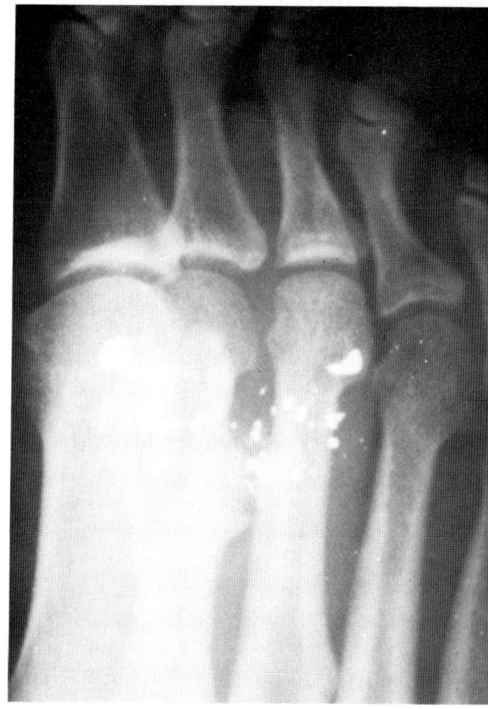

Figure 10.30. High-velocity gunshot wound.

Staged management of combat-type wounds with delayed closure is advocated. Appropriate IV antibiotics are used when there are suggestions of infection.

Complications secondary to foot and ankle trauma include swelling, skin bulla and infection, limitation of movement at the ankle, posttraumatic arthritis, nerve and tendon impingement, Sudeck's atrophy, nonunion and delayed union of fractures and posttraumatic calcifications of tendon and ligaments.

Regarding swelling, patients are encouraged to begin active flexion/extension exercises at the toes and knee joint while still in a cast. Doing so facilitates venous and lymphatic return, increases metabolic demand to augment blood supply and minimizes stiffness and vascular stagnation at the injured areas. After the cast is removed, heat with active and passive exercise is indicated to facilitate joint motion. Because they lead to venous congestion, warm whirlpool baths are counterindicated in edematous extremities. Post-traumatic skin blebs or bullae, whether they are caused by a new shoe or a crushing insult, must be managed with the utmost care. Aseptic technique is essential in preventing secondary infection. Nerve entrapment can occur. Most commonly the posterior tibial nerve is involved in cases of medial foot and ankle injury. The resultant tarsal tunnel syndrome presents very few objective findings. The patient has subjective complaints of paresthesia progressing to hyperesthesia. Tinel's sign is usually positive. Exploration of the nerve usually results in an abatement of symptoms.

Oloff et al. (53) present a review of 49 patients with a mean age of 45 who had electrodiagnostically confirmed tarsal tunnel syndrome; 24 of these patients had bilateral involvement. In addition to direct or indirect trauma, local etiologic factors included varicosities, aneurysms, arteriovenous malformations, soft tissue or bone tumors, abnormal subtalar pronatory problems and congenital anomalies. Oloff found a 34.7% incidence of systemic disease associated with tarsal tunnel syndrome. Concomitant diseases included diabetes mellitus, severe flatfoot deformity, inflammatory arthritis, foot and ankle injury, venous disease, neurofibromas, previous surgery, thickened laciniate ligament, hypothyroidism, plantar fibromatosis, anomalous flexor digitorum longus tendon and iatrogenic injections.

Tendon entrapment by fibrous or scar tissue or exuberant callus formation from a healing fracture is uncommon, but does occur. The long flexor tendons to the toes can become bound down as a result of a healing posterior malleolar fracture. Sudeck's atrophy, a vasomotor response initiated by pain impulses, initially presents with a warm, perspiring, indurated, diffusely painful foot. There is a limitation of motion at the ankle, subtalar joint, and me-

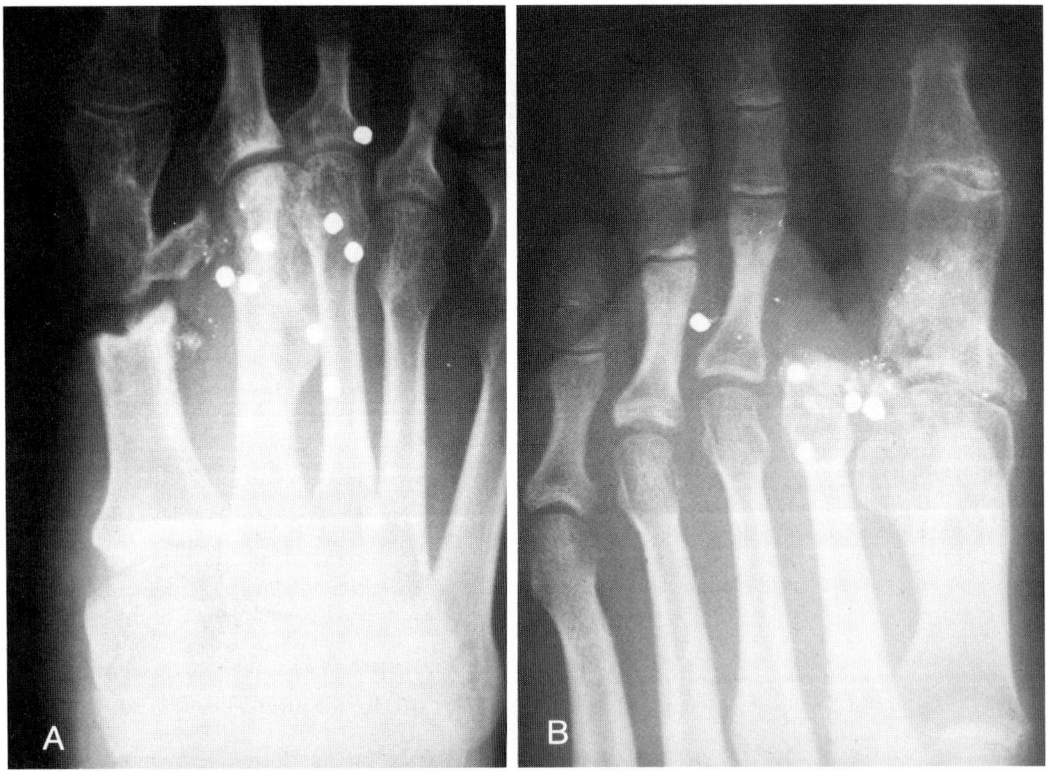

Figure 10.31. *A* and *B*. 12-gauge shotgun wounds.

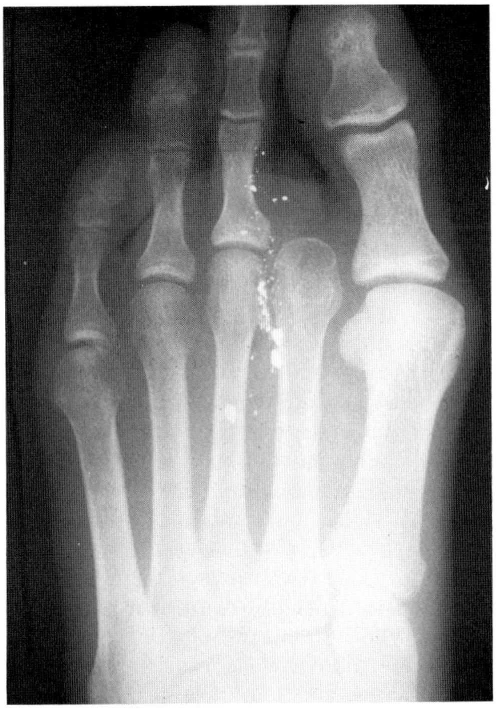

Figure 10.32. Fragmentation wound.

tatarsophalangeal joints. The patient cannot bear weight. X-rays reveal excessive spotty deossification involving the tarsals and metatarsals (Fig. 10.33).

Imanuel et al. (54) review the literature concerning Sudeck's atrophy and present a staged approach to diagnosis and treatment. Descriptions of Sudeck's atrophy include reflex hyperemic deossification, traumatic reflex osteodystrophy, posttraumatic osteoporosis and reflex sympathetic dystrophy. In stage I a constant, severe, burning, aching pain is experienced at the site of trauma. There is a nonpitting edema, and the foot is dry and hyperemic. Deossification takes 4–8 weeks to develop. Treatment consists of local anesthetic infiltration and rest. Stage II develops after 3 months, with pain becoming more severe and diffuse. There is a larger area of edema, and the skin may become cold, pale, gray, and sometimes cyanotic. Hair growth is diminished. The nails become brittle and ridged, there is muscle atrophy, and the foot joints become stiff and restricted in their range of motion. Sympathetic blocks, including periarterial anterior and posterior tibial blocks, are utilized for treatment. The foot joints are mobilized, and cool hydrotherapy treatments are instituted. Stage III Sudeck's atrophy results in intractable pain, severe muscle atrophy and restriction of the range of joint motion. Neurolysis has been recommended for treatment. Other treatment recommendations during all three stages include vasodilators, dilatol, padutin, Echinacin (a vegetable extract), x-ray therapy, androgenic hormones, calcium, phosphorus, ultra-sound and psychiatric consultation.

Delayed or nonunion of fractures is caused mechanically, by infection or by impaired circulation. Mechanical causes include inadequate immobilization and severed periosteum (Fig. 10.34). Three types of electrical stimulation have been used in the treatment of nonunion fractures. The two invasive types involve implantation of the electrode across the nonunion site and insertion of K-wire cathodes under local anesthesia and fluoroscopic visualization. In the third noninvasive type of electrical stimulation two electromagnetic induction coils are placed over the nonunion site (55). Walter and Pressman (56) discuss the use of an

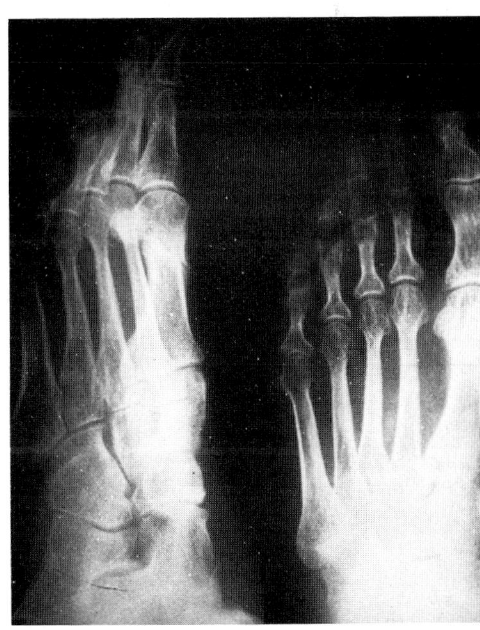

Figure 10.33. Sudeck's atrophy secondary to first metatarsal fracture.

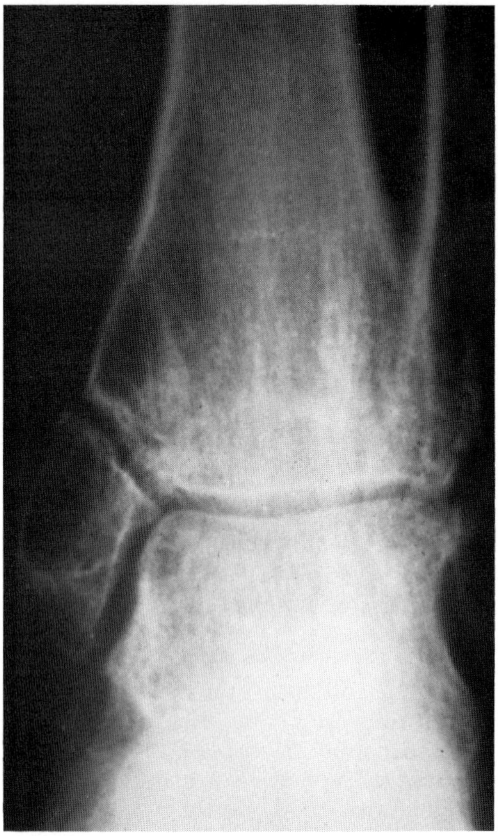

Figure 10.34. Nonunion medial malleolar fracture.

external compression device for treatment of nonunion fractures. If a pseudoarthrosis has formed, fibrocartilage must be resected prior to bone graft and/or fixation. Posttraumatic calcification of tendons and ligaments can be needled. Usually they become asymptomatic after the acute stage.

Chemical and Thermal Burns

Burns are divided into first, second, and third degree. A first-degree burn involves rubor and pain with no skin loss. In second-degree burns, blistering of the skin, marked rubor and pain with the opportunity for secondary infection occur. Third-degree burns involve deep destruction of tissue with fluid loss and, because of severe damage, severe pain or anesthesia. Primary first- and second-degree burn care consists of covering the wound, minimizing contamination and applying cool water. The second-degree burn wound is cleaned with bland soap and warm water. Under sterile conditions all dirt and dead tissue along with detached pieces of epidermis are removed. A copious amount of water is used when debriding chemical burns. If the burn victim has had a tetanus booster within the last 4 years, one-half cc of tetanus toxoid is administered subcutaneously. If the toxoid has not been administered within the last 4 years, 250 u of human immune globulin is administered intramuscularly.

In the first- and second-degree burn cases that the podiatrist sees, blood and fluid replacement are usually not required. If the burn area is dirty, prophylactic antibiotics may be used. Nutritional intake must be enhanced, and minimal narcotic analgesics should be prescribed. Topical treatment consists of aseptic surgical debridement followed by the use of 1% silver sulfadiazine cream (Silvadine), 10% mafenide acetate cream (Sulfamylon), one-half percent aqueous silver nitrate solution, or Vasaline-impregnated gauze.

Cold Injury

Cold injury ranges from pernio (chilblains) and trench foot or immersion foot to frostbite. Pernio is a cold injury that does not lead to death of tissue. Skin lesions, typically seen at the plantar aspects of the toes, appear as intradermal hemorrhages with violaceous borders. Avoiding the cold, use of vasodilating medication and occasional periarterial sympathetic nerve block lead to healing in 4 to 6 weeks. The use of a heating pad beneath the umbilicus is also helpful. Trench foot is commonly seen during wartime, with immobility and dampness being the predisposing factors. The feet become edematous and painful. When removed from the cold to a warm environment, reactive hyperemia ensues, which may predispose to future Raynaud's phenomenon occurence. Paresthesias and hypersthesia are prevalent. Pedal pulses are patent. Superficial areas of gangrene may be seen. Treatment is supportive and consists of elevation, a warm environment, rest, nonnarcotic analgesics and vasodilating drugs.

Frostbite is a severe cold injury with actual freezing that may result in tissue necrosis. Frostbite is classified in four stages, depending upon the severity of tissue damage. The four degrees of frostbite are similar to the three degrees of burn damage. In first-degree frostbite mild swelling and skin erythema with puritis occur. Second-degree frostbite involves blister formation with a pregangrenous base. Third-degree frostbite results in tissue necrosis, deep swelling and pain leading to local gangrene. Fourth-degree frostbite leads to severe tissue necrosis, edema, gangrene and resultant loss of the affected part.

Foreign Bodies

Foreign bodies found in the foot may vary from the lead of a pencil to the fragment of a mine, mortar, or grenade. It is not unusual for a patient with plantar pain and no history of trauma to have a dog hair implanted beneath the skin. Hairdressers, dog groomers and owners of wire-haired dogs are prone to foreign body hair implantation. Foreign bodies with metallic density, such as pins, nails and leaded glass, are readily identified on radiograph (Fig. 10.35) (5) Wood, unless unusually dense, thorns, cactus and sea urchin spines are not easily identified radiographically. Jeffrey (58) reviews the problems encountered in surgically removing different foreign bodies from the foot. Techniques of localizing foreign bodies and a new method for foreign body removal are discussed. Right-angle paper clips, single needle, triangle needle, fluoroscope-television (59), indelible marking, and a new type location method for foreign body removal in the foot are presented.

References

1. Byers W: Trauma syllabus. Oakland, CA, Highland General Hospital, 1966.
2. Laurich W, Witt CS, Zielsdorf LM: Treatment of fractures of the fifth metatarsal bone. *J Foot Surg* 22:207–211, 1983.
3. Smith H, Green AL: Cerclage wiring of metatarsal fractures. *J Am Podiatry Assoc* 73:25–26, 1983.

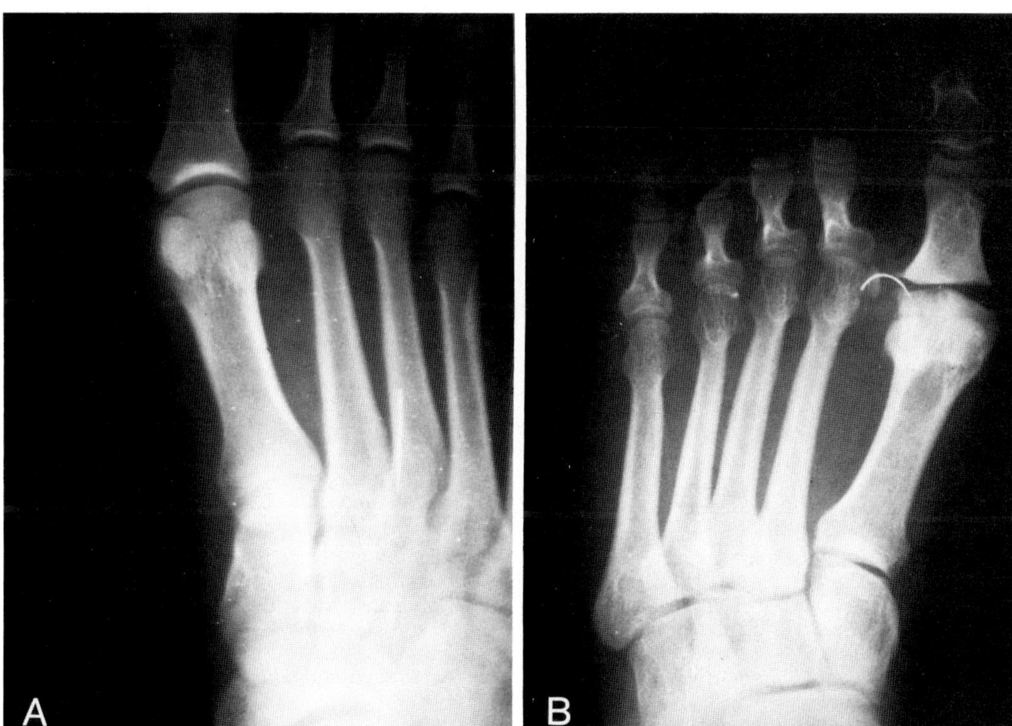

Figure 10.35. *A.* Broken sewing needle in foot. *B.* Surgical needle left in foot after "Keller" bunionectomy.

4. Spector FC, et al.: Lesser metatarsal fractures (incidence, management, and review). *J Am Podiatry Assoc* 74:259–264, 1984.
5. Maxwell JR: Open or closed-treatment of metatarsal fractures. *J Am Podiatry Assoc* 73:100–106, 1983.
6. Smith JS, et al: Fracture and disclocation of the middle cuneiform—A case report. *J Am Podiatry Assoc* 74:406–410, 1984.
7. Ochwat GF, Hugar DW: Fractures of the neck of the talus: A review of the literature based on Hawkins[1] classification with two case presentations. *J Foot Surg* 23:308–313, 1984.
8. Ganel A, et al: Subtalar dislocation. *J Foot Surg* 20:142–144, 1981.
9. Kavros SJ, Schoenhaus HD, Joy RM: Fracture of the posterior process of the talus (A case report). *J Am Podiatry Assoc* 73:421–422, 1983.
10. Portillo, RL: Osteochondritis dissecans of the talus: Diagnosis, treatment, and case report. *J Foot Surg* 20: 239–242, 1981.
11. Duddy RK, et al: Anterior calcaneal process fractures—recognition and treatment. *J Am Podiatry Assoc* 74:398–401, 1984.
12. Moss A, Modad AG: Ultrasonic assessment of stress fractures. *Br Med* 286:1479–1480, 1983.
13. Yale JF: A statistical analysis of three thousand six hundred and fifty seven consecutive fatigue fractures of the distal lower extremities. *J Am Podiatry Assoc* 66:739–748, 1976.
14. Lauge-Hansen N: Fractures of the ankle: Analytical historical recovery as the basis of new experimental roentgenologic and clinical investigations. *Arch Surg* 56:259, 1948.
15. Weiss L, Docks G, Freedland JA: Lauge-Hansen classification: A clockwork injury. *J Foot Surg* 22:192–197, 1983.
16. Freer DH: The treatment and evaluation of ankle sprains. *J Am Podiatry Assoc* 73:337, 1983.
17. Heller AJ, Vogler HW: Ankle joint arthroscopy. *J Foot Surg* 21:23–29, 1982.
18. Dowling JW, Oloff LM, Jacobs AM: Radiologic diagnosis and assessment of lateral ankle ligamentous injuries. *J Foot Surg* 18:135, 1979.
19. Hice GA, Solomon W, Faschad P: The plaster-synthetic cast. *J Am Podiatry Assoc* 73:427–431, 1983.
20. Canglialosi CP: Ruptured anterior talofibular ligament: A simplified procedure for late repair. *J Foot Surg* 20:224–226, 1981.
21. Ransom RA, Dailey JM: The plantaris tendon: A lateral ankle stabilization procedure (A case report). *J Am Podiatry Assoc* 74:295–299, 1984.
22. Kaplan EG, et al: A triligamentous reconstruction for lateral ankle instability. *J Foot Surg* 23:240–247, 1984.
23. Gächer A, et al: Clinical application of unwoven carbon fibers for a scaffold in ligament surgery. *Aktuel Probl Chir Orthop* 26:124–6, 1983.
24. Visser HJ, Oloff LM, Jacobs AM: Lateral ankle stabilization procedures: Criteria and classification. *J Foot Surg* 19:74–84, 1980.
25. Reinherz RP, Sharon SM and Knudsen HA: Surgical repair of lateral ankle instability by modification of traditional approaches. *J Foot Surg* 17:12–15, 1978.
26. Knudsen HA, et al: Ankle fracture classification with approaches to surgical repair by AO-ASIF techniques. *J Foot Surg* 22:145–152, 1983.
27. Skinner HA: *The Origin of Medical Terms*. New York, Hafner Publishing Co, 1970, p. 36.
28. Gamble FO, Yale I: *Clinical Foot Roentgenology*. 2nd Ed. Krieger, Melbourne, FL, 1975, p. 56.
29. Yale JF: Growth center injuries of the foot. *Arch Pod Med & Foot Surg* 1:129–140, 1973.
30. Rogers LF: The radiography of epiphyseal injuries. *Radiology* 96:289–299, 1970.
31. Frances CC: The appearance of centers of ossification from 6 to 15 years. *Am J Phys Anthropol* 27:127, 1939.
32. Frances CC: Factors influencing appearance of centers of ossification during early childhood, *Am J Dis Child* 57:817, 1939.
33. Frances CC, Werle PP: The appearance of centers of ossification from birth to 5 years. *Am J Phys Anthropol* 24:273, 1939.
34. Harsha WN: Effects of trauma upon epiphyses, *Clin Orthop* 10:140–147, 1957.
35. Aitken AP: The end results of the fractured distal radial epiphysis, *J Bone Joint Surg* 17:302–308, 1935.
36. Slater RB, Harris WR: Injuries involving the epiphyseal plate. *J Bone Joint Surg* 45-A:587–622, 1963.
37. Holland CT: A radiological note on injuries to distal epiphyses of the radius and ulna. *Proc Roy Soc Med* 22:23–28, 1929.
38. Nordentoft EL: Experimental epiphyseal injuries. *Acta Orthop Scand* 40:176–92, 1969.
39. Wicks MH, et al: Tendon injuries about the foot and ankle in children. *Aus NZ J Surg* 50:158–161, 1980.
40. Reinherz RP: Management of flexor hallucis longus tendon injuries. *J Foot Surg* 23(5):366–369, 1984.
41. Thompson TC: Spontaneous rupture of tendon achilles: A new clinical diagnostic test. *J Trauma* 2:126–129, 1962.
42. Bruce RK, Hale TL, Gilbert SK: Ultrasonography evaluation for ruptured Achilles tendon. *J Am Podiatry Assoc* 72:15–17, 1982.
43. Lee RB, Smith L: Rupture of the Achilles tendon nonsurgical treatment. *Clin Orthop Relat Res* 60:115–168, 1968.
44. Lindholm A: A new method of operation in subcutaneous rupture of the Achilles tendon. *Acta Chir Scand* 117:261, 1959.
45. Kirschenbaum SE, Kelman C: Modification of the Lindholm procedure for plastic repair of ruptured Achilles tendon: A case report. *J Foot Surg* 19:4–11, 1980.
46. Yale JF: DuVries Modification of Kelly's wedge bone graft for chronic anterior peroneus longus dislocation (A case report). *Arch Pod Med & Foot Surg* 2:285–288, 1975.
47. Goldman F: Snapping of the tibialis anterior tendon. *J Am Podiatry Assoc* 73:29–30, 1983.
48. Kwada GT, Schoberth J: Evaluation of Achilles tendon rerupture. *J Foot Surg* 23:340–343, 1984.
49. Hosey T, Werthheimer S: A retrospective study on surgical repair of the Achilles tendon. *J Foot Surg* 23:1984.

50. Crenshaw AH (ed): *Campbell's Orthopedics,* ed 5. St Louis CV, Mosby CO, 1971.
51. Marcus SA, Block BH (ed): *Complications in Foot Surgery, Prevention and Management. American College of Foot Surgery,* ed 2. Baltimore, Williams & Wilkins, 1984, pp. 45–47.
52. Binson DR, et al: Treatment of open fractures: A prospective study. *J Trauma* 23:25–30, 1983.
53. Oloff LM, Jacobs AM, Jaffe S: Tarsal tunnel syndrome: A manifestation of systemic disease. *J Foot Surg* 22:302–307, 1983.
54. Imanuel HM, et al: Sudeck's atrophy: A review of the literature. *J Foot Surg* 20:243–246, 1981.
55. Mahan KT: Electrical stimulation of bone. *J Am Podiatry Assoc* 73:86–92, 1983.
56. Walter JH, Pressman MM: External fixation in the treatment of metatarsal nonunions. *J Am Podiatry Assoc* 71:297–301, 1981.
57. Byron TJ: Foreign bodies found in the foot. *J Am Podiatry Assoc* 71:30, 1981.
58. Jeffrey JI: Surgical excision of foreign bodies. *J Am Podiatry Assoc* 74:229–232, 1984.
59. Puhl RW, et al: The use of fluoroscopy in the detection and excision of foreign bodies in the foot. *J Am Podiatry Assoc* 73:514–517, 1983.

Suggested Readings

Arner O, Lindholm A, Grell SR: Histologic changes in subcutaneous rupture of the Achilles tendon. *Acta Chir Scand* 116:484–490, 1958.

Arner O, Lindholm A, Lundvall N: Roentgen changes in subcutaneous rupture of the Achilles tendon. *Acta Chir Scand* 116:496–500, 1958.

Byron RJ: Soft tissue trauma of the foot. *J Foot Surg* 15:134–142, 1976.

Carlino J: Removal of a penetrating foreign body, a case report. *Cur Podiatry* 2:13–14, 1971.

Gilchrist AK: Surgical care of the traumatized foot. *J Am Podiatry Assoc* 65:816, 1975.

Graziano TA, et al: Crush and avulsion injuries of the foot: Their evaluation and management. *J Foot Surg* 23:445–450, 1984.

Hunt TK, Dunphy J (eds.): *Fundamentals of Wound Management.* New York, Appleton Century Crofts, 1979, pp. 364–455.

Johnson JB, Cavallaro DC: Post-traumatic reflex sympathetic dystrophy. *J Am Podiatry Assoc* 67:870–873, 1977.

Kazin F, McCarthy DJ, Sims J, et al: The reflex sympathetic dystrophy syndrome. I. Clinical and histological studies: Evidence of bilaterality, response to corticosteroids and articular involvement. *Am J Med* 60:321, 1976.

Kelikian H, Kelikian A: *Disorders of the Ankle.* Philadelphia, WB Saunders Co, 1985.

Lang AG, Peterson HA: Osteomyelitis following puncture wounds of the foot in children. *J Trauma* 16:993–999, 1976.

LaPorta G (ed.): *Osteosynthesis in Foot and Ankle Surgery. Clinics in Podiatry.* Philadelphia, WB Saunders, Co, 1985.

Meyerding HW, Stuck WG: Painful heels among children (apophysitis). *JAMA* 102:1658–1660, 1934.

Mozena JD, Kroepel LR: Digital fractures in children, *J Am Podiatric Med Assoc* 75:288–292, 1985.

Nuzzo JJ: Gunshot wounds of the foot. *J Foot Surg* 15:76–79, 1976.

Page JA: Painful feet syndrome among war prisoners in the Far East. *Br Med J* 2:709, 1946.

Pickett NJ: Gun shot wound in the heel. *Chirop Rec* 22:27–29, 1939.

Randolph TJ, Vogler H: Nonunions and delayed unions. *J Foot Surg* 24:62–67, 1985.

Scurran BL (ed): *Osseous Trauma of The Foot, Clinics in Podiatry.* Philadelphia, WB Saunders, Co, 1985.

Thompson TC: A test for rupture of the tendo achilles. *Acta Orthop Scand* 32:461–465, 1962.

Yablon IG, Segal D, Leach RE: *Ankle Injuries.* New York, Churchill Livingstone, 1983.

11

Podiatric Surgery

This chapter, which reflects podiatric surgical experience of the past 50 years, emphasizes preoperative, intraoperative and postoperative principles. The surgical principles and techniques discussed in this chapter are podiatric surgical refinements of procedures described over the past 200 years in the general surgical and orthopaedic literature. In treating the podiatric problem, the foot surgeon must not lose sight of other areas of pathology and underlying systemic disease. Medical and surgical specialist consultation augments patient care through a team approach.

Before discussing surgical principles pediatric foot surgery is briefly reviewed. Vomiting and aspiration of vomitus, aspiration pneumonia and postoperative ileus are of special concern when operating on the feet of infants and children. The upper outer quadrant of the buttocks is to be avoided when using intramuscular medications so as to avoid sciatic palsy. Rather, the lateral thigh or deltoid areas should be used. Because aspirin may stimulate the CNS and cause hyperventilation, diaphoresis and vomiting in the neonate, it should be used with caution in young infants. Aspirin also competes with bilirubin for protein binding, which may result in kernicterus. Acetaminophen is less toxic and better tolerated. Be alert for respiratory depression when using narcotic analgesics. Morphine is used orally as paregoric and subcutaneously or intramuscularly by injection in children. Promethazine may be used to potentiate narcotic analgesics. Prophylactic antibiotics are used in newborns because of the hazard of postoperative pneumonia. Care must be exercised when administering chloramphenicol to the pediatric patient because of its toxic effect. Tetracyclines may cause temporary shortening of fibular growth rate in newborns and may lead to permanent tooth discoloration. Sulfa drugs my cause hyperbilirubinemia because of the newborn's inability to detoxify the drug (1). There are problems with using a specific reference, such as Clark's, Fried's or Young's rule, for determining pediatric drug dosage. The physical and physiological differences between children and adults, including weight, body surface area and metabolic rate, make following a specific rule unwise (1).

When treating the foot articulations, the podiatric surgeon deals primarily with synovial joints. An appreciation of the anatomy and physiology of joint capsule, hyaline cartilage, synovium and synovial fluid is essential. Care must be taken to be atraumatic in the handling of articular and periarticular tissues. Preservation of the neurovascular supply to synovial joints is mandatory. Respect for synovial tissue and fluid pH, temperature and integrity is crucial to the surgical approach to foot joint pathology. Interference with synovial tissue and fluid integrity will interfere with joint lubrication and cartilage nutrition.

Joint shape and movement must be evaluated in the overall context of the surgical procedure contemplated. Proper surgical technique dictates differing approaches to the ellipsoid metatarsophalangeal joint as compared to the uniplane intermetatarsal joint. An appreciation of the dynamic interrelationship of synovial joints is essential to the foot surgeon.

The complex process of hyaline cartilage repair, although not totally understood, suggests that prudent mobilization of the postoperative joint may be more beneficial than strict immobilization (2). Podiatric surgeons have found this to be clinically evident over the past 50 years.

Preoperative Principles

The muscle-tendon complex must be functional in order to achieve the desired result from arthroplasty procedures. Surgical attention to pathological joints must be preceded by attention to the joint function mechanism, i.e., the muscle-tendon complex. The surgically reconstructed joint must be able to function, and the muscle-tendon complex must be preserved and strengthened (3). Joint fusion in the foot is a last resort. Surgical joint reconstruction based on sound biomechanical principles is mandatory. Control of adverse mechanical forces through the use of foot orthotic devices is an integral part of postoperative care (4–7).

Cosmetic surgery of the feet has only rare application. Only in cases of extreme psychological overlay should cosmetic surgery for the nonpainful, nondebilitated foot be considered. Rather, surgical approach is determined by the patient's subjective complaints, deformity, adverse function, inability to wear protective footgear, debility and predictable debility. Although it is difficult to predict the impact of adverse function on foot deformity, it is important to appreciate the interrelationship of structure and function (5–11).

In most cases it is to the patient's benefit that multiple forefoot surgical procedures be performed during the same surgical session. Long-term morbidity is essentially the same with lesser risk and cost factors related to anesthesia and facilities, respectively.

Laboratory assessment is of little value in choosing a specific surgical procedure. However, blood, urine and synovial tissue and fluid analysis are essential to correct diagnosis and medical management.

The medical condition of the patient must be taken into consideration as well. Primary and secondary anemia, hyperuricemia and hypertension must be medically evaluated and controlled. Roper et al. (2) review the preoperative, intraoperative and postoperative management of the gouty patient. Caputi et al. (13) present an excellent discussion of the diagnosis, clinical manifestations and surgical management of sickle cell anemia with an emphasis on pedal pathology. Chronic anemia associated with collagen disorders is not a contraindiction to surgery. The questions of the amount of local oxygen perfusion and the inability of oxygen to get to the surgical site have not been answered satisfactorily. Surgery is not advised during acute exacerbations of unerlying systemic disease, including but not limited to rheumatoid arthritis, systemic lupus erythematosus and gout. Foot joint surgery is contraindicated in the presence of an infected bursa or infected tophaceous deposit. Surgery is not recommended through areas of skin associated with psoriasis, contact dermatitis, neurodermatitis, dermatomycosis, monilia, excessive scar formation, ulcerations, fissures, sinus tracts, acute vasculitis and the skin lesions associated with diabetes and Reiter's syndrome.

Obtaining standardized angle of stance in gait radiographs of the feet and ankles is an integral part of the preoperative evaluation procedure (9, 14). Measurement of angular relationships is a prerequisite to proper foot surgical approach (15–18).

Hip, knee, ankle, subtalar, midtarsal, tarsal, metatarsal and phalangeal joint position, stability, quality and range of motion must be evaluated. Structural and torsional lower extremity bony involvement must be determined (11). Intrinsic and extrinsic muscular, neurological and vascular status must be assessed. Foot type; digital and metatarsal length pattern, parabola and angulation; interphalangeal angle; and lesser tarsal angle must receive studied evaluation prior to operating on the deformed foot (2, 9, 10, 17–20).

Vascular analysis utilizing Doppler or plethysmographic studies is important. All vascular parmeters should be assessed, including skin color, texture and temperature; hair and nail growth; capillary and venous filling time; and pedal pulses (21). Special care should be exercised with patients having a history of deep or superficial phlebitis. The benefits derived from the use of low-dose heparin in general surgery do not seem to affect foot surgical procedures (22). Patients who smoke should be encouraged to stop or, if they cannot, to limit the number of cigarettes smoked per day 1 week before surgery.

The neurological status of the patient is of major importance in the preoperative evaluation. Neurotrophic arthritis secondary to the sensory loss found in diabetes, leprosy and lues requires thorough evaluation. Upper and lower motor neuron involvement needs to be assessed. The impact of a neurological or sensory deficit on foot surgery is profound (21).

Careful attention should be paid to the nutritional status of any person with rheumatoid or other form of arthritis. People with rheumatoid arthritis are predisposed to undernourishment and deficiencies of metals, vitamins, amino acids and other nutrients. Undernourishment in the arthritic patient may be a result of the patient's inability to use the hands, wrists, elbows and shoulders to cut and eat foods. The arthritic process may interfere with chewing as well. General fatigue and difficulty in preparing meals may also be contributing factors (23). It appears that arthritis affects diet, rather than diet affecting arthritis.

From a surgical point of view, it is important that nutritional deficiencies be reversed before surgery. A generally healthy and well-nourished patient is certainly preferable to the undernourished debilitated patient. Obese patients should be encouraged to lose weight. However, this weight loss should not be attempted in the hospital during recovery from surgery.

Preoperative management of the foot surgery patient includes medical control of systemic disease, muscle strengthening and stretching exercises, active and passive joint motion exercises and the use of foot orthotic devices (4, 11, 24). Hypertensive patients taking diuretics must be evaluated for electrolyte inbalance. Other medications, including aminoglycoside antibiotics, digitalis, anticoagulants, insulin and oral contraceptives, predispose the surgical patient to perioperative complications. Haber et al. (25) and Lowe (26) review the course and treatment of malignant hyperthermia. The authors stress the importance of early recognition and treatment of this defect in regulation of intracellular calcium in skeletal muscle, induced by certain inhalation anesthesia-related agents. Obese patients, the elderly, alcoholics and those with a past history of phlebitis, venous or arterial insufficiency, congestive heart failure, myocardial infarction and angina present a greater surgical risk. Insulin-dependant diabetics should have their blood sugar controlled before surgery. Insulin should be used perioperatively for diabetics being treated with oral hypoglycemic agents. Hypoglycemic agents should be discontinued 3 to 4 days before surgery and the institution of the use of insulin. The insulin-dependent diabetic should receive one-half the usual insulin dose before surgery and the other half when oral intake is resumed after surgery. When thyroid dysfunction is suspected, a free T_4 index screening test should be performed preoperatively.

The psychosocial history of the patient is an important and vital part of patient assessment. Family history and marital, and employment status affect the surgical approach. The so-called rheumatoid personality is predisposed to acute anxiety states, denial and neurotic behavior patterns (3). Understanding, patience and informed consent are the hallmarks of the good doctor-patient relationship.

It is essential that the surgeon fully inform the patient about the specific surgery to be performed, risks involved, possible complications and prognosis. Same-day foot surgery is counterindicated unless the problem is emergent. Proper examination, study and informed consent dictate that sufficient time be given to both physician and patient. The doctor should make a special effort to enable the patient to understand thoroughly the progressive nature of any underlying systemic disorder.

Intraoperative Principles

The skilled surgeon is not born, but rather develops over a period of many years. It is imperative that those podiatrists operating on highly specialized foot structures be adequately trained and experienced. Perceptual motor skills necessary in the skillful surgeon can be acquired only through repetitive clinical practice (27). Gibbons et al. (28) conducted a "flexibility of closure" test utilizing 39 podiatric surgical residents. The test is designed to measure special skills and is correlated with the skills needed in most podiatric surgical procedures. A significant correlation was found between test scores and consensus faculty ratings of technical surgical skills.

As in the case with most surgery, an aseptic environment is essential. Foot surgery may be performed in a properly equipped outpatient office (29, 30), surgical center (31) or hospital environment. Pre- and postoperative angle of stance in gait X-ray evaluation is utilized to monitor initial joint position and later bone healing. Podiatric surgical patients admitted for elective surgery spend an average of 4 days in the hospital (57).

Local nerve block or regional or general anesthesia may be used depending on the skill and judgment of the surgeon and the presurgical assessment. In a study involving 2 million injections of 1:100,000 and 1:200,000 epinephrine-containing local anesthetic agents into the toes, the incidence of significant tissue necrosis or gangrene was well within acceptable therapeutic limits (32). Analysis of associated data has shown that, after adequate medical, peripheral vascular and neurological assessments, the use of epinephrine-containing anesthetic agents in foot surgery is safe and effective (32, 33). The use of epinephrine in local anesthetics provides local vasoconstriction at the injection site and delays absorption of the anesthetic agent, which results in more profound anesthesia for a longer period of time. There is no vasoconstriction distal to the site of a local anesthetic containing epinephrine nerve block; the distal blood vessels dilate. This sympathetic response is utilized therapeutically by posterior tibial periarterial local anesthetic injections for distal ischemia. The use of epinephrine in local anesthetics is contraindicated in patients with coronary artery disease (angina, with or without a previous myocardial infarction), hypertension, arrhythmias, congestive heart failure, peripheral organic arterial occlusive or spastic disease; in pregnant patients; during or following general anesthesia; and in patients taking β-blockers or monoamine oxidase inhibitors. A debilitated patient with liver disease should be given one-half the recommended adult dose of a 1% local anesthetic solution.

Available local anesthetics include

1. Esters of para-aminobenzoic acid: procaine, chloroprocaine, butethamine
2. Esters of benzoic acid: piperocaine, hexylcaine, meprylcaine, propoxycaine, tetracaine
3. Esters of meta-aminobenzoic acid: metabutoxycaine, metabutethanine, isobucaine
4. Amides: dibucaine, lidocaine, mepivocaine, prilocaine, bupivacaine

Howard et al. (34) describe the local anesthetic use of diphenhydramine hydrochloride in patients who are allergic to the "caine" drugs. Because of a narrow margin of dosage safety, caution is advised.

Unless contraindicted, tourniquet control providing a bloodless operating field is desirable. An Esmarch bandage or pneumatic cuff tourniquet may be used at the midfoot, rearfoot, above the ankle or the proximal thigh level. Care must be taken to ensure that the tourniquet does not produce false deformity through application of pressure to tendon or muscle. Vasculitis as a result of small vessel disease may accompany collagen disorders in a minority of cases, and care must be taken to minimize tourniquet and surgical trauma in areas of vasculitis or superficial varicosities. Adequate padding between the tourniquet and the extremity is essential in order to avoid local skin, nerve and vascular damage.

Although there has been no conclusive evidence relating the postoperative complications of phlebitis, vascular embarrassment or nerve injury to less than 2 hours of tourniquet time, in forefoot surgery an experienced foot surgeon should rarely have to exceed 1½ hours surgical time per foot (35, 36). A roll of Webril padding should be placed beneath a proximal thigh or distal leg tourniquet. The proximal thigh and distal leg tourniquet may be elevated from 60 to 100 mm Hg pressure higher than the patient's systolic blood pressure, up to 350 mm Hg, in order to achieve necessary hemostasis. The greater the leg circumference, the greater the pressure needed. Contrary to recent reports (37, 38), the author finds less complications with the use of a properly applied midfoot Esmarch bandage tourniquet with sterile Webril padding or a folded towel beneath the tourniquet compared with the use of a proximal thigh tourniquet (39). It would seem logical that the more distal the tourniquet application the less tissue will be subjected to ischemic changes thereby resulting in fewer complications (35, 40).

Skin preparation and draping technique are accomplished according to accepted principles and the desire of the surgeon. Care must be exercised not to traumatize the skin mechanically.

If surgery is to be performed under general inhalation anesthesia, a long-acting 0.25% marcaine regional nerve block may be performed to assist postoperative comfort. Two minums of a short-acting steroid not to exceed a total of 0.5 cc, such as dexamethasone (4 mg/cc), may be used at each ostectomy site (41, 42). A steroid is not to be used directly at an osteotomy site requiring bone healing or internal fixation. When implant surgery is being performed, prophylactic antibiotic irrigant solutions, such as 1 cc neomycin sulfate (Neosporin GU) dissolved in 500 cc of normal saline or Ringer's lactate solution, may be used (19).

Indications for podiatric antibiotic prophylaxis include (a) implantation of foreign materials; (b) pre-, intra- and postoperatively in patients with systemic diseases interfering with the natural mechanism of host defense, e.g., diabetes, rheumatic heart disease, corticosteroid therapy, etc; (c) acute trauma, (d) patients who have had a previous infection or surgery at the same site; (e) patients over 70 years of age; and (f) those cases where prolonged surgical time is anticipated (43).

First-generation cephalosporins are recommended both parenterally and orally. Oral administration is initiated 24 hours preoperatively and continued 24 hours postoperatively. Parenteral dose is administered 30 minutes preoperatively and intraoperatively, if the procedure lasts longer than 1½ hours. Intraoperative antibiotic flush of kanamycin (1 G to 500 ml of saline or Ringer's lactate solution) and povidone-iodine (Betadine with equal amounts of saline) are the two most commonly used antibiotic-antiseptic flushes used. Povidone-iodine flush is not recommended during implant surgery (43). Frequent irrigation with cool saline or Ringer's solution is suggested during all foot surgical procedures (35).

An adequately sized and properly placed incision is necessary to ensure correct exposure and healing. As a rule, linear incisions following skin lines are most effective in minimizing trauma to soft tissue, nerve and blood supply. Hodor and Dobbs (44) review incisional approaches to metatarsal head resection and introduce a five-incision, dorsal longitudinal approach. Incisions should not be directed over or under a bony prominence or through marginal skin. The plantar of the heel and the lateral plantar aspect of the foot should be avoided. Incisions over the navicular tuberosity and fifth metatarsal base should also be avoided.

Minimal or small incision surgery has application for ablation of medial, lateral and dorsal interphalangeal joint osteophytes (Fig.11.1). Traversing of deeper tissues, with high-speed instrumentation and without adequate visualization, often predisposes to further arthritic changes in an already arthritically compromised joint.

Meticulous atraumatic handling of tissues is of vital importance (45). The initial skin incision should traverse entire skin thickness. Separate no. 15 blades should be used for the skin and soft tissues, and the blades should be changed as frequently as needed. Skin edges should not be subjected to crushing by thumb and finger forceps. Small one-tooth Adson forceps may be used 2 cm or more inside the incision line to invert the skin. Skin hooks or blunt catspaw retractors with little tension application may be used to retract skin and soft tissues. Skin hooks and retractors should be in contact

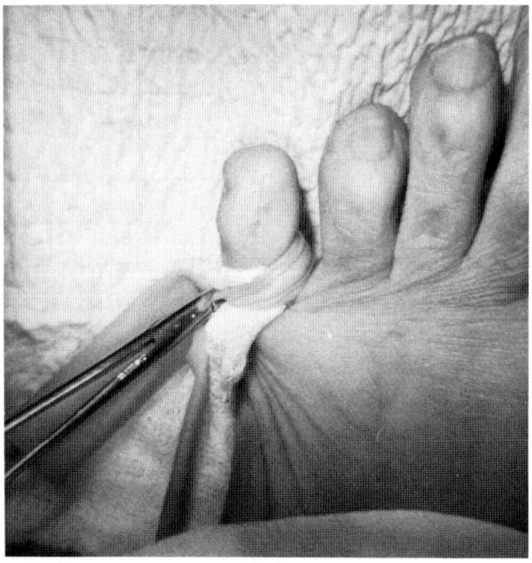

Figure 11.1. Minimal incision surgery for ablation of medial distal phalangeal exostosis fifth toe.

with subcutaneous fat and superficial fascia, not with the skin. Soft tissues should be handled with care. Controlled sharp dissection along tissue planes is preferred over blunt dissection of the soft tissues. Handling of the tissues in an injudicious manner may cause postoperative acute exacerbation of an underlying arthritic process. Superficial nerves should be avoided and surrounded with fat prior to closure. Avoid multiple ligatures and electrical cautery of superficial veins in the forefoot.

Marcinko et al. (46) discuss the use of the Shaw electric scalpel as an improved tool for sealing severed blood vessels. The authors state that this device offers an improved method of surgical hemostasis without the muscle stimulation and tissue damage of conventional electrosurgical units. Always cut toward the pathological bone being excised. Stryker, Storz, Richards, Ritter or 3 M or Zimmer nitrogen- or electric-powered instrumentation is preferred. Hand instruments tend to fragment bone to a greater degree than power instruments. Rasp away from viable hyaline cartilage at joint surfaces so as to avoid microcartilagenous fissuring.

Tissue closure should be along tissue planes. The smallest gauge suture and atraumatic needle should be used to produce the desired tissue closure, e.g., 3, 4, or 5-0 Dexon (polyglycolic acid), PDS (polydioxanone) or Vicryl (polyglactin 910) for forefoot joint capsule and soft tissue closure; 5-0 Dermalon (nylon) for skin closure. Avoid the use of chromic and plain catgut suture materials. When forefoot fusion procedures are performed, internal fixation by means of through-and-through wire (2-0 monofilament stainless steel), small compression screws or fine nonthreaded Kirschner wire may be used (47). Intraoperative x-ray evaluation is utilized as needed.

External fixation may be accomplished by the use of plaster or fiberglass casts or splints, or plastic, Celastic or adhesive tape splints depending on healing requirements (Fig. 11.2). The joint distal and proximal to the fusion procedure should be externally immobilized. Short leg plaster cast immobilization is rarely indicated in forefoot surgery. Appropriate internal fixation and external splinting, which allow greater maneuverability, seem to be of greater overall benefit to the patient recovering from foot surgery.

DiGiovanni and Martin (48) catalogue the various uses of wires and pins in foot surgery. They discuss the use of one hole, two hole, three hole, and figure of eight wiring techniques, as well as staples, Kirschner wires and Steinman pins for osteotomy, fusion, bone graft and fracture fixation procedures. Floyd et al. (49) present an overview of bone healing with regard to tension and compression; they discuss the use of Richards scaphoid compression staple as an effective form of fixation for closing abductory base wedge osteotomies of the first metatarsal. Cast immobilization is indicated in those fusion procedures when splinting is impossible or impractical. Tarsal joint fusion procedures require strict immobilization for proper healing. Areas of tendon graft or repair must be immobilized as well in order to allow satisfactory healing. The long extensor tendons may be temporarily aligned and immobilized proximal to a lengthened area or proximal to an operated joint by means of a single absorbable suture attachment to the soft tissues.

When skin closure is complete, Adaptic and sterile gauze are applied to the surgical site. Betadine solution-soaked gauze sponges may be used. When dry they have a splinting effect. Two layers of eight-ply 3

× 3 inch gauze sponges are applied to dorsal incision sites and covered by one roll of 3-inch Kling dressing. Digital incision sites are dressed with one 3 × 3 inch gauze sponge opened and folded lengthwise, which is applied over and around the digit. A recurrent 1-inch Kling dressing is used to reinforce the digital dressing with the toes being held in anatomically correct alignment. Adhesive tape splinting is used to reinforce the dressing material. Care must be exercised to ensure that the dressings are not too tight and that the adhesive tape does not come into contact with the skin. If external splinting is required, a Celastic or prenyl splint may be incorporated around this dressing by means of an additional roll of 3-inch Kling dressing reinforced with adhesive tape splints (Fig. 11.2).

Postoperative Principles

The overall medical and functional status of the patient should be of concern postoperatively, as well as the surgical healing process. Concomitant medical control of systemic disease is essential. Encourage coughing and deep breathing. Note how analgesics affect breathing. Adverse intrinsic muscle function around deformed and/or limited range of motion joints leads to muscle atrophy. A postoperative physical therapeutic regimen is of prime importance to enable the patient to gain as much muscle strength and joint range of motion as possible (see Chapter 13, Podiatric Treatment). It may begin on the first postoperative day with the patient doing active and passive range of motion exercises while in bed for those lower extremity joints not surgically involved. Forefoot joints undergoing reconstruction may be actively exercised (off weightbearing) 1 week postoperatively. The operated extremity is elevated for the first 48 hours. Ice bags are applied to the surgical sites intermittently (on 3 hours/off 1 hour) for the first 48 hours after surgery.

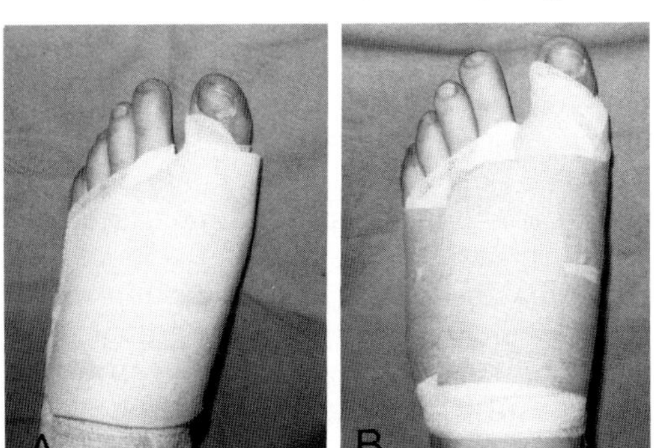

Figure 11.2. A, Celastic splint application following first metatarsal proximal metaphyseal abductory wedge osteotomy with through-and-through wire fixation. B, Celastic splint covered with Kling and adhesive tape.

Postoperative discomfort is controlled with appropriate narcotic and/or nonnarcotic analgesic medication. A typical postoperative pain-relieving order is one oxycodone HCL (Percocet) tablet, with 1 tablespoon of a nonmagnesium-containing antacid of choice, every 4 to 6 hrs as needed for postoperative discomfort. Rarely are injectable narcotic medications required following forefoot surgery. For severe postoperative pain, meperedine HCL (Demerol) IM may be prescribed in doses ranging from 25—100 mg every 3 to 6 hr (not to exceed 400 mg in any 24-hour period), depending upon the weight of the patient. Meperedine is poorly absorbed orally. Promethazine HCL (Phenergan) may be used concomitantly to potentiate meperedine and for its antiemetic and sedative effect. Triazolam (Halcion) in a 0.25- or 0.5-mg tablet may be used at bedtime as needed for sleep.

Cornell et al. (50) studied the postoperative course of 65 foot surgical patients who had transcutaneous electrical nerve stimulation (TENS) administered for pain relief. The authors report an overall analgesic reduction of 74.9% in those patients receiving both oral and intramuscular analgesics. A significant reduction was seen in the use of oral analgesics and, to a lesser extent, intramuscular analgesics. Lanham et al. (51) report the use of hypothermia initiated 6 hours preoperatively and continued up to 48 hours postoperatively, together, with TENS, which was initiated in the recovery room and continued for 48 hours postoperatively; this procedure decreased morbidity after podiatric surgery in 69 patients who underwent 380 foot surgical procedures. The authors report a decrease in narcotic analgesic use as well. There is no mention of intraoperative steroid use to lessen postoperative discomfort. Wittenberg et al. (52) found no difference between ibuprofen and acetaminophen-codeine in a double-blind, randomized and multidose trial as far as daily pain level, number of tablets taken, use of additional medications, side effects or reasons for termination in postoperative foot patients.

Assisted limited weightbearing ambulation wearing a wooden-soled surgical shoe is allowed the first postoperative day. Early active and passive mobilization of joints are encouraged. However, care must be taken to ensure that mobilization is not too strenuous; it should not be so great as to exacerbate the usual inflammatory response to healing. Residual swelling is dissipated by active and passive range of motion exercises while the extremity is elevated. In most instances the patient is ambulatory within 24–48 hours with the use of postoperative wooden-soled shoes, internal and/or external fixation devices in place and the use of crutches or a walker for added stability as needed.

It is not unusual for the postoperative patient to experience an elevation in body temperature during the first 48 hours. This elevation may be a normal physiological response to the surgery or anesthetic used or be due to constipation, medication, urinary or respiratory tract infection or anesthetic hepatitis (53, 54). One should suspect surgical wound infection when temperature elevation exceeds 100° F and inflammatory response is greater than normally expected.

Infection must be distinguished from normal wound healing, incisional dehiscence and hematoma formation (53). Diagnosis of postoperative infection includes gram stain and aerobic and anaerobic culture and sensitivity studies of the offending organism. Tissue space infection is the most common, followed by infection of the tendon sheaths, fascial spaces, muscles, bone and lymphatic channels. Local infection may progress to bacteremia and septicemia (53). A red, poorly localized infection with little or no exudate may be due to *S. pyogenes*. A foul-smelling localized infection with little surrounding inflammation may be due to pseudomonas, whereas abscess formation with creamy, yellow, odorless pus might be caused by *S.aureus*. One should suspect gram negative organisms including *C.perfringens* and *E.coli* when tissue crepitus is found. Chronic indurated skin infection may be due to a deep mycosis, whereas a chronic paronychia may be aggravated by a superficial mycotic infection (54). Incision and drainage with use of an appropriate antibiotic are indicated. A broad spectrum antibiotic, such as dicloxicillin or a first-generation cephalosporin, may be prescribed IV, IM, or orally prior to receiving conclusive organism identification results. If clinical response is positive, changing the antibiotic to conform to culture and sensitivity study results is not necessary.

Osteomyelitis is an uncommon sequela to foot surgery. This bone inflammation secondary to infection may be caused by direct inoculation or may spread through the blood stream (hematogenous). Hematogenous osteomyelitis is seen mostly in children. The osteomyelitic process is divided into acute, subacute and chronic stages. Radiographic lytic changes do not appear until 10 to 14 days after initiation of infection. Technetium-99m phosphate and gallium citrate-67 bone scans may be helpful in early diagnosis. Gallium has an affinity for polymorphonuclear leukocytes. However, treatment should be instituted well before radiographic changes are evident. Bone infection leads to a formation of dead bone (sequestrum), new reactive bone formation (involucrum) and intraosseous channels (cloaca) sometimes coursing through the soft tissues as sinus tracts. Treatment of osteomyelitis is based on thorough surgical debridement with concomitant administration of appropriate organism-sensitivity-tested IV antibiotics (55). Delayed primary closure may be necessary. Ingress-egress saline or Ringer's solution may be used along with necessary antibiotics in a closed suction irrigation system after surgical debridement. In the early stages of osteomyelitis appropriate IV antibiotics usually are effective. Once bone destruction has taken place, it is almost always necessary to intervene surgically (Fig. 11.3). Schwartz and Marcinko (56) describe construction and utilization of the Blajwas-Schwartz drain®. This closed-suction irrigation drainage

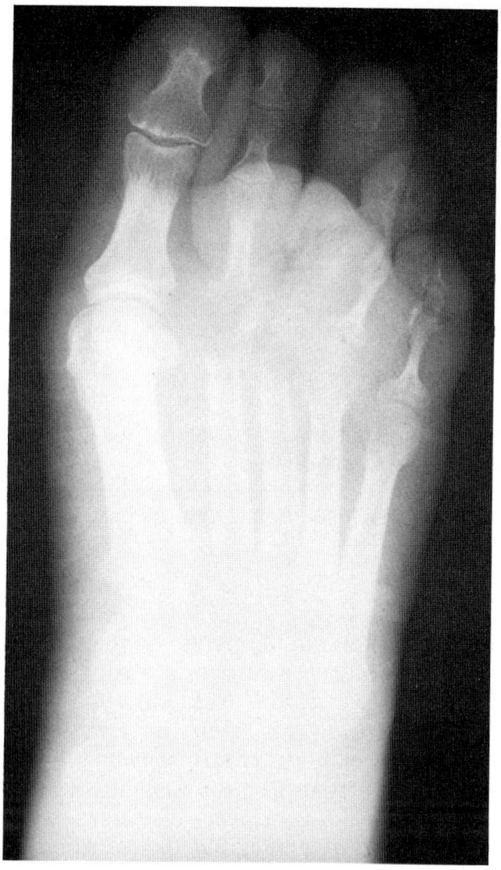

Figure 11.3. Osteomyelitis of the right forefoot; note the extensive bone destruction.

system is designed to be dependable, self-cannulizing and useful in the treatment of contaminated wounds and infected body parts.

The first postoperative redressing is done 4 or 5 days after elective surgery. An appropriate office setting is more desirable for this purpose than a hospital setting because antibiotic-resistant organisms are found to a much greater degree in a hospital than in an aseptic office environment. Adhesive tape splinting over the gauze dressings is utilized for 3–5 weeks.

Suture removal is performed just past the middle of the proliferative or repair phase of healing, from 11 to 15 days postoperatively (45). Urethane molds and other materials have been utilized effectively for postoperative splinting while mobilization of joints is taking place (58). Splinting is continued into the remodeling phase of healing, which begins after 3 weeks.

Within 3 weeks of forefoot arthroplasty procedures, impressions are taken for the construction of foot orthotic devices (6, 17, 18, 59). These are dispensed 4–5 weeks after surgery. Semirigid balanced orthoses with rearfoot control are recommended (60).

Postoperative Complications

Surgical treatment cannot be performed without danger and risk. However, postoperative complications may be minimized by adhering to the principles discussed earlier in this chapter. Complications encountered in foot surgery include phlebitis, atalectasis, infection, hematoma, devitalization and necrosis of tissues. Phlebitis, deep venous thrombosis and pulmonary embolism are rare complications of foot surgery. Care is taken not to irritate superficial varicosities by injudicious tourniquet application and to encourage active flexion and extension, immediately postoperatively, of those joints not involved in the surgical procedure. Patients with superficial varicosities may be instructed to wear support hose during the recuperative period. Ace bandages are sometimes used from the forefoot distally to just below the knee proximally. Settlemire and Beneson (61) present an overview of the pathophysiology, diagnosis, treatment and prevention of deep venous thrombosis and its major sequela, pulmonary embolism, in the podiatric surgical patient.

The patient is encouraged to breathe deeply while bedridden so as to ensure full lung expansion and avoid atalectasis, pneumonitis and upper respiratory distress. The smoker is advised to either stop smoking 1 week before surgery or, if this is not possible, to decrease the number of cigarettes smoked during this period. Patients with pre-existing pulmonary disease must be evaluated preoperatively with arterial blood gases, spirometry and chest x-ray. Prophylactic pre- and postoperative respiratory therapy may be helpful in those patients with compromised pulmonary status.

The problems in surgical technique noted in Table 11.1 predispose to an ex-

Table 11.1.
Postoperative Complications[a]: Causal Relationships[b]

1.	Multiple improper and inappropriate skin, capsular and soft tissue incisions
2.	Unnecessary and excessive handling of tissues during procedure
3.	Surgical trauma through sharp and blunt retraction of skin and soft tissues, e.g., the use of multitooth forceps on skin and soft tissues
4.	The use of heavier and greater numbers of suture material than are necessary to repair the surgical site adequately, e.g., ligature of superficial forefoot veins
5.	Retention of surgical debris within the surgical site
6.	Allowing tissues to become dry
7.	Allowing irrigation solutions to become too warm
8.	Excessive use of electrical cautery, e.g., for control of bleeding from superficial veins in the forefoot
9.	Improper dressings, e.g., too tight around bony prominences or too loose around the operative site
10.	Inadequate postoperative care, e.g., too much movement or not enough movement, not using ice for the first 48 hours, in-hospital redressing and exposure to infection

[a] Skin, soft tissue and bone infection, phlebitis, atalectasis, necrosis, hematoma, chronic edema, vascular impairment, anatomical instability and deformity.
[b] From references 3, 81, 157–159.

traordinary inflammatory response. In the arthritic patient this response is manifested to a greater degree, as inflammation leads to tissue compromise with a greater chance of bacterial infection. Subsequent loss of vascularity, devitalization and tissue necrosis ensue (Fig. 11.4). Excessive swelling, limitation of joint motion, fibrosis and recurrence of deformity are often directly attributable to poor surgical technique (19).

Causalgia and Sudeck's atrophy are an uncommon sequelae of foot surgery. Care must be taken not to operate on the patient with causalgia or Sudeck's atrophy (see Chapter 10, Foot and Ankle Trauma).

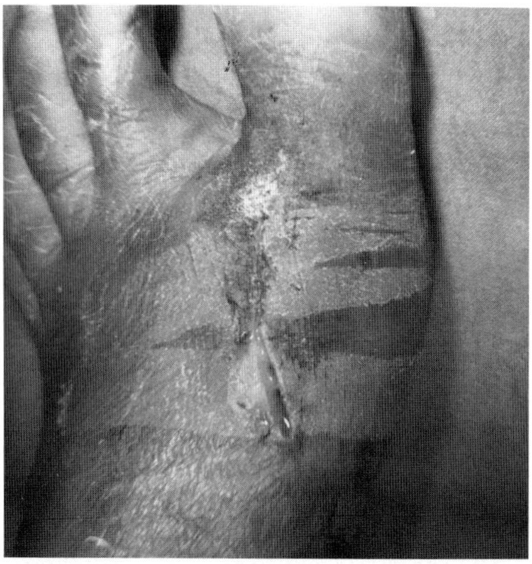

Figure 11.4. Skin dehiscence secondary to excessive trauma to the skin margins intraoperatively.

Malposition, malunion, nonunion, regeneration of bone and the occurrence of an arthritic painful pseudoarthrosis may complicate foot surgery. Reinherz et al. (62) cite proper surgical technique, age and sex of the patient and latent trauma as factors affecting postoperative bone regeneration. The authors advise application of bone wax to the stump of the remaining phalanx in digital arthroplasty procedures as an aid in preventing bone regeneration. Avascular necrosis is a rare postoperative complication (see Chapter 10, Foot and Ankle Trauma).

Special postoperative problems and complications with the use of implant materials in joint reconstruction are listed in Table 11.2.

Special Considerations in Arthritic Foot Surgery

The evolutionary nature of collagen disease is such that the clinical course of the disease involves acute exacerbations and remissions. Infrequently, the disease may involve few acute exacerbations, with no progression of the disease process, or it may have continuous acute exacerbations with rapid progression of deformity.

The podiatric surgeon and internist

Table 11.2.
Postoperative Complications: Implant Surgery

1. Infection (157, 160)
2. Delayed healing (157)
3. Excessive inflammation and chronic swelling due to bone detritus, Silastic chards, reactive synovitis, foreign body reaction and soft tissue hyperplasia (19, 157, 161, 162)
4. Rejection of implant (157, 160)
5. Failure of the implant material (58, 102, 103, 114, 137, 161, 163, 164) (Fig. 11.5)
6. Stress fracture of the involved bone or adjacent bone (15, 157)
7. Erosion of the juxtapositional articular surface when using a hemi-implant (58, 102, 103, 114, 160, 163)
8. Proliferation of bone around implant base (63, 102, 103, 114, 161, 165) (Fig. 11.6)
9. Dislocation of implant (157) (Fig. 11.7)
10. Avascular necrosis (157)
11. Sudeck's atrophy
12. Lymphadenitis (166)
13. Pseudocyst formation (juxta and periarticular)
14. Surgical technique error (164)

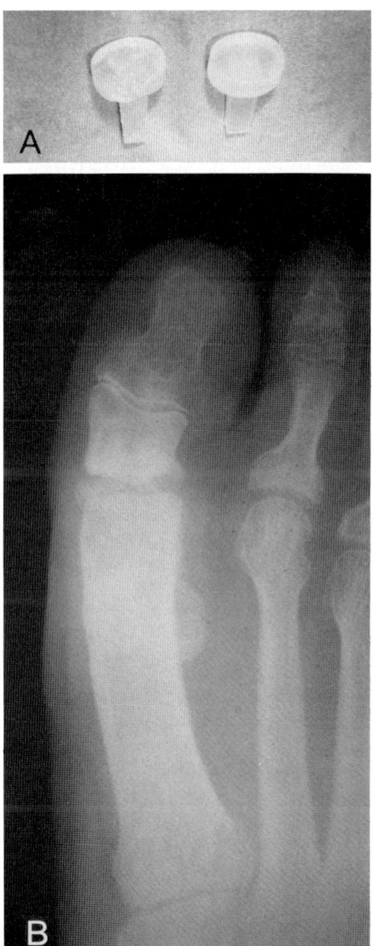

Figure 11.5. *A.*(left) Swanson design hemi-implant degeneration after 7 years in vivo; (right) new Swanson design hemi-implant. *B.* Swanson design hemi-implant degeneration 3 years after insertion for inappropriate "Keller" bunionectomy.

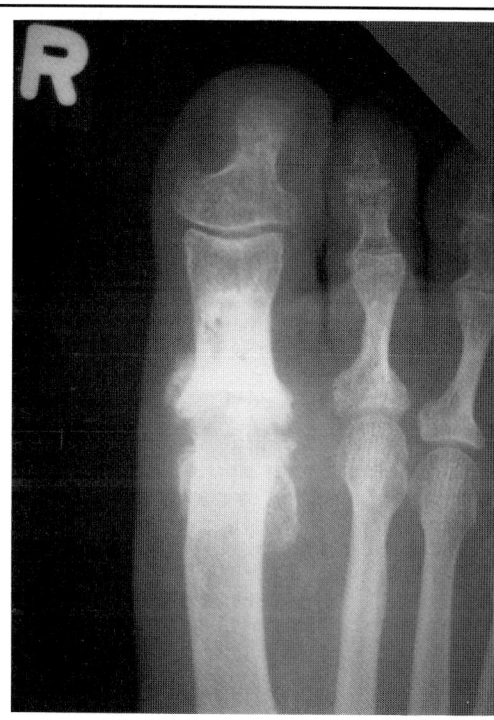

Figure 11.6. Proliferation of bone around Swanson design hemi-implant base 5 years after insertion.

(rheumatologist) must work together. The collagen diseases affect glandular and organ function, as well as joints, synovia, tendons, muscles, nerves and blood vessels. Potential occurrence of adrenal insufficiency in those patients receiving steroid medications mandates steroid coverage before, sometimes during and usually after surgery. Various dosage regimens have been recommended (45). Doubling

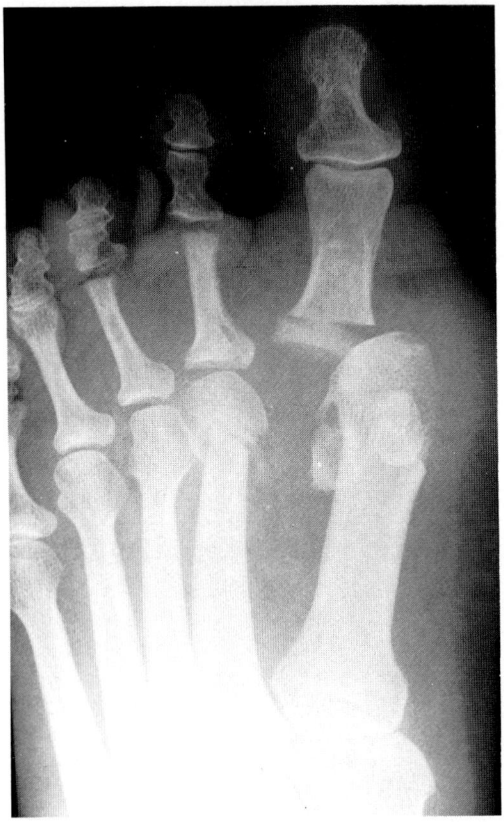

Figure 11.7. Great toe and implant lateral dislocation.

the usual steroid dose the day before surgery, prescribing 1½ times the usual dose the evening of the day of surgery, and then resuming the usual dose the day after surgery is typical of the recommended steroid coverage dosage regimens. Patients receiving steroid medications have a greater predisposition to infection, osteoporosis and avascular necrosis. Patients receiving penicillamine are predisposed to wound dehiscense due to interference with collagen synthesis. The anticoagulant effect of long-term salicylate therapy may predispose to hematoma formation.

The primary aim of all foot surgery is to facilitate pain-free function with the minimal amount of structural change needed to produce the desired result. Surgery for the arthritic patient, as with surgery for the nonarthritic, cannot and must not be "cookbook" in outlook or performance. Years of experience coupled with good surgical judgment are essential. Because of the evolutionary basis of all the arthritides, it is of the utmost importance that the podiatric surgeon have a background in dealing with the somatic disease entity and the psychologically distinct elements of the various disease states. Because arthritic disorders are evolutionary, surgical procedures appropriate at one stage of the disease may not be appropriate at another. Psychological variables, such as fear, pain, anxiety, and age, play an important role in the behavioral outcome of podiatric surgery. Dealing with these and other psychological factors is essential to the healing process (63).

Individualization of surgical approach is required. Indications and approach depend upon a sound biomechanical didactic and experiential base (5, 7, 9, 10, 17, 18, 45). A deep and detailed understanding of podiatric biomechanics is essential to the primary surgical aim, i.e., pain-free function. Without training and experience in podiatric biomechanics, the surgeon does a disservice to the arthritic patient about to undergo an operation.

Deformity results from a combination of disease process, multiple minimal trauma and inefficient function (7, 64). Relief depends on correction of the deformity and control of inefficient function (24, 65). Deformity correction is achieved surgically, and control of function is achieved biomechanically (7). The obviation of inappropriate mechanical forces can only be attained through control of inefficient function (7, 11, 24). The construction of appropriate foot orthotic devices is a postoperative necessity (4, 6). Concomitant with deformity, the collagen disorders affect the microcirculation to bone, joints, soft tissue and skin. Resultant neuroangiopathy requires the greatest diligence, experience and judgment on behalf of the surgeon. It has been reported that 20% of the rheumatoid arthritic population has extraskeletal manifestations of the disease (66). Because cardiopulmonary and cervical spine disease secondary to the rheumatoid disease state are prevalent, postoperative respiratory therapy and preoperative evaluation of cervical spine status in those patients receiving general inhalation anesthesia are indicated (66). Special care should be exercised in patients with Raynaud's phenomenon. Postoperative posterior tibial periarterial local anesthetic injection procedures may be helpful.

Acute stage changes in rheumatoid arthritis involve the synovia, with a predilection for areas subject to multiple minimal trauma, e.g., beneath metatarsal heads and areas of tendon insertion. An area that is frequently involved is the insertion of the Achilles tendon. A more profound early synovitis and/or late nodular formation may be found at the insertion of the Achilles tendon in the presence of gastrocnemius or gastrocnemius/soleus equinus. Multiple peritendinous steroid injections may lead to spontaneous rupture of the Achilles tendon (see Chapter 10, Foot and Ankle Trauma). Greater soft tissue pathology is found beneath a plantarflexed first metatarsal ray. The plantar aspect of the great toe interphalangeal joint is more readily involved with synovitis leading to painful nodular formation when there is limitation of dorsiflexion at the first metatarsophalangeal joint. Excision of painful rheumatoid nodules that interfere with function is the preferred treatment (67). Attention to function is mandatory. Later cartilage and bone involvement with pannus formation, subchondral cystic formation and cystic changes at chondro-osseous joint margins, accompanied by great pain and debility, may require surgical intervention for relief.

Fibular deviation of the toes with concomitant rearfoot valgus occurs insidiously. This deviation does not seem to correspond with the disease process alone. There appears to be a greater correlation with the foot becoming or remaining, through compensation to the disease process, a mobile pronatory adaptor throughout the stance phase of gait through propulsion (5, 6). Compensatory inefficient function, which allows the foot to adapt to the substrate to a greater degree, may avoid discomfort initially. However, the adverse affects of inefficient function over a period of time lead to greater pain and pathology (7, 64). Therefore, foot orthosis control is just as essential in the early presurgical stage (4). Concomitant medical management is essential at the time of surgical indication. Although rest, salicylates and physical therapy remain the basis of medical treatment in the acute stage rheumatoid arthritic, foot orthotic devices and intra-articular steroid injection (no more than three over a 3-week period in any 6-month period) are of continued benefit. Surgical intervention is rarely indicated in the acute stages. However, synovectomy in select cases can be of major benefit in terms of comfort and function (3, 68). Synovectomy does not appear to slow the pathological process.

Foot surgery is contraindicated in the acute, quick-progression arthritic stage and in the elderly patient and others with primary or secondary neurovascular impairment. Foot surgery in the nonacute phase, medically stable, and nonvascularly compromised arthritic patient may be performed under regional nerve block, i.e., ankle block local anesthesia, as well as general inhalation anesthesia as indicated by surgical experience and judgment. Foot surgery should precede upper extremity corrective procedures (3). Deformity is not the only criteria for surgical intervention. Pain and adverse function are of greater importance. One must pay attention to the psychological position of the patient in order for the surgical treatment plan to be successful. Severe osteoporosis is a contraindication for implant arthroplasty.

Gouty arthritic foot joints are amenable to surgical correction. Excision of painful tophaceous deposits is indicated when the soft tissue deposit is subjected to chronic irritation from shoes or adverse function. Occasionally, a tophus may become infected or develop a chronic bursa or draining sinus from shoe or mechanical pressure. After the infection has been successfully treated, excision of the tophus, bursa and/or sinus is indicated. Rarely does involvement of the first metatarsophalangeal joint require excision of the first metatarsal head. Surgical procedures should be oriented toward preservation of functional joint integrity.

Surgery is contraindicated during an acute attack of primary or secondary hyperuricemia. Medical control of the gouty process is mandatory. Acute attacks at the first metatarsophalangeal joint, ankle joint and the calcaneal insertion of the plantar fascia and Achilles tendon must be properly diagnosed. Pre- and postoperative use of nonsteroidal anti-inflammatory medications (NSAIDs) is important in minimizing the stimulation of an acute gouty attack by surgical trauma. Pre-, intra- and postoperative hydration of the gouty patient is essential. Intraoperative use of a short-acting steroid in the involved area is of benefit.

Acute pyogenic arthritis affecting the foot presents special difficulties. Pyogenic arthritis is more prevalent in times of combat. However, a local puncture wound or hematogenous source may be implicated. The sequela of injury from mines, mortars, grenades and gunshots may result in an acute pyogenic arthritis progressing to osteomyelitis. Appropriate organism-sensitive systemic and local ingress-egress antibiotic therapy are essential. Delayed primary closure, after the infective process has been eliminated, is necessary to ensure a positive result (69).

Myopathies and neuropathies, which affect the distal lower extremities and are associated with muscle imbalance and motor and sensory loss, may result in adverse joint function and subsequent traumatic or neurotrophic arthritis. Interdigital neuroma, tarsal tunnel syndrome and other nerve entrapments are prevalent in the arthritic patient. Chronic inflammation and deformity predispose to multiple levels of nerve entrapment. Spinal cord lesions, tabes dorsalis, diabetic neuropathy, Friedrich's ataxia, Charcot-Marie-Tooth disease, amyotrophic lateral sclerosis and paralysis may lead to adverse foot joint function and arthritic disorders. The neurotrophic-insensitive foot must be approached with caution. Bony prominences, preventing healing of under- or overlying ulcerations, may sometimes have to be surgically excised. Fusion procedures are sometimes necessary to prevent further joint deterioration. Often, accompanying large vessel, small vessel and basement membrane disease adversely affect a favorable result. The surgical approach must be individualized to fit the overall criterion of pain-free function. Foot, ankle and leg orthotic and bracing devices are often indicated pre- and postoperatively.

Tubercular and gonococcal infections, though rare, do occasionally affect foot joints with resultant arthritic changes. It is important that a diagnosis be made prior to surgery and that medical treatment be instituted.

With the exception of the most severe cases of neurotrophic arthritis, amputation of the toes or foot is rarely indicated for treatment of an arthritic joint or joints.

Surgical Approach to Foot Joints

The surgical approach to foot joints depends on the ability to control abnormal pronation postoperatively (5, 6, 17, 18, 70). The abnormally pronated foot predisposes to posttraumatic arthritic changes due to joint instability (7, 24). Resultant digital, metatarsophalangeal, tarsal, and ankle joint deformity involve arthritic changes (64, 65).

Abnormal limitations of efficient subtalar and midtarsal joint function, as seen in anterior, posterior, global, and combined cavus foot deformity, predispose to lateral ankle arthritis and instability and/or traction exostoses at the base of the fifth metatarsal, medial navicular tuberosity, and plantar and posterior calcaneus. The ability to control abnormal mechanical forces through muscle stretching and strengthening exercises and foot orthotic devices affects surgical procedure selection and surgical result. Intrinsic muscle atrophy and/or denervation of specific intrinsic muscles also alters the surgical approach. Posttraumatic arthritis of foot joints is aggravated by gastrocnemius, gastrocnemius-soleus and ankle equinus (71).

Sesamoids

Sesamoid involvement in osteoarthritis is seen between the sesamoid and the first metatarsal head. Osteophytic changes may predispose to plantar skin lesions. Aquino et al. (72) report a study of 26 tibial sesamoid planing procedures for intractable plantar keratoma. The subjective success rate was 88.8%, and the objective success rate was 76.9%. The authors recommend not performing this procedure when there is a first metatarsal declination angle of more than 8°. The procedure was not found to alter the biomechanics of the first ray. Rheumatoid arthritic changes may progress from sesamoid deformity to fusion of both sesamoids. Normally misshapen, broad unipartite, bi- and tripartite sesamoids must be differentiated from the pathological (15). As toes contract, the submetatarsal head fat pad moves distally in the osteoarthritic foot. The rheumatoid foot exhibits fat pad atrophy, severe rearfoot valgus, fibular deviation and dorsal contraction of the toes and the metatarsophalangeal joints with secondary plantarflexion of the lesser metatarsals, pronation of the fifth rays, adduction of the first rays, extension at the distal interphalangeal joints and flexion at the proximal interphalangeal joints. Osteoarthritis of the sesamoids must be differentiated from posttraumatic sesamoiditis, synovitis and osteochondritis. Sesamoidal osteochondritic symptoms precede radiographic changes by several months. Removal of a painful medial sesamoid is effective (18). Care must be taken not to interfere with flexor hallucis longus function and to repair the medial limb of the flexor hallucis brevis (73). Troy (74) reports on the use of a Downing cartilage knife for excision of the tibial sesamoid in 16 cases. The author believes there to be a lesser incidence of flexor hallucis longus injury utilizing this technique. Lateral sesamoidectomy is commonly performed during joint arthroplasty procedures.

Plantar hallux interphalangeal joint sesamoids either may be bony and easily visualized on x-ray or may be fibrocartilagenous and not identifiable on x-ray. The author has seen feet with multiple (2–4) fibrocartilagenous plantar hallux interphalangeal sesamoids. The sesamoid, which is usually invested on the dorsal surface of the flexor hallucis longus tendon, often predisposes to distal phalangeal extensus and painful plantar tyloma. Hallux interphalangeal joint extensus may lead to hallux toenail pathology secondary to shoe pressure. Incisional approaches include the "U"-shaped, transverse linear and medial. The transverse approach may encompass the presenting skin lesion, as well as a section of flexor hallucis longus, which when repaired corrects the soft tissue extensus. This procedure may be accomplished prior to dorsal contracture. Care must be taken to repair the flexor hallucis longus whatever the surgical approach. Painful involvement of periarticular lesser metatarsophalangeal joint sesamoids sometimes requires surgical excision of the involved sesamoid.

Phalanges

Phalangeal surgery is indicated for resection of tumor, exostosis and angular correction. Osteoid osteoma of a phalanx must be differentiated from unicameral and aneurysmal bone cyst, fibrous dysplasia and osteomyelitis. Salicylate ingestion results in abatement of osteoid osteoma pain. Partial amputation (distal Syme procedure) may be required to eradicate the lesion totally (75). Subungual exostosis and osteochondroma are best approached by a distal transverse incision with reduction of the lesion by means of hand or power instrumentation. If a total matricectomy is to be performed, the bone lesion may be resected through a distal midline incision from the transverse matricectomy incision. Pinch callus, affecting the hallux and associated with improper function or increase in the hallux abductus angle, may be treated effectively by excising the offending distal medial plantar aspect of the proximal phalanx or the proximal medial plantar aspect of the distal phalanx and/or correcting abnormal great toe position. Adductory osteotomy of the proximal phalanx at the proximal or distal metaphyseal level or excising a section of proximal phalanx may be indicated to correct abnormal great toe abduction, eversion or length pattern (76, 77) (Fig. 11.8).

Interphalangeal Joints

Arthritic involvement of the interphalangeal joints is a common finding. Heberden's nodes are pathognomonic of osteoarthritis involving the distal interphalangeal joints of the fingers and toes. Psoriatic arthritis often affects the distal interphalangeal joints. "Swan-neck" deformity at the distal interphalangeal joint level is commonly found in the toes of patients with systemic lupus erythematosus, rheumatoid arthritis and other collagen disorders. Proximal interphalangeal joint involvement is frequently seen in the multiple minimal cumulative trauma-induced arthritic hammertoe deformity seen in the abnormally functioning, osteoarthritic and rheumatoid foot (78).

The progressive approach to digital sur-

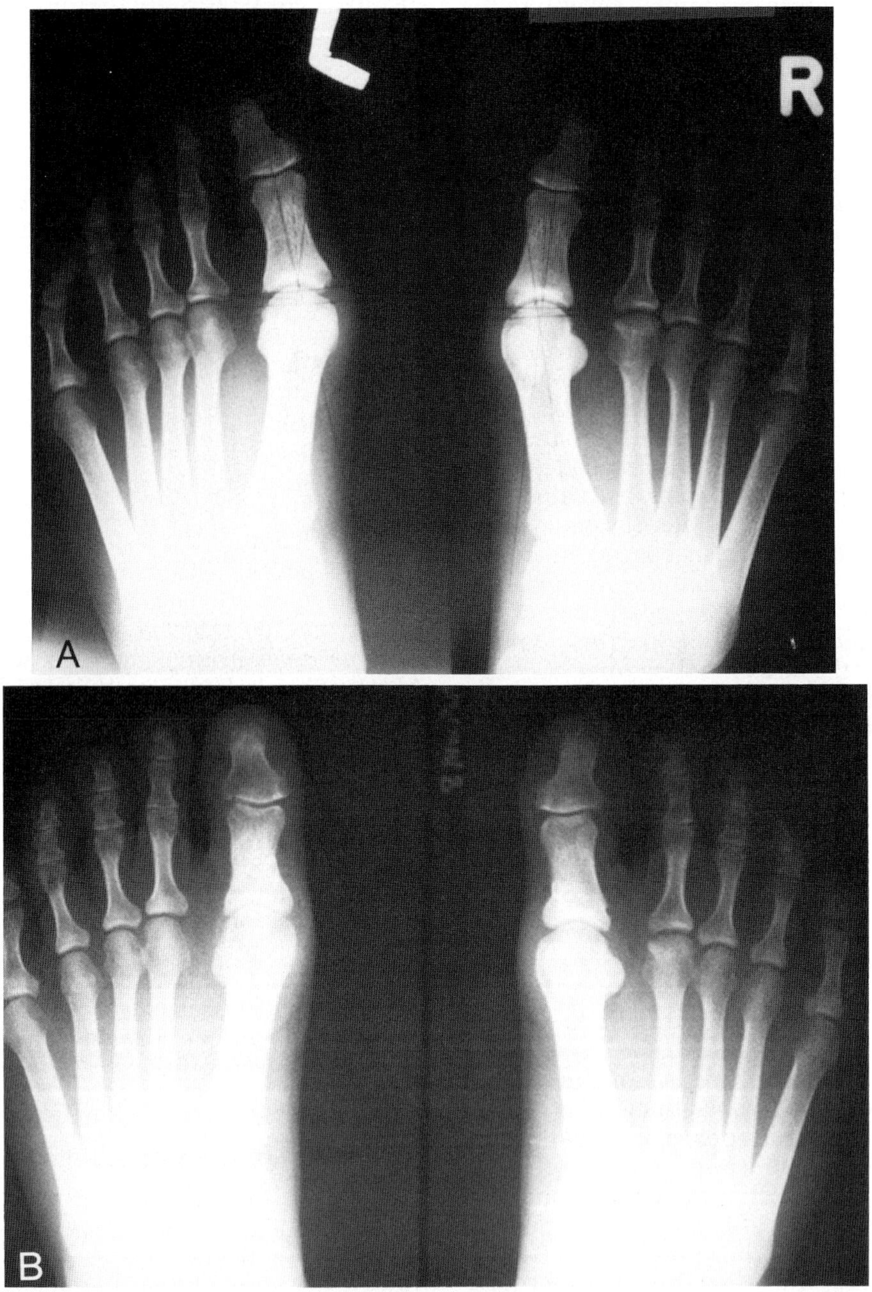

Figure 11.8. *A*, Preoperative view of pathological distal articular set angles bilaterally. *B*, Postoperative view 7 months after proximal metaphyseal great toe proximal phalanx adductory wedge osteotomies with wire fixation bilaterally.

gery (79) is a rational, functionally oriented approach to the arthritically involved toe. Proximal and/or middle phalangeal head resection, middle phalangectomy, extensor hood recession or release, extensor tendon lengthening or tenotomy proximal to the metatarsophalangeal joint, flexor tenotomy, metatarsophalangeal joint capsulotomy (dorsal medial and dorsal lateral), plantar metatarsophalangeal joint capsular release and fusion of the proximal and/or distal interphalangeal joint are useful procedures for correction of digital arthritic deformity (80, 81) (see Chapter 9) (Fig. 11.9). The experienced use of the transverse surgical approach across interphalangeal joints is recommended. Care must be taken to preserve the dorsal medial and dorsal lateral neurovascular anatomy. The small cartilagenous disk found on the underside of the dorsal aponeurosis over interphalangeal joints is excised along with a transverse section of dorsal aponeurosis. Closure through this approach results in a straighter alignment of the digit. If the great toe interphalangeal joint is operated on, this joint must be fused because arthroplasty has not proved to be of long-term benefit (82). When the base of a lesser toe proximal phalanx must be removed as an independent procedure, syndactyly to an adjoining toe is necessary to provide length and stability. (Fig. 11.10) Combinations of procedures may be indicated in order to correct digital subluxations (45, 78).

Johnson and Hugar (83) provide an excellent review of the surgical procedures described for a congenital digiti quinti varus (hyperextension of the fifth toe; overlapping fifth toe; overriding fifth toe; elevated, contracted and varus fifth toe). When discovered soon after birth, treatment includes stretching and manipulation with adhesive strapping of the fifth toe into abduction and plantar flexion. In the Lantzounis procedure the long extensor tendon is transferred through the surgical neck of the fifth metatarsal. The Lapidus procedure is performed by transferring the long extensor tendon insertion to the lateral aspect of the head of the proximal phalanx into the conjoined ten-

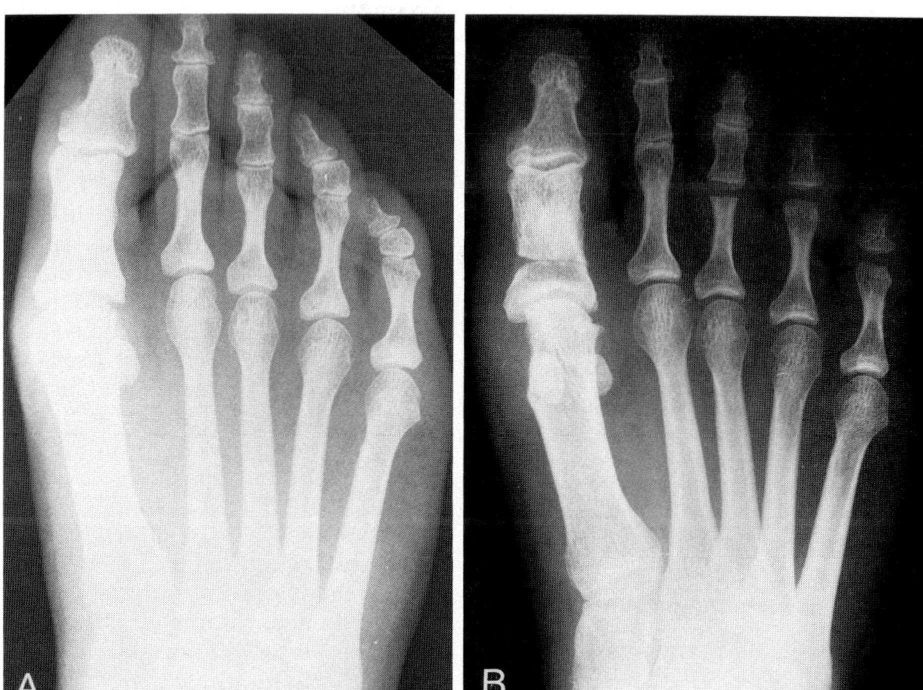

Figure 11.9. *A,* Preoperative painful digital deformities. *B,* Postoperative correction utilizing a functional surgical approach to digital deformity.

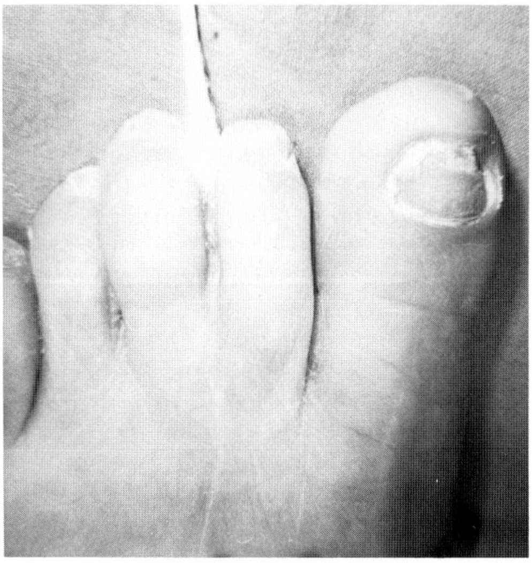

Figure 11.10. Surgical syndactyly of unstable second toe to third toe.

dons of the flexor digiti quinti brevis and abductor digiti quinti. Goodwin and Swisher perform a "Y" skin plasty, dorsal capsulotomy at the fifth metatarsophalangeal joint and "Z" plasty lengthening of the long extensor tendon. For the pediatric patient, Wilson advises a V-Y elongation of the tight skin folds dorsally at the fourth toe web space. Kelikian (84) removes the proximal phalanx and syndactylizes the fifth to the fourth toe, and Butler performs a racquet-shaped incision around the fifth toe with capsulotomy and long extensor tenotomy. Other procedures include plantar incision on the fifth digit, dorsal medial soft tissue release and "Z" plasty incision with or without partial or total proximal phalanx excision.

Depending upon the degree of deformity contracture the author prefers utilizing a plantar skin tuck, partial or total proximal phalangeal excision with syndactyly to the fourth toe, long extensor and capsular release through "Z" plasty skin incision and middle phalangectomy if that is the level of deformity (Fig.11.11).

Metatarsophalangeal Joints

The metatarsophalangeal joints, specifically the first metatarsophalangeal joint, have received a great deal of attention in the surgical literature (17, 84). First metatarsophalangeal joint arthritis and deformity are most commonly caused by multiple minimal cumulative trauma brought on by inefficient function (7, 45). This joint and the lesser metatarsophalangeal joints may have rheumatoid, gouty, osteoarthritic, and other arthritic involvement as well. When cartilage is intact and the joint is not fully dislocated, the joint can usually be left intact. Medial, dorsal and lateral first metatarsal head and proximal phalangeal base osteophytes are excised (17, 85, 86). In the case of a dorsiflexed or long first metatarsal with dorsal bony proliferation and intact joint cartilage, the dorsal distal aspect of the first metatarsal head is excised at an angle (17, 87). Drago et al. (88) and Cohn and Kanat (89) present excellent reviews of hallux limitus etiology, clinical and radiographic findings and surgical treatment. Metatarsal and phalangeal torsional and/or length abnormalities may have to be corrected to obtain a better functional result (76, 77).

Rzonca, Levitz and Lue (90) describe the three stages of hallux equinus, which they equate with the development of hallux limitus and hallux rigidus. The first stage occurs secondary to pronatory disorders and presents with no bony pathology. There is only soft tissue contracture. Treatment is through foot orthotic devices. The second stage involves both osteophytic changes and soft tissue contracture and is treated with orthoses and surgical chielectomy. The third stage presents as hallux rigidus and requires either orthotic devices or shoe modification to redistribute weight or first metatarsophalangeal joint arthroplasty with or without implant.

Spinner (91) describes the pathomechanics of the hallux abductus deformity and proper radiographic technique to interpret relationships. Evaluation of the proximal articular set angle (PASA), distal articular set angle (DASA), interphalangeal angle, hallux abductus angle and metatarsus primus adductus angle is essential to determining which procedure should be performed for hallux abductus and hallux abductovalgus deformity (92). Foot and joint type, sesamoid position, metatarsal and digital length pattern, age of patient and associated foot, ankle, knee, and hip deformity and disease must also be taken into consideration (17, 93). Care should be exercised not to incise or interfere with the secondary tendon slip from the extensor digitorum longus inserting into the medial dorsal aspect of the first metatarsophalangeal joint capsule. This extensor hallucis capsularis tendon seems to act as the great toe is dorsiflexed to pull the capsule away from the joint.

Over 100 surgical procedures for first metatarsophalangeal joint deformity have been described in the literature (84). Almost all have been discarded, with the exception of the Mayo, Hueter, Silver, McBride, Reverdin, Peabody, Hohmann, Mitchell, Austin, Lapidus, Logroscino, Akin, Trethowan, and McKeever procedures and their many variations and refinements. (17, 84). The formulation of podiatric criteria in first metatarsophalangeal joint surgery has greatly progressed in terms of avoiding confusion about this important area of foot surgery (94). McCarthy (95, 96), through application of cryomicrotomy, reviews the surgical anatomy of the first metatarsal ray along with the common surgical procedures used for correction of hallux abductovalgus deformity.

Congenital and acquired hallux varus, because of functional interference or pain, may require surgical correction. (Fig. 11.13). The step-wise surgical approach to acquired hallux adductus or hallux varus is a rational means of attaining the desired correction. Medial first metatarsal head capsulotomy and/or abductor hallucis tenotomy, mobilization of the medially displaced medial sesamoid to its proper location, excision of the medially displaced medial sesamoid, tightening of the lateral first metatarsal phalangeal joint capsule, extensor digitorum longus lengthening and resection of the base of the great toe proximal phalanx, in the order of achieving correction, are the preferred approaches (Fig. 11.14). Wood (97) describes a total joint stripping procedure (TJR) for total release of all medial soft tissues used for correction of iatrogenic hallux varus. If discovered within the first 3 weeks after surgery when the medial sesamoid is not

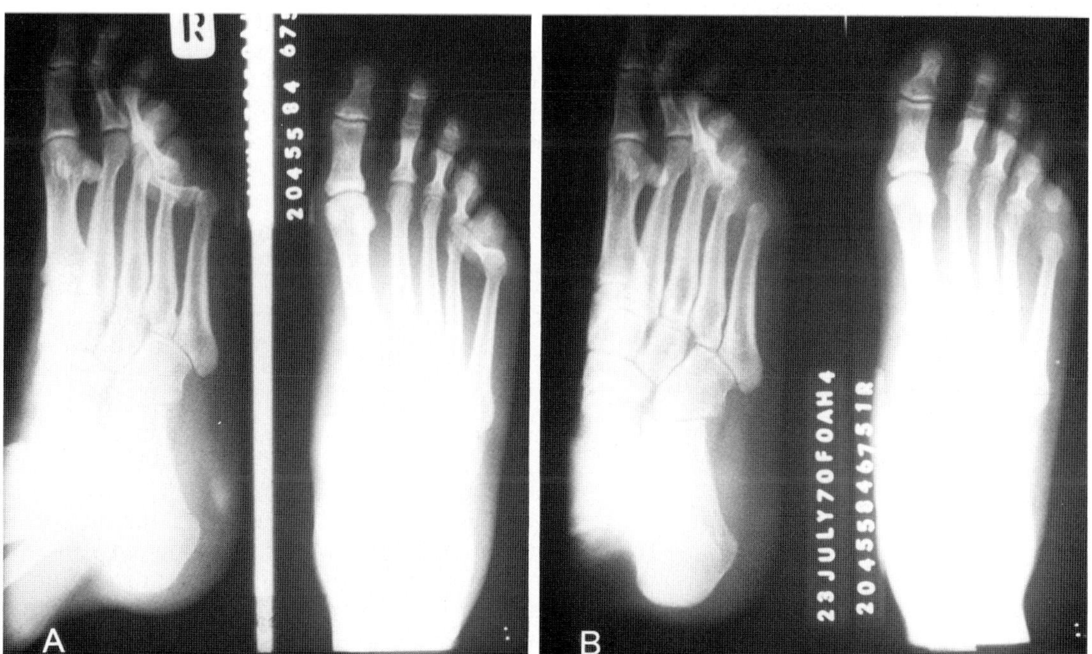

Figure 11.11. *A,* Preoperative severe digiti quinti varus. *B,* Postoperative proximal phalangectomy and syndactyly to fourth toe.

lodged medial to the first metatarsal head, a dynamic elastoplast sling may be used to force the great toe into a more abducted position.

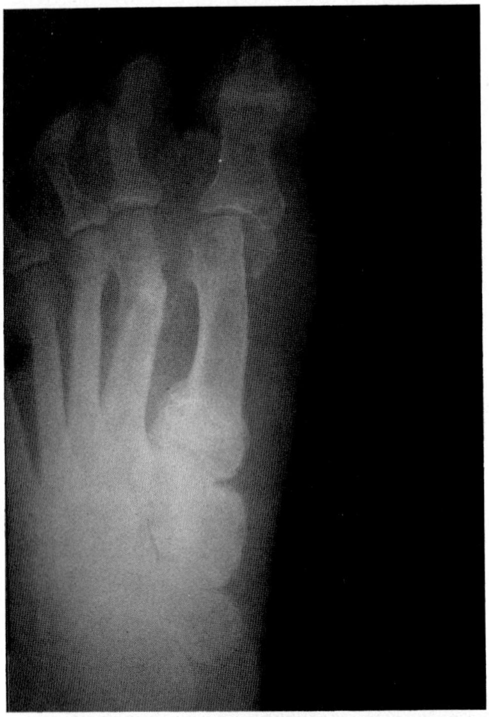

Figure 11.13. Iatrogenic hallux varus secondary to excessive reduction of metatarsus primus adductus angle. Note medial sesamoid location medial to the first metatarsal head.

When the arthritic process has resulted in joint destruction, various first metatarsophalangeal joint arthroplasty procedures have been recommended (17, 84, 97, 98). It is important not to remove too much bone from the base of the great toe proximal phalanx when performing the Keller procedure as doing so leads to a poor functional result. Rather than dealing with eponyms to describe a surgical procedure specifically, the experienced surgeon should do what is necessary according to preoperative and intraoperative evaluation and postoperative biomechanical, psychological and living requirements.

Arthroplasty and/or fusion procedures for nonarthritic or arthritic interphalangeal and metatarsophalangeal joints are performed in conjunction with indicated metatarsal and phalangeal angulation, shortening and lengthening procedures. Procedures or combinations of procedures are determined by entire lower extremity biomechanical evaluation, leg length differential, intrinsic joint pathology and angular bone measurement differentials (5, 14, 17, 19) (Table 11.3).

Fusion of the first metatarsophalangeal joint should be avoided in the stable foot (27, 60). This procedure invariably leads to traumatic arthritis of the great toe interphalangeal joint (100). Although non-

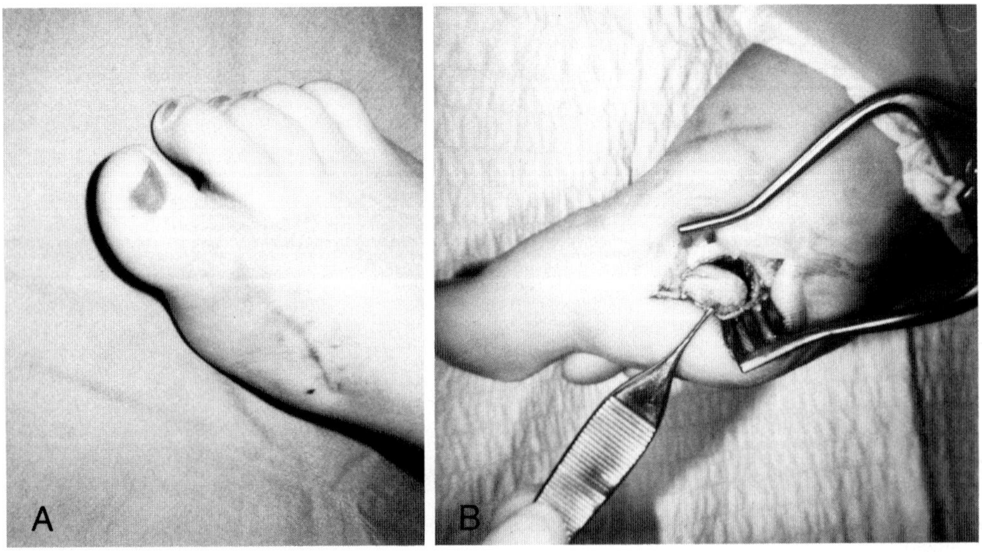

Figure 11.14. *A,* Surgically induced hallux varus, *B,* Excision of medially displaced medial sesamoid.

weightbearing metatarsal heads are the primary goal when operating on a rheumatoid arthritic forefoot, indicated excision of lesser metatarsal heads and/or proximal phalangeal bases should be performed in such a manner as to maintain a functional metatarsal protrusion, parabola and length pattern (80, 101). More bone should be removed plantarly than dorsally when excising the second, third and fourth metatarsal heads. The fifth metatarsal head should be excised in such a way as to ensure more bone removal laterally and plantarly. The incidence of bone regeneration dictates excision of more, rather than less, bone in rheumatoid arthritic foot surgical procedures (66). Because the fifth metatarsal has an independent axis of motion, there are few functional complications (45) associated with fifth metatarsal head excision in an arthritic fifth metatarsophalangeal joint. (Fig. 11.15).

The surgical approach to tailor's bunion

Table 11.3.
Metatarsal and Phalangeal Angulation, Shortening and Lengthening Procedures

1. Dorsiflexory wedge osteotomy (extension osteotomy) (18)
2. Plantarflexory wedge osteotomy (flexion osteotomy)
3. Adductory wedge osteotomy (open or closed wedge) (17)
4. Abductory wedge osteotomy (open or closed wedge) (17, 167) (Fig. 11.12)
5. Two-plane wedge osteotomy (sagittal and frontal plane (18)
6. Step-down osteotomy (17, 124)
7. Chevron "V" osteotomy (18, 125)
8. Crecentric osteotomy (18, 168)
9. Extension osteoarthrotomy (18)
10. Collectomy (18)
11. Plantar condylectomy (70, 18)
12. Horizontal "V" osteotomy (169).

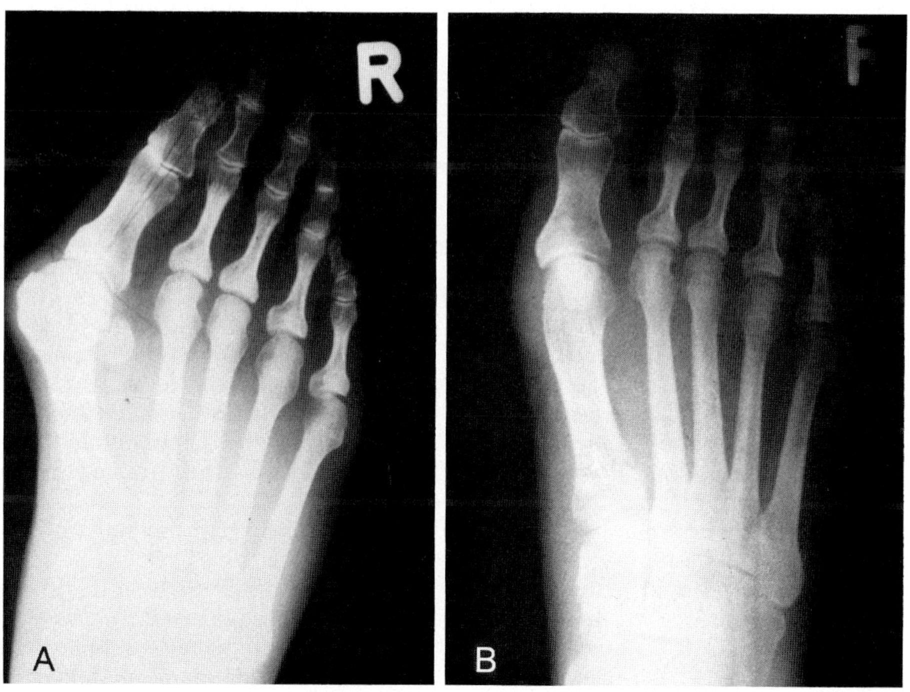

Figure 11.12. *A,* Preoperative, hallux abductovalgus with metatarsus primus adductus, *B,* Postoperative, reduction of deformity.

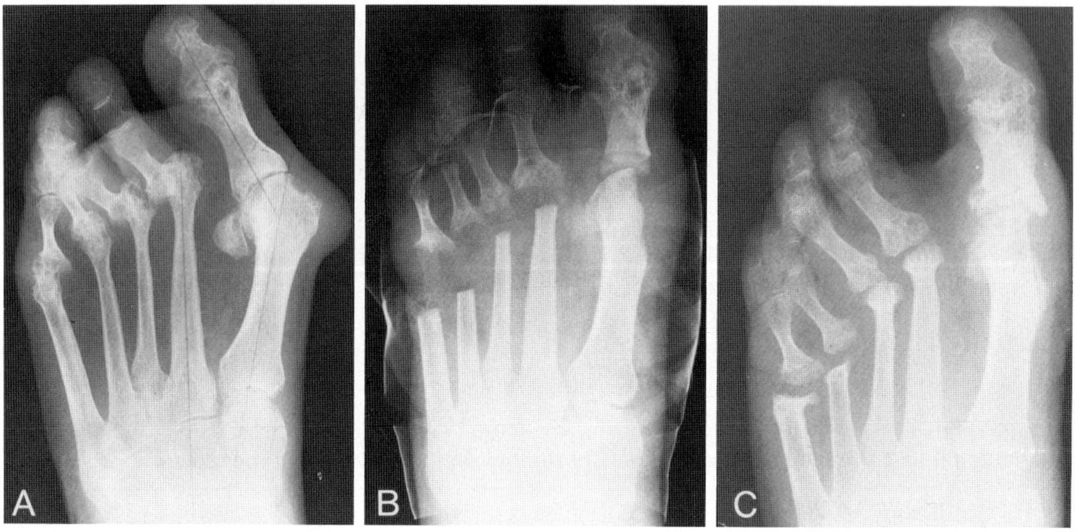

Figure 11.15. *A*, Preoperative painful rheumatoid arthritically involved metatarsophalangeal joints. *B*, Postoperative result of combination lesser metatarsal head and great toe phalangeal base resection with Silastic implant. *C*, Same patient 4 years later. Note partial regeneration of metatarsal heads and proliferation of bone around implant base.

and fifth metatarsal pathology depends on function, the level of deformity and associated arthritis, concurrent fifth toe deformity and presence or absence of intractable plantar or lateral tyloma or bursitis. Deformity may present in the head, neck or fifth metatarsal shaft. A pronated or abducted fifth ray may present alone or in combination with a splay foot or digiti quinti varus deformity. Plantar prominence of the fifth metatarsal head may be a result of forefoot varus or cavus foot deformity. Surgical treatment of fifth metatarsal pathology ranges from removal of an enlarged fifth metatarsal head to an extension-adduction biplane osteotomy at the level of the surgical neck for plantar and lateral prominence (Fig 11.16). A proximal metaphyseal adductory wedge osteotomy with wire fixation may be performed for an abducted fifth metatarsal. Plantar condylectomy and dorsal tilt-up osteotomy or metatarsal head excision may be performed for intractable plantar tyloma. Lateral condylectomy with or without osteotomy may be performed for distal metatarsal bowing, tailor's bunion and painful bursitis (Fig. 11.17). Concurrent fifth toe deformity may be corrected. Removing the weightbearing capability of the fifth metatarsal head in forefoot varus and cavus foot deformity predisposes to transfer lesion beneath the fourth metatarsal head.

Keating et al. (102) report on a study of 25 oblique fifth metatarsal neck osteotomies performed for tailor's bunion in which there was a 56% success rate. Symptomatic transfer lesions occurred in 36% of the feet operated on. Proper clinical and radiographic evaluation, taking into consideration postsurgical functional requirements, is essential (9, 45).

Joint implantation has progressed rapidly in the past 20 years (19, 107). First metatarsophalangeal joint implant arthroplasty is indicated for relief of pain, reduction of deformity and restoration of digital length, weightbearing and range of motion. The use of Silastic single- and double-stem joint implants, angulated or straight, has resulted in remarkable progress in restoring first metatarsophalangeal joint function (19, 78, 81, 103–106, 108). Tissue-compatible medical-grade silicone (Silastic) has been used successfully for partial or total replacement of arthritically destroyed first metatarsophalangeal joints over the past 12 years (19). Combinations of metatarsal head and phalangeal base resection have been advocated for rheumatoid arthritically involved joints (68, 84). In a retrospective study of 165 foot operations, published in 1979, Swanson et al. note encouraging results with the use of single-stem and flexible hinge-implants for arthritic first metatarsophalangeal joints (109). Cracchiolo et al. (110) and Borovoy et al. (111) in 1983 note similar favorable results with the use of a double-stem silicone implant for replacement of destroyed first metatarsophalangeal joints in rheumatoid patients and in patients who previously had destructive first metatarsophalangeal joint arthroplasties. Lipscomb (112) in 1981 advocates proximal phalangeal base resection, plantar

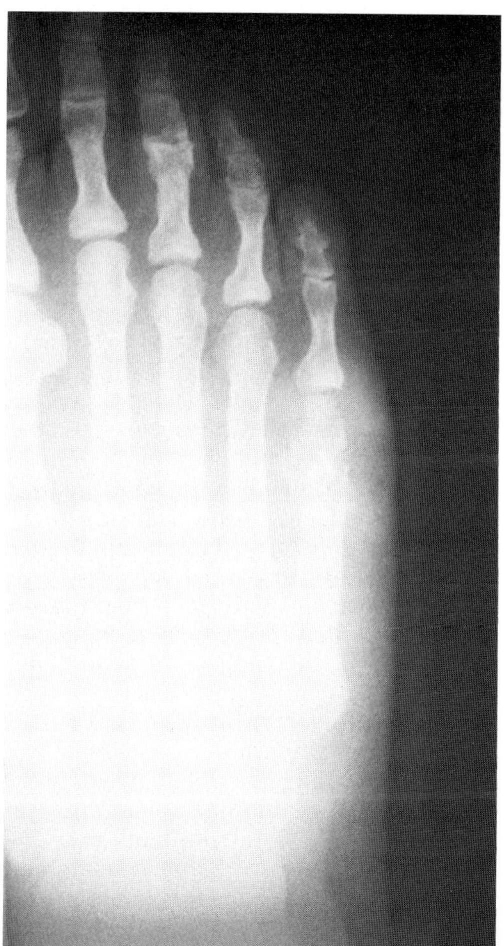

Figure 11.16. Extension-adduction biplane osteotomy of fifth metatarsal distal metaphysis 4 weeks postoperative.

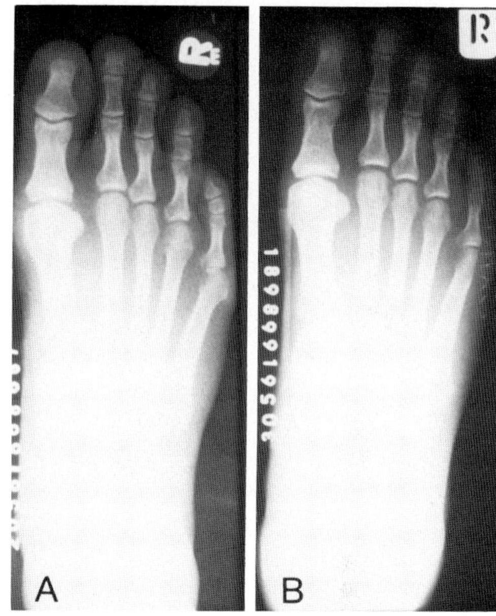

Figure 11.17. *A,* Preoperative, tailor's bunion. *B,* Postoperative, lateral condylectomy.

metatarsal head condylectomies, extensor tenotomies, arthrodesis of the first metatarsophalangeal joint and early talonavicular fusion for correction of the rheumatoid forefoot. It is interesting to note that Lipscomb cites the need for a team approach in treating the rheumatoid arthritic patient, but fails to mention the podiatrist as an integral part of that effort. Vahvanen et al. in 1980 completed a follow-up study of surgery performed on 179 rheumatoid forefeet and recommended that first metatarsophalangeal joint arthrodesis be performed for destroyed first metatarsophalangeal joints (113).

As early as 1976, LaPorta et al. reported on 536 procedures using a Silastic intramedullary-stemmed implant for arthritic first metatarsophalangeal joints (9). The author's criteria and results in over 270 first metatarsophalangeal implant arthroplasties utilizing the Swanson design Silastic intramedullary-stemmed implant closely correlate with those of LaPorta's study. (Figs. 11.18 and 11.19). Care should be exercised to ensure reattachment or retention of the flexor hallucis brevis and abductor hallucis tendons to the base of the great toe proximal phalanx (45). Long-term effects of great toe hemi-implants in

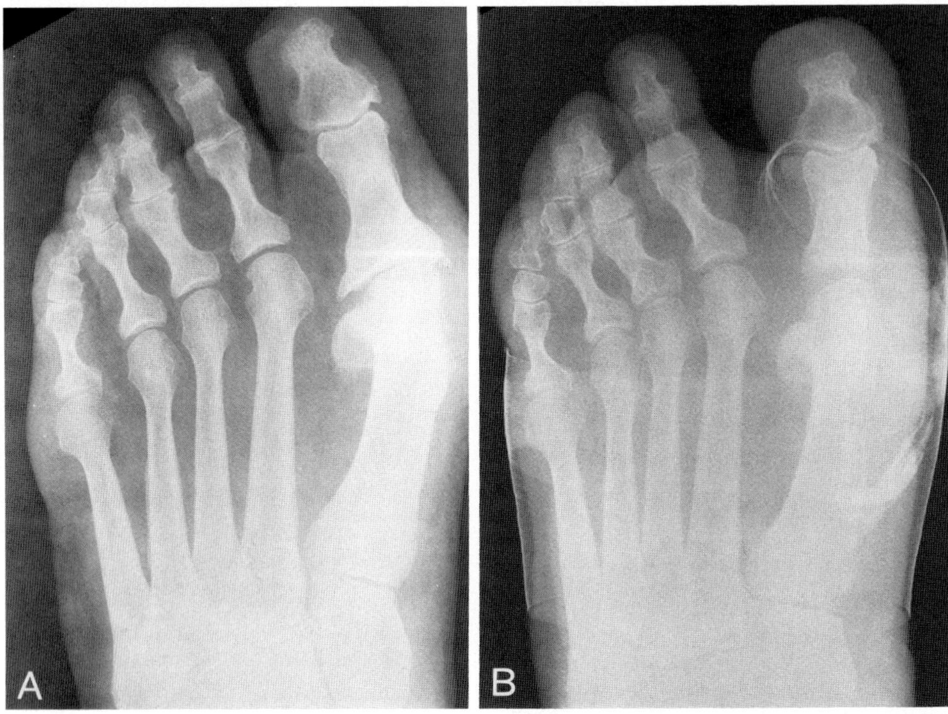

Figure 11.18. *A,* Preoperative painful limited range of motion posttraumatic arthritis of the first metatarsophalangeal joint secondary to previous surgery. *B,* Postoperative Swanson design Silastic hemi-implant arthroplasty.

the presence of metatarsus primus elevatus have been questioned (114). Revision of the anterior distal first metatarsal head is advised. The resulting "jamming" may lead to implant failure and deposition of Silastic particles in bone and soft tissue. The author has found the use of a drain and cast immobilization to be unnecessary. Limited ambulation, wearing a postsurgical wooden-soled shoe, is begun within 24 hours after surgery.

Since podiatric surgeons have developed the selective criteria for implant surgery the success rate has been high. Thousands, if not hundreds of thousands, of implants have been inserted in hallux joints that have undergone degenerative joint disease and rheumatoid arthritis. With careful evaluation of the deformity, maintenance of capsular and flexor hallucis brevis integrity, good judgment and surgical expertise, the percentage of favorable results has been encouraging from both a structural and functioning standpoint (9).

Weil et al. (48) report on long-term results in 484 cases of a total first metatarsophalangeal joint replacement in hallux valgus and hallux rigidus. The authors advise that extreme caution be used when contemplating use of Silastic hinge great toe or similar implants in the young active athlete. Advantages of the Swanson total first metatarsophalangeal joint implant include the ability to correct the proximal articular set angle, built-in correction of the abductus deformity, built-in range of motion within the hinge and stems and resultant good hallux purchase.

Favorable long-term results and sufficient documentation are not available regarding lesser metatarsophalangeal joint and interphalangeal joint implant surgery (115–119). Finger joint implants and ulnar head implants are being used to replace destroyed toe joints and lesser metatarsophalangeal joints (115, 117). However, long-term results have not been sufficient to warrant their standard use (115).

Lanham (48) reports results attained from over 1,000 digital implants since 1977. Included in this study are 124 Weil design implant (Dow) cases and 109 Sgarlato design implant (Sutter) cases. The author recommends digital implant use in selected cases as an alternative to resection arthroplasty or digital arthrodesis. Sgarlato (48) reports his 6 to 30 month, 384 case experience with the Sgarlato design implant (Sutter). The author concludes that the use of this implant warrants an expanded evaluation over a longer time period.

Arthroplasty of an arthritic lesser metatarsophalangeal joint might range from removal of loose bodies of bone and cartilage and revision in cases of adult symptomatic Freiberg's infraction (120) to complete removal of a metatarsal head in cases of severe rheumatoid arthritis.

Many studies fail to approach arthritic foot surgery from a biomechanical perspective (100, 112, 113, 121). The choice of surgical procedure must take into consideration lower extremity biomechanics (7, 9–11, 17–20). Foot and lower extremity pathology and its effect on structure and function must be thoroughly evaluated prior to selecting the appropriate surgical procedural approach (5, 7, 19).

Surgical approach to the intractable plantar keratosis or tyloma is determined after a thorough evaluation of foot type and function and after conservative treatment has been found to be ineffective. Often sufficient pressure beneath a metatarsal head or heads is relieved by a functional and/or accommodative foot orthotic device. Control of adverse lower extremity function and resultant shearing forces to the skin beneath the affected metatarsal head or heads is necessary preoperatively and postoperatively. Correction of associated digital deformity is often indicated. Functional versus positional deformity must be differentiated. An increase in ankle dorsiflexion may be indicated through conservative stretching-flexibility exercises or surgical methods. Gerbert et al. (18) present detailed criteria for surgical treatment of intractable plantar tyloma. Goforth et al. (122) describe a single distal metatarsal osteotomy for painful plantar keretosis beneath a lesser metatarsal head in a retrospective study. Berkun et al. (123) describe a distal tilt-up osteotomy for correction of intractable plantar tylomas beneath the lesser metatarsal heads with a report of 25 osteotomies and an 8–20 month follow-up. The author reports a 60% success rate with a patient satisfaction rate of 92%. If the metatarsal head is excessively elevated, the incidence of transfer lesion development beneath an adjacent metatarsal head is increased.

Plantar metatarsal head tyloma may be caused by subtalar joint pronatory problems, such as forefoot varus with callus forming beneath the fifth metatarsal head or beneath the fourth metatarsal head in the presence of a hypermobile fifth ray. Intractable plantar tyloma may be found secondary to hallux abductovalgus beneath the second metatarsal head or beneath the tibial sesamoid in the presence of a rigid plantar flexed first ray. The lesion may also be seen beneath the first and fifth metatarsal heads in cavus deformity. Localized surgical procedures include excision of the lesion superficial to the superficial fascia with a small bone curette or through two semielliptical incisions with suture placement. An inclusion cyst

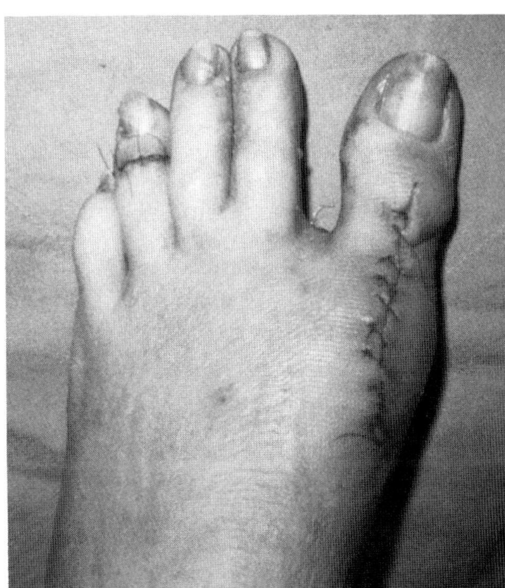

Figure 11.19. Two weeks postoperatively hemi-implant first metatarsophalangeal joint and arthroplasty fourth toe.

or adventitious bursa is often identified beneath the skin lesion. Surgical procedures involving metatarsal bone include plantar condylectomy (29), extension osteotomy (18), step-down osteotomy (124), Chevron "V" osteotomy (125), extension osteoarthrotomy (18), collectomy (18), and tilt-up osteotomy (123) and their numerous variations in technique. If more than one metatarsal osteotomy is indicated, it is best to vary the osteotomy site on adjacent metatarsals from distal to proximal.

Tarsometatarsal, Intertarsal and Ankle Joints

Tarsometatarsal, intertarsal and ankle joint arthritis may be idiopathic, caused by infection or systemic disease, may result from multiple minimal cumulative trauma, or may manifest in a joint or joints that were previously traumatized. Surgical procedures may be divided into joint salvage and joint destructive approaches. If cartilage is intact, joint salvage procedures are recommended. If joint cartilage is pathological and destroyed, joint destructive procedures, including fusion or replacement, are indicated. Often, pain and adverse function of these joints may be controlled through medical and mechanical means. If conservative treatment fails to control painful symptoms, surgical intervention is indicated.

Painful osteoarthritic or posttraumatic arthritic involvement of the first metatarsocuneiform-second metatarsal joint interface responds well to fusion. Dorsal arthritic "spurring" at the first metatarsocuneiform joint may result from a hypermobile first metatarsal ray, plantar flexed first metatarsal, or other intrinsic and extrinsic mechanical inefficiencies causing jamming at this joint (7). If symptomatic, the osteophytes are excised at an oblique angle (Fig.11.20). Smith (126) discusses the rational and surgical techniques associated with navicular, calcaneal and first metatarsocuneiform hyperotosis resection.

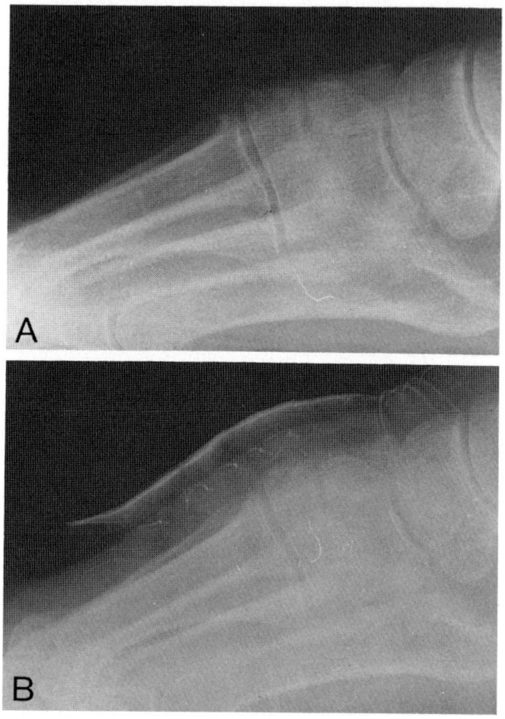

Figure 11.20. *A,* Painful dorsal arthritic "spurring" at the first metatarsocuneiform joint. *B,* Osteophyte excision at an oblique angle.

Control of adverse foot function is a mandatory postoperative requirement (6). Tarsometatarsal fracture dislocation or Lisfranc's fracture dislocation with the dislocation force lateral and dorsal may result in separation of the first and second metatarsal bases. This painful posttraumatic arthritic result responds to fusion. Traumatic arthritic involvement of the talonavicular joint secondary to adverse function, tarsal coalition or forced dorsiflexion injury may be treated by surgical arthroplasty with removal of painful osteophytes and loose bodies (15, 65). Swiontkowski et al. (127) report on a surgical study involving 40 patients with calcaneonavicular coalition (44 feet) and talocalcaneal coalition (13 feet). The use of interpositional fat or muscle was advocated after tarsal coalition resection. The authors suggest that the presence of a talar beak is not always indicative of degenerative joint disease and does not always require triple arthrodesis. They further suggest that the periarticular talar beak may be a traction exostosis at the insertion of the talonavicular ligament. In the author's experience, resection of a tarsal synchondrosis, syndesmosis or synostosis almost always predisposes to posttraumatic arthritis of the involved joint or joints. In the case of peroneal spastic flatfoot associated with a tarsal coalition, orthotic device control of foot function after the spasm has been reduced is almost always effective. Arthritic changes caused by chronic excessive subtalar pronation associated with an os tibiale externum accessory bone and the medial plantar navicular tuberosity may require removal of the os tibiale externum. Care should be taken to ensure proper intraoperative repositioning of the tibialis posterior tendon beneath the navicular. The arthritic subtalar joint, secondary to chronic adverse function or crush injury, must be fused in order to control painful symptoms. Foot orthosis control is mandatory following subtalar or ankle joint fusion. The long-term impact on midtarsal, ankle, knee and hip joint function makes subtalar fusion and/or triple arthrodesis a poor prognostic choice (128).

Occasionally, severely deformed and symptomatic flatfeet require surgical intervention in order to relieve symptoms and/or to restore functional integrity. Dollard et al. (129) report on a 3-year, 36-case (50 feet) experience with the Evans calcaneal osteotomy for flexible flatfoot syndrome. They conclude that the procedure restores functional integrity to the medial longitudinal arch and reestablishes the midtarsal joint locking mechanism. It is important that flatfoot surgery not be performed until and unless every conservative treatment modality has been shown to be ineffective and unless the patient continues to suffer a significant degree of pain and disability.

Smith (130) and Lundeen (131) discuss the technique of subtalar arthroereisis utilizing a small peg (Stapeg) of polyethylene implanted into the dorsal surface of the calcaneus just anterior to the posterior facet and fixed with polymethylmethacrylate. This procedure, performed to limit subtalar pronation in children with flexible flatfoot over age 6, holds the heel vertical and the subtalar joint neutral. It is reported to produce optimal osseous alignment, preserve flexibility, allow for normal function and create the potential for preventing secondary deformities.

Marcinko et al. (132) review the indications, counterindications, bone grafting techniques, postoperative care and complications of the Silver opening wedge calcaneal osteotomy used to correct excessive heel valgus and to realign the heel under the weightbearing surface of the tibia in flexible flatfoot. This technique is used in combination with other procedures as needed (133). Preliminary results in ten cases over a 3-year period have been favorable.

Cavuoto (134) and Grumbine and Chesler (135) review and discuss the diagnosis and surgical treatment of the cavus foot deformity. An anterior cavus deformity may require osteotomy of the first metatarsal and plantar fascial release, whereas a posterior cavus deformity may respond well to Dwyer osteotomy and a combined cavus deformity may require midtarsal joint osteotomy. Sudmann et al. (136) studied 118 clubfoot cases over a 10-year period in very young babies treated both operatively and nonoperatively. The authors recommend early tenotomy of the tibialis anterior and posterior and suggest that these muscles are the dynamic features affecting the resistant rearfoot deformity in congenital clubfoot.

Talar impingement arthritis is found in football linemen, basketball players and gymnasts. It results from repetitive jamming of the anterior distal tibia into the neck of the talus. The resulting dorsal talar neck exostosis and anterior distal tibial osteophytes respond well to resection (15, 137). Forced plantar flexion injury with resultant os trigonal and/or posterior talocrural joint arthritis respond well to os trigonum and osteophyte excision (138) (Fig. 11.21). Osteochondral fractures and osteochondritis dissecans of the talar trochlea, if not responsive to conservative management, respond well to surgical curettage. If the medial trochlear surface of the talus is involved, an osteotomy of the tibia is sometimes necessary to gain adequate exposure (see Chapter 10, Foot and Ankle Trauma).

Arthroscopic surgery for osteochondral fractures, loose bodies, synovial and other arthritic manifestations in the foot and ankle are becoming more readily available as fiberoptic and microsurgical instrumentation is further refined (139). To date, total ankle joint implant arthroplasty

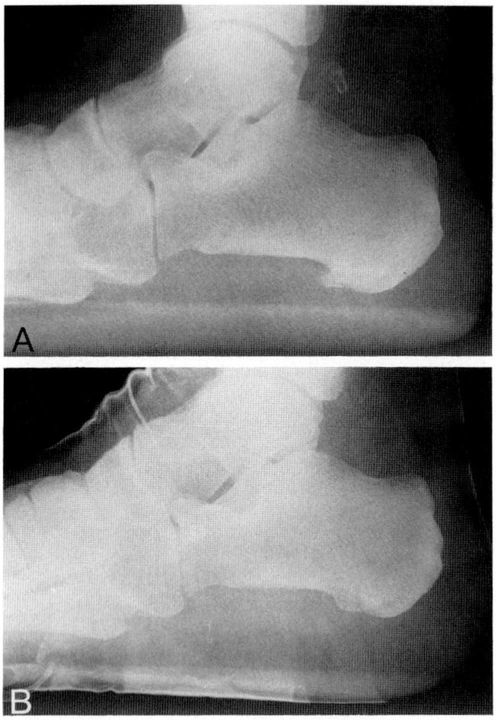

Figure 11.21. *A,* Painful posterior talocrural joint arthritis and unilateral plantar calcaneal exostosis secondary to 20 years of occupationally induced (foot pedal) forced ankle plantar and dorsiflexion. *B,* Postoperative result of osteophyte and exostosis excision.

(140) has not resulted in lasting benefit (15); however, with the development of more suitable materials, this salvage procedure for severe ankle joint arthritis may have greater long-term benefit. Triple arthrodesis and arthrodesis of the ankle joint are recommended in only the most symptomatic and severe progressive foot deformities (141) and arthritic feet (15, 142, 143). It has been the author's experience that subtalar and/or ankle arthrodesis leads to multiple minimal cumulative traumatic arthritis of the distal foot joints, hip and, to a lesser extent, the knee (Fig. 11.22).

Smith (144) reviews the use of bone grafts in foot surgical fusion procedures, particularly cortical and cancellous graft and autograft and allograft healing. The lateral aspect of the calcaneus has been utilized as a donor site for cancellous bone used in foot arthrodesing procedures. Homologous cadaver bone grafts have been used in flatfoot surgery.

Rothstein (145) reviews the use of skin grafting technique. The selection of a proper graft, recipient bed preparation and timing of graft placement, as well as a description of graft healing and major causes of graft failure, are discussed. Larger amounts of split thickness skin may be obtained from the upper outer or inner leg. Small amounts of split or full thickness skin may be obtained from the lateral dorsal aspect of the foot, just below and anterior to the lateral malleolus or the nonweightbearing area of the medial longitudinal arch (146). The author has used skin from these sites to cover digital deficits left after nevus, mucous cyst or soft tissue tumor excision.

In the geriatric patient, surgical treatment of osteoarthritis of the ankle, subtalar and midtarsal joints is rarely indicated (147). Davis and Millis (148), in a retrospective study of 48 patients who underwent ankle arthrodesis for a traumatic arthritis, established that the most prevalent problem was a limitation of motion and pain in the subtalar joint. Relief was accomplished in most cases by subtalar or triple arthrodesis. However, a high incidence of infection was also present. Although the surgery seemed to be helpful, the use of appropriate foot orthotic devices prior to surgery may have obviated the need for surgical intervention.

Arthritic soft tissue and extra-articular tarsal bony involvement may require surgical intervention. Heel spur syndrome; tarsal tunnel syndrome; insertional plantar fasciitis; peroneus brevis; tibialis posterior, flexor and extensor tenosynovitis; and Achilles tendonitis may be caused by functional inefficiency, one of the arthritides or a combination of both conditions (15, 149). Manifestations of psoriatic, gouty or rheumatoid arthritis, Reiter's syndrome or hyperlipidemia are commonly present as one or more of the above inflammatory processes (45). Surgical treatment consisting of synovectomy, neurolysis and exostectomy is indicated when medical and biomechanical measures fail to control pain and dysfunction (Fig. 11.23).

Often it is necessary to resect the prominent posterior superior aspect of the calcaneus. This normal anatomical varient (Haglund's deformity or disease) may lead to overlying skin and soft tissue inflammation with irritation of the anatomical bursa and/or development of a painful adventitous bursa (Fig 11.24). The skin and soft tissues are further irritated by abnormal movement of the calcaneus in the shoe due to a compensated rearfoot varus or forefoot valgus or by the shoe counter itself (150). Medial, lateral, linear and transverse posterior approaches have been described. The lateral approach must ensure the integrity of the sural nerve. Linear and transverse posterior approaches may predispose to painful scar formation and subsequent shoe irritation (151), chronic Achilles tendon fibrosis and inflammation or loss of Achilles tendon insertion. A hockey-stick shaped medial approach just anterior to the Achilles tendon and posterior to the neurovascular bundle seems to afford the best surgical approach. Care must be taken not to interfere with the medial calcaneal branch of the posterior tibial nerve or the insertion of the Achilles tendon. Other procedures have included a slide osteotomy through the calcaneus with the posterior aspect of the calcaneus moved into a more dorsal and anterior position (152, 153). A traction exostosis due to a long-standing gastrocnemius or gastrocnemius-soleus equinus may be present. Calcification of the Achilles tendon may be visualized in hyperlipidemia, coronary artery disease or collagen disorder.

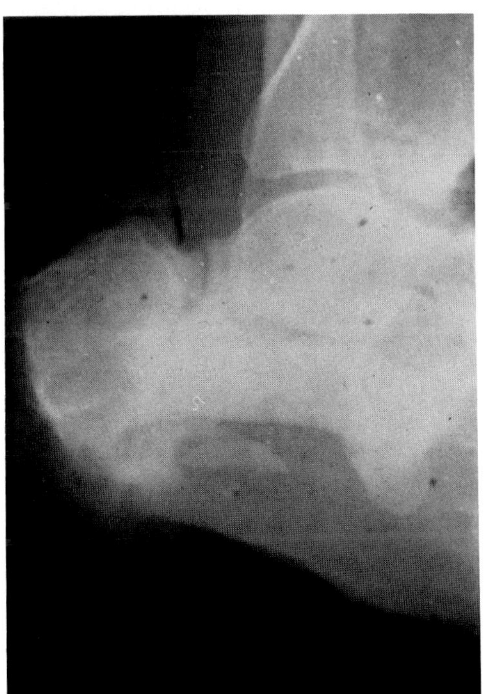

Figure 11.22. Painful subtalar joint arthritis secondary to crush injury requiring fusion.

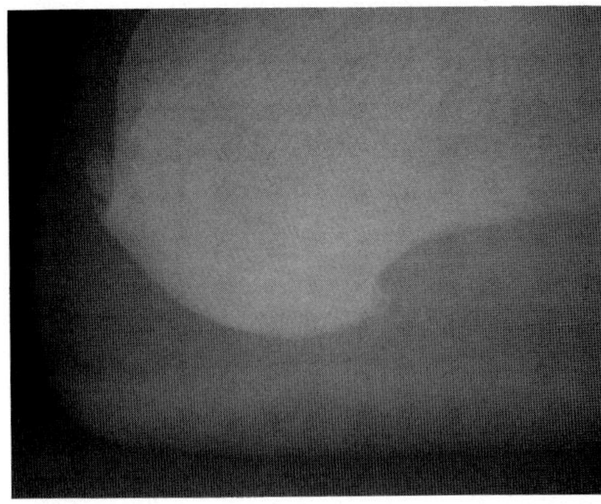

Figure 11.23. Plantar and posterior calcaneal exostoses in patient with hyperlipidemia and gastrocnemius-soleus equinus.

Shama et al. (154) report on a study involving the review of 1,000 random foot radiographs for the presence of plantar calcaneal exostosis (heel spur). Of the radiographs, 13.2% revealed signs of heel spur. Sixty-one percent of those people with radiographic evidence of heel spur were asymptomatic, with 62% showing evidence of abnormal subtalar pronation and 81% reporting painful heel spur symptoms. A causal relationship between abnormal foot pronation and painful plantar calcaneal exostosis was established.

In most cases painful heel spur syndrome can be managed conservatively. Foot orthotic devices designed to lessen the insertional stress of the plantar fascia have been universally effective. In the less than 10% incidence of painful heel spur syndrome that does not respond to nonsurgical treatment, surgical intervention is indicated. Often heel spur syndrome is complicated by an adventitious bursa,

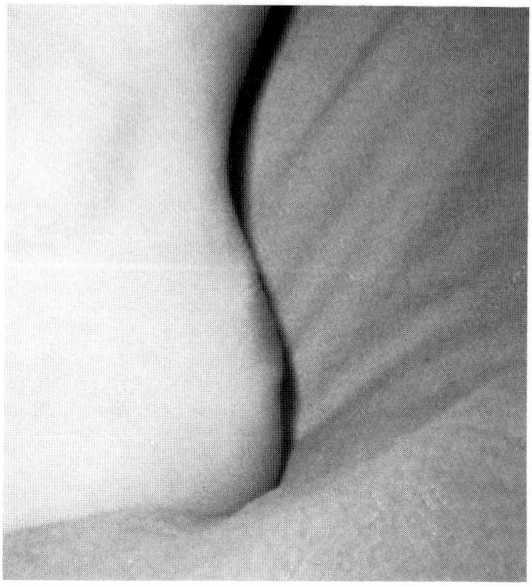

Figure 11.24. Haglund's deformity with overlying skin and soft tissue inflammation.

neuroma, obesity, the occupational necessity to walk on hard, flat, man made surfaces or underlying systemic disease. The medial surgical approach to the heel spur results in better visualization of the involved anatomy and complicating soft tissue tumors, if present. A small disposable meniscus knife is used to detach the plantar fascia and intrinsic muscle origin from the plantar calcaneal tubercle. The plantar calcaneal exostosis is excised from medial to lateral with hand or power instrumentation with the denuded bone rasped smooth. A primary and often secondary plantarly declined exostosis is also excised. McCarthy et al. (155) performed a cryomicrotomy rearfoot anatomical study with findings correlated to podiatric literature over the past 10 years. The study identifies structures at risk during surgery to the rearfoot and provides an historical appreciation of the evolutionary development of podiatric rearfoot surgery.

Tendon lengthening, shortening, transposition and transfer in the foot are often indicated as independent procedures or in combination with other procedures. Achilles tendon lengthening (TAL) by means of slide technique and "Z" plasty have been used in the treatment of gastrocnemius and gastrocnemius-soleus equinus. Gastrocnemius recession has been advocated as a more lasting and beneficial technique for lengthening of the triceps surae group. Fenton et al. (156), in a retrospective study involving 306 procedures in 286 feet, review commonly performed major tendon transfers in the foot and compare the justification for performance of these procedures to published recommendations. The criteria used in this study were found to be compatible with previously published criteria. Commonly lengthened foot tendons include the long extensors for digital dorsiflexion deformities and the peroneus longus for flexible plantar flexed first ray. Short and long flexor and extensor, abductor and adductor hallucis, lumbricale and interrosseous tenotomies have been performed alone or in combination with other procedures for digital deformity. Tibialis anterior and posterior, extensor hallucis and digitorum longus and peroneus longus tendon transfers have been utilized in correction and stabilization procedures for paralytic, congenital and traumatic foot deformity.

References

1. Petrich RJ: Considerations in pediatric surgery. *J Am Podiatry Assoc* 74:445–449, 1984.
2. Sokoloff L: Repair mechanisms of articular cartilage. *J Am Podiatry Assoc* 72:228–232, 1982.
3. Nicolle FV, Dickson RA: *Surgery of the Rheumatoid Hand (A Practical Manual).* Chicago, Year Book Publishers Inc, 1979.
4. Sedar JI: Management of foot problems in arthritis. *Cleve Clin Q* 37:111, 1974.
5. Sgarlato TE: *A Compendium of Podiatric Biomechanics.* San Francisco, California College of Podiatric Medicine, 1970.
6. Burns MJ: Orthotic control following surgical correction of hallux abducto valgus. *J Foot Surg* 18:89, 1979.
7. Root ML, Orien WP, Weed JH: *Normal and Abnormal Function of the Foot.* Los Angeles, Clinical Biomechanics, 1977.
8. Lemont H, Gibley CW, Jr: Prevalence of osteoarthritis of the foot. *J Am Podiatry Assoc* 72:214–216, 1982.
9. Gamble F, Yale I: *Clinical Foot Roentgenology.* Huntington, NY, RE Krieger, 1975.
10. Root ML: *Biomechanics Examination of the Foot.* Los Angeles, Clinical Biomechanics, 1971.
11. Jones CL: The damaging effects of a disaligned musculoskeletal system (conservative vs. surgical management of foot disorders). *Symposia Specialists.* pp. 251–269, 1972.
12. Roper RB, et al: The perioperative management of the gouty patient. *J Am Podiatry Assoc* 74:168–172, 1984.

13. Caputi R, Jacobs AM, Oloff LM: Sickle cell anemia in podiatric surgery. *J Foot Surg* 23:135–145, 1984.
14. LaPorta GA Melillo T, Olinsky D: X-ray evaluation of hallux abducto valgus deformity. *J Am Podiatry Assoc* 64:545, 1974.
15. Yale JF (ed): *Yearbook of Podiatric Medicine and Surgery.* Mt. Kisco, NY, Futura Publishers, 1981, p. 381.
16. Whitney AK: Radiographic charting technique. Philadelphia, Pennsylvania College of Podiatric Medicine, 1978.
17. Gerbert J, Mercado OA, Sokoloff T: *The Surgical Treatment of the Hallux Abducto Valgus and Allied Deformities.* Mt. Kisco, NY, Futura, 1973.
18. Gerbert J, Melillo T, Sokoloff TN, Spector E, Whitney A: *The Surgical Treatment of the Intractable Plantar Keratoma.* Mt. Kisco, NY, Futura, 1974.
19. LaPorta GA, Pilla P, Jr, Richter KP: Keller implant procedure. A report of 536 procedures using a Silastic intramedullary stemmed implant. *J Am Podiatry Assoc* 66:126, 1976.
20. Donick I, Berlin S, Block L, Costa A, Fox J, Martorana V: An approach for hallux valgus surgery—Fifteen-year review, Part I. *J Foot Surg* 19:113, 1980.
21. Yale I: *Podiatric Medicine,* ed 2. Baltimore Williams & Wilkins, 1980.
22. Hatch DJ, Magnusson PG, DiGiovanni JE: Minidose heparin prophylaxis for high-risk patients in podiatric surgery. *J Am Podiatry Assoc* 70:73–83, 1980.
23. Grant R: Management of the rheumatic patient in the community. *Practitioner* 205:641, 1970.
24. Yale JF: Firm footings for the athlete (a preventive injury and self-help guide for those athletes involved in the running sports). Ansonia, CT, 1981.
25. Haber J, Hammer DJ, Butler B: Malignant hyperthermia (a review and case report). *J Am Podiatry Assoc* 73:422–426, 1983.
26. Lowe MK: Malignant hyperthermia. A surgeon's nightmare. *J Foot Surg* 24: 139–141, 1985.
27. Lauf E, LeCompte G: Manual dexterity (Its importance in podiatry). *J Am Podiatry Assoc* 72:291–298, 1982.
28. Gibbons RD, Gudas C, Gibbons SW: A study of the relationship between flexibility of closure and surgical skill. *J Am Podiatry Assoc* 73:12–16, 1983.
29. DuVries HL: *Surgery of the Foot.* St. Louis, CV Mosby Co, 1959.
30. Wood WA, Wayne J: Office-based surgery in podiatry. *J Am Podiatry Assoc* 71:591–594, 1981.
31. Hugar DW, Salvino FA: Experience in delivering ambulatory surgical services. *J Am Podiatry Assoc* 70:609–613, 1980.
32. Roth RD: Utilization of epinephrine-containing anesthetic solutions in the toes. *J Am Podiatry Assoc* 71:189, 1981.
33. Kaplan EG, Kashuk K: Disclaiming the myth of use of epinephrine local anesthesia in feet. *J Am Podiatry Assoc* 61:335, 1971.
34. Howard K, et al: Diphenhydramine hydrochloride as a local anesthetic. *J Am Podiatry Assoc* 74:240–242, 1984.
35. Fox IM, Mandracchia V, Jassen M, Chu J: The pneumatic tourniquet in extremity surgery. *J Am Podiatry Assoc* 71:237, 1981.
36. Martin WJ, et al: Tourniquet use in sickle cell disease patients. *J Am Podiatry Assoc* 74:291–294, 1984.
37. Arenson DJ, Weil LS: The uses and abuses of tourniquets in bloodless field foot surgery. *J Am Podiatry Assoc* 66:854, 1976.
38. Cohen RS, Kaplan EG: Use of the pneumatic tourniquet. *J Foot Surg* 18:96, 1979.
39. Maurer NH: Non-cardiac circulatory overload secondary to pneumatic thigh tourniquet. *J Am Podiatry Assoc* 73:589–592, 1983.
40. Chu J, Fox I, Jessen M: Pneumatic ankle tourniquet: Clinical and electrophsiologic study. *Arch Phys Med Rehab* 62:570–575, 1981.
41. Locke RK, Strauss H: The reduction of postoperative pain and edema in foot surgery through instillation of corticosteroids. *J Am Podiatry Assoc* 58:169, 1968.
42. Curda GA: Postoperative analgesic effects of dexamethasone sodium phosphate in bunion surgery. *J Foot Surg* 22:187–191, 1983.
43. Till KE, Solomon MG, Kerwan B: Indications and use of prophylactic antibiosis in podiatric surgery. *J Foot Surg* 23:166–172, 1984.
44. Hodor L, Dobbs BM: Pan metatarsal head resection (A review and new approach). *J Am Podiatry Assoc* 73:287–292, 1983.
45. Hara B (ed): *Complications in Foot Surgery. American College of Foot Surgeons.* Baltimore, Williams & Wilkins, 1976.
46. Marcinko E, Field N, Barnett, L: Use of the Shaw scalpel in podiatric surgery. *J Foot Surgery* 23:460, 1984.
47. Vega MR, Wisniew J, Johnson TE: Johnson Tucker: Instrumentation for better fixation. *J Foot Surg* 23:121–122, 1984.
48. Weil LS (ed): *Clinics in Podiatry—Implants in Foot Surgery.* Philadelphia, W B Saunders Co, 1984, p. 211.
49. Floyd EJ, et al: The scaphoid compression staple: An effective form of fixation. *J Foot Surg* 23:56–59, 1984.
50. Cornell PE, et al: Pain reduction with transcutaneous electrical nerve stimulation after foot surgery. *J Foot Surg* 23:326–333, 1984.
51. Lanham RH, Powell S, Hendrix BE: Efficacy of hypothermia and transcutaneous electrical nerve stimulation in podiatric surgery. *J Foot Surg* 23:152–158, 1984.
52. Wittenberg M, et al: Comparison of ibuprofen and acetaminophen-codeine in postoperative foot pain. *J Am Podiatry Assoc* 74:233–237, 1984.
53. Marcus SA, Block BH (eds): *Complications in Foot Surgery. American College of Foot Surgeons.* Baltimore, Williams & Wilkins, 1984, p. 495.
54. Miller SJ: Temperature regulation and postoperative fever (a preliminary study). *J Am Podiatry Assoc* 74:373–379, 1984.
55. Bravo AB, et al: A review of osteomyelitis with

case presentation. *J Am Podiatric Med Assoc* 75:83–99, 1985.
56. Schwartz NH, Marcinko DE: Suction irrigation. *J Am Podiatry Assoc* 74:216–221, 1984.
57. Parrot DL: Profile of hospital podiatry. *J Am Podiatry Assoc* 71:646–656, 1981.
58. McGlamry ED, Kitting RW: Postoperative urethane molds. *J Am Podiatry Assoc* 58:169, 1968.
59. Yale JF: Foot impression technique (F.I.T.): An accurate moderate weight bearing technique. *Arch Podiatr Med Foot Surg Annual Sports Medicine Edition;* pp. 117–119, May 1979.
60. Yale JF: Complications of Keller-implant arthroplasty secondary to the stress of golf: A case report. *Arch Podiatr Med Foot Surg Annual Sports Medicine Edition:* pp. 83–92, May 1978.
61. Settlemire WE, Beneson DE: Deep venous thrombosis and pulmonary embolism. *J Am Podiatry Assoc* 74:268–283, 1984.
62. Reinherz R, Marks M, Winters G: Bone regeneration in podiatric surgery. *J Foot Surg* 23:131–134, 1984.
63. Marcinko DE, Carlson R: Psychological considerations of the surgical patient—an emerging issue. *J Am Podiatry Assoc* 74:441–443, Sept. 1984.
64. Shields MH, Wards JR: Treatment of related knee-ankle foot deformity in rheumatoid arthritis. *J Am Phys Ther Assoc* 46:1101, 1966.
65. Yale JF: Surgical and biomechanical approach to the talonavicular joint. *J Am Podiatry Assoc* 63:247–254, 1973.
66. Jacobs A: Surgical management of the arthritic patient. Pathfinders Lecture Series, 75th Annual Meeting of the American Podiatry Association, Boston, Massachusetts, August 20, 1983.
67. Greenberg AJ: Rheumatoid nodules. *J Am Podiatry Assoc* 72:84–88, 1982.
68. Raunio P, Laine H: Synovectomy of the metatarsophalangeal joints in rheumatoid arthritis. *Acta Rheumatol Scand* 16:12, 1970.
69. Yale JF: Foot and ankle trauma. Address given to the 49th Annual Meeting of the American Podiatry Association, San Francisco, August, 1970.
70. Kruger FJ, Valmassy RL: The use of rigid orthoses in a surgically corrected clubfoot patient. *J Foot Surg* 21:202–205, 1982.
71. Melillo TV: Gastrocnemius equinus—Its diagnosis and treatment. *Arch Podiatr Med Foot Surg* 2:159, 1975.
72. Aquino M, DeVincentis AF, Keating SE: Tibial sesamoid planing procedure: An appraisal of 26 feet. *J Foot Surg* 23:226–230, 1984.
73. Kaiman ME, Piccora R: Tibial sesamoidectomy: A review of the literature and retrospective study. *J Foot Surg* 22:286–289, 1983.
74. Troy TV: New instrumentation for removal of the fibular sesamoid. *J Foot Surg* 23:248–249, 1984.
75. Kahn MD, et al: Osteoid osteoma of the great toe. *J Foot Surg* 22:325–328, 1983.
76. Yale JF: Non-joint destructive procedure for long great toe with abductus deformity. *J Foot Surg* 14:114–115, 1975.
77. Yale JF: Non-joint destructive procedure for long great toe with abductus deformity (a retrospective study). *J Foot Surg* 18:7–9, 1979.
78. Moeller F: *Surgical Treatment of Digital Deformities.* Mt. Kisco, NY, Futura, 1975.
79. Green D: The progressive approach to digital surgery. Lecture given to Connecticut Podiatry Association Seminar, Woodbridge, Connecticut, May 26, 1982.
80. Schubert DA: *Techniques of Foot Surgery.* Ann Arbor, MI, J Thaddeus, 1965.
81. Buckholz JM, Vogler H W (eds): *Yearbook of Podiatric Medicine and Surgery (Surgery section).* Mt. Kisco, NY, Futura, 1981.
82. McGlamry ED: Unfavorable long-term results in the Jones metatarsal suspension. *J Am Podiatry Assoc* 65: 479, 1975.
83. Johnson CP, Hugar DW: A literature review of congenital digiti quinti varus: Clinical description and treatment. *J Foot Surg* 22: 116–120, 1983.
84. Kelikian H: *Hallux Valgus: Allied Deformities of the Forefoot and Metatarsalgia.* Philadelphia, W B Saunders Co., 1965.
85. Mosher MR: Modified stone bunionectomy. *J Am Podiatry Assoc.* 61: 207–211, 1971.
86. Feldman RS, Hutter J, Lapow L, Pour B: Cheilectomy and hallux rigidus. *J Foot Surg* 22: 170–174, 1983.
87. Spinelli J, Taylor P: Stone procedure evaluation: Two years postoperatively. *J Foot Surg* 12: 39, 1973.
88. Drago JJ, Oloff L, Jacobs AA: A comprehensive review of hallux limitus. *J Foot Surg* 23: 213–220, 1984.
89. Cohn I, Kanat IO: Functional limitation of motion of the first metatarsophalangeal joint. *J Foot Surgery* 23: 477–484, 1984.
90. Rzonca E, Levitz S, Lue B: Hallux equinus: The stages of hallux limitus and hallux rigidus. *J Am Podiatry Assoc* 74: 8: 390–393, 1984.
91. Spinner SM: Radiographic criteria in the assessment of hallux abductus deformity. *J Foot Surg* 23: 25–30, 1984.
92. Gerbert J (ed), Sokoloff TH (assoc ed): *Textbook of Bunion Surgery.* Mt. Kisco, NY, Futura, 1981.
93. Fox IM, Smith SD: Juvenile bunion correction by epiphysiodesis of the first metatarsal. *J Am Podiatry Assoc* 73: 448–455, 1983.
94. Donick II, et al: An approach for hallux valgus surgery—fifteen year review: Part I. *J Foot Surg* 19: 113–126, 1980.
95. McCarthy DJ: The surgical anatomy of the first ray (Part I: the distal segment). *J Am Podiatry Assoc* 73: 111–121, 1983.
96. McCarthy DJ: The surgical anatomy of the first ray (Part II: the proximal segment). *J Am Podiatry Assoc* 73: 244–255, 1983.
97. Wood WA: Acquired hallux varus: A new corrective procedure. *J Foot Surg* 20: 194–197, 1981.
98. Clayton MD: Surgery of the forefoot in rheumatoid arthritis. *Clin Orthop* 16: 136, 1960.
99. Hoffman P: An operation for severe grades of contracted or clawed toes. *Am J Orthop Surg* 9: 441, 1912.
100. Fitzgerald JAW. A review of long-term results of

arthrodesis of the first metatarsophalangeal joint. *J Bone Joint Surg* 51B: 488, 1969.

101. Costa AJ, Rubin L: Surgical indications and discussion of the Hoffman-type Pan metatarsectomy and a report of cases. *J Foot Surg* 12: 66, 1973.
102. Keating SE, et al: Oblique fifth metatarsal osteotomy: A follow-up study. *J Foot Surg* 21: 104–107, 1982.
103. Teich LJ, Frankel JP, Lipsman S: Silicone hinge replacement arthroplasty. *J Am Podiatry Assoc* 71: 266, 1981.
104. Zlotoff H: Swanson flexible hinge toe implant: A preliminary report. *J Am Podiatry Assoc* 73: 347–355, 1983.
105. Kalish SR, McGlamry ED: The modified Keller hallux valgus repair utilizing Silastic implants. In McGlamry ED (ed): *Reconstructive Surgery of the Foot and Leg*. New York, Intercontinental Medical Book Corporation, 1974, p. 39.
106. Miller RJ, Rattan N, Sorto L: The geriatic bunion: Correction of metatarsus primus varus and hallux valgus with the Swanson total joint implant. *J Foot Surg* 22: 263–270, 1983.
107. Seeburger RH: Surgical implants of alloyed metal in joints of feet. *J Am Podiatry Assoc* 54: 391, 1964.
108. Weil, LS (ed): *Implants in Foot Surgery. Clinics in Podiatry*. Philadelphia, WB Saunders Co., 1984.
109. Swanson AB, Lumsden RM, Swanson GD: Silicone implant arthroplasty of the great toe. A review of single stem and flexible hinge implants. *Clin Orthop Relat Res* 142: 30–43, 1979.
110. Cracchiolo A, Swanson A, Swanson GD: The arthritic great toe metatarsophalangeal joint: A review of flexible silicone implant arthroplasty from two medical centers. *Clin Orthop Relat Res* 157: 64–69, 1981.
111. Borovoy M, Gray W, Rinker A: Total replacement of the first metatarsophalangeal joint. *J Foot Surg* 22: 159–164, 1983.
112. Lipscomb PR: Surgery of the rheumatoid foot: Preferable procedures. *Rev Chir Orthop* 67: 375–382, 1981.
113. Vahvanen V, Piirainch H, Kettunen P. Resection arthroplasty of the metatarsophalangeal joints in rheumatoid arthritis. A follow-up study of 100 patients. *Scand J Rheumatol* 9: 257–265, 1980.
114. Jacobs A: Intraoperative Complications of Implant Arthroplasty. Pioneers Lecture Series, 75th Annual Meeting of the American Podiatry Association, Boston, Massachusetts, August 22, 1983.
115. McGlamry ED, Ruch JA: Status of implant arthroplasty of the lesser metatarsophalangeal joints. *J Am Podiatry Assoc* 66: 155, 1976.
116. Kaplan BR, Cohen SJ: The use of the Calnan-Nicolle prosthesis for metatarsophalangeal joint replacement. A preliminary study. *J Am Podiatry Assoc* 66: 165, 1976.
117. Tintocalis CA: Nicolle finger joint prosthesis: A preliminary study of total joint replacement for lesser metatarsophalangeal joints. *J Foot Surg* 21: 57–60, 1982.
118. Sgarlato TE: Implants for lesser toes. *J Foot Surg* 22: 247–250, 1983.
119. Silberman J, Kanat IO: Total joint replacement in digits of the foot. *J Foot Surg* 23: 207–212, 1984.
120. Kehr L: A new surgical technique for the correction of Freiberg's deformity. *J Am Podiatry Assoc* 72: 130–134, 1982.
121. Delagoutte JP: Endoprosthesis in surgery of the rheumatoid foot. *Rev Rhum Mal Osteoartic* 47: 135–137, 1980.
122. Goforth PW, et al: Distal metatarsal osteotomy—a retrospective study. *J Am Podiatry Assoc* 74: 402–405, 1984.
123. Berkun RN, et al: The tilt-up osteotomy for correction of intractable plantar keratoses. *J Foot Surg* 23: 52–55, 1984.
124. Mitchell CL, Fleming JL, Allen R, Glenney C, Sanford GA: Osteotomy-bunionectomy for hallux valgus. *J Bone Joint Surg* 40: 41, 1958.
125. Davidson MR: V-osteotomy for correction of metatarsal head pathology. *J Foot Surg* 13: 23, 1974.
126. Smith TF: Resection of common pedal prominences. *J Am Podiatry Assoc* 73: 93–99, 1983.
127. Swiontkowski MF, Scranton PE, Hansen S: Tarsal coalitions: Long term results of surgical treatment. *J Pediatr Orthop* 3: 287–292, 1983.
128. Wolf EW: Case records of the California Podiatry Hospital: A clinicopathologic exercise. Traumatic arthritis of the subtalar joint. *J Foot Surg* 68: 437, 1978.
129. Dollard MD, et al: The Evans calcaneal osteotomy for correction of flexible flatfoot syndrome. *J Foot Surg* 23: 291–301, 1984.
130. Smith SD, Wagreich CR: Review of postoperative results of the subtalar arthrodereisis operation: A preliminary study. *J Foot Surg* 23: 253–260, 1984.
131. Lundeen RO: The Smith Sta-Peg operation for hypermobile pes planovalgus in children. *J Am Podiatric Med Assoc* 75: 177–183, 1985.
132. Marcinko DE, Lazerson A, Elleby DH: Silver calcaneal osteotomy for flexible flatfoot: A retrospective preliminary report. *J Foot Surg* 23: 191–198, 1984.
133. Johnston WB: A literature review of calcaneal osteotomies in the treatment of valgus deformities. *J Foot Surg* 21: 139–142, 1982.
134. Cavuoto JW: Foot surgery in Charcot-Marie-Tooth Disease. *J Foot Surg* 9: 130–134, 1980.
135. Grumbine NA, Chesler SM: An evaluation for compensated anterior cavus. *J Foot Surg* 19: 142–147, 1980.
136. Sudmann E, Hald JK, Skandfer B: Features resisting primary treatment of congenital clubfoot. *Acta Orthop Scand* 54: 850–857, 1983.
137. Subotnick SI: Anterior impingement exostosis of the ankle: A hazard to the athlete. *J Am Podiatry Assoc.* 66: 958, 1976.
138. Krusch RS: Excision of a large os trigonum: A case report. *J Foot Surg* 11: 77–78, 1972.
139. Weil LS: Arthroscopy. Address given to the Annual Meeting of the American Academy of Podiatric Sports Medicine, Sheraton Center, New York, June 13, 1982.
140. Arancia LJ, Rinaldi FT: *Atlas of Rearfoot Surgery*. Mt. Kisco, Futura, NY, 1978.

141. Fenton CF, et al: Surgical considerations in the presence of Charcot-Marie-Tooth Disease. *J Am Podiatry Assoc* 74: 490–498, 1984.
142. Sharpe DA: A comprehensive look at triple fusions of the tarsal bones of the human foot. *Arch Podiatr Med Foot Surg* 2: 235–253, 1975.
143. Kaplan EG, Kaplan GS: Triple arthrodesis. *J Foot Surg* 15: 93–98, 1976.
144. Smith TF: Bone graft physiology. *J Am Podiatry Assoc* 73: 70–74, 1983.
145. Rothstein AS: Skin grafting techniques. *J Am Podiatry Assoc* 73: 79–85, 1983.
146. Souther SG: Skin grafts from the sole of the foot: Case report and literature review. *J Trauma* 20: 163–165, 1980.
147. Tisa VN: *Podiatric Surgical Consideration of the Aging Patient (Clinical Podogeriatries) Baltimore, Williams & Wilkins, 1981, p. 77.*
148. Davis RJ, Millis MB: Ankle arthrodesis in the management of traumatic ankle arthrosis: A long-term retrospective study. *J Trauma* 20: 8; 674–678, 1980.
149. Wilds AH: Surgical treatment of the foot and ankle in rheumatoid arthritis. *J Foot Surg* 8: 31–32, 1969.
150. Berlin D, et al: Surgical approaches to Haglund's disease. *J Foot Surg* 21: 42–44, 1982.
151. Michetti ML, Jacobs SA: Calcaneal heel spurs: Etiology, treatment, and a new surgical approach. *J Foot Surg* 22: 234–239, 1983.
152. Ruch JA: Haglund's disease. *J Am Podiatry Assoc* 64: 100, 1974.
153. Berun D, Coleman W, Nickamin A: Surgical approaches to Haglund's disease. *J Foot Surg* 21: 42, 1982.
154. Shama SS, Kominsky SJ, Lenart H: Prevalence of non-painful heel spur and its relation to postural foot position. *J Am Podiatry Assoc* 73: 122–123, 1983.
155. McCarthy DJ, et al: The surgical anatomy of the rearfoot (Part I: the greater tarsus). *J Am Podiatry Assoc* 73: 607–619, 1983.
156. Fenton CF, et al: Criteria for selected major tendon transfers in podiatric surgery. *J Am Podiatry Assoc* 73: 561–568, 1983.
157. Girlando J, Berlin S: Complications of Keller bunionectomy and Keller with Swanson hemi-implant. *J Foot Surg* 20: 148, 1981.
158. Carrel JM, Davidson DM: Venous thrombosis. *J Foot Surg* 13: 8, 1974.
159. Johnston WB, Golda KR: Venous thromboembolic disease. *J Am Podiatry Assoc* 71: 254, 1981.
160. Jay RM, Schoenhaus HD: Complications in implant arthroplasties for the osteoarthritic joint. *J Am Podiatry Assoc* 72: 248–255, 1982.
161. O Keefe RG: A classification of complications of implant arthroplasties. Pioneers Lecture Series, 75th Annual Meeting of the American Podiatry Association, Boston, August 21, 1983.
162. Weinstock RE, et al: Osseous engulfment of a silicone prosthesis with foreign body reaction. *J Am Podiatry Assoc* 74: 80–88, 1984.
163. Krauette MA, Baker GI: The Swanson arthroplasty of the great toes: A prospective study. *J Foot Surg* 17: 155, 1978.
164. Vanore J, O'Keefe R, Pikscher I: Silastic[R] implant arthroplasty—complications and their classifications. *J Am Podiatry Assoc* 74: 423–433, 1984.
165. Nenad DR: Postoperative osteophytic activity: A case report. *J Foot Surg* 17: 31, 1978.
166. Lim WT, Landrum K, Weinberger B: Silicone lymphadenitis secondary to implant degeneration. *J Foot Surg* 22: 243–246, 1983.
167. Gerbert J, Melillo T: A modified Akin procedure for the correction of hallux valgus. *J Am Podiatry Assoc* 61: 132–136, 1971.
168. Rosenthal DC, Callahan Df: Distal transverse crecentic osteotomy for correction of hallux abducto-valgus. *J Am Podiatry Assoc* 74: 411–414, 1984.
169. Austin DW, et al: A new osteotomy for hallux valgus: A horizontally directed "V" displacement osteotomy of the metatarsal head for hallux valgus and primus varus. *Clin Orthop* 157: 25–30, 1981.

Suggested Readings

Adams E: Surgery with special reference to podiatry. *J Int Coll Surg* 45: 339, 1932.

Addante J: Metatarsal osteotomy as a surgical approach for the elimination of plantar keratosis. *J Foot Surg* 8: 36–38, 1969.

American Podiatry Association: Model screening criteria for the review of surgical procedures and associated care rendered by podiatrists: Contract No. HSA 105-BQA-48(4) DHEW. *J Am Podiatry Assoc* 65: 1143–1180, 1975.

Anderson GS, Katz JH, Zier BG: Bacterial endocarditis—clinical considerations and prophylaxis. *J Am Podiatric Med Assoc* 76:332–336, 1986.

Axler DA, Dziarski R: Bacteria causing podiatric infections, and processing of clinical specimens. *J Am Podiatric Med Assoc* 75: 1–12, 1985.

Bailey H: Infections of the foot. *J Int Coll Surg* 27: 475–482, 1957.

Borovoy M, et al: Laser surgery in podiatric medicine—present and future. *J Foot Surg* 22: 353–357, 1983.

Boyce-Smith G, Scherer PR: Unexplained hepatitis after podiatric surgery with halothane anesthesia. *J Am Podiatric Med Assoc* 75: 23–27, 1985.

Burns, AE (ed): Digital Surgery. *Clinics in Podiatry.* Philadelphia, WB Saunders, Co, 1986.

Cangialosi CP (ed): *Symposium on Minimal Incision Surgery. Clinics in Podiatry.* Philadelphia, WB Saunders, Co, 1985.

Curtin JW: Functional surgery for intractable conditions of the sole of the foot. *Plast Reconstr Surg* 59: 806–811, 1877.

Delaney HN, Travis LO: A clinical evaluation of one hundred cases of infection of the lower leg and foot in military personnel. *Milit Med* 130: 184–190, 1965.

Dintcho A: Procedures to correct hallux abducto valgus and metatarsus primus adductus. *J Foot Surg* 15: 15–21, 1976.

Drucker WR, Hubay CA, Holden WD, et al: Pathogenesis of postraumatic sympathetic dystrophy. *Am J Surg* 97: 454, 1959.

Farley RD: Medial arthroplasty for correction of heloma. *J Am Podiatry Assoc* 61: 473–476, 1971.

Fenton CF: Postoperative management following digital surgery. *J Am Podiatric Med Assoc 75*: 36–40, 1985.

Frankel JP, et al: Surgery for tophaceous gout. *J Foot Surg* 23: 440–444, 1984.

Friend G: Correction of elongated underlapping lesser toes by middle phalangectomy and skin plasty. *J Foot Surg* 23: 470–476, 1984.

Freeman DW: Prolonged local anesthesia in chiropody. *J Am Podiatry Assoc* 44: 28–34, 1954.

Gamble FO: *Applied Foot Roentgenology.* Baltimore Williams & Wilkins, 1957.

Geller SD: Foreign body removal with the aid of a metal locator. *J Am Podiatry Assoc* 51: 502–503, 1961.

Greenfield LJ (ed): *Complications in Surgery and Trauma.* Philadelphia, JB Lippincot Co, 1984.

Gumbine, NA (ed.): Plastic Surgery. *Clinics in Podiatry.* Philadelphia, WB Saunders, Co, 1986.

Hubay CA: Sesamoid bones of the hands and feet. *Am J Roentgenol Radium Ther* 61: 500–505, 1949.

Keck C: The tarsal tunnel syndrome. *J Bone Joint Surg* 44-A: 180, 1962.

Kravette MA: Peripheral nerve entrapment syndromes in the foot. *J Am Podiatry Assoc* 61: 457–472, 1971.

Krevitz HM, Sokoloff T: Tarsal tunnel syndrome. *J Am Podiatry Assoc* 65: 825–840, 1975.

Kuwada GT: Ankle stabilization and primary repair with a peroneus brevis tendon graft. *J Foot Surg* 25:139–145, 1986.

Landry JR, Schilero J: The medical/surgical management of gout. *J Foot Surg* 25:160–175, 1986.

LaPorta, G (ed.): Osteosynthesis in Foot and Ankle Surgery. *Clinics in Podiatry.* Philadelphia, WB Saunders, Co, 1985.

Lendir JL: A perspective focus on the indicated surgical treatment of resistant clubfoot in the infant. *South Med J* 69: 837–843, 1976.

Levitus IM, Scheimer OM: Gout as a complication. *J Natl Assoc Chirop* 28: 36–38, 1938.

Levy, LA (ed.): Systemic Diseases Affecting the Foot. *Clinics in Podiatry.* Philadelphia, WB Saunders, Co, 1985.

Lowy A, et al: Sinus tarsi syndrome: A postoperative analysis. *J Foot Surg* 24: 108–112, 1985.

Malek N, Beneson DE: Cardiac arrhythmias during the perioperative period. *J Am Podiatric Med Assoc* 75: 17–22, 1985.

Mann R (ed.): *Surgery of the Foot,* ed 5. Princeton, CV Mosby, 1986.

McGlamry, ED, McGlamry R (eds): Doctors Hospital Podiatric Education and Research Institute Fourteenth Annual Surgical Seminar, Stamford, CT, April 18–21, 1985.

McGlone JJ: The tarsal tunnel syndrome. *J Am Podiatry Assoc* 58: 435, 1968.

McGregor RR: New stretch nylon shoe lace as a therapeutic aid. *J Am Podiatry Assoc* 51: 497–500, 1961.

Nealon F: *Fundamental Skills in Surgery.* Philadelphia, W B Saunders Co., 1979.

Olson AC, Collis S: Bacterial study on surgical scrub techniques. *J Am Podiatry Assoc* 67:255–258, 1977.

Perrone MA: *Podiatric Nail and Bone Surgery.* Canton, OH; The Webber Dental Manufacturing Co, 1972.

Pressman D: Ambulatory condylectomy for intractable plantar keratosis. *Curr Podiatry* 11–12, 1971.

Purgett DL: Surgical correction for dislocated joint. *Chirop Rec* 21: 52, 1938.

Raj PP (ed): *Handbook of Regional Anesthesia.* New York, Churchill Livingstone, 1985.

Rutherford RB: *Vascular Surgery,* ed 2 Philadelphia, W B Saunders Co, 1984.

Rutledge BA, Green AL: Surgical treatment of plantar corns. *U S Armed Forces Med J* 8: 219–234, 1957.

Tillman K: Surgical treatment of the foot in rheumatoid arthritis. *Reconstr Surg Traumatol* 18: 195–204, 1981.

Sabiston DC, Jr (ed): *Davis-Christopher Textbook of Surgery,* vol. I and II, ed. 12. Philadelphia, W B Saunders Co, 1981.

Wolf E, Federbusch MJ: Perioperative fever: etiology and treatment. *J Foot Surg* 24:272–274, 1985.

Yale I: Foreign bodies in the foot. *Conn Chiropodist* 10: 3–4, 1954.

12

Sports Medicine

Aerobic capacity—the maximum amount of oxygen the body can consume and transport to striated muscle during a measurable period of time—is the best overall index of physical fitness. It depends on the ability to breathe rapidly, the ability to deliver forcefully large volumes of blood throughout the cardiovascular system and the ability to deliver oxygen throughout the body. An aerobic exercise is heart- and lung-stimulating exercise that is sufficiently intensive to produce beneficial change in the body (1). The resultant aerobic conditioning, which is attained by participation in many varieties of exercise, results in a lower heart rate resulting in less cardiac workload. Aerobic conditioning in conjunction with genetic and dietary factors has been shown to lessen the incidence of coronary artery disease and to increase emotional stability and mental alertness (2).

The vast majority of aerobic exercises involve the lower extremities (3). Defining exercise parameters and indigenous lower extremity movements in each sport remains a challenge to the podiatric physician. Specific injuries due to macrotrauma (overt injury) and microtrauma (multiple minimal cumulative injury) are presented to the podiatrist. Biomechanically and training-induced "overuse syndromes" due to microtrauma are discussed in this chapter. (Chapter 10, Foot and Ankle Trauma, provides a more detailed discussion of injuries due to a sudden traumatic event.) A cross-section of individual sports are discussed, and related areas of interest, including diet, footgear, training techniques and sport psychology, are described.

A warm-up period before engaging in aerobic or anaerobic exercise is essential. This period, which may last from 5–30 min, is utilized to stretch myotendinous tissues, increase joint range of motion, allow the body to adjust slowly to an increased cardiovascular workload and to lessen the risk of injury. A cool-down period after aerobic exercise is also of prime importance. It may also last from 5–30 min and differs in every sport. This period of continued use of the muscles involved in the aerobic activity allows time for pooled blood to return to the heart and enhances joint range of motion through stretching-flexibility exercises.

Running

All sports utilizing the lower extremities incorporate running to some degree. Walking, sprinting, waggeling (a cross between walking and jogging), jogging, middle-intermediate and long-distance running are the precursors of most individual and team sports. Whether involved in a racquet sport or a sport requiring special equipment, such as skiing or bicycling, lower extremity functional ability is essential.

Preparation

Preparation for sprint running differs from preparation for the 26-mile, 385-yard marathon. Studies show that there is a decrease in performance level as well as an increase in physical damage sustained by marathon runners, with full recovery taking up to a week to achieve. It is possible to monitor the damage and rate of recovery by measuring serum levels of creatine kinase, maximum heart rate, ventilations per minute, and VO_2 maximum. Muscle biopsies may also indicate degree of damage and predict recovery rate.

Proper conditioning of appropriate muscles is mandatory. Stretching, flexibility and strengthening exercises should be performed before and after running. Running too fast, running too soon and running too long are the "quicksand" of all those engaged in the running sports. Common sense is the key to avoiding problems. Warm-up exercises should be performed slowly. When returning to running after a prolonged absence one must begin at a lower level of activity. Proper clothing and shoes and a proper diet are essential.

There is nothing more dangerous to personal health than the "weekend athlete" who overstresses his or her body. It is important to follow an organized and consistent training program to avoid injury. This program is determined by the age, weight and past podiatric and medical history of the beginning athlete. It is dangerous for a middle-age person to engage initially in vigorous exercise for more than 30 minutes for 5 days a week. Rather, it is realistic to engage in vigorous exercise for progressively longer time limits over a 6 month period. Goodyear and Blair (4) evaluate the incidence of orthopaedic injury in 1,837 healthy runners and 693 nonrunners, 43 years old or older, who were seen in a large preventive medicine clinic. Upper body injury rates did not differ between the two groups. Lower extremity injury rates were significantly higher ($P<.05$) in runners than in nonrunners. However, the absolute rate of injuries in long-term runners was relatively low. Sohn and Micheli (5), in a survey of 498 runners and 287 swimmers, with an average follow-up of 42 years from years of competition, found no relationship between running at moderate levels (below 25 miles per week) and the development of osteoarthritis of the knee or hips. Neither number of years running nor heavy mileage seemed to increase the incidence of osteoarthritis. Pagliano and Jackson (6) examined 3,000 long-distance runners (2,173 males and 912 females ages 10 to 75 years) over a 5-year period. A low incidence of disabling injuries was found. The most common injuries were to the plantar fascia and medial and lateral aspects of the knee due to microtraumatic overuse.

Proper shoes are a necessity for the athlete, whether he or she is a neophyte or a professional. Clothing should be loose fitting. It is essential to protect the exposed parts of the body in both summer and winter. A warm-up suit and ski mask protect from exposure in cold weather. A light-weight hat may be necessary for protection from the sun. Dressing in layers maintains warmth and prevents dehydration. A firm supportive brassiere is necessary for female athletes.

Runners should attempt to stay away from hills initially. Running uphill can aggravate Achilles tendon, hamstring and low back problems. Level surfaces are important to all the running sports.

Body style and form should be what is most comfortable and natural for the individual. Hands should be relaxed when running. Overstriding may lead to stress and injury.

Proper dietary habits are encouraged. Eating within 3 hours of athletic participation is not wise. Adequate fluid intake is important to minimize the possibility of becoming dehydrated.

If pain in the lower extremities does not go away with rest or if difficulty in breathing or chest pain is experienced, immediate medical attention is necessary.

Style and Form

The correct running style is the style that feels right for the individual. However, these guidelines should be followed. Run faster by running easier. Breathe through the mouth, not the nose. Stand up straight. Look straight ahead, not at the feet. Do not overstride.

Sprinters land on their toes; their heels may never touch the running surface. In contrast, the distance runner contacts the surface with the heel first. Occasionally, the forepart of the foot strikes the surface first, followed immediately by heel contact. Initial surface contact is on the outside of the foot across the forepart of the foot and forward through the great toe. Runners should not land on their toes while training. Foot contact with the ground should be on the outside of the heel or flatfooted.

Foot plant should be directly under the knee. The beginner should use a short low stride and avoid hills. Alterations of this pattern may have detrimental effect on the lower extremities.

An unbending elbow is the most common upper extremity fault. Elbows and wrists should not be held in a rigid position. Fists should be loosely closed, with wrists and hands in line with the arms and the palms facing the body. Shoulders and head should be kept level. Jaw, neck and face muscles should be relaxed and not tight.

Training plays an important role in preparing the athlete to participate in a running sport. Principles of athletic training are of prime importance to all those interested in maintaining tip top fitness (Table 12.1.).

The training programs should be specific for each individual, with consideration given to age, weight, past history and sport undertaken. For example, the "four corner drill" is recommended for badminton players, but would not be used for baseball players. The athlete should not smoke. Smoking causes arterial narrowing

Table 12.1.
Athletic Training Principles

1. **Stress:** The stimulus that provides a training response. Too much stress overtaxes the body and causes breakdown. Too little stress is of insufficient help in maintaining fitness. Stress must be strong and regular to provide beneficial effects. Other stress factors to consider include weather, dietary and psychological.
2. **Overload:** Stressing in a selective manner. Overloading is not overworking. Selective stress, enough to produce the desired training response without exhaustion, is what is meant by overloading. The training load must be frequent, severe and intense enough to cause the body to adapt to its fullest to a selected activity.
3. **Specificity:** The concept that one trains in a specific sport in order to participate maximally in that sport. A swimmer trains through swimming and a runner through running. The body adapts in specific ways to specific exercise patterns. There are even different specific training patterns in sprinting and distance running.
4. **Regularity:** Performance depends on a regular training schedule. Without training 4 out of 7 days, the runner could not hope to perform well. Conditioning cannot be maintained by irregular training patterns. When the regularity of training is interrupted speed disappears first, followed next by endurance.
5. **Progression:** Training progress takes place most rapidly at the beginning of training and slows down as the maximum fitness level is reached. The more improvement one makes, the harder it is to continue to improve. There are slow periods of improvement separated by periods of no improvement. It is important to appreciate this fact and not become frustrated by a lack of progress.
6. **Lesser Returns:** The longer one trains, the less one receives in return. The first part of a training period produces the greatest benefit in conditioning and fitness. The athlete must work harder and harder for less and less improvement as he or she draws closer to maximal individual fitness.
7. **Recovery:** Constant stress without rest leads to exhaustion. Rest is essential for recovery. Physical and psychological relaxation are necessary during training and in between training periods. Continual effort without alternating periods of rest and recovery diminishes fitness.
8. **Participation:** An athlete should not participate in a chosen event every month all year round. It is important to take time to recoup and restore the body's reserves. One cannot participate to the maximum on an everyday basis without harmful effects. There is a season for maximal training and a season for recovery.
9. **Pacing:** The average rate at which a distance is traveled. The kind of pace the athlete maintains on a weekly and monthly basis helps determine the training response. The faster and harder a person trains, the shorter the distance traveled. The faster the pace, the quicker the end. The slower the pace, the longer it takes to reach the end.
10. **Individualization:** One training schedule must not be followed rigidly by all athletes. There is no one training plan that fits the needs of everyone. Each training program must take into consideration individual needs. Blindly following a written schedule is unwise.

and a decrease in oxygen-transport ability.

Training programs vary depending on the specific running sport. Long-slow distances (LSD) are often recommended for the endurance athlete. Interval training consisting of running a slow 220 yards, a moderately fast 440 yards, a slow 220 yards, followed by a very fast 440 yards builds stamina. The optimal program combines weight training, stretching, interval training and long-slow distance running. A variety of terrain is essential for the experienced long-distance runner.

Training Instrumentation and Equipment

Professional equipment, instruments and training aids have proliferated in recent years. Their variety and application for specific uses are most helpful to the athlete for training, rehabilitation, physical fitness and stress management.

Equipment is available both for generalized conditioning and for specific sports conditioning. Cybex, Universal Gym and other fitness equipment afford the athlete the diversity of isotonic, isometric and isokinetic muscle exercise training and rehabilitation. Specific sport training equipment includes cardiovascular exercisers with a smooth, rhythmic cross-country skiing motion; rowing machines; various motorized and nonmotorized treadmills; electric bicycle ergometers; and progressive resistance exercisers with adjustable tension. Heart monitors, muscle tension monitors, skin fold calipers, flexometers, arthropometric tape measures, goniometers, weight belts, ankle weights, knee, foot and ankle orthoses and braces and biofeedback systems are available to assist the athlete in training, conditioning and rehabilitation.

Stretching and Strengthening Exercises

Specific exercise programs can be tailored to the individual according to functional requirements and deficits.

Joint manipulation and mobilization helps enhance the range of motion of foot joints. Apply traction to each toe by slowly pulling each toe forward, then moving it up, down and side to side to the point of feeling tension. The midpart of the foot and ankle may be moved in the same manner. Movements are performed with the hands.

The following six important stretching and strengthening exercises should be performed while wearing shoes before and after participation in running sports. They should take no longer than 15 min to perform.

Gastrocnemius Stretch (Fig. 12.1) Stand with legs internally rotated (toes pointing toward nose) about 3 feet from the wall. Touch hands to wall. Lean in until your chin touches the wall, keeping your knees locked, heels on the floor, legs straight and "back side" in. Hold this position for 10 sec. Slowly return to an upright position. As you lean toward the wall you should feel a pulling sensation below and behind your knees and/or in the back of your lower leg. If this does not occur, move away from the wall. If your heels come off the ground move closer to the wall. Repeat the exercises, increasing slowly over a period of time to a maximum of 15. Start slowly. Do not bounce. If your gastrocnemius muscle contracts, you are being too forceful.

In order to stretch the soleus, repeat this exercise with knees slightly bent. The leg being stretched should be away from the wall. The leg not being stretched should be close to the wall. This exercise may be done with the elbows against the wall in-

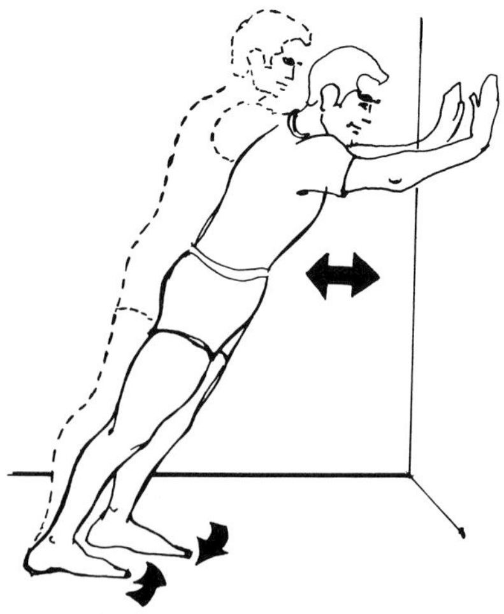

Figure 12.1. Calf stretch.

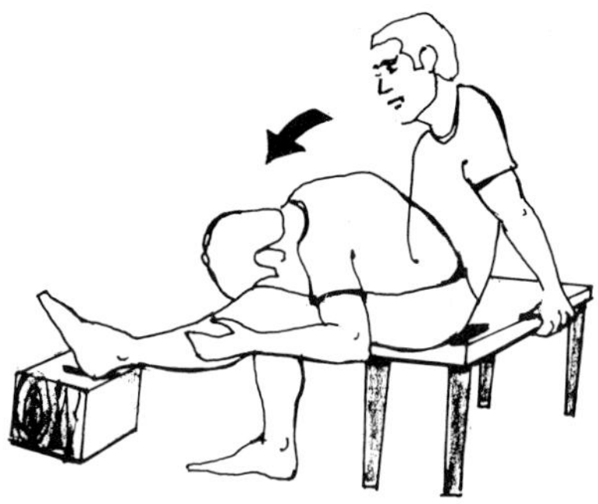

Figure 12.2. Hamstring stretch.

stead of with outstretched arms, if that position is more comfortable.

Hamstring Stretch (Fig. 12.2) Put your straight leg to be stretched with knee locked on a footstool; later it can be placed on a chair and finally a table as you improve. From a sitting position (later while standing), bring your head toward the knee of the extended leg until a pulling sensation occurs at the back of the upper leg. Hold this position for 10 sec. If you experience pain or discomfort behind your knee, bend your knee slightly.

Repeat the exercise by extending the opposite leg in the same manner. Repeat the exercise, increasing slowly over a period of time to a maximum of 15 stretches for each leg.

Low Back and Hamstring Stretch (Fig. 12.3) Lie on a soft yielding surface, such as grass. Bring straight legs with knees locked over your head, and try to touch the surface with your toes. When you feel a pulling sensation behind your upper legs and low back, hold the position for 10 sec. Flex the knees to your ears and relax for 5 sec. Repeat the exercise, increasing slowly and gradually over a period of time to a maximum of seven stretches.

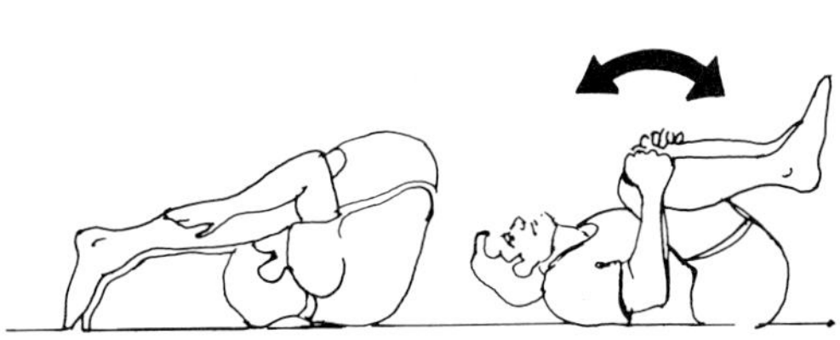

Figure 12.3. Low back and hamstring stretch.

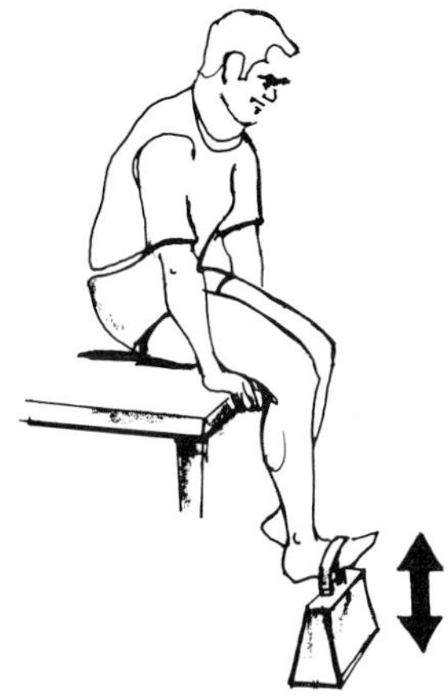

Figure 12.4. Tibialis anterior and extensor digitorum longus strengthening exercise.

This exercise should not be performed if a sharp pain is experienced in the neck, shoulder or upper and lower back or while recovering from an irritation of the sciatic nerve.

Tibialis Anterior and Extensor Digitorum Longus (Fig. 12.4) Sit on a table with the legs hanging down. Attach a 3-lb weight to one foot. (Socks filled with sand may be used.) Move your foot up toward your leg and hold for 5 sec. Relax. Repeat the exercise, increasing slowly over a period of time to a maximum of 15 each foot.

Quadriceps Muscles (Fig. 12.5) Sit on a table with the legs hanging down. Attach a 3-lb weight to one foot. With your knee flexed approximately 15° and leg externally rotated approximately 25° raise your entire leg from the hip and hold for 5 sec. Relax. Repeat the exercise, increasing slowly over a period of time to a maximum of 15 for each leg.

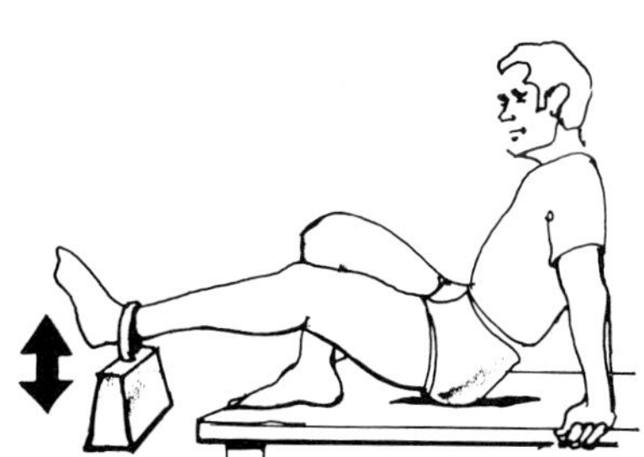

Figure 12.5. Quadriceps (vastus medialis) strengthening exercise.

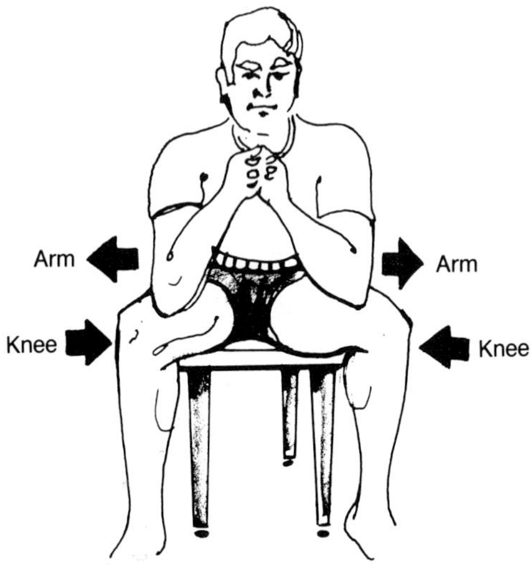

Figure 12.6. Miller exercise.

Miller Exercise / Adductors (Fig. 12.6) Sit on the front of a chair with feet flat on the floor and 6–9 inches apart. Knees should be at a 90° angle and 12–15 inches apart. Clasp your hands together and place your elbows inside the thighs just above the knees (bend forward at the waist to do this.) Now, try to bring the knees together while simultaneously resisting this motion by exerting force outward with the elbows. Slowly let the knees push your elbow in until the elbows touch. Then, without relaxing, let the elbows push the knees out until the knees are back to their original separation. Repeat this maneuver 10–12 times without resting between repetitions. Each repetition should take about 20 sec.

Shoes

A running shoe has more features built into it than most other shoes.

All shoes are made over foot-shaped forms called lasts. The last is a wooden or plastic model of a foot. Traditionally, last makers spent days carving wooden lasts over which millions of shoes were constructed. These lasts were designed in a very unscientific way. The last maker would often try to model the foot last after a family members' foot. One can imagine what occurred when millions of shoes were made over a last patterned after a deformed foot. Today, many lasts are plastic foot models designed by computers.

The upper part of a shoe is designed by a pattern maker. Lace shoes have two basic designs: Bal and Blucher. The bal pattern shoe is laced up from a V with no overhanging leather. The blucher pattern shoe laces up from two overhanging pieces of leather on each side of the tongue of the shoe.

The upper part of the shoe may be made of leather, nylon, suede, plastic or other man-made material. It is important that this material be able to breathe enabling moisture to escape. This is the major difficulty with solid man-made upper materials, such as Corfam.(R) After the upper of the shoe is stitched together it is applied to the last and a midsole is attached. This process is called lasting.

There are three basic lasting techniques: slip lasting, board lasting and combination lasting. The slip-lasted shoe is placed on the last and stitched together in a mocassin-like pattern and then attached to the midsole. Shoes constructed by this method have no support and do not absorb shock. In board lasting, the upper is stretched over the last, and the midsole is attached and glued to a piece of cardboard or other more firm material. This shoe has stability, but it is not flexible and is a poor shock absorber. However, the board-lasted shoe is beneficial for the heavy overpronating runner. The third lasting technique is a combination between slip and board lasting. Combination lasting results in a shoe with the back part being firm (board lasting) and the forepart of the shoe being soft and flexible (slip lasting). The shoe constructed over a combination last is usually the most supportive and comfortable for most feet.

Lasts or foot models, as are feet, may be straight or curved. Until recently most shoes were constructed over inflair lasts, although most feet are outflair feet. This resulted in rubbing and blister or heloma formation on the last two toes. Today, shoe companies are beginning to manufacture straighter lasted shoes to accommodate the majority of feet.

After the upper and/or cardboard is attached, the midsole is glued to the bottom of the shoe. The midsole is designed to control motion and at the same time absorb shock. Midsole materials used for running, tennis and other sports-related shoes have improved greatly in recent years. The midsole in a running shoe consists of multiple layers of different densities. The material used is either EVA (ethylene vinyl acetate) or polyurethane. The midsole is usually made thicker in the heel area to absorb more shock at heel contact. Some manufacturers make multidensity midsoles with softer material at the outer heel edge or the inner heel edge. Softer outer midsole heel material with harder inner midsole heel material is helpful for the overpronating, compensated rearfoot varus foot; the opposite combination is beneficial to the under pronating cavus rigid foot. In a nonrunning shoe, such as an Oxford or a ½-inch heel pump, there is no midsole. A plastic, wooden or metal shank, beginning beneath the heel and running forward to just behind the metatarsal heads is placed between the cardboard and the outersole.

After the midsole is applied to the shoe a heel wedge or heel counter support may be applied to give the heel of the shoe more stability. The heel wedge may be soft at its outer edge to absorb shock and firmer at its inner edge for support. The heel counter support is a collar of thermoplastic material applied around the outer heel edge to help maintain the heel's stability. The heel counter itself may be either flexible or stiff. The stiffer and firmer the heel counter, the more motion control it provides. Motion control is essential for the overpronated flatfoot. The heel counter is made more stable with various thermoplastic materials between the inner shoe heel material and the outer shoe heel leather or other material and may be extended medially along the inner side of the foot.

Running and other athletic shoes have a padded ankle collar designed for fit and comfort and a heel tab at the back of the collar to prevent irritation to the Achilles tendon.

To complete shoe construction, the outersole is now applied. In most athletic shoes the outersole is glued to the midsole. In well-constructed mens' Oxfords, the outersole is stitched (Goodyear welt) to the shoe. The outersole in a running shoe is constructed of compressed EVA, blown rubber, rubber interspersed with air or hard rubber. Rubber, leather and synthetic materials are used in nonathletic shoe outersole construction. Often a heel plug is placed at the outerside of the heel. The bottom of the outersole may have a waffle, nubbed, ripple, banded or herringbone pattern. Waffle soles are better suited for running on yielding surfaces, such as grass or sand. Ripple-soled shoes are better suited for running on hard flat surfaces, such as asphalt or cement. The innersole or sockliner of a running shoe may be made of foam, Spenco, Sorbothane or other material or may be a removable insert. There may be a rubber or synthetic arch support present. If this aggravates the foot it is easily removed.

If a shoe insole is not present, Spenco insoles may be inserted. For those who use foot orthotic devices, it is often necessary to remove the innersole and replace it with the foot orthoses.

The following shoe characteristics are recommended for overpronating foot types: board or combination lasting, rigid shank (if available), a firm dual-density midsole, a straight last shoe, a rigid firm heel counter and outside heel counter support. Qualities that exacerbate overpronation include a slip-lasted shoe with a soft heel counter, a curved last shoe with inflair and a shoe with a soft compressible midsole or outersole.

Runners who have underpronating foot types should look for a slip-lasted shoe with outer heel counter support, soft mid- and outersoles and a shoe constructed over a curved last to conform better to the shape of the foot. Shoe qualities that exacerbate underpronation include board or straight lasting, firm extended medial counters and firm mid- or outersoles.

Shoes should be bought at the end of the day when the feet are larger. If orthotic devices are being used, shoes should be fitted with the devices inserted (Fig. 12.7). The shoe should have an easily removable arch support or no additional inside padding in order to accommodate the orthotic device. Do not buy shoes according to numerical size. Shoes manufactured of the same size by different companies may or

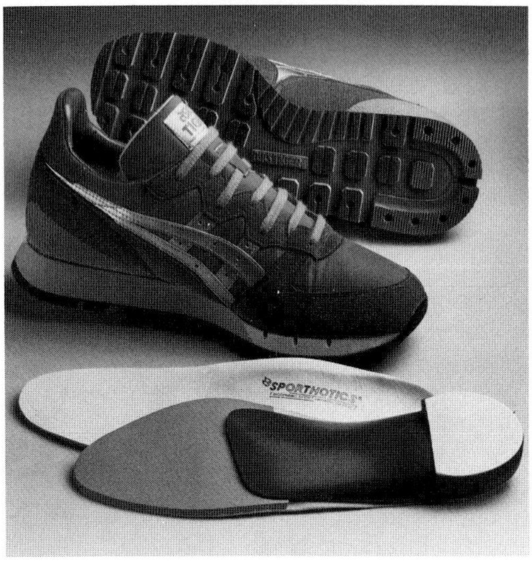

Figure 12.7. Tiger prescription athletic shoe designed to accommodate foot orthotic devices.

may not fit the same. Do not buy mail-order shoes. Try both shoes on. If the shoes are not comfortable initially, they should not be bought. Check to ensure that the shoes are level and balanced and do not lean to one side or the other. Training shoes should be used for running (Fig. 12.8). Avoid racing flats (7).

No one shoe is adequate for everyone because there are many foot types requiring a variety of shoes. The scientific evaluation of an athletic shoe must first take the individual sport with its indigenous movements into consideration. Within a functional context other areas of evaluation should include rearfoot impact and control, forefoot impact and control, flexibility, sole wear and traction and shoe weight.

Many of the shoes made for the running sports are constructed with little or no

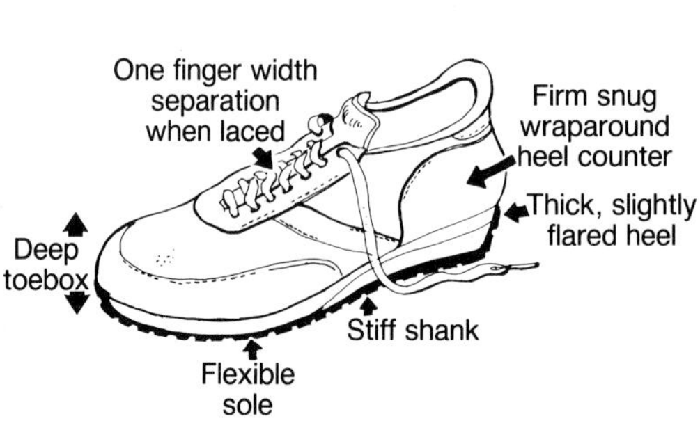

Figure 12.8. Runner's training shoe.

concern for the way the foot functions. Some shoes may help foot function, whereas others may interfere with efficient foot function. The sport, running surface, participation time and age, weight, lower extremity function and foot structure of the individual must be considered in selecting the proper athletic shoe.

Heel cushioning, lift, support and width are of great importance. Training on flat, hard surfaces requires a good shock-absorbing heel. The tendency toward tight triceps surae muscles requires a running shoe heel that is a little higher than work shoes. The heel counter should be firm and fit snugly around the heel to help stabilize the heel. If the bottom of the heel is too narrow, the calcaneus has a tendency to rotate. The heel of the shoe should be wider on its bottom than at the area where it attaches to the upper part of the shoe. Flared heels are helpful when running on trails and uneven surfaces. The shank should be firm or stiff for adequate support.

The forepart of the sole should be flexible, not easily compressible and not stiff. The shoe must have the ability to bend forward at the metatarsophalangeal joint level for efficient foot function. Cavus foot types need more shock absorption; planus foot types need more rearfoot control and support.

The toebox should be deep enough and long enough to accommodate toe size and length. The end of the shoe should be one thumbnail's length beyond the tip of the longest toe. With the shoe on, the eyelets should not be pulled together. Nor should they be wide apart. A finger's width between the eyelets is appropriate when the shoe is laced.

The normal shoe shows wear on the outside of the heel as opposed to the inner area of the heel (Fig. 12.9). This wear should take place gradually and should progress along the outside of the sole, across the lesser metatarsal heads and out through the big toe. When attempting to repair worn heels and soles, be sure that the repair material is not used to excess or applied higher than the original heel or sole level. Individuals running over 50 miles a week should own several pair of

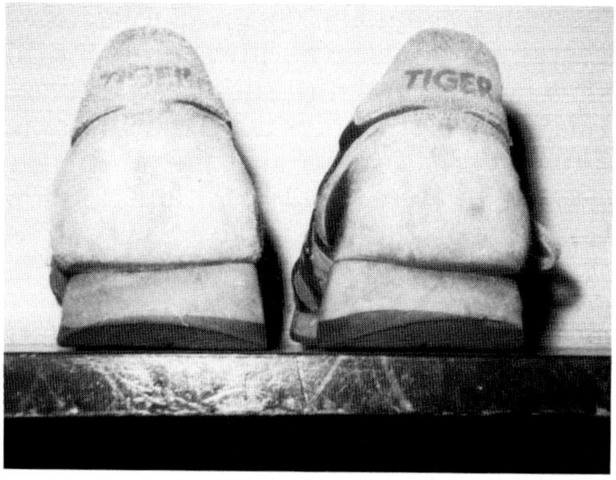

Figure 12.9. Normal heel wear.

shoes. Excessive heel wear on the outer side or on the inner heel and/or sole indicates abnormal function requiring further investigation.

Diet

Athletes function best on a high complex carbohydrate, low-fat, low-protein diet. Because digestive and other metabolic factors may interfere with performance, a meal should not be eaten within 3 hrs of sports participation. It is essential to drink a good amount of water before participating in all running sports. Liquid replacement is necessary on hot and humid days to avoid dehydration. Symptoms of dehydration include a tired listless feeling, lightheadedness and extreme thirst. An electrolyte- and mineral-containing drink is helpful before, during and after participation in all running sports. Although drinking beer in moderation may be an effective liquid replacement, alcohol in excess is to be avoided. Leg cramps, common to the distance runner, are usually caused by dehydration and salt loss. The daily requirement of salt approximates 50–100 mg. A diet high in carbohydrates, such as bread, cereals, potatoes, fruits, vegetables, spaghetti and honey, leads to an increase in stored glycogen in the muscles and liver. Glycogen is essential in the endurance athlete. Heavy red meats should be discouraged and chicken, veal and fish encouraged. Large amounts of animal and vegetable fats and food high in cholesterol should be avoided.

Vitamins E, C and B complex are beneficial to the speed and endurance athlete. The B complex vitamins are dependent upon each other for effective interaction. Alcohol destroys vitamin B_2 (riboflavin). Natural B complex sources include liver and brewer's yeast (3 tablespoons/day). Iron (27 mg/day) and zinc (22.5 mg/day) help the healing process following injury. Average daily vitamin requirements for a 150-lb athlete include 6 mg vitamin A, 8 mg niacin, 500 mg vitamin C (ascorbic acid), and 200 IU vitamin E. Daily intake of an all-inclusive natural multiple vitamin of choice—not necessarily high potency—is recommended for all athletes involved in the running sports. An additional 500 mg of vitamin C and 200 IU of vitamin E may be beneficial (7).

Running Program for the Beginner

A running program for the beginner should be organized in a rational manner. The beginning runner under the age of 30 should have had a general physical examination within the past year. The beginning runner over 30 years old should have a general physical examination, including an ECG. If there is a family history of heart disease, a stress test is advised. Kirby and Valmassy (8) describe a case history evaluation of the runner patient. A helpful question list is utilized in obtaining a runner's history before the physical examination.

A running sports program should not be embarked upon solely in order to lose weight although an overweight individual may engage in a running sports program if he or she is especially careful not to exceed his or her limits. Excess weight puts additional stress on both the cardiopulmonary vascular system and the lower extremities. Running while pregnant may be beneficial; advice from an obstetrician familiar with athletic medicine is mandatory.

The beginner should run 4–6 days each week. The running surface should be flat with no obstacles. Level cinder tracks, packed dirt, trails or flat roads are the most common surfaces. Avoid running on the sides of slanted roads or on soft shoulders. If running on roads, run facing traffic. The time of day chosen for running is an individual preference. However, running toward the end of a busy work day can be psychologically and physiologically beneficial. There is less chance of injury when running at the end of the day.

One goal of engaging in any running sport from a medical standpoint is to lower one's resting pulse. Doing so puts less stress on the heart-lung-blood vessel system. It is not uncommon for an athlete to lower the resting pulse from the 70s and 80s to the 40s after consistent exercise. In order to achieve a lowered resting pulse the athlete must endeavor to almost double the resting pulse during exercise and to keep it at that rate for a period of time, usually 10–12 min for 1–6 days a week. This period varies as training progresses (1).

The beginning runner should not train at double the resting pulse for long periods of time. On the contrary, he or she should spend between 10 and 15 min walking 1–6 days a week initially. The runner should next proceed to a slow jog. This activity should be accomplished in a steady, even fashion without excessive exertion. The beginning runner should be able to carry on a conversation while training without becoming tired and/or strained. The easier and slower the pace the farther the beginner can go. It is important that the beginner not overstress. Building of endurance at one's own pace is the important goal, and the time taken to do so is unimportant. An initial 10–15 minute daily fast walk proceeding to a jog should carry the runner approximately 1 mile. A runner's training, besides lowering the resting pulse, results in fat loss, a greater capacity for the lungs to take in oxygen and a reduction of blood pressure.

Once the beginning runner is able to run 15 min/day (meeting the above criteria without becoming tired or strained) and has done so for 1 week, he or she is now ready to progress to 20 min/day. However, the runner should not attempt to run the 15 min in competitive record time. Instead, alternate every other day of the 4–6 day running week with runs of 15 min one day and 20 min the next. Speed will increase as the runner becomes better conditioned. When the beginner is running 20 minutes every training day, an additional 5 minutes should be run on alternate days, thereby gradually building up running time. Training limits should not be exceeded on consecutive days. If continuous pain is experienced, the runner is cautioned to *STOP*. An attempt should not be made to run through pain.

Participation of Children and Teenagers in Sports

There are various methods to assess the athletic potential of children and adolescents; no single test can predict the future athletic success of a child. Variations of growth and development are such that the early physically mature child may be initially successful, only to be surpassed by the later developing child. The American Academy of Pediatrics recognizes three factors that determine athletic performance: physical characteristics and abilities, skill and mental attitude. The physical characteristics and abilities of the child are for the most part determined on a hereditary basis. Athletic skill depends on repetitive practice and some hereditary contribution. The skill must be learned properly through effective coaching. However, in order to develop and maintain any skill, practice is important. This is just as true for the foot surgeon as it is for the developing athlete. Proper mental attitude involves one's ability to accept instructions, desire to win, ability to sacrifice, self-control and a positive self-image. The ability to take instructions and accept advice is crucial to skill development in the young athlete.

The strong desire to win shows itself in enthusiastic assertive participation. Desire is inbred; it cannot be taught. The athlete has to want to achieve in order to do so. Self-control is also a major advantage of the developing athlete. The ability to think clearly and perform well often depends on maintaining one's self-control during sports participation. Self-control can be developed, but only if the athlete realizes the benefits of that quality. Poor examples shown by other athletes and adult role models have a negative effect on the development of self-control.

Whether one succeeds or fails in athletics and in life is often determined by the ability to maintain self-confidence. Having confidence in yourself as a person and in your ability to win can be crucial to success.

Although the exceptional child or adolescent athlete is a familiar figure to many professionals, one may never have considered the impact that success has on a child. How should parents relate to the exceptional child athlete who becomes the star of the soccer team or the major hitter on the All-Star Little League Team? Often the child lacks the maturity to deal with the pressures of success. Therefore, it is important to stress the basic worth of the child and not his or her achievements. Recognizing the child as a person without regard to athletic success or achievement is important. Children must be reminded that they are loved for themselves, not for what they can or cannot achieve athletically or academically.

Early physical development may enable a youngster to outshine his or her contemporaries on the athletic field. When the child's peers catch up with the early physical development of the exceptional child athlete, the earlier ability to outshine others may not be able to be sustained. At this point, it is of the utmost importance to emphasize the individual worth of the child without regard for athletic success. Doing so helps the early maturing child to develop a healthy value system, rather than a distorted self-centered image and/or a distorted view of the meaning of sports participation.

The pediatrician and podiatrist are often asked the question at what age should the child begin participating in team sports. There is no set time during the development of each child when he or she is better equipped to participate in a team sport. Expressed interest by the child (not an adult) and individual development determine when a child is ready to participate with others in team sports. Although children begin to compare themselves and their skills with other children at about age 6, late maturing children should refrain from contact sports until they are able to withstand its rigors.

The important factor to consider regarding participation in team sports is the real reason why the child wants to participate. Some of the more common motivating factors include wanting to be like Mom, Dad or other role models; interest in sports-related hobbies, such as collecting baseball cards; the desire to be noticed and to attract attention; the need to feel a part of a group; and the desire to wear the uniform of a winning team. No child should be pushed into participation in any sport. The more a child is pushed, the least likely he or she is to succeed.

"Little League syndrome" is a condition that presents itself in parents with children participating in team sports. It is overaggressiveness on behalf of parents and sometimes coaches. Those parents and coaches who push, push, push children to win at any cost, emphasizing winning at the expense of fun and enjoyment, suffer from "Little League syndrome." In recent years many professionals involved in sports-related programs have learned to recognize the extraordinary number of young athletes who have given up athletics because of adult pressure and intimidation. In the past this phenomenon was attributed to too much training at too fast a pace at too young an age. The realization is now growing that psychological pressure to win at any price is most unhealthy to children. The obsession of some parents to push their children to compete and set age group records in running sports, such as the marathon, often at the price of serious injury, is both foolish and dangerous. *Runner's World Magazine* has taken a stand on this issue by refusing to accept or maintain records for runners under the age of 12. The magazine states, "We do a disservice to our youngsters when we set them out at such a tender age in pursuit of meaningless standards" (9).

From a physical point of view, there is no reason why a child cannot run long distances or participate in other individual or team sports. The fear that the growing child will injure the growth centers of the bones of the feet, ankles, knees, legs and hips has proven to be unfounded. No significant increase in growth center injuries has been reported in the noncontact sports, and injuries have actually decreased in the contact sports, such as football, due to better training methods and equipment.

In fact, the possibility of a child incurring a physical injury is not as great as the chance a child has of sustaining psychological or emotional injury. It is the environment in which sports activity takes place, not the activity itself that is cause for concern. Youth sports should be tailored to the needs of children, not the needs of parents. Of major importance is the environment surrounding the athletic child. Jack Wilmore, Ph.D., an exercise physiologist, has written, "If the climate is such that winning is the only goal . . . the child will be likely to have a negative experience. If competition is organized . . . to satisfy the needs of the child and not the adult, the experience should be positive and facilitate sound emotional growth and psychological development" (10).

Parents often ask the pediatrician and podiatrist whether they should let their child quit the Little League or the soccer team. Although it is important not to let a child develop a pattern of quitting whenever a situation becomes stressful, it is sometimes better for the child to quit a team, than to remain in an unhealthy situation.

Being patient and understanding while determining the facts behind the child's desire to terminate participation is essential. Talking to the child, without reacting in a negative manner, helps elicit the child's feelings. There are valid reasons why a child should stop participating in a team sport, the most valid one being the risk of physical injury and/or repeat injury. Sometimes, it is necessary for the doctor to recommend that a certain sport be curtailed in the best interests of the child's health. If the child is experiencing stress-related symptoms, including but not limited to diarrhea, vomiting, nausea or headaches, then there is a valid reason to allow a child to quit a sport. A coach who is abusive in language or physically is not in the child's best interests. If a parent or a coach is so overly competitive as to cause the child to be fearful of failure, thereby affecting the child's personality and everyday life patterns, the child may have ample reason to quit a sport.

One should consider physical maturation and the child's physique when attempting to predict the success of the young athlete. In turn, inherited characteristics, exercise, hormonal influences, nutrition and overall health of the child influence the physique of the child. These factors should be taken into account when determining the potential ability of a child to participate in sports activities.

The inherited characteristics of height, shape and functional foot type are examples of factors that influence physical characteristics and ability. Although the height and shape of grown children usually is close to that of their parents, weight is not always as predictable because it is often determined by the caloric intake of the child. Exercise has a major influence on muscle development, joint movement and bone strength by allowing the body to develop fully. Hormonal influences affect individual maturation, fat distribution, strength and endurance. Individual physique is influenced by the hormones released during early childhood and adolescence. Nutritional factors influencing body type and physique are present from the time of conception through intrauterine development, after birth and into childhood. The nutritional status of the mother influences the birth weight and early development of the child. The nutritional needs of the pregnant woman and the young child affect the ultimate size of the individual. The overall health of the child is of paramount importance in the child's developing physique. A malnourished child will not develop fully. The growth of a child with a chronic medical disorder affecting the heart, lungs, or kidneys will almost always be altered or stunted.

There is virtually no physical handicap that will prevent participation in sports activity. Interest and participation in sports are beneficial for those children born with physical handicaps from both a psychological and a physical standpoint. The basketball player with one arm and the skier with one leg illustrate that the physically handicapped child or adult can achieve beyond what might be imagined.

The handicapped child who desires to participate in athletics should be encouraged to do so unless the specific sports activity has the potential of harming the youngster. Sometimes the child wants to participate in a sport that is inappropriate because of his or her handicaps. For example, it is inappropriate for a child with a bleeding disorder to participate in contact sports. Nor would it be advisable for a child with a severe uncorrectable flatfoot condition to participate in long-distance running events. Despite these cautions, the level of participation in any appropriate activity should be left to the child. The podiatrist can assess any handicaps affecting the feet of a child and recommend an appropriate physical fitness program. Consultation with the pediatrician or other medical specialist is advisable concerning physical handicaps involving other areas.

The quadriceps muscles should be stretched as well as strengthened in the young. Tight quadriceps in a teenage runner may lead to injury of the proximal tibial apophysis. To stretch the quadriceps, weight is applied on both hands behind with feet on the ground as if getting ready for a sprint. The knee is pointed straight ahead as the runner leans back. A stretching sensation will be experienced in the quadriceps mechanism. This position is held for 5 seconds and released. This exercise should be performed 15 times before and after participation in a running sport.

Hip pain in children and teenagers requires immediate attention. Some conditions, if not treated adequately, may lead to osteoarthritis of the adult hip.

Active children from ages 8 to 13 commonly irritate the calcaneal apophysis. This inflammation may be self-limiting. Use of an M/F heel cup, a ¼-inch sponge heel seat and rest usually results in a lessening of painful symptoms. A short Achilles tendon, gastrocnemius or gastrocnemius-soleus equinus may be the etiologic factor.

Children may also injure the metatarsal or phalangeal epiphyses. Spenco insoles may help. Stress fracture, nerve impingement, tendonitis and capsulitis should be ruled out.

As a general rule children below age 12 should refrain from running over 10 miles at a time. Teenagers below age 15 should not participate in marathon events.

Medical Sports Injuries in Adolescents

Medical sports injuries and diseases in the adolescent include epilepsy, mononucleosis syndromes, viral diseases, diabetes, athletic heart syndrome, congenital heart disease, exercise-induced bronchoconstriction (asthma), exercise-induced anaphylaxis, postexercise hematuria, proteinuria, menarche and menstruation delay, heat-related illnesses, hypothermia and drug-related problems (11).

The insulin-dependent diabetic athlete must be well controlled, and insulin dosage may have to be altered. Dilute glucose solutions are used when participating in endurance sports.

Athletic heart syndrome presents with a large heart bradycardia and a systolic murmur. ECG abnormalities are seen and are reversible upon detraining. Athletes with congenital heart disease and epilepsy are restricted on the basis of functional evaluation by a cardiologist.

Exercise-induced bronchoconstriction (asthma) occurs 5–10 min after exercise begins. Breathing cool dry air initiates the reaction. Bronchoinhalers help control the constriction.

On rare occasions, exercise-induced anaphylaxis occurs. Caused by immunologic stimuli triggered by unknown agents, this condition may result in sudden death.

Postexercise hematuria secondary to bladder wall trauma and inadequate rehydration is not uncommon. If serial urinalysis results are negative for blood, no treatment is necessary.

Proteinuria in the athlete is of little concern unless a repeat urinalysis after 48 hours of no exercise is positive. A trace to 1+ proteinuria is common in the athlete. Referral for an orthostatic test to a urologist is indicated if proteinuria persists despite rest.

There is a 4-month delay on onset of menarche for every year the girl has participated in endurance exercise. Training increases oligoamenorrhea.

Heat-related illnesses, cramps, syncope, exhaustion (water depletion, salt depletion) and stroke are seen in untrained or underconditioned athletes.

Hypothermia is seen in athletes who are in poor physical condition, advanced in age or are not acclimatized to the locality of training. Cold urticaria has been described by McCain and Kanat (12).

Drug-related problems often result from the athlete's attempts to achieve greater levels of success. Abuse of antidepressants, tranquilizers, sedatives, β-blockers, adrenocorticosteroids, NSAIDs, vitamins, and anabolic steroids have been reported. Subotnick (13) has described dimethylsulphoxide (DMSO) dehydration of the foot.

Injuries: Their Prevention and Treatment

This important section is devoted to common injuries associated with the running sports. The universal treatment for an acute athletic injury is rest, ice, compression and elevation (RICE). Many problems affecting the feet, ankles, knees, hips and back are caused by inefficient function, which results in overuse of various parts of the body followed by injury.

Skin and Nail Problems

Blisters The skin is not accustomed to the friction and pressure from athletic shoes and the repetitive movements of the running sport, and blisters commonly occur. Precautionary measures include wearing well-fitting shoes that fit snugly (not tightly) in the heel and across the instep. The toebox must be deep enough and long enough to allow freedom of movement of the toes. Cotton, wool or cotton-wool blend socks should be worn. Shoes should not be worn without socks. If blisters continually form, wearing a thin synthetic sock beneath the usual athletic sock is recommended. Ordinary commercial cornstarch is sprinkled between the two pair of socks. Tincture of benzoin compound may be applied at sites of irritation twice daily to toughen the skin. Vaseline applied to the skin may limit blister formation. Spenco insoles may be used to absorb friction stress. If a blister occurs in the inner arch area of the foot, remove any built-in sponge arch raise from the shoe. When blisters do occur, drain the blister at one side in a clean manner, wiping with alcohol first. Leave the overlying skin, apply merthiolate and cover with a clean dry gauze dressing. Avoid applying adhesive tape to the skin. Construction of a protective pad or correction of a deformity may be indicated in order to minimize the potential danger of infection and pain.

Mycotic Infections Fungus infections are caused by four major families of fungus. Keeping the feet clean and dry helps prevent these infections. Exposure to the air is helpful. The use of a fungistatic powder on the feet and between the toes absorbs moisture. The itching and blistering associated with the acute phase of mycotic infections is controlled with appropriate medication after proper microscopic and/or culture evaluation. Running should be curtailed until the infection is under control (see Chapter 6).

Contact Dermatitis It is not unusual to experience a contact dermatitis to one or more of the materials or chemicals used in the manufacture of athletic socks or shoes. If small blisters, a rash and/or itching occur, change sock and shoe materials. Appropriate microscopic and/or culture examination is performed. Saline or Burow's Solution soaks are prescribed, and topical steroids are utilized. Rarely are systemic steroids indicated (see Chapter 6).

Helomas and Tylomas Corns and calluses are a build-up of dead cells of the stratum corneum. The stratum corneum builds up as a result of long-term friction and pressure over or under a bony prominence and usually secondary to poor function. Helomas form on or between the toes, whereas Tylomas usually form on the plantar or the medial or lateral surfaces of the feet. These areas may be protected and friction and pressure minimized with nonmedicated pads or Spenco insoles. A pumice stone may also be used. Construction of a protective pad or foot orthotic device or correction of a deformity may be indicated in order to minimize the potential danger of infection and pain.

Small black capillary hemorrhages may form around the outside and bottom of the heels. There may be an associated pinching sensation. The cause of this condition is sudden friction and pressure on the areas of skin at the junction of where the sole of the shoe stops and the upper part begins. Ensure careful fit of both shoes and socks. Shock-absorbing heel cups and a ⅛-inch heel raise sometimes help. Occasionally shoes must be changed (see Chapter 6).

Ingrown Toenails When the nail is involuted on one or both sides and/or aggravated by shoe pressure or abnormal function, there is a tendency to form a local infection. This infection usually affects the big toes, but can develop at the sides of any of the toenails. Prevention includes cutting the nails straight across and not down on the sides. A piece of cotton may be wedged beneath the side of the nail. Scrubbing with a mild soap and soft-bristled tooth brush may remove the dead skin in this area. If the side of the nail becomes red, hot, painful or begins to drain, surgical excision and drainage are indicated. A phenol-alcohol procedure can be performed to prevent the reoccurrence of an infected ingrown toenail without losing more than 2 or 3 days of running participation (see Chapter 6).

Biomechanical Disorders

Runner's Toe Most often the second toe is longer than the other toes. This often leads to jamming of the second toenail into the tip of the inside of the shoe, which results in a subungual hematoma. The multiple jamming of the toe and toenail may cause permanent nail deformity and may lead to inflammation of the toe joints as well.

This condition has been called "runner's toe" or "tennis toe." It is very common because it is difficult to find an adequate shoe that can accommodate a long second toe. Often the blood must be drained from beneath the nail to relive the pressure and pain. Sometimes the nail itself has to be removed.

Care should be taken to ensure that the athletic shoe is long enough and deep enough to accommodate a long second toe.

Turf Toe (Strain of the hallux by overextension) In this condition pain and swelling of the great toe joint are usually caused by running up hills in very flexible athletic shoes. It is also commonly seen in football linemen who, when charging, extend their great toe to extremes. Early treatment consists of rest, ice massage and aspirin therapy. If the condition recurs, rule out arthritic problems of the big toe joint.

Inflammatory Disorders

Bursitis A bursa is a sac-like structure found over joints or bony prominences. It may be present at birth (anatomical) or may be formed by the body (adventitious) to protect underlying structures. When the bursa is irritated it fills with fluid and swells. Although designed to protect the underlying structures from injury, a bursal sac can be quite painful. Bursae are found at various areas in the lower limbs, such as the dorsum of the toes, the great toe joint bunion, the heel, superior and inferior to the knee joint and anterior and lateral to the hip. One should suspect a bursitis over a bone or joint that becomes larger when irritated. If the toes are involved, a better-fitting shoe with a deeper toe box may be all that is needed. If the "bunion joint" is involved, a wider shoe or latex shield may alleviate the problem. Hallux abductovalgus deformity may have to be surgically corrected.

If a bursa on the posterior of the heel is inflamed, the basic treatment consists of a soft counter in a better-fitting shoe. A wider-flared shoe heel may limit the heel movement when the heel strikes the ground, and a ⅛- to ¼-inch heel lift in the shoe often relieves posterior heel pain. Stretching exercises for the calf muscles are helpful. If pain persists there may be a calcific deposit or underlying bony deformity. Swollen bursae superior and inferior to the knee respond well to ultrasound, ice massage, aspirin therapy and rest. Occasionally a steroid injection is needed. Stretching for flexibility and strengthening exercises are helpful and important. Bursitis involving the hip is treated in a similar manner. Crossover or scissoring running style should be avoided. Foot orthoses may be used to limit the irritation from abnormal motion in the area of a hip bursa.

Neuroma and Nerve Entrapment

When a neuroma is found in the athlete, the mass is usually a result of chronic irritation of the involved nerve. Symptoms include a shooting-type pain, tingling, burning and numbness. When these symptoms are found between the third and fourth toes the condition is called Morton's neuroma. A wider shoe and a temporary foot support may relieve the symptoms. If the symptoms persist, the neuroma must be removed. These symptoms may also occur on the top of the foot radiating into the big toe and/or second toe. If this occurs, suspect that pressure from the shoe over the first metatarsocuneiform joint is irritating the medial dorsal cutaneous branch of the superficial peroneal nerve. Make sure the sock is not bunched up over this area. If the shoe has metal eyelets, remove the eyelet over the prominent area. Skip an eyelet over this area when lacing the shoes, cut the shoe where it crosses the foot in this area or advise the patient to get a new deeper and/or wider shoe. When these symptoms occur just below and to the inside of the ankle or heel, suspect posterior tibial nerve entrapment. Foot orthoses are of tremendous benefit. Excision of a neuroma, freeing of a trapped nerve or removal of a dorsal bony prominence is sometimes necessary (see Chapter 7, Soft Tissue Tumors and Cysts).

Knee Problems

Knee pain accounts for a significant percentage of complaints associated with running. Hollander (14) describes a practical knee evaluation for athletes involved in the running sports. "Runner's knee," patello-femoral syndrome or chondromalacia is an irritation of the cartilage on the undersurface of the patella that occurs when the patella fails to glide properly along the groove of the femur. A grinding sensation with or without pain may be experienced beneath or around the patella. There may be mild swelling or a feeling of fullness. Often the knee aches and is stiff after a period of rest. The most common cause of "runner's knee" is abnormal subtalar pronation at the propulsive phase of gait. Quadriceps weakness, a small or high-riding patella (patella alta), pronated foot gear, flexibility and running style contribute to this condition. Patellar cartilage degeneration with fibrillation proceeding to basal degeneration occurs. An increased Q angle predisposes to subpatellar cartilage damage due to increased internal tibial rotation. The Q angle, measured from the anterior superior iliac spine through the bisection of the patella as compared with a line bisecting the anterior tibial tubercle, should not exceed 10–15°. If the Q angle is greater than 20°, an excessive amount of lateral patellar movement results in subpatellar cartilage damage. Patello-femoral syndrome must be differentiated from meniscal injury, synovial plica, lateral patellar subluxation, pes anserinus bursitis, patellar tendonitis and iliotibial band syndrome. If the knee locks or gives way, suspect internal derangement.

Clark's apprehension test is often helpful in diagnosing subpatellar cartilage damage. With the patient lying on a table with the knee extended, the examiner pushes down on the patella as the patient contracts the quadricep muscles. Subpatellar cartilage damage results in pain upon proximal movement of the patella. Crepitus may also be felt upon active as well as passive movement of the patella against the femur. The patient may experience pain in the knee when squatting or while sitting (movie sign).

Abnormal pronation has a number of different causes, including running on slanted surfaces, unequal leg lengths, tight triceps surae and hamstring muscle groups and a limitation of motion in various joints. Abnormal pronation may also cause strain of the medial collateral knee ligaments. An abnormal cavovarus foot may cause strain of the lateral collateral ligaments. Knee problems are more commonly found on the shorter extremity when there is a lower limb shortage.

The medial and lateral femoral condyles are not equal when there is dysfunction. If the extremity is functioning inappropriately, the patella does not glide properly, unequal stresses are placed on the knee and the menisci—for example, positional genu valgum—may predispose to meniscal pressure by the femoral condyles. The following knee integrity testing procedures have been described.

1. *Anterior Drawer Sign:* The patient sits with the lower leg hanging over the table. The lower leg is held and moved anteriorly and posteriorly. If the anterior excursion is pronounced as opposed to the opposite leg, this signifies a disruption of the anterior cruciate ligament. This movement is repeated with the leg fully extended. A similar maneuver may be used to evaluate the soft tissue integrity of the anterior ankle.
2. *McMurray Test:* The patient is supine with the knee flexed. While the knee is passively moved by the examiner from flexion to extension, the leg is passively internally rotated to test for lateral meniscus tear and externally rotated to test for medial meniscus tear. One hand is placed over the knee while the examiner moves the leg through the range of motion noted above. If there is a meniscal tear, a painful clicking sensation may be palpated over the lesion. As with other examination techniques, the absence of a positive response does not totally rule out meniscal injury.
3. *Apley's Test:* The patient is prone with the lower leg placed at right angles to the knee that is in contact with the table. The lower leg is rotated and moved up and down relative to the knee as the examiner attempts to palpate a torn meniscus.
4. *Pyer's Test:* The patient sits in the lotus position. When pressure is placed on the medial knee, pain results in the face of a meniscal injury.

Iliotibial band syndrome occurs in muscular individuals with a tight fascia lata and often weak abductors. The iliotibial band, coursing along the lateral aspect of the upper leg and attaching to the lateral tibial tubercle (Gerdey's tubercle), head of the fibula and lateral collateral ligaments, may be responsible for both lateral knee, and lateral hip pain. The iliotibial band may become irritated in the presence of an uncompensated rearfoot varus or genu valgum. Abnormal excessive subtalar pronation may cause it to tighten as a result of internal rotation and adduction of the tibia, with resulting irritation and pain as the tight band moves over bony prominences. Treatment includes stretching exercises, control of abnormal pronation, abductor strengthening exercises, rest, ice massage, aspirin therapy, NSAID therapy, ultrasound and steroid injection.

Synovial plica syndrome causes pain along the lateral aspect of the patella. Synovitis at the anterior aspect of the parapatellar bursa may lead to a synovial plica interposing between the femur and patella. Upon examination, a popping sensation is felt at 30° of extension as the plica moves between the patella and the femur. Treatment is directed toward the synovitis and the plica itself (15). Patellar tendonitis may be caused by tight hamstrings or quadriceps, unequal leg lengths, equinus, overstriding or pronatory abnormalities. Popliteus muscle syndrome with pain just anterior to the lateral collateral ligament may be aggravated by inefficient function. Patellar fat pad syndrome may result from supinatory problems—uncompensated cavus—equinus or unequal leg length.

Inflammation of the tendons or ligaments superior, inferior, medial and lateral to the knee may be treated by rest, ice massage, aspirin therapy, quadriceps strengthening and hamstring stretching exercises. Abnormal pronatory problems may be controlled with appropriate foot orthoses.

The treatment for "runner's knee" must be directed toward the cause of the improper glide of the patella. Foot orthoses may have to be prescribed to control abnormal pronation. Flexibility exercises for triceps surae and hamstring muscles are essential for relief of discomfort. The vastus medialis should be strengthened. Various knee braces such as ChoPat, may be prescribed to limit adverse lateral patellar movement and to improve patellar tracking. Good training shoes with a firm shank, shock-absorbing heel and multilayered soles are essential for rehabilitation. A shoe lift to accommodate a leg shortage may be necessary. Running surfaces should be flat, and running down hills should be avoided.

Achilles Tendonitis

One of the most common areas in the lower extremity to suffer from inefficient function and overuse is the Achilles tendon. This tendon arises from the gastrocnemius and soleus muscles and attaches to the middle third of the posterior surface of the calcaneus plantarward to become functionally confluent with the plantar fascia.

Athletes engaged in the running sports must use their gastocnemius and soleus muscles to a greater degree, leading to overdevelopment of these muscles. In turn, overdevelopment leads to a shortening of these muscles and tightening of the Achilles tendon. When body weight glides over the foot, the foot dorsiflexes and the Achilles tendon is stretched, often to the point of tearing. An inflexibility of the gastrocnemius-soleus complex or a short leg is often the cause of excessive stretching of the Achilles tendon. This usually causes tendonitis with resultant inflammation of the paratenon. A variety of foot and leg disorders can cause abnormal movement of the calcaneus. Because the Achilles tendon inserts into the abnormally moving calcaneus, it may become excessively stretched. This also can result in Achilles tendonitis.

Proper stretching exercises may be the only treatment needed to clear up this condition. Application of ⅛ to ¼-inch heel lifts into the shoes may help. A one-sided heel lift to accommodate a leg shortage may be necessary. Ice massage, aspirin therapy and contrast baths are beneficial. Appropriate foot orthoses may be needed to control abnormal calcaneal motion. Soft surfaces, such as sand, and running up hills should be avoided. Occasionally tenolysis and posible bone or bursal excision is necessary (16).

Stress Fractures

The forefoot is often overused and abused by runners. Improper weight transfer may lead to metatarsal stress or fatigue fracture. Being overweight, a significant mileage increase over a short period of time, running on hard uneven surfaces and poor shock-absorbing shoes predispose to stress fracture.

If swelling and pain occur at the distal second or third metatarsal metaphyseal areas, on either side of the calcaneus, directly over the distal or proximal metaphysis of the tibia, fibula or femur, suspect stress fracture (17). Most stress fractures occur after the athlete exceeds his or her trained limits. There is no history of direct injury. Noncalcaneal tarsal stress fracture is rare (17, 18).

A slight soreness may be present during and immediately after running. The next morning, upon arising, the area is usually quite painful. Often this type of fracture does not show up on x-ray examination until the osteoblastic healing response is visualized. Bone scan is the most valuable diagnositc aid (19).

If stress fracture is suspected, proper treatment should be instituted. Usually a plaster cast is not necessary (see Chapter 10, Foot and Ankle Trauma).

Morton's Foot

"Morton's foot" (Morton's syndrome) is commonly associated with forefoot problems. This foot type includes a short hypermobile first metatarsal ray and a long second toe.

The Morton's foot associated with a varus forefoot may lead to a number of common foot complaints in runners, including plantar calcaneonavicular ligamentous strain, plantar fasciitis and heel spur syndrome. Compensated forefoot varus, if uncontrolled, may result in bunion formation and painful plantar tylomas. Treatment must include the proper positioning of the foot in the shoe to provide for normal function. Foot orthotic devices should be prescribed.

Metatarsalgia and Sesamoiditis

Metatarsalgia may be caused by a number of factors. An unusually long metatarsal may have to bear more weight than the others, causing pain. The foot may be in an improper position during each stride, causing undue stress on one or more metatarsal bones. There may be a limitation of movement at the ankle joint leading to too much weight being borne too soon and for too long on one or more metatarsals. Abnormal foot pronation, as well as anterior, posterior and global cavus feet, may predispose to pain beneath one or more metatarsal heads. An arthritic process or stress fracture may be present as well.

Sesamoiditis may be caused by continual irritation from running on hard surfaces, pivoting and turning or an abnormality in the bones themselves. Often this condition is associated with a cavus foot type with a more prominent sesamoid area or a plantar flexed first ray.

Treatment for metatarsalgia and sesamoiditis consists of removing as much pressure from the forefoot as possible. Good, multilayered, shock-absorbing soled shoes and triceps surae stretching may be beneficial. Spenco insoles help absorb shock. If swelling is observed, a stress fracture must be suspected, and x-ray examination may be indicated. Appropriate shoe padding and/or construction of a balancing orthotic device may be necessary. Rest, aspirin therapy, ice massage and contrast baths may be helpful (see Chapter 8).

Shin Splints

Pain along the attachment by Sharpey's fibers of the tibialis anterior into the tibia may result from muscle imbalance. This condition is called anterior shin splints. Faulkner (11) maintains that normal physical activities can injure skeletal muscle fibers. Stiffness and discomfort may last for several days. Considerable variability exists among individuals sustaining this type of injury, the circumstances necessary to cause injury and the extent of injury.

Over a period of time, as the tibialis anterior attempts to dorsiflex the foot, the muscle attachments begin to pull away from the periosteum, causing the pain of anterior shin splints, which must be differentiated from tibial stress fracture and acute anterior compartment syndrome requiring immediate decompression.

Posterior shin splints or pain along the tibialis posterior attachment to the medial posterior aspect of the tibia may also result from muscle imbalance. Typically, this occurs between 3 and 6 inches above the medial malleolus. A limitation of ankle joint and/or subtalar joint motion may be an aggravating factor. The tibialis anterior and extensor digitorum longus muscles are weak. The opposing triceps surae muscles are strong and tight. The tight triceps surae muscles prevent the foot from dorsiflexing to the degree necessary for efficient function, causing the tibialis anterior to work "overtime."

Triceps surae muscle stretching exercises and tibialis anterior and extensor digitorum longus muscle strengthening exercises help prevent anterior shin splints. The runner should be instructed to run on softer surfaces, to stay away from hills and to wear good shock-absorbing heeled shoes. In addition to muscle imbalance, posterior shin splints may be caused by the inability of the foot to function as a rigid lever at propulsion. Strengthening of the tibialis anterior and extensor digitorum longus and stretching of the triceps surae are essential. Running on soft sand and on sides of roads and slanted tracks should be avoided. Foot orthoses are almost always beneficial. A leg shortage must be ruled out. Treatment for the acute painful problem requires rest, physical therapy and anti-inflammatory medication.

Ankle Problems

Ankle ailments in runners usually result from strains or sprains. Uncompensated rearfoot varus and forefoot valgus predispose to ankle strain and sprains, especially when running on slanted surfaces, such as the side of the road.

Stretching of the ankle ligaments (ankle strain) and tearing of the ankle ligaments (ankle sprain) are common injuries experienced by basketball, tennis, raquetball and football players. Because of the side movements common to these sports and the foot's tendency to invert, lateral ankle ligamentous injuries result. A chronic subluxating peroneus longus tendon may develop as well. Runners may develop an anterior ankle impingement exostosis. This condition is more often seen in basketball players due to multiple forced dorsiflexion injuries. When symptomatic, the anterior distal tibial and/or superior talar exostoses must be removed surgically.

Ankle strain is frequently caused by inadequate or badly worn shoes. The shoe heel may be too narrow and unstable or too soft and compressible. Physical fitness, flexibility, adequate wider-heeled shoes and flat surfaces take care of most ankle complaints in runners.

Prevention of strain or sprain may require an adhesive tape ankle strap and wider-heeled shoes. Initial treatment consists of rest, ice, compression and elevation. Depending on the severity of the strain or sprain, an x-ray examination is performed, and a soft or hard cast is applied. Foot orthotic devices are necessary to control abnormal motion (see Chapter 10, Foot and Ankle Trauma).

Heel and Medial Longitudinal Arch Pain

Arch and heel problems are among the painful problems associated with all running sports. The plantar fascia often becomes strained. This strain at first may feel like a dull ache. It may progress to plantar pain upon arising in the morning and finally to constant pain while walking.

Under severe strain, the plantar fascia may tear along its course. Faulty foot function over a period of years may cause low-grade irritation at the fascial attachment to the medial plantar calcaneal tubercle, which leads to what is known as "heel spur syndrome." There is pain on arising after a period of rest. After a few steps the pain eases, only to return as one continues to walk or run. Initial treatment consists of rest for 2 weeks, ice massage and contrast baths.

If ignored too long, a plantar calcaneal exostosis may develop and have to be injected or removed surgically to relieve pain. Orthotic devices may be beneficial. It is important to perform proper stretching exercises for the posterior leg group muscles. Strain of the plantar fascia and heel spur syndrome are commonly found in cavus feet and in feet that pronate excessively just prior to the foot leaving the ground during the running cycle.

Snider (20) et al. reported on plantar fascial release for chronic plantar fasciitis in runners in 11 cases. They discussed the use of "flexible leather arch supports" with medial heel posts, oral anti-inflamatory agents and local steroid injections. There was no mention of appropriate presurgical biomechanical examination; conservative biomechanical therapy, such as low Dye and longitudinal metatarsal pad strapping; shoe therapy; or medical evaluation to rule out the seronegative spondyloarthopathies, gout or hyperlipidemia. The question arises as to whether treatment of the primary biomechanical etiology of the chronic plantar fasciitis would have resulted in relief of symptoms. It has been the author's experience in treating thousands of patients, including hundreds of runners, over 20 years of practice that rarely is plantar fascial release necessary for relief of chronic plantar fasciitis of biomechanical etiology.

Feet with excessive pronation often develop strain of the plantar calcaneonavicular ligament and the abductor hallucis. Treatment is based on muscle balance, flexibility, leg length equalization, good shock-absorbing shoes and control of excessive pronation. Either a temporary foot orthosis or a permanent orthotic device is made for the patient.

Groin Pain

The most common cause of groin pain in runners is strain of the adduction muscles. This may occur after a sudden stretch of the area caused by the sudden outward movement of the leg. The discomfort may be mild at first, progressing to chronic pain. Ice therapy, aspirin and rest are of immediate help. Strengthening and stretching exercises are of later benefit. It is important that the presence of a stress fracture be ruled out.

Hip, Hamstring and Triceps Surae Muscle Pain

Hip and hamstring muscle pain are often foot-related. Pulled hamstrings are seen in sprinters, football and basketball players. Hamstring muscle spasm is seen in long-distance runners. If symptoms persist it is important that a stress fracture be ruled out. Trochanteric bursitis, degenerative joint disease and iliotibial band syndrome must be appreciated when lateral hip pain occurs.

Soreness in the buttocks radiating down the backs of the legs may often be due to irritation of the sciatic nerve, which may be caused by pressure from the piriformis muscle or discogenic disease.

A difference in leg lengths may cause sciatic nerve irritation with pain, numbness and sometimes tingling. In the runner with sciatic nerve irritation and a leg length differential, the construction of an orthotic device to help equalize the leg lengths often results in relief. The majority of hip problems are seen on the long extremity side.

Lower extremity limb length may be measured from the anterior superior and posterior superior iliac spine to the ground (with the subtalar joints in neutral) and then compared. One screening procedure involves placing a level on the patient's knees while the patient is sitting and the feet, with subtalar joints neutral, are on the ground. This test measures lower leg length differential. With the patient kneeling on a level surface and bending forward, the posterior superior iliac spine level may be determined. It is difficult to evaluate sacroiliac etiology in lower extremity limb length differential. Functional and structural limb length discrepancies may be found alone or combined.

Triceps surae pain in runners is almost always caused by a tight group of muscles. Many runners, especially weekend runners, neglect proper warm-ups and stretching exercises.

The efficient functioning foot must have the ability to dorsiflex approximately 10° beyond a right angle with the leg. A limitation of this essential motion is usually due to a tight triceps surae muscle group or to a bony ankle equinus. Stretching exercises are essential prior to and after running to help stretch the muscles and to improve their ability to function under stress. A 1/8 to 1/4-inch heel lift may be beneficial. Resection of an anterior distal tibia or superior talar bony block may be indicated.

Low Back Pain

Low back pain can be caused by inflexibility of the posterior leg muscles. Low back muscle spasm may result from favoring the tight muscle groups. Flexibility stretching exercises are recommended. If a leg shortage is present, a shoe lift and/or orthotic device may be beneficial (21).

Bent and straight leg sit-up exercises to strengthen the abdominal muscles and stretch the lower back muscles are essential to good function.

Spondylolysis or spondylolisthesis of the lumbosacral vertebra, functional or structural scoliosis, a narrowed disk space, irritation of the sciatic nerve and/or a ruptured disc must be suspected if back pain symptoms persist.

Treatment. *Ice Massage* is used to bring a greater flow of blood to the areas being treated. A styrofoam or paper cup is filled with water and frozen. The ice is applied to the area being treated in a sweeping flowing fashion. A larger area than is painful is covered. The ice is not allowed to rest on any one small area for more than 5 seconds. As the ice melts, the styrofoam or paper is peeled back to expose more ice. At first a cold sensation is experienced, which is followed by tingling, burning, aching and finally a numb feeling. Ice massage should be continued for no more than 5 minutes and should be discontinued when the skin is observed to become reddened. The area is dried with a towel prior to stretching.

Aspirin Therapy Aspirin is not to be used solely as an analgesic; it is also recommended for inflammation. Aspirin therapy should not be used if there is a history of sensitivity to aspirin or aspirin products. Nor should aspirin be taken if there is a history of asthma or stomach ulcer or if the patient is taking anticoagulants. Aspirin should not be taken with alcohol as doing so irritates the gastric mucosa. Studies indicate aspirin therapy may be harmful when sports participation takes place in extremely hot weather.

Finally, aspirin therapy is not to be used for children.

In aspirin therapy two 5 grain aspirin tablets are taken every 6 hours for 5 days. Each 5 grain aspirin tablet contains 325 mg. The two aspirin tablets are taken with water, meals, whole milk, or a nonmagnesium-containing antacid of choice. Aspirin combined with other ingredients, such as caffeine or phenacetin, should not be taken. An antacid containing magnesium sometimes causes diarrhea. This therapy is continued for 5 days only. At the first sign of stomach upset, nausea, vomiting, skin rash, dizziness, ringing in the ears, chest pain, hay fever or attack of asthma, the aspirin therapy is discontinued. Overuse of aspirin may cause hearing loss, ulcerative colitis, gastrointestinal bleeding, kidney damage and aplastic anemia.

Contrast Baths are used to stimulate healing by alternately causing the blood vessels to contract and to dilate. The effect on nerves is to break up the pain cycle.

A pan of warm water (approximately 100°F) and a pan of cold water (approximately 55°F) are prepared. Beginning with the warm water and ending with the cold water, the feet are immersed for 60 sec in each, back and forth for a total of 6 min. Three min are spent in each contrasting temperature water for 1 minute at a time. The feet are dried thoroughly, and cornstarch is applied between the toes and on the plantar surface of each foot.

Helpful Hints

Runners must learn to listen to their bodies. There are many days they will not feel well when starting to run. If they feel better while running, the workout can continue. However, if the runners feel worse while running, they should go home. Additionally, if local tenderness develops, the workout should immediately be curtailed.

A frequently asked question is whether a runner should run with a cold or when feeling ill. Forced workouts never accomplish anything. A runner must learn to accept forced days off. Running in training should be fun, and the person who listens to his or her body will get the most out of a jogging program. The older the runner, the longer an injury will take to heal. Therefore, it is better to do less, rather than too much.

Recreational runners should run for 15 minutes four times a week. Do not bother with distance. Train, don't strain. Effect is important, not speed. Run at a comfortable pace. The runner should be able to carry on a conversation while running. The runner should wear shock-absorbing and motion-controlling running shoes, not spikes or running flats.

When running on trails or uneven surfaces, a shoe with a wide heel should be worn. Stretching and strengthening should be done prior to and after running. Bouncing while stretching should be avoided; stretching should be accomplished in a steady even fashion.

If the front of one's legs and/or knees hurt, stay off hills and do not run faster than 8-minute miles. The runner should try to run on flat surfaces. Remember that the side of most roads slant away from the center. Alternate sides. If a runner experiences repeated injuries on one side of the body, suspect a lower limb shortage on that side. If a runner suffers posterior lower leg muscle pain he/she should do stretching exercises and have the heels on the shoes repaired.

If he or she suffers from Achilles tendonitis, the runner should stretch (over ice) and check the back of the shoes for excessive heel wear.

The runner should be cautioned not to stop suddenly after running. The cool-down walking period should be for a minimum of 3–5 min. Stopping suddenly may cause syncope.

When resuming running after 1 to 3 weeks of inactivity, the runner should begin at 50% of the previous participation. After 3 to 6 weeks of inactivity, the runner should begin at 25% of previous participation. After 6 weeks nonparticipation, the runner should start at the beginning level again.

The runner should be cautioned to run to pain, not through pain. If pain persists, the runner should STOP!

Racewalking

Racewalking differs from running in several ways. The racewalker has one foot on the ground at all times and has a straight leg, with no knee bend, as the body passes over the foot in contact with the ground. Proper style and technique are most important to proper racewalking.

Poor posture, arm swing, foot contact, leg movement and foot toe off position can and often do lead to inefficiency, energy loss and overuse injuries.

The pushoff position of the foot is very important. The toes must point straight ahead and not out at an angle. If pushoff is at an angle the leg rotates inward leading to stress on the medial knee, medial slip of the plantar fascia and the medial longitudinal arch of the foot. Over a period of time the improper toe off position can also lead to "runner's knee", poplateus tendonitis, anterior and posterior shin splints and sciatica. A foot orthotic device is sometimes necessary to control abnormal function.

Running is a pushoff sport. The posterior leg muscles become strong and sometimes overdeveloped. In racewalking the muscles behind and in front of the legs are used and strengthened. This involves a pushing and pulling activity. Also, there is a slight stretch to the hamstrings with each forward extension of the leg.

Because the rules for racewalking require the leg to be straight as the body passes over and one foot to be on the ground at all times, one may have the impression that the hips are swiveling. However, if observed carefully, in racewalking there is very little side-to-side movement of the hips. The good racewalker pushes his or her hip forward as the leg is extended to its maximum just before heel contract. The idea is to minimize side-to-side and extra up-and-down motion.

The racewalker must function in the smoothest efficient manner possible. The extended leg must be perfectly straight as the edge of the heel touches the ground. Toes must be pointed straight ahead. The upper body must be erect with shoulders level with the ground. As the quadriceps pull the body over the extended leg, weight is transferred from the outer heel edge across the outer area of the foot, then across the area behind the toes onward through toe pushoff. As this is happening the posterior leg muscles are pushing off for greater forward thrust.

Arm motion is critical to the good racewalker. As forward speed increases, the bent arms move rhythmically. Each arm swings forward with the opposite leg. The arms begin a pumping movement with the lightly clenched fists ending chest high. This pumping acting results in greater forward thrust and movement efficiency. Because racewalking is an aerobic sport the heart-lung mechanism is strengthened. Breathing should be coordinated with each step. Inhaling and exhaling take place as a full stride is completed. The racewalker inhales as contact is made with first the left, then the right foot. He or she exhales as contact is made the next time around with both feet.

Racewalking can be fun, enhance cardiovascular fitness and help the serious runner in training.

Skipping Rope

Few exercises can match the cardiovascular benefits supplied by rope skipping. According to Dr. Kenneth Cooper in his book, *The Aerobics Program for Total Well Being,* just 10 minutes of skipping rope is equivalent to 1 mile of jogging (22). One would have to ski for 30 minutes to obtain the same health benefits as skipping rope for 10 minutes. Tom Morris of Australia holds the world record. He skipped rope for 1,264 miles along the eastern coast of Australia.

Rope skipping sharpens footwork, improves coordination and concentration and is an ideal form of aerobic training. It is convenient and inexpensive and can be done in a minimum amount of time.

A proper rope may be a sash cord made of cotton, polyethylene or nylon. Average rope lengths are 7 to 10 feet. While stepping on the middle of the rope, the ends should reach to the chest, the desirable length. Select a flat-cushioned surface, such as a mat or rug, in a room with a high ceiling or jump rope outdoors. Proper shoes with good forefoot stability and impact protection are essential. Either an aerobic dance shoe or runner's training flat is ideal. A Spenco or Sorbothane insole may be inserted to lessen impact shock further.

The first week of rope skipping exercise should involve endurance hopping. Start out with 100 hops the first day and add 10 to 20 hops each day thereafter for the first week. Doing so allows the participant to become accustomed to the feel of the hopping surface and to the rhythms of hopping. After the first week the rope skipper is ready to use the rope. Keeping the elbows slightly bent and close to the body and wrists about waist level and with the rope just barely touching the ground, rotate the wrists so that the rope swings forward. As the rope hits the ground, hop. This may be an awkward feeling at first. Controlling the rope can be difficult, and there is no way to avoid tangling the rope. However, success will be achieved with practice and patience. The rope skipper must look straight ahead, stand straight and try to relax. If the body tightens up, tangling may become more likely.

Use the wrists only. Increased arm movements increase the speed of the rope and should be reserved for more advanced training. Jump just high enough to clear the swinging rope.

There are several types of hops useful for beginners. The one-footed gallop hop is the easiest. It involves stepping over the rope, one foot at a time. A second useful hop for the beginning rope skipper is the two-footed hop. With this hop the feet land slightly ahead of where the person started, necessitating a quick step back after each hop. As rope skippers become more proficient, they will land where they started and will not have to take a step back. Remember to land on the balls of the feet and slowly roll back until the heels make contact with the ground.

Rope skipping may be utilized to train for almost any running sport from football to tennis. The athlete must remember never to overdo this activity. Skipping in cadence to music helps maintain rhythm. Aerobic skipping for endurance might begin with two 3 min sessions with a 1 min rest in between. Aim for approximately 140–160 skips per minute. Gradually decrease rest periods and raise the knees higher over the next several weeks. Three-min sessions are gradually increased up to 6 min. Because everyone is different and there is no set way of skipping rope for everyone, the person skipping rope will have to experiment with different styles in order to determine which is best. If anterior shin splints develop, decrease rope skipping sessions and increase session time more slowly.

Aerobic Dance

The benefits derived from aerobic dance include a decrease in heart rate, improved muscle tone and endurance, a decrease in blood pressure and an overall feeling of fitness (23). After a 5 to 10 min warm-up period consisting of stretching/flexibility exercises, sit-ups and a warm-up dance performed at a gentle walk pace, the aerobic phase of the dance process begins. This aerobic dance phase, timed sufficiently long enough to produce beneficial effect, lasts for 30–45 min. Dance routines are choreographed to popular music, each lasting from 3–3½ min (2). The dance routines incorporate standard movements of rhythmic jogging, skipping, hopping, twisting and jumping, as well as ballet reaches, bouncing kicks, knee lifts, jumping jacks and lunges. With one goal being to increase heart rate to 75–80% of the maximal, heart rate may be self-monitored throughout the aerobic dance phase. The aerobic dance phase should be repeated a minimum of three times per week in order to maintain aerobic conditioning. A 5 to 10 min cool-down period consisting of slower dance routines and stretching exercises completes the aerobic dance program.

Cushioned gymnastic mats or wood over air are ideal surfaces for aerobic dance. Proper straight last shoes with a stable rigid counter, flexible smooth tread forefoot sole, slightly elevated heel and an adequate toebox are essential. Dancers with uncompensated forefoot valgus or uncompensated rearfoot varus may require a ⅛ to ¼ inch felt lateral heel pad placed into the shoe, a ¹⁄₁₆ to ⅛ inch lateral heel wedge placed on the heel sole and/or a slightly flaired lateral heel so as to prevent ankle inversion injury during the dance routine. At the same time, it is essential to minimize the pronatory effect of the lateral heel modifications during midstance and into propulsion by adding an appropriate medial longitudinal ¼-inch felt pad to the aerobic dance shoe. A semirigid foot orthotic device may incorporate these modifications in order to prevent injury.

Cotton socks are used to absorb moisture. A thin nylon or rayon sock beneath the cotton sock may help prevent blister formation. Typical overuse injuries seen in aerobic dancing include blisters, plantar fasciitis, inversion ankle injury, subungual hematoma, Achilles tendonitis, anterior shin splints, bursitis and stress fracture (24). Anterior shin splints may be avoided by encouraging less forefoot contact and more heel contact.

Water Skiing

Although water skiing is not an aerobic sport, it is important that the water skier condition himself or herself properly prior to participation. Other aerobic sports, such as swimming, help in the conditioning of a water skier. Proper upper and lower extremity conditioning exercises are a necessity prior to water skiing. Development of fast twitch pale muscle fibers and slow twitch red muscle fibers is necessary. Fast twitch muscle fibers come into play when attempting multiple quick turn maneuvers, and slow twitch muscle fibers are utilized while following in the boat's wake.

The biomechanics of water skiing, with the weightbearing foot operating in a closed kinetic chain, includes a very complex integration of muscle and joint interactions. Compensatory movement of the midtarsal joint, allowing for improved weight distribution and fine tuning to maintain balance and better ski control, is very important to the water skier.

Muscle spasm and tenosynovitis, as well as ankle and knee ligamentous injury, are seen in the water skier. Sudden jerking motions and shearing forces predispose to epiphyseal injuries in children. Twisting type falls predispose to spinal injury. Adductor muscle strain, tendonitis or avulsion may occur when a skier has lost control of an abducted ski. An exaggerated lean may predispose to trochanteric bursitis, an iliotibial band syndrome, or knee ligament or meniscus injury. Damage to the peroneal, tibialis anterior and posterior and Achilles tendons is possible. Warm-up and cool-down exercise routines help avoid injury. Adhesive tape or neoprene sleeve immobilization, deep friction massage and ultrasound are important treatment modalities (25).

Boxing

Boxers, trainers and physicians have all but ignored lower extremity equipment, training and treatment needs. Yet, few sports subject the foot to as many combinations of vertical, lateral and rotary stresses. Training techniques include rope skipping and foot movements attendant to shadow boxing, including the use of light and heavy bags and sparring.

Correct stance is of prime importance. Although no one stance style is appropriate to all boxers, the classic straight-up stance is most often used. The right foot is placed 12–18 inches behind the left foot, which is held in a slight intoe position with the subtalar joint supinated. The posteriorly placed right forefoot is in contact with the surface as most of the body weight is concentrated on the anteriorly placed left foot (26).

Because there are several biomechanical considerations unique to boxing, there is increased medial and lateral hip rotary stress and lateral knee stress. Adequate ankle and first metatarsophalangeal joint dorsiflexion is essential. Boxers wear light-weight leather high-top lace shoes with leather or rubber soles. Some boxers wear heavy boots as a training method out of the ring. Because the aerobic exercise of running is utilized most often for training purposes, the boxer is subject to the variety of lower extremity overuse syndromes. Rarely are the lower extremities injured while boxing. However, a fighter with an uncompensated rearfoot varus or forefoot valgus is predisposed to lateral ankle injury while in the ring. To avoid overuse syndromes from running, a running shoe specific to the boxer's foot type and weight should be worn. Ankle weights and heavy boots should be avoided. Stretching flexibility exercises should be encouraged (27).

Ice Skating

Ice skating develops overall fitness and a knowledge of an intricate art, as well as a keen sense of balance, upright stance and musical appreciation. Children with physical disabilities and adults engaged in rehabilitation programs have found skating to be beneficial. Figure skating, speed skating and ice hockey comprise the three categories of ice skating. Each type of skating requires different types of blades and boots.

Figure skating, which is classified into single skating, ice dancing and pair skating, demands total flexibility. Poise, grace and flexibility are achieved through a dance training program. Ballet exercises strengthen and stretch those muscles used for skating. Skating exercise programs involve the entire body. Head, neck, arm, torso, hip, thigh, leg and foot stretching and strengthening exercises are essential. One such foot exercise involves holding the side barrier on the ice while extending one leg rearward with the foot extended. The top of the toebox should be in contact with the ice with the foot in the drag position. With the opposite leg positioned over the third toe, the rearward extended leg is bent slowly. There is a resulting anterior muscle stretch of the backwardly extended leg and foot (28). Skating becomes easier as conditioning improves.

Speed skating also requires intensive training and conditioning. The speed skater's skate consists of a flat, straight, thin blade 12 to 18 inches long and $\frac{1}{32}$ inch wide. The boot is cut low and is light weight. Skaters use the entire blade surface and bend their knees to the maximum in order to obtain a longer stroke resulting in a more powerful pushoff. Speed skating techniques depend on balance, strength and drive. Other training techniques for speed skaters include swimming, weight lifting, cycling, rope skipping and roller skating.

Hockey skating, one of the fastest growing sports in the United States, requires a totally different muscle conditioning than the running sports. In the running sports the leg propels the body forward or backward by raising the heel and transferring weight to the forefoot. In skating, posterior leg group muscle strength is not that essential. Hockey skating is 80% anaerobic and 20% aerobic.

Overdevelopment of nonskating muscles, combined with underdevelopment of skating muscles, leads to groin, knee and ankle injuries, making pre- and postskating conditioning programs essential. Bruises, discoloration, abrasions and fractures are among the lower extremity injuries seen in hockey skaters (29). Ankle dorsiflexion is essential to the skater. Ligamentous knee injuries and hip avulsion fractures occur frequently.

Badminton

Lower extremity motion, quick movements, speed and racquet stroke are conducive to foot stress and strongly predispose to the development of foot pathology. In badminton, the bird or shuttlecock is hit back and forth over the net, racquet to racquet, on an average of once every 0.7 to 0.8 sec. A power shot may leave the racquet at speeds in excess of 140 mph and can reach the other racquet in less than 0.5 sec. Or the bird can be hit softly and take a long time to traverse the net and come down. Superb reflexes and a sprinter's speed are required to accommodate a constant change of pace and movement, more than in any other racquet sport. During a typical singles match a player may run a mile, change direction 200–300 times and hit the bird 400 times (30).

All footwork should take the player quickly and fluidly to the bird, allowing him or her to stroke the bird properly and in a mechanically efficient position. Badminton requires an extremely rapid forward and backward movement. A change of direction in a relatively confined space is challenging to the most skilled players. They need excellent balance, superspeed and the ability to make a quick recovery.

The badminton player must be in superb physical condition. The nature of this sport requires optimum strength and a good range of motion in body joints. Pre- and postplay conditioning are important in limiting the athlete's risk while engaging in the sport. Preplay conditioning should not focus solely on elevating the pulse and heart rate, but rather should center around maintaining the greatest active and passive range of motion across lower extremity joints. Those muscle groups used the most—that is, the triceps surae and hamstrings—should be stretched. Their antagonist muscle groups, the lower leg anterior compartment and quadriceps, should be strengthened (31).

The "four-corner drill", a dynamic conditioning exercise performed between five and ten times according to the condition of the player, is described below. Initial speed is moderate and increases gradually as the number of repetitions increase.

The following sequence is advised, beginning with home base in the ready position.

1. Forward to right forehand net corner
2. Return to base position
3. Forward to left backhand net corner
4. Return to base position
5. Backward to forehand right baseline corner
6. Return to base position
7. Backward to left backhand or around the head corner
8. Return to base position

Initially, this sequence is performed five times at a moderate pace; then the speed is increased. Gradually the player works up to ten repetitions as speed is increased. The sequence can then be changed to the following:

1. Forward to right forehand net corner
2. Return to base position
3. Backward to left backhand net corner
4. Return to base position
5. Forward to left backhand net corner
6. Return to base position
7. Backward to forehand right baseline corner
8. Return to base position

Efficient footwork begins with an alert, ready-to-move starting position. A stiff upright stance should be avoided. The exact ready position varies slightly with individual players, depending on their body build, quickness and often the stroke they prefer to play. The ready position also depends on what the player has done immediately before assuming that position. For example, a player takes a different position after receiving than before receiving the serve—and a different position between rallies.

The ready position after serving one high single serve and between rallies is described below. Keep the feet nearly parallel. The position may vary slightly with one foot just in front of the other. The legs are spread a little wider than the shoulders. A more narrow stance has an unstable influence and a wider stance allows too much stability and a lesser ability to respond quickly. The knees should be bent 15–20° with weight being borne on the forefeet (metatarsal heads). Subtalar joints should not be fully supinated or pronated anticipatory to quick forward or back movement. The racquet should be held up and slightly on the backhand side. The left hand is held up, bent at the elbow, at the same height as the racquet hand.

The ready position waiting to receive a serve is described below. The feet are placed in the diagonal stride position. The left foot is placed slightly in front of the right. It is easier to move forward and back in this position. The legs are spread a little wider than the shoulders. The left knee is bent slightly more than the right. In singles play, the weight is borne on the metatarsal heads of the left or nonracquet foot. The left subtalar joint should be slightly supinated for a quicker pushoff backward. The right subtalar joint should be slightly pronated so as to be able to adapt quickly to forward or backward movement. In doubles play, most serves are short and low. Therefore, the receiver's weight is borne on the metatarsal heads of the left foot. Most players lean forward in anticipation of moving forward. The receiver's partner stands in a more parallel position. Weight is borne evenly on both feet anticipatory to sideward movement. The racquet should be held up and on the forehand side. The left hand is held up, bent at the elbow, at the same height as the racquet hand (31).

Forward, backward and sideway movements involve footwork indigenous to badminton. The player with an uncompensated rearfoot varus foot type is predisposed to inversion ankle injury, peroneus brevis tenosynovitis and Achilles tendonitis. Uncompensated forefoot valgus and plantar flexed first ray predispose to sesamoiditis and forefoot instability. The excessively pronated compensated forefoot and rearfoot varus foot type predispose the badminton player to plantar fasciitis, heel spur syndrome, Achilles tendonitis, periarticular fibrocitis of the second metatarsophalangeal joint and tibialis posterior tenosynovitis-myositis (posterior shin splints.)

Attention must be directed toward stretching the posterior leg muscle groups and strengthening the anterior leg muscle groups. Badminton shoes should provide a firm shank and heel counter, flexible rubber sole, shock-absorbing heel and adequate toebox.

A slight laterally flared heel may be of benefit to the player with a rigid uncompensated rearfoot varus foot type. One-quarter-inch felt longitudinal metatarsal padding, applied to the badminton shoe, is helpful to the player with an overpronating foot type. Semirigid foot orthotic devices with shock-absorbing heel seats can assist the badminton player in functioning to the optimum level.

Tennis

According to Rosenthal (32), a fit tennis player is one who can play aggressive and defensive tennis on a continuous aerobic basis for 90–120 minutes in a daily workout program. By concentrating on playing with appropriate bending and lifting positions coordinated with proper foot position, the tennis player excels at his or her sport.

A tennis conditioning program should consist of on-court stretching exercises and an off-court exercise program to increase stamina, flexibility, agility and muscle strength. Specific exercises might include leg and back stretch, Achilles tendon stretch, wind sprints, jumping rope and jogging. Shadow tennis, a shadow boxing through an imaginary point, and the coin footwork drill, running toward a coin with the back foot landing on the coin while the body is turned toward the net, enable the tennis player to take shuffling steps and to prevent hitting the ball while on the wrong foot (33).

Skipping and leaping exercises are another form of training for the serious tennis player. These bounding exercises involve high and low knee action. They improve leg strength and lift, which leads to improved speed and agility. These exercises should not be done on hard surfaces; grass is an ideal surface for bounding exercises. One leaping exercise consists of running slowly while lifting each knee up toward the chin as high as one can. This high-knee exercise should be done for 20–30 yards and repeated three times. Land on the balls of the feet, not the heels. Another bounding exercise consists of keeping the knees low and moving the feet up and down rapidly. A third bounding exercise involves skipping, either skip with the knees low or elevate the knees as high as possible. This may be done for 20–30 yards as well. These bounding exercises, coupled with speed and endurance running exercises, performed twice a week should improve conditioning and court play.

Although lower extremity tennis injuries are not as common as upper extremity injuries, indigenous tennis movements, including cuts, jumps, leaps, turns, shuffles, slides, twists and pivots, predispose to a number of lower extremity injuries. Common lower extremity tennis injuries include "tennis toe" (subungual hemorrhage beneath great or second toenail), blisters, heloma, tyloma, avulsion fracture of the fifth metatarsal base, Achilles and plantaris tendon rupture, medial origin of the gastrocnemius rupture, anterior and posterior shin splints, muscle cramping, patellar-femoral syndrome, Osgood Shlatter's disease seen in young teenagers, ankle strain and sprain, second and third metatarsal stress fracture, calcaneal periostitis, plantar fasciitis, heel spur syndrome, calcaneal apophysitis in children and superficial peroneal nerve entrapment secondary to shoe lace tightness in an anterior, posterior, or global cavus foot type.

The tennis shoe is of singular importance. The rolled posterior heel allows shock absorption at heel strike when the leg is stretched forward. A firm motion-controlling heel counter, supporting side strips, a reinforced pivot point under the first metatarsal head and a deep toebox with reinforced toe bumper to absorb the wear of serving are important features of a good tennis shoe. Uppers are available in leather, canvas and nylon mesh. Leather is heavy and has poor breathability, but is better supporting. Canvas is light weight and has excellent breathability, but gives little support and loses shape. Nylon mesh seems to combine the best qualities of leather and canvas (32). Soles are of gum rubber, air-injected rubber, Radial and polyurethane construction. Injected rubber works well on clay courts, but wears out quickly on cement. Radials and polyurethane have poor shock-absorbing qualities, but are better for traction. Sport socks help cushion shock, are better supporting and absorb perspiration (32).

Cross-Country (Nordic) and Downhill (Alpine) Skiing

There are three types of cross-country or Nordic skiing: jumping, mountaineering and ski touring. Ski jumpers have the lowest injury rate. Mountaineers perform well with high-top, cable-binding boots, and those who ski tour use low-cut boots with pin bindings that allow freedom and mobility but less control of the skis (34).

Cross-country skiing is a demanding sport combining cardiopulmonary fitness with endurance to serve as an excellent wintertime conditioning sport of runners and cyclists (35). Recent studies show cross-country skiers have one of the highest maximum oxygen uptake levels (VO_2 maximum of greater than 80 mg/Kg/min) of any competitive athlete (34).

It has been reported that the risk of injury from collisions or falls is less than 0.5 per 1,000 in cross-country skiing and 1 to 13 per 1,000 in downhill skiing (36). Lower extremity injury from falls occurs from an external rotation-abduction force, internal rotary force or from a forward fall. External rotation usually associated with abduction is the most frequent source of injury (37). It occurs when the ski becomes fixed while the skier is still in motion. Resultant injuries include fracture of the lateral malleolus, spiral fracture of the tibia and fibula, and various sprains of the knee and ankle (35). Internal rotation injuries commonly affect the beginning skier who tends to cross the ski tips. Specific injuries include ankle sprain, medial malleolar fracture and, on occasion, tibial fracture (37). The forward fall may result in boot-top tibial fracture and/or Achilles tendon rupture. Only 5% of injuries are associated with collisions (36). Downhill skiing is responsible for the great majority of boot-top fractures. Ankle joint fractures, ankle ligamentous injuries and tarsal and metatarsal injuries are less common when Alpine boots are used compared to cross-country boot use.

Other injuries common to cross-country and downhill skiers include blisters, nerve compression, frostbite, Achilles and patellar tendonitis and dehydration.

Skiers can condition themselves for their sport by running or jogging during the off-season. Adequate stretching, especially of the posterior leg muscle groups, is essential prior to and after Nordic and Alpine skiing. For the recreational skier, a conditioning exercise program should be performed for about 20–30 min 3 days a week (38). A conditioning program might include isometric exercises composed of quad sets and resistive exercises for the hamstrings, foot inverters and everters, shoulder extensors and hip flexors. Active exercises might include weight lifting, abdominal and low back strengthening, wall sitting, bicycle riding, rope jumping and running (38).

The same socks worn while skiing should be worn when being fitted for ski boots. Boots should fit tightly without undue pressure on the first and fifth metatarsal heads, and there should be plenty of toe room. Cross-country boots should have enough side-to-side rigidity to prevent twisting. They should have a firm heel counter and an adequately deep toebox.

The following easy recommendations are designed to ensure a well-fitting cross-country ski boot (38).

1. With the boot unlaced, slide your foot forward so the toe touches the front of the boot. If you can slide your finger between the counter and your heel, the boot is not too tight and fit is good.
2. Lace up the boot and stand up. Now raise up onto the ball of your foot. If the crease formed across the top of your toes hurts or rubs, try a larger size.
3. Stand on a downhill incline with boots laced. If your feet slide forward in the boot, try on a smaller size.

The following downhill ski boot fitting and binding safety recommendations have been formulated by Dr. Lloyd Nesbit (Canadian Podiatric Sports Medicine Academy) (39). Possible ski boot modifications include the use of heating elements, casts, inboot padding, modification of the liner, skims, orthoses, heel lifts and heating the outer shell in order to mold it around a deformity. As a rule, rear entry boots provide a better fit, while front entry boots provide better performance.

Initial Considerations

1. Try to be flexible about your choice of boots. Various makes or models fit differently, so try not to have a preconceived idea about buying one specific pair of boots.
2. Plan to spend enough time in the shop to make sure the fit is correct. Trying on different makes and sizes gives you an idea of the range of comfort that you can expect.
3. By taking your ski socks with you when you go to shop for boots, you can expect a more precise fit.

Trying Boots On

1. When placing your foot in a boot, your first impression may be that the boot is small. This may change once you have fastened the boot and flexed your ankle forward.
2. (a) Stand and flex your knee and ankle in order to get your heel into the heel pocket. Kicking back your heel does not help because the heel tends to bounce forward because of the foam in the boot. (b) The heel pocket should be firm enough to hold the heel but not too tight as to cause excessive pressure.
3. The top flap of the boot should not cause abrasions or tightness to the front of your ankle. (Make sure your socks are pulled up smoothly so that they do not have wrinkles that would cause pressure points).
4. (a) Buckling of the boot should not cause "hot spots" or tightness in the area of the buckles. The pressure should be evenly spread while the foot is held firmly. (b) New buckling systems require less pressure to close them, so watch that you do not over tighten them, which is very easy to do.
5. (a) There should not be too much pressure at the inside or outside edges of the ball of the foot. (b) If the boot is too narrow at the ball of the foot, do not necessarily go to a larger size. With larger sizes the length may be too long and the fit improper. Try a different boot model that fits wider.
6. There should be room for the toes to wiggle, but the forefoot should not slide from side to side. Your toes may almost touch the end of the boot, but note how they move back as the knees flex.
7. The forward tilting at the ankle joint, which is increased in boots for advanced skiers, should not cause excessive discomfort in the calf muscles or Achilles tendon area. If even a beginner's boot causes this pain, you may wish to have a podiatrist check your ankle joint motion. Stretching exercises may be necessary.
8. Boots should not be too tight in the ankle area as this can cause a decrease in circulation, cold feet, numbness or pain with skiing.
9. Boots should be able to flex forward in the ankle area when they are buckled. This smooth flex gets stiffer and should stop just when the knees are forward of the toes.
10. Note that most ski boots get a little bigger (about ¼ size) after they have been used for a little while. This is because the lining compacts somewhat.
11. In the shop, try to simulate skiing by doing some knee bends. Be sure that the boots do not hurt before you make your final decision!

By taking these pointers into consideration you should be off to a good start. If you have the best possible fit and your feet still feel loose or you feel that something just is not right, you may have a foot imbalance.

Abnormal foot mechanics is a common cause for complaints regarding boot fit. A foot imbalance can also cause foot and lower leg pain during skiing. Some other problems in skiing that may be due to a foot imbalance are (1) having to hop before initiating turns, (2) frequently catching the outside edge of your skis, and (3) having to jam the "downhill" knee behind the "uphill" knee in order to edge the downhill ski.

If you are in doubt about the nature of your foot structure and are having problems with boot fit, ski edge control or pain in your feet, consider seeing a sports-minded podiatrist. A prescription for an orthotic device to be worn in the ski boot may be required in order to control your foot mechanics and reduce symptoms. Arch pads and supports are nonspecific and usually inefficient.

The function of a binding is to hold the ski during normal maneuvers, but to release the ski when injury-producing loads are encountered.

From the standpoint of safety, the binding is

the most important factor in causing or preventing acute downhill skiing injuries. Its function depends on many variables that must all be carefully controlled to avoid injury. Skiers must realize that failure to care for their bindings properly can cause severe injuries.

Safety Tips

1. Studies show that the most expensive bindings produced by each manufacturer have resulted in the lowest injury rates. Therefore it is false economy to buy an inexpensive binding model. This especially holds true for children!
2. Do not presume that a binding will function properly simply because it is present on the ski.
3. Have binding service checks performed by a qualified ski shop at the beginning of the ski season. Test and maintain the bindings frequently thereafter, especially if you are doing a good deal of skiing during the season. This is your responsibility!
4. Be certain that the ski shop you select has a certified technician. (The technician's diploma should be on the wall).
5. Try using soft covers for your bindings while they are on your car ski rack. This will help keep out salt and debris that can cause corrosion and malfunction.
6. Purchase new bindings every few years to keep up with the state-of-the-art equipment.
7. The more attention you pay to the details of proper binding function, the less likely you are to sustain an acute lower extremity injury.
8. All bindings function best when set at their midrange. Ask your ski shop technician what settings would be right for you and your bindings.
9. Have "AFD's" replaced yearly (at a minimum). These are the "anti-friction devices" or plates behind the toe piece of the bindings.

The following self-test ensures a safe low setting for a binding when competent safety inspection by a qualified shop is not available.

With your ski boot buckled, ensure that there is no ice or debris on the boot sole before placing it on the binding. Then do the following.

1. Put on one ski only!
2. Step into the binding.
3. Do the toe test. Bend you knee slightly, and twist the foot inward, with a smooth twisting motion (not a sudden jerking motion). Your boot should come out of the binding. (The outward twist is hard to do.)
4. Do the heel release. Place the boot in the binding. Bend the knee forward and try to kick up your heel at the same time. (Do not have anyone stand on back of ski!) The heel of the boot should come out of the binding.
5. Repeat for the opposite boot and ski.

It is helpful to try both twisting out at the toe and pulling your boot heel out several times.

Baseball

Although the sports medicine aspects of baseball center on injuries to the throwing arm, lower extremity injuries include all those seen in other running sports. Injuries to the lower extremity may occur from sliding into a base or diving after a ball, from sudden bursts of speed necessary to steal a base or to chase down a fly ball and during training drills (40). Because baseball is a running sport, running conditioning programs are incorporated into the training regimen. Common lower extremity injuries seen in baseball include spike injuries, abrasions and contusions; hamstring, quadriceps, adductor and triceps surae muscle strain; ankle sprains; meniscal tears; and others. The many overuse problems in baseball players are usually seen during the conditioning period prior to competition. Common overuse injuries include shin splints, plantar fasciitis, heel spur syndrome, Achilles tendonitis, blisters and patellofemoral syndrome. Biomechanical inefficiencies predisposing to overuse injury are controlled with foot orthotic devices in combination with stretching-strengthening exercise programs. Indigenous stance positions of the batter, catcher, umpire and field player can often be enhanced by control of faulty foot function.

Various forms of a base running drill may be utilized within the baseball conditioning program. The base running drill prepares the athlete for quick starts and 90-foot sprints. Running through first base, stealing second base, taking a lead off second and scoring on a base hit are examples of various base running drills. A series of these drills may be repeated four to six times, providing aerobic training specific to the sport. Sliding drills with spikes removed help prevent injury during a game. Baseball shoes should have a stable heel counter, a deep toebox, rigid shank and flexible sole.

Flexibility, strength, speed, coordination, agility, endurance, concentration, balance and vision are requirements of the successful baseball player.

Soccer

Soccer is one of the most popular sports in the world. Only soccer shoes, a ball and a playing field are required to play. Of the 11 players on the team, only the goalie is allowed to use the hands. Players are characteristically of average build and possess the ability to run fast, skill and knowledge of the game and agility.

There are several types of kicks and ball control skills indigenous to soccer. The inside of the foot kick is used for accuracy. The ball makes contact with the medial aspect of the foot at the level of the navicular tuberosity. The instep kick has two versions: the lofted kick for long distances and the low-drive kick for hard shooting at the goal. These kicks are similar except for slight differences in body positioning. The foot makes contact with the ball, with the toes pointed forward at the level of the dorsal lesser metatarsal heads or just medial to the second metatarsal head. Chipping is a variation of the lofted kick with the foot kept parallel to the ground and the knee forcefully extended. The toes are forcefully extended at ball contact in order to kick the ball over the opponent's head. The foot is inverted and the hip is internally rotated while moving into abduction during the outside of the foot kick. In backheeling the ball is kicked with the back of the heel. Other skills requiring lower extremity movement include dribbling with the inside and outside of the forefoot, trapping the ball between both feet and volleying with the ball making contact with the feet while it is still airborne (41).

Players must be ready to move quickly. Weight is transferred to the toes with knees slightly flexed in the ready position. Balance is essential to the soccer player. Pregame conditioning, including a suitable warm-up to raise muscle temperature and facilitate function, is required. There is some evidence that speed, strength, and efficiency of muscle contractions are enhanced by a rise in temperature to the 102–105°F range. The only efficient way of raising muscle temperature is by the work of the muscle itself (42). With increased muscle, tendon, ligament and nerve conduction function the chance for injury decreases (41).

Basmajian (42) described five areas of concern to be addressed in optimal strength training:

1. The speed of exercise movement must not be fast or slow. It should take a shorter period of time to lower a weight than to raise it.
2. To prevent injury the strengthening exercise should be isokinetic and carried out over the greatest possible range of motion.
3. The exercise movement should be started from a prestretched position to bring into play the greatest percentage of muscle.
4. The load must be heavy enough to require a maximum intensity of contraction. At least ten repetitions must be performed, and sufficient time should be allowed for total recovery.
5. Exercise should begin with the largest muscle groups in order to provide the greatest growth stimulus.

During a game the soccer player may run 5–10 miles. Soccer involves both anaerobic and aerobic activity. Interval training is specific to the needs of the soccer player. If anaerobic training is continuous with short rest periods, an aerobic training effect is achieved (43). A period of stretching during warm-up and cool down is necessary in order to avoid injury. Most injuries involve strains, sprains, contusions and abrasions (44). Inversion ankle injuries are most common. Knee injuries are more commonly seen in soccer players wearing cleated shoes. Shin guards are worn to help prevent contusions and abrasions. Other lower extremity overuse injuries common to the soccer player are plantar calcaneonavicular ligamentous strain, subungual hemorrhage, plantar fasciitis, Achilles tendonitis, anterior and posterior shin splints and heel spur syndrome. Appropriate soccer shoes include a snug, rigid controlling heel counter, firm shank, rubber cleats, flexible forefoot sole and a 6 to 8 eyelet lacing system.

Ballet

Ballet requires rigorous conditioning in order to perform at the maximal level. The professional ballet dancer is one of the best conditioned of all athletes. Stretching flexibility exercise routines must be performed on a daily basis. The warm-up period may last up to twice as long as the performance. Every muscle group should be stretched. Male ballet dancers, because they are called upon to lift their female counterpart, often participate in weight training.

Indigenous movements in ballet predispose to specific injury, mostly in the lower extremities. The ballet dancer with a compensated rearfoot or forefoot varus or uncompensated rearfoot valgus does not function well. The dancer with a supinated foot is best able to perform (45). Clarkson and James (46) found that a simple auditory feedback system reduced foot pronation, thereby accelerating the learning of correct foot placement in classical ballet.

The skill of going "en pointe" is acquired over a long period of time. A common mistake made by instructors and dancers is encouraging this movement at too young an age. The forefoot must be plantar flexed while the rearfoot is supinated and the leg externally rotated to obtain the pointe position. Although inversion ankle injuries occur in young ballet dancers who are undergoing growth spurts, the older dancer suffers tendonitis and muscle tears. The ballet dancer's pointe slipper has a toebox that is flattened distally. When going en pointe the first and fifth metatarsal heads contact the weightbearing surface, predisposing to a functional plantar flexed first ray. Adventitious bursae may develop beneath these areas of friction and pressure. An elastoplast sling strap with an appropriately skived ¼-inch felt pad may be incorporated over the ballet dancer's foot for greater stability and protection. Although the ballet dancer suffers the majority of overuse injuries attendant to poor conditioning and function, other injuries, including flexor hallucis longus tenosynovitis, anterior and posterior ankle impingement, iliotibial band syndrome, contusions, helomas, tylomas, incurvated toenails, os trigonum syndrome and stress fractures, may occur. Hard training surfaces and worn-out shoes may predispose to further injury. Wood surfaces over air are best. A cement surface is the worst (47).

Basketball

The basketball player must have excellent coordination and be mentally alert. Body balance, muscular power, endurance, speed, and good timing are essential.

In the basic stance, a basketball player has one foot forward and the other back. This so-called boxer stance enables body weight to be distributed evenly beneath the forefeet while heel contact is maintained (48). The knees are flexed and the body bent forward in order to maintain a ready position. From this ready position the basketball player may quickly turn to either side. The body's center of gravity is maintained at a lower level through the game with the exception of shooting and some throwing techniques. Various basket shots, including the lay-up, hook, jump, and overhead, involve specific upper and lower extremity placement and movement. Some of these movements predispose to injury of both extremities. The basketball player with an uncompensated rearfoot varus or cavus deformity is predisposed to lateral ankle sprain and fifth metatarsal base fracture when descending from a jump shot.

It is common practice for the trainer or coach to tape the ankles of a basketball player prior to a game. Doing so serves to stabilize the ankle and subtalar joints and minimize ankle injury. There is some question as to whether this practice predisposes to lateral knee injury.

Pregame conditioning of the basketball player includes stretching flexibility exercises, on-court drills and specific muscle group strengthening, e.g., the peroneals. The wooden court surface must be smooth, clean and free from splinters. The sidelines and net areas should be free of obstacles (48).

Although the most common basketball injury is the lateral ankle sprain, other lower extremity injuries include fifth metatarsal base fracture, patellar tendonitis, patellofemoral syndrome (patellar chondromalacia), tibial and metatarsal stress fracture, Achilles tendonitis, plantar fasciitis, heel spur syndrome, plantar calcaneonavicular ligamentous strain, blisters, sesamoiditis, and anterior ankle impingement exostosis. Thirty-nine percent of injuries occur during rebounding (7).

The high-top basketball shoe is designed to help stabilize the foot and ankle. A thick shock-absorbing heel and sole are important features. Cushioning, forefoot flexibility, light weight (less than 550 g), ankle support, motion control, and energy return are important (30). The lacing systems should not interfere with circulatory or neurological function. Metal eyelets should be discouraged. The heel counter should be rigid, and the heel should fit snugly in the shoes. A deep toebox with a wide vamp is important.

Bicycling

Although it is beyond the scope of this book to describe the qualities in a good 10-speed bicycle, it is important to be aware of the many factors affecting safety and health. Some of these factors include the bicycle's frame, stem, handlebar; saddle; wheel height, size and type; tire pressure; rim type; and pedal type.

The preferred pedal type is light-weight forged aluminum alloy with "rattrap cages" allowing for foot insertion with a minimum of slippage (49). A toe clip and strap are often incorporated into the pedal for stability and efficiency. Hlavac (7) describes a three-plane adjustable pedal designed to allow the cyclist more efficient function with less expenditure of energy (Fig. 12.10).

The cycling shoe is critical to proper technique. It is designed to be lighter weight with snug, ventilated leather uppers, thin reinforced grooved soles and a steel shank. By using cleats that fit over

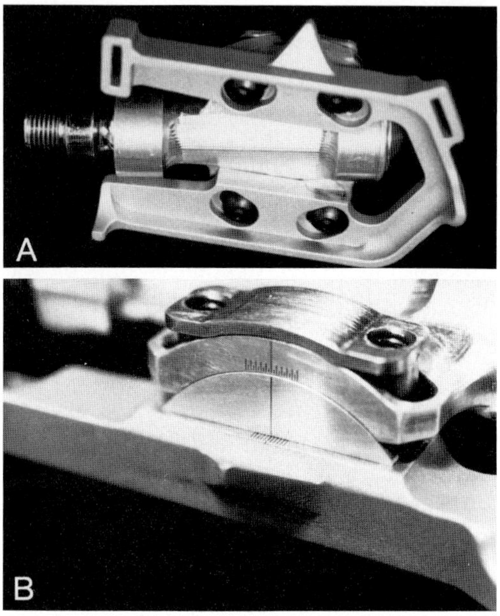

Figure 12.10. *A,* The Biopedal[R] is adjustable in three planes to support any structural or functional imbalance of the foot. *B,* The Biopedal[R] may be prescribed by a podiatrist or self-adjusted and fixed in the position of optimum performance. (Courtesy of Biosports, Inc, Mill Valley, CA 94941.)

the "rattrap cage" bridge one foot may be pulled up while the other is depressed. This increases pedalling efficiency up to 40% (49).

The foot is placed in the pedal with the ball of the foot on the pedal axle (spindle) and with the foot in the same position as the basic angle of stance in gait—straight, turned in or out. Most experienced cyclists use some form of toe clip and strap in order to position the foot accurately as was mentioned previously. This allows a more efficient and comfortable pedal stroke. Novice cyclists tend to place their midfoot above the spindle leading to inefficient function. The toe clip allows the tibialis anterior, gastrocnemius, biceps and rectus femoris to function for a longer period of time during each pedal cycle (48). External tibial torsion is the "cyclist's curse" (7).

Pedal rate or cadence, measured in RPMs, is important to good cycling technique. Cadence depends on individual conditioning and skill. Cyclist posture and weight and bike weight and gear size also affect cadence. It is important to maintain constant pedal pressure and to pedal rapidly against little resistance in order to find the natural cadence. After an individual's natural cadence is attained less gear shifting is required.

Adjustment of the bicycle position is extremely important and involves seat height, seat position (fore and aft), pedal position, stem length and frame size. When straddling the bike, the frame should be 1 inch lower than one's crotch. The seat height should be measured by pedaling backwards with the heels on the pedals and seat raised until one's buttocks begin to rock side to side. At this point the seat is moved downward approximately ¼-½-inch. The knee will now be flexed on the down stroke.

The fore and aft position is measured by using a plumb bob. With pedal position at 3:00 o'clock, a plumb bob is dropped by the center of the outside of the knee; it should fall to the spindle of the pedal. If it is too far forward or backward, the seat is moved forward or backward accordingly.

The stem length is based on the rider sitting on the seat and resting on the brake hoods. A plumb bob dropped from the tip of the nose should bisect the center of the handlebars. Many bicycle shops now have a "fit kit" that is used to set up all the basic adjustments needed.

Bicycling is an aerobic sport requiring superb conditioning and adequate pre- and postride warm-up and cool down periods. A 10-min stretching program should precede and follow cycling. Cycling training programs include aerobic strength training to strengthen the upper body, as well as the lower extremities. Other on-cycle training methods include interval training and long steady distance training.

Although adequate strength and flexibility are key to injury prevention, overuse syndromes due to poor function are the cause of most cycle injuries. Nonlower extremity injuries range from saddle burns to nerve compression to lumbar muscle spasm. Twenty-five percent of cycling problems involve the knee (7). Lower extremity injuries include popliteal and patellar tendonitis, lateral collateral knee ligamentous strain, bursitis, patellofemoral syndrome (patellar chondromalacia), hip pain from altered pedal stroke and/or limb length discrepancy, metatarsalgia due to soft cycle shoe soles, nerve compression injuries to the superficial peroneal nerve branches and around the ischial tuberosity and blisters from ill-fitting shoes.

In-shoe orthotic devices, cants and blocks attached to pedals and three-plane adjustable pedals are used to control abnormal function and prevent injury.

Weight Lifting

Weight lifting is utilized both as a training method and as a sport. Weight lifting is not recommended for children. Training with weights is used by many athletes to strengthen their muscles and provide overall conditioning.

Weight lifting as a sport concentrates on specific muscle groups in order to participate in either powerlifting or Olympic lifting (17). There is little technique in power lifting. However, a great deal of strength is required. Olympic lifting requires strength, coordination and technique (50).

Equipment includes barbells, dumbbells and Universal, Nautilus or Cybex weight machines. Their use depends on individual training program needs. Lower extremity muscular strength is enhanced with the use of squats, lunges, toe raises, and off-weightbearing extension and flexion weight lifting exercises.

Weight lifting shoes must provide protection from the floor and foot press apparatus of a weight machine, as well as cushioning and adequate support (50). Forefoot sole flexibility is important. A steel shank helps support the weight of both the lifter and the load. High-supporting wool or cotton wool blend socks are recommended. Because the weight lifter stands on flat surfaces and competitors stand on flat wooden square platforms, weight is transmitted equally through each lower extremity.

Weight lifting technique requires pretraining flexibility exercise routines and a gradual warm-up period. Bouncing when lifting is to be avoided because of the possibility of muscle strain and tear. Plantar fascial strain, plantar calcaneonavicular ligament strain and Achilles tendonitis can be avoided by pretraining stretching and by using adequate, well-supporting shoes.

Swimming

Swimming is one of the best aerobic sports. The four strokes used in competition are freestyle, butterfly, backstroke and breaststroke. Each stroke involves different lower extremity function. The frog kick has been replaced by the whip kick in the breaststroke. The whip kick has been replaced by the flutter kick in the backstroke. The butterfly developed out of the breaststroke utilizing the dolphin kick instead of the frog or whip kick (51).

Training aids utilized by swimmers include hand paddles, pull buoys, kickboards and swim fins. The kickboard is used to strengthen the anterior leg muscle groups. Swim fins help develop thigh, calf and abdominal muscles and enhance foot and ankle joint flexibility. The precompetitive swimming conditioning program includes weight training in order to add strength necessary for speed and endurance. The training program is designed to work on specific muscles used in the various strokes and kicks by means of high-repetition, light-resistance weight training. Weight training is performed four to five times a week, decreases to three times a week and tapers off prior to competition (51).

Stretching flexibility programs are essential to the swimmer. The breaststroker must stretch the groin area, which can be strained from the outward motion of the kick, and the triceps surae muscle group in order to allow maximum dorsiflexion of the foot, an important part of the breaststroke kick. Backstrokers, butterflyers, and freestylers need to stretch the anterior lower leg muscle groups so as to allow maximal foot plantar flexion during the flutter kick.

In-water training includes anaerobic and aerobic regimens. Training includes marathon, Fartlek, interval, repetition, and sprint swimming. Aerobic marathon training is designed to produce a training effect of 60% of the target heart rate. The target heart rate is determined by subtracting the age of the swimmer from 220 and taking 60% of the remainder. In Fartlek training, fast and slow laps are alternated without rest in order to develop speed and endurance. Interval training involves a series of repeat swims at a set distance with short rest periods in between. Repetition training also involves a series of repeat swims at a set distance. However, unlike interval training, which is swum at 70% of the heart rate target, repetition training is swum at 100% of the heart rate target with long rest periods in between. Sprint training consists of short fast swims performed at maximum speed with long rest periods in between. The warm-up, comprising 20% of the workout, consists of long relaxed swimming that slightly elevates the heart rate. The main set, comprising 70% of the workout, consists of a variety of the before-mentioned training methods and is performed at 70% of the heart target rate. The cool down, comprising 10% of the workout, allows the body to relax and the heart rate to return slowly to its normal resting state (52).

Injuries associated with swimming include swimmer's shoulder, apprehension shoulder, breaststroker's knee and tenosynovitis of the foot extensors (52). Breaststroker's knee, inflammation of the medial collateral ligaments, is best treated by correcting kick technique. A decrease in yardage doing the whip kick, anti-inflammatory medications, ultrasound, ice and local heat may be beneficial. Foot extensor tenosynovitis is caused by hyperextension of the foot during the flutter and backstroke kicks, which leads to irritation of the tendon sheaths. Change from a 6-beat to a 2-beat kick may be beneficial (51). Local ice applications, steroid injection or a short course of a NSAID may be helpful.

The author has attempted in this chapter to present a variety of sports from a lower extremity sports medicine perspective. Space does not permit the inclusion of the many dozens of additional athletic endeavors requiring lower extremity function. Needless to say, the list is exhausting and the variety staggering. Additional sports not included in this chapter include football; paddle-, racquet-, and handball; most field events, such as the javelin throw, hammer and discus throw;

high, broad and long jumps; hurdle events; lawn and alley bowling; rowing; gymnastics; riflery; wrestling; street hockey; wind and water surfing; golf and tournament marbles. Each sport and its many varieties include indigenous lower extremity movements requiring specialized podiatric medical appraisal. Totally effective injury management cannot be accomplished without specialized knowledge of podiatric biomechanics and treatment methods. Individuals participating in these and other sports deserve the best medical care available.

References

1. Cooper K: *The New Aerobics.* Bantam, 1980.
2. Hancock AL: Aerobic dancing. Quinnipiac College, Hamden, CT, Principles of Sports Medicine, Masters in Health Sciences Program, 1981.
3. Dobbins B, Sprague K: *Gold's Gym Weight Training Book.* New York, Berkley Publishing Co, 1980, p. 222.
4. Goodyear NN, Blair SN: Incidence rates and risk of orthopedic injuries in healthy middle aged runners and nonrunners. Address given to American College of Sports Medicine (ACSM) Annual Meeting, San Diego, CA, May 23, 1984.
5. Sohn RS, Micheli LJ: The effect of running on the pathogenesis of osteoarthritis of the hips and knees. Address given to American College of Sports Medicine (ACSM) Annual Meeting, San Diego, CA, May 23, 1984.
6. Pagliano J, Jackson DW: A clinical study of 3000 long distance runners. Address given to American College of Sports Medicine (ACSM) Annual Meeting, San Diego, CA, May 24, 1984.
7. Yale JF: *Firm Footings for the Athlete* (a preventive injury and self-help guide for those athletes involved in the running sports). Ansonia, CT, 1981, pp. 4–5.
8. Kirby KA, Valmassy RL: The runner patient history. *J Am Podiatry Assoc* 73:39–43, 1983.
9. *Runner's World Magazine,* Mountain View, CA, World Publications..
10. *Runner's World Magazine.* Mountain View, CA, World Publications.
11. Faulkner J: Exercise-induced injury of skeletal muscle fibers. Address given to American College of Sports Medicine (ACSM) Annual Meeting, San Diego, CA, May 23, 1984.
12. McClain J, Kanat IO: Cold urticaria. A podiatric consideration. *J Am Podiatric Med Assoc* 75-245–248, 1985.
13. Subotnick SI: Dimethyl sulfoxide dehydration of the foot. A case history. *J Am Podiatric Med Assoc* 75-263–265, 1985.
14. Hollander J: The practical knee examination. Amer. Academy of Podiatric Sports Medicine Annual Scientific Seminar, San Francisco, July 29, 1984.
15. Zanoli Z, Piazzai E: Synovial plica syndrome of the knee: Pathology, differential diagnosis, and treatment. *Ital J Orthop Traumatol* 241–250, 1984.
16. Taunton JE, et al: Achilles tendonitis in runners. Address given to American College of Sports Medicine (ACSM) Annual Meeting, Nashville, TN, May 27, 1984.
17. Jarrell S: *Working out with Weights.* New York, Arco Publishing Co, Inc, 1978.
18. Campbell G, Warnekros W: A tarsal stress fracture in a long distance runner (a case report). *J Am Podiatry Assoc* 73:532–535, 1983.
19. Matheson O, et al: Characteristics of tarsal stress fractures in athletes. Address given to American College of Sports Medicine (ACSM) Annual Meeting, Nashville, TN, May 27, 1984.
20. Snider MP, Clancy WG, McBeath AA: Plantar fascia release for chronic plantar fasciitis in runners. *J Am Podiatry Assoc* 11:215–219, 1983.
21. Blake RL, Fettig MH: Chronic low back pain in a long-distance runner (a case report). *J Am Podiatry Assoc* 73:598–601, 1983.
22. Cooper K: *The Aerobics Program for Total Well Being,* New York, Evans Co, 1982.
23. Bzdyra B: Coronary heart disease and aerobic dancing. Quinnipiac College, Hamden, CT, Principles of Sports Medicine, Masters in Health Science Program, 1981.
24. Garrick JG, et al: The epidemiology of aerobic dance injuries. Address given to American College of Sports Medicine (ACSM) Annual Meeting, Nashville, TN, May 27, 1984.
25. Hawes L: Water skiing, Quinnipiac College, Hamden, CT, Principles of Sports Medicine, Masters in Health Sciences Program, 1981.
26. Cokes C: *The Complete Book of Boxing.* Palm Springs, CA ETC Publications, 1980, p. 46.
27. Rimillor RW: Sports medicine and boxing, Quinnipiac College, Hamden, CT, Principles of Sports Medicine, Masters in Health Sciences Program, 1981.
28. Spicer RF: Ice skating. Quinnipiac College, Hamden, CT, Principles of Sports Medicine, Masters in Health Sciences Program, 1981.
29. Gerberich S, et al: An epidemiological study of high school hockey injuries: Implications for prevention. Address given to American College of Sports Medicine (ACSM) Annual Meeting, Nashville, TN, May 27, 1984.
30. Rutledge A, Friedlich J: *Beginning Badminton.* Belmont, CA, Wadsworth Publishing Co, 1969.
31. Yale JF, McGuire, R: Badminton—The fastest Racquet Sport. *Arch Podiatric Med Foot Surg: Annual Sports Medicine Edition, Part I,* May, 1980.
32. Rosenthal AI: Tennis. Quinnipiac College, Hamden, CT, Principles of Sports Medicine, Masters in Health Sciences Program, 1981.
33. Branden V: *Vic Brandens Tennis for the Future.* Boston, Little, Brown and Co 1977.
34. Lyons JW: Cross-country ski injuries. *Physician Sports Med:* 1:67, 1980.
35. Emple TJ: Cross-country skiing: Implications for sports medicine. Quinnipiac College, Hamden, CT, Principles of Sports Medicine, Masters in Health Sciences Program, 1981.
36. Westlin NE: Factors contributing to the production of skiing injuries. *Orthop Clin* 7:1976.

37. Ellison AE: Skiing injuries. *Clin Symposium.* 29:1977.
38. Cota CJ: Cross-country skiing. Quinnipiac College, Hamden, CT, Principles of Sports Medicine, Masters in Health Sciences Program, 1981.
39. Nesbit L: Canadian Podiatric Sports Medicine Academy: *Tips on Buying Ski Boots and Binding Safety.* Toronto, Ont, 1983.
40. Swiderski JR: Baseball and sports medicine Quinnipiac College, Hamden, CT, Principles of Sports Medicine, Masters in Health Sciences Program, 1981.
41. Kulas E: Soccer: a sports medicine approach. Quinnipiac College, Hamden, CT, Principles of Sports Medicine, Masters in Health Sciences Program, 1981.
42. Basmajian JV (ed): *Therapeutic Exercise,* ed 3. Baltimore Williams & Wilkins, 1978, p. 452.
43. Dominguez RH: *The Complete Book of Sports Medicine.* New York, Warner Books, 1979, p. 14.
44. Dahl E, Maehlum S: Types and frequency of injuries in youth soccer. Address given to American College of Sports Medicine (ACSM) Annual Meeting, Nashville, TN, May 27, 1984.
45. Marr SJ: The ballet foot. *J Am Podiatry Assoc* 73:124–132, 1983.
46. Clarkson PM, James RJ: The effect of auditory feedback on foot pronation during a classical ballet exercise. Address given to American College of Sports Medicine (ACSM) Annual Meeting, San Diego, CA, May 25, 1984.
47. Werter R: Dance floors. A causative factor in dance injuries. *J Am Podiatric Med Assoc* 75:355–358, 1985.
48. Doto EM: Basketball. Quinnipiac College, Hamden, CT, Principles of Sports Medicine, Masters in Health Sciences Program, 1981.
49. Buteau J: Bicycling—The machine and the sport. Quinnipiac College, Hamden, CT, Principles of Sports Medicine, Masters in Health Sciences Program, 1981.
50. Fleischman GF: The effects of weight lifting on the lower extremity. Quinnipiac College, Hamden, CT, Principles of Sports Medicine, Masters in Health Sciences Program, 1981.
51. Davidowicz MF: Competitive collegiate swimming. Quinnipiac College, Hamden, CT, Principles of Sports Medicine, Masters in Health Sciences Program, 1981.
52. Kennedy JC, et al: Orthopaedic manifestations of swimming. *Am J Sports Med* 6:309–322, 1978.

Suggested Readings

American Academy of Podiatric Sports Medicine: Syllabus 1972–1980.

Archives of Podiatric Medicine and Foot Surgery: *Sports Medicine* 78 Mt. Kisco, NY, Futura, 1978.

Archives of Podiatric Medicine and Foot Surgery: *Sports Medicine* 80. Mt. Kisco, NY, Futura, 1980.

Blair SN, Caspersen CJ: Running injuries: Rates, risk factors, and prevention. ACSM Annual Meeting, Nashville, TN, May 26, 1985.

Blake RL, Denton JA: Functional foot orthoses for athletic injuries. A retrospective study. *J Am Podiatric Med Assoc* 75:359–362, 1985.

Blustein SM, D'Amico JC: Limb length discrepancy. Identification, clinical significance, and management, *J Am Podiatric Med Assoc* 75: 200–206, 1985.

Brandt A: Badminton: Fastest birds in play. *NY Times Mag* 6:154–164, December 2, 1979.

Cantu RC: *Clinical Sports Medicine.* Lexington, MA, Collamore Press, 1984.

Carsen, JM: *Winning Boxing.* Chicago, Contemporary Books, Inc, 1980.

Conway DH: An introduction to podiatric sports medicine. *J Am Podiatry Assoc* 65:495–499, 1975.

Councilman JF: *The Complete Book of Swimming.* New York, Atheneum, 1980.

Cyriax J: *Textbook of Orthopedic Medicine,* vol. 2. ed 11. London, Baillière Tindall, 1984.

D'Amico JC, Rubin M: The influence of foot orthoses on the quadriceps angle. *J Am Podiatric Med Assoc* 76:337–340, 1986.

Eads WJ: Non-specific tendonitis of flexor longus hallucis tendon. *J Am Podiatry Assoc* 44:32–44, 1954.

Falknor GW: All-weather track syndrome. *J Am Podiatry Assoc* 62:435–439, 1972.

Fancy footwork: Selecting cleated shoes. *Bicycling.* September/October; 164–172, 1985.

Faria, I: *Cycling Physiology for the Serious Cyclist.* Springfield, IL, Charles C Thomas, 1978.

Fixx JF: *The Complete Book of Running.* New York, Random House, 1977.

Frederick EC (ed): *Sports Shoes and Playing Surfaces.* Champaign, IL, Human Kinetics Publishers, Inc, 1984.

Frenette JP, Jackson DW: Lacerations of the flexor hallucis longus in the young athlete. *J Bone Joint Surg* 59:673–676, 1977.

Gazivoda P, Rzonca EC, Schiraldi, F: Soccer Injuries: Types, locations, etiologies, and preventive measures. *J Am Podiatric Med Assoc* 76:109–111, 1986.

Hice GA, Kendrick Z, Weeberk, Bray J: The effect of foot orthoses on oxygen consumption while cycling. *J Amer Podiatric Med Assoc* 75:513–516, 1985.

Hlavac H: *The Foot Book.* Mountain View, CA, World Publications, 1977.

Hoover JA: Exertional anterior compartment syndrome with fascial hernias. *J Foot Surg* 22:271–272, 1983.

Hunter R, Broccoletti P: *Shape up for Soccer.* South Bend, IN, Icarus Press, 1981.

Inman VT: *The Joints of the Ankle.* Baltimore, Williams & Wilkins, 1976.

Isaacs ND: *All the Moves,* Philadelphia, JP Lippincott Co, 1975.

Katz J: *Swimming for Total Fitness.* Garden City, NY, Doubleday and Co, 1981.

Kerner JA, D'Amico JC: A statistical analysis of a group of runners. *J Am Podiatry Assoc* 73:160, 1983.

Kirschenbaum, SE: Boxing and its role in podiatric sports medicine. In Archives of Podiatric Medicine and Surgery (ed): *Sports Medicine 80,* Mt Kisco, NY, Futura, 1980, pp 99–110.

Kuprian W (ed): *Physical Therapy for Sports.* Philadelphia, WB Saunders, 1982.

Kuritz HM: Anterior entrapment syndromes. *J Foot Surg* 15:143–148, 1976.

Landry M, Zebas CJ: Biomechanical principles in common running injuries. *J Am Podiatry Assoc* 75:48–52, 1984.

Matsen F, III, Clawson DK: The deep posterior compartmental syndrome of the leg. *J Bone Joint Surg* 57A: 43–37, 1975.

McGown IA: Boxing safety and injuries. *Physician Sports Med* 3:1979.

McLeod WD, Hunter S: Biomechanical analysis of the knee. *J Am Physical Therapy Med Assoc* 12:1561–1564, 1980.

Mirkin G: The prevention and treatment of running injuries. *J Am Podiatry Assoc* 66:881–884, 1976.

Mishalanie MA: Recurrent anterior tibial compartment syndrome in an athlete. *J Am Podiatry Assoc* 73:157, 1983.

O'Donoghue DH: *Treatment of Injuries to Athletes* ed 4. Philadelphia, WB Saunders, 1984.

Oflin HF, Kempi V, Van Der Linden W, Ringquist I: Effect of flow material ski boots on foot circulation. *Orthop Clin North Am* 7:151–157, 1976.

Root ML, Orien WP, Weed JH: *Normal and Abnormal Function of the Foot.* Los Angeles, Clinical Biomechanics Corp, 1977.

Root ML, Orien WP, Weed JH, Hughes RJ: *Biomechanical Examination of the Foot, vol. I.* Los Angeles, Clinical Biomechanics Corp, 1971.

Ross CF, Schuster RO: A preliminary report on predicting injuries in distance runners. *J Am Podiatry Assoc* 73:275, 1983.

Roy S, Irvin R: *Sports Medicine, Prevention, Evaluation, Management, and Rehabilitation.* Englewood Cliffs, NJ, Prentice Hall, Inc., 1983.

Ruland DN, et al: Tennis injuries: Prevention and treatment. *Amer J Spts Med* 7: 1979.

Runner's World Magazine, Beginning running. September, 1972.

Runner's World Magazine, Athletes' feet, 1974.

Runner's World Magazine, Interval training, August, 1975.

Runner's World Magazine, The runner's diet. 1977.

Sanders W: *The Bicycle Racing Book.* Chicago, Domas, 1979.

Schuster RO: Podiatry and the foot of the athlete. *J Am Podiatry Assoc* 62:465–468, 1972.

Sgarlato TE: *A Compendium of Podiatric Biomechanics.* San Francisco, California College of Podiatric Medicine, 1970.

Sharkey BJ: *Physiology of Fitness,* ed 2. Champaign, IL, Human Kinetics Publishers, 1984.

Smith LS, Clarke TE, Hamill CL, Santo Pietro F: The effects of soft and semi-rigid orthoses upon rearfoot movement in running. *J Am Podiatric Med Assoc* 76:227–233, 1986.

Southmayd W, Hoffman M: *Sports Health.* New York, Quick Fox, 1981.

Sprague K: *The Athlete's Body.* Los Angeles, J P Tarcher, Inc, 1981.

Stones CN: Air stirrup management of ankle injuries in the athlete. *Amer J Orthop Med* 8:360–365, 1980.

Strauss RH: *Sports Medicine,* Philadelphia, W B Saunders, 1984.

Strauss R (ed): *Sports Medicine and Physiology.* Philadelphia, W B Saunders, 1979.

Subotnick SI: The biomechanical basis of skiing. *J Am Podiatry Assoc* 64:54–66, 1974.

Subotnick SI: Compartment syndromes in the lower extremities. *J Am Podiatry Assoc* 65:342–348, 1975.

Subotnick SI: *Podiatric Sports Medicine,* Mt. Kisco, NY, Futura, 1975.

Subotnick SI: *Cures for Common Running Injuries.* Mountain View, CA, World Publications, 1979.

Watkins WL, Cobb S, Finesinger J, Brazier M, Shands SH, Pincus G: Psychiatric and physiologic studies on fatigue. *Arch Phys Med* 28:199–206, 1947.

Wolpa ME: *The Sports Medicine Guide: Treating and Preventing Common Athletic Injuries.* West Point, NY, Leisure Press, 1982.

Yale I: Foot protection device for use in athletic shoes. *J Am Podiatry Assoc* 48:53–56, 1958.

Yale JF: Surgical and biomechanical approach to the talonavicular joint. *J Am Podiatry Assoc* 63:247–254, 1973.

Yale JF: Growth center injuries of the foot. *Arch Podiatric Med Foot Surg* 1:129–140, 1973.

Yale JF: A statistical analysis of 3657 consecutive fatigue fractures of the distal lower extremities. *J Am Podiatry Assoc* 66:739–748, 1976.

Yale JF: Complications of Keller-implant arthroplasty secondary to the stress of golf (A case report), *Arch Podiatric Med Foot Surg:* Annual Sports Medicine Edition, 1978.

Yale JF: Foot impression technique (F.I.T.): An accurate moderate weight bearing technique. *Arch Podiatric Med Foot Surg:* Annual Sports Medicine Edition, 1979.

13

Podiatric Treatment

Biomechanical foot disorders result in abnormal weight distribution with secondary alterations in supporting structures. The stress on an affected part is capable of disturbing structure beyond physiological limits and creating pathological changes in the skin, subcutaneous tissue and bony architecture. Many times the resultant pathology is not reversible or correctable. Yet, the patient requires relief from pain. This can often be accomplished by a thorough study of the problem followed by an evaluation of what is and what is not amenable to treatment (Fig. 13.1). Foot and ankle radiographic examination is mandatory.

The day-to-day practice of podiatric medicine includes the construction of orthoses, molds, shields, and other devices to accommodate and correct abnormal structure and function. Prosthetic devices may be constructed in laboratories by technicians in accordance with the podiatrist's instructions. Some prosthetic devices are made by the podiatrists themselves in the office laboratory, and proper construction requires highly specialized skills. Podiatrists must construct, reconstruct and correct orthotic devices in their offices if they are to practice their profession to the fullest. In order to do this they must be well trained and well supplied with quality materials and equipment. To this end, they are dedicated to seeking improved techniques and materials that lend themselves to quality foot care.

The type of orthotic devices constructed for the patient is only limited by the skill, ingenuity and creativity of the podiatrist who makes corrective and accommodative orthotic devices, molds and shields. For the purpose of this chapter, the term *orthosis* refers to any device of sufficiently rigid construction to maintain the foot and its superstructure in a more efficient functional state in stance and in gait. Orthosis also refers to any device constructed of a flexible or semirigid material, the purpose of which is to control adverse function, accommodate a foot deformity or lesion and limit pain. A *mold* is an orthosis that is molded over a foot or a part of the foot. It may also be constructed over a cast of the foot or a last. A *shield* is a protective device constructed of any flexible or moldable material over the foot, the toe or a model of the foot or toe for the purpose of limiting pressure, friction and extrinsic irritation.

Foot Orthotic Devices

The purpose of orthotic devices is to relieve stress from strained or injured soft tissues, bony prominences, deformed bones and joints, rheumatoid nodules, inflamed or chronic bursae and dermatologic lesions secondary to deforming arthritis or biomechanical abnormality.

Dynamic orthotic device—Molded in the shoe by the functioning foot. Materials—removable moldable silicone (MPC), rubber, cork or synthetic compounds, liquid latex and felt.

Static orthotic device—Molded and ground out to fit plaster cast of the foot, ankle and/or lower leg. Materials—leather, felt, latex, rubber, sponge, foam, Celastic, PPT, hardwood dust, plastic, cork, cork dust, monks cloth, Rohadur, Korex, Plas-

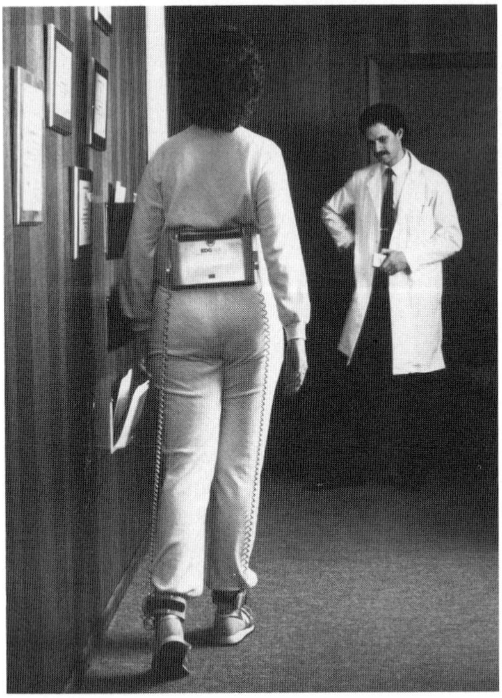

Figure 13.1. The Langer Electrodynogram (EDG) System 1184 is a portable, computerized force data acquisition/gait analysis system that measures and analyzes the forces affecting key segments of the foot during the gait cycle. A printout compares force data to normal ranges and indicates probable clinical conditions with therapeutic considerations.

tazote, Aliplast, Sorbothane, Novalite, molo, S-Ortholen and a variety of substances capable of being shaped, fixed and ground (Figs. 13.2 and 13.3).

Dynamic Orthotic Device

Most foot disorders require accommodation for the deformities that develop secondary to disease. The joints of the feet are basically concerned with stance and locomotion. The foot should serve as a structurally competent member of upright posture biomechanics. The destruction taking place in arthritis is not only damaging to the joints but secondarily creates a variety of functional disabilities. The pathology of the chondro-osseous margins and periarticular tissues results in deforming prominences, outgrowths and calcareous deposits, as well as structural and anatomical malpositions. The podiatrist deals with these problems by evaluating the patient's complaints, functional needs and essential accommodations. From this study of structure and function, clinically and radiographically, an orthotic device is designed and fabricated.

In the severely deformed foot greater pain relief may be obtained by prescribing a dynamic orthotic device in a reasonably well-fit shoe. The orthoses may be constructed of any one or a combination of moldable materials. Some are made of compressible rubber compounds, liquid latex combined with fine cork or hardwood dust, felt and latex, as well as a variety of new plastic materials.

The moldable material is placed in the patient's shoe, and the weightbearing foot shapes the material to the contours of the functioning foot.

Techniques for Dynamic Foot Orthotic Device Fabrication First, all plantar excrescences, tylomas, helomas, plantar verrucae, bursae, nodules, prominent bone enlargements, deformities, etc are marked off on the foot using an indelible skin pencil or ballpoint pen.

Next, the shoe is prepared to accept the material to be inserted. Ordinary talcum powder is adequate if the material is dry and moldable. However, where liquid latex is being used the insole and side walls of the heel seat, waist and forepart of the shoe are best covered with Saran Wrap or other thin-gauge plastic.

The author prefers either of the following techniques:

1. Synthetic liquid latex and ground cork or wood flour (hardwood dust)
   a. Pour latex into a rubber or plastic bowl (begin with 1 pint and gradually add more as needed).
   b. Slowly pour and gently mix the ground cork or wood flour into the latex until a firm paste is developed. Rapid whipping of the material will cause it to expand, creating an air-filled, lighter mixture.
   c. Cut out and place #115 thin-gauge Celastic or thin leather in the shoe for testing shape and size. Allow for cupping about the heel and medial and lateral sides. Remove the Cel-

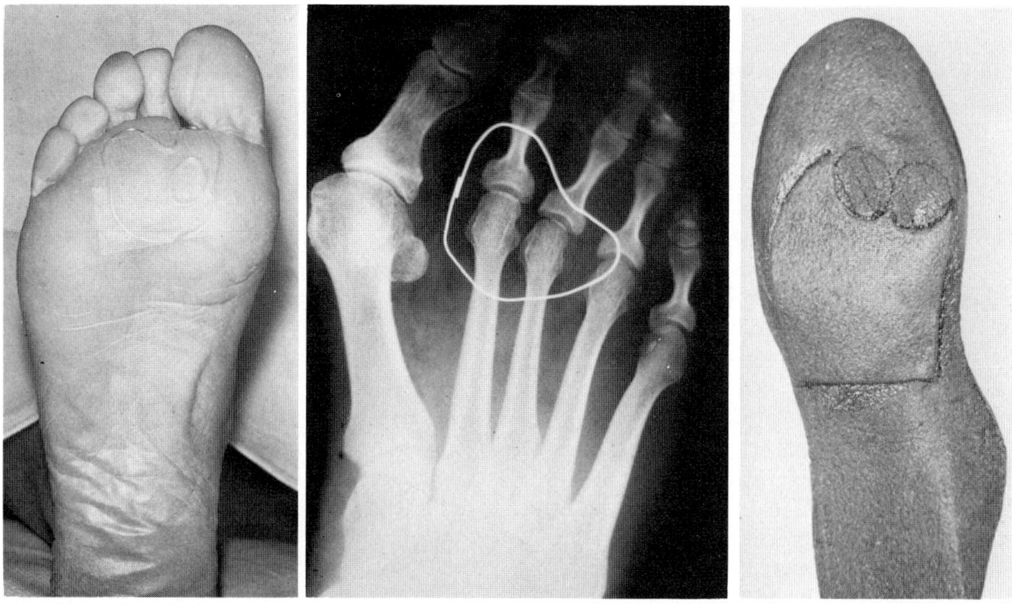

Figure 13.2. Wire technique to isolate skin lesion prior to diagnostic radiography. Wire shaped to size of lesion and attached with plastic tape. (*Center*) Radiograph depicting site of lesion. (*Right*) A Molo insole is constructed to remove pressure from the offending part. (Courtesy of L Hymes.)

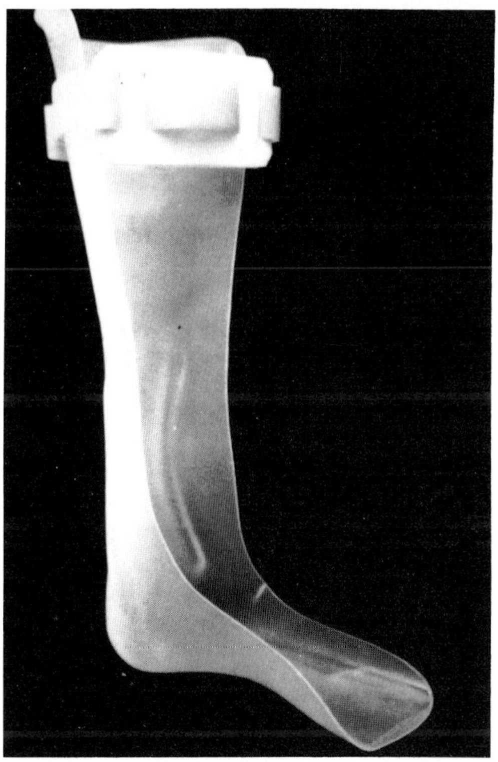

Figure 13.3. Type 670 Below knee Orthosis (BKO) is a lightweight polypropylene Drop Foot Brace trimmed high in the malleolus area. This gives exceptional medial-lateral stability and prevents plantarflexion. It is recommended as an immediate post cerebral vascular accident training brace when medial-lateral stability is paramount. Malleolus fitting may be required. Will fit in user's normal shoe. (Countesy of Ali-Med. Inc, Boston.)

astic insole and apply rubber cement for about 1 inch around the top edge of the Celastic.

d. Dampen the Celastic on its undersurface lightly with acetone or alcohol to provide for molding. It may be dipped and hung to dry partially, then molded into the shoe when not tacky.
e. Apply the mixture, by spatula, about 1/4–1/2-inch thick on the top surface of the previously molded Celastic or leather, taking care to feather the edges.
f. A finely woven monk's cloth is applied over the mixture on the Celastic and lightly pressed on the edges to create an envelope-like unit.
g. This envelope-like unit is placed in the shoe and powdered. Laces are opened wide and the patient's bare foot is gently placed in the shoe on the mixture covered with monk's cloth.
h. The patient is instructed to stand and walk on this application until he or she retires. The material will shape to all the contours in the weightbearing areas of the deformed foot, allowing for a broad distribution of weight.

i. The shoe is removed carefully upon retiring and dusted with talcum powder. If the patient is comfortable he or she does not have to return to the office laboratory for 5–7 days. However, the patient should be advised to call the office the following day to report any evidence of irritation.

j. The orthotic device formed by this method is removed from the shoe at the next visit. The entire device is trimmed by scissors, and a grind wheel is used to feather all edges. Further accommodative materials may be applied to the device. If the patient is comfortable, a thin leather or plastic top cover is applied.

2. Synthetic liquid latex and felt

a. Precut an insole out of ⅛-inch cotton and wool felt providing for heel cupping and medial and lateral flanges. Skive felt edges. Cut (⅛-inch) felt to size or place an indelible pencil mark over painful joints, arthritic prominences or skin excrescences on the plantar surface of the foot. Skin elevations will create a displacement of the moldable material to provide an impression.

b. The felt insole pattern is dipped in liquid latex (saturated and gently squeezed out). Use plastic gloves for handling.

c. The saturated felt is placed between layers of Saran Wrap and put in the shoe. The patient gently slips into the shoe and walks about the office. If comfortable, the shoe is not removed until retiring.

d. Upon returning for the next visit in 1–5 days the affected tender or painful weightbearing sites are marked off and the patient bears weight on the latex-impregnated felt in the shoe, which is now dry and shaped, void of the Saran material. The pressure points will be transferred to the felt.

e. The mold is left at the office for cutouts, elevations or whatever alterations the doctor deems necessary to obtain relief of the foot pathology.

f. The entire mold is covered with a fine soft leather, and all edges are feathered before dispensing it to the patient.

Note that no corrective forces are being used in these techniques. Dynamic orthotic devices provide accommodation and a broad distribution of weightbearing. The term "dynamic orthotic device" is used to indicate that it is shaped and constructed during stance in gait.

Plastazote for Dynamic Accommodation of Foot Lesion Plastazote, an expanded polyethylene, may be used without plaster cast models of the foot. The polyethylene appliance is constructed by making an outline of the foot on the sheet material (3/16, 5/16, or ⅜ inch in thickness). This is cut out, allowing for a medial flange. The polyethylene is heated over a flame or hot plate and molded into a shoe. The foot is placed in the shoe, and weightbearing for a few minutes provides an image of the dynamic foot. The shaped insole is trimmed and serves as a base for a permanent foot orthosis. Corrections may be added to the Plastazote as needed. Cellulose acetate may be rubbed into the material to provide additional firmness. Rigidity is accomplished through the use of successive layers of gauze and cellulose acetate. When dry, leather or synthetic coverings may be adhered to top and bottom surfaces. Silicone gel may be used instead of cellulose acetate for a semirigid sturdy construction.

Dynamic Plantar Mold The vinyl foam insole is used primarily to give more depth to the mold. It also smooths the inner sole of the shoe and can be used as the finishing undercover of the mold. Such thermoplastics as Neolite and several rubber compounds are useful.

A vinyl foam insole is placed in the shoe, and the heated thermoplastic material is placed on top of the vinyl. the patient then puts his or her foot into the shoe and walks around. If a metatarsal raise is to be incorporated in the mold, place a rubber pad of an individual design on the insole of the shoe before the vinyl foam insole is placed into the shoe. The pad will make a convexity into the plantar mold; the rubber metatarsal pad can then be removed.

If an excrescence on the foot is to be accommodated, place a ¼-inch piece of felt, cut to the size of the excrescence, on the excrescence. Put on the stocking and have the patient walk about on the heated insole. When the patient walks, the felt will make an indenture in the thermoplastic material. The felt piece is removed from the foot after about 10 to 15 min when the thermoplastic becomes firm.

The procedure for duplicating an existing comfortable pad or shield on the foot is as follows. Outline the pad on the foot with an indelible pencil. Then moisten the inside of the shoe and have the patient walk barefooted in the shoe for a few minutes. The indelible outline will appear in the shoe. Remove the pad or shield from the foot and place it into the shoe within the outline. The pad can be held in place with a piece of adhesive tape. Place the vinyl foam and warm insole into the shoe and have the patient walk about in the shoe. The pad will make a convexity in the mold. Remove the mold and pad from the shoe and adhere the pad to the underside of the mold in the concavity with cement. Adhere the vinyl foam to the thermoplastic mold covering the pad on its undersurface.

Inlite, a heat-molded insole that is durable and resistant to multiple long-term compressive forces for accommodation of plantar excrescences, is similar to Plastazote in its uses. For long life, a 3⁄16-inch thick material may be cut to suitable size and shape for placement in a shoe. The undersurface is ground down to fit the shoe without crowding the toes. The edges are feathered. The bottom is heated with a heat gun or any suitable heat-dispensing blower. When the material is malleable, it is placed in the shoe, and the stocking-covered foot is put in the shoe for immediate weightbearing. Care should be exercised to avoid nylon hose or too hot an insole. Cotton or woolen hose are adequate for a good mold. After molding the insole in the above manner, the shell is trimmed and corrected for comfort. Plantar excrescences are marked off with lipstick or a skin pencil. The foot is inserted into the shoe, and the markings will imprint on the insole. Cutouts are made, and raises can be cemented on the undersurface to provide a fulcrum or to remove pressure. Cover with leather.

Static Orthotic Device

The static foot orthotic device is used to control function and to accommodate structural deformities. The term "static" is used to differentiate it from the orthoses created by the dynamic foot in the shoe as previously described. Static is used to note that the orthotic device is constructed over a plaster cast of a partially, full, or non-weightbearing, nonfunctioning foot. Various casting techniques have been used. The author prefers the foot impression technique (FIT). This technique is performed with the foot in a partial weightbearing position. The following techniques have been used in combined practice for over 60 years with a high degree of success in the treatment of foot, ankle and lower extremity pathology. From a strictly orthopaedic approach one would discuss function and structure from an anatomical, physiological and biomechanical perspective. The author's primary concern here is with dynamic and static as they relate to the impressions, design and construction of a foot orthotic device.

The finished plaster of paris cast, over which the foot orthotic device is to be constructed, should present the outline of excrescences and bony prominences. The following techniques involve construction of flexible, semirigid and rigid foot orthotic devices.

Flexible Orthotic Device A ⅛ inch thick piece of felt is cut to fit the plaster cast about the heel, medial and lateral sides and forward under the toes. It is dipped in synthetic liquid latex, squeezed out and molded on the plaster cast. If the orthotic device is to be flexible, ⅛–¼-inch thickness variations of longitudinal and metatarsal pads are designed out of felt. These pads are soaked in the latex, squeezed and applied to the previous felt latex overlay on the cast to provide the greatest benefits for the specific structural and functional disability. The felt raises may encompass cutouts under bony prominences or may gently force function. Later one may wish to add Sorbothane, Novalite, soft foam, PPT or rubber to relieve shock. The felt, impregnated with latex buildups, is rubbed smoothly into the existing felt latex to feather the edges and to provide a firm adhesion, resulting in a single unit.

The material is allowed to dry on the cast for at least 24 hr. The entire felt-latex construction is removed in the dry state and trimmed with a scissors for shape and design. It is then ground down to a feather edge or ground out beneath prominent bones. Additions and subtractions are made to the orthoses to balance and/or remove stress from prominent parts. Rubber cement is brushed over the top of the orthotic device, and a leather covering is applied. The techniques of grinding and balance are as intricate and productive as applying elevations. All podiatrists or their technicians are skilled in constructing these devices. Special commercial laboratories can fabricate orthoses to the doctor's specifications. Podiatrists have well-equipped laboratories to adjust discrepancies in construction. The well-equipped office laboratory has a variety of materials to work with, as well as technical personnel to follow the doctor's prescription.

Not all foot specialists have the time or skill to construct the type of device necessary for all foot disabilities. However, the podiatrist's judgment and training provide the "know-how" necessary to order orthotic devices by prescription. Great progress in research and design is being made by commercial professional podiatric laboratories. They are able to construct devices suitable for relief and control of most foot deformities on prescription by the knowledgeable doctor.

The construction of orthotic devices by podiatric laboratories is only as accurate as the impressions supplied, as well as the information they require to understand fully the foot problem being treated. Professional laboratories provide an excellent product, scientifically accurate and of quality materials. Some sample illustrations are herewith presented. They have been constructed, on prescription by the foot specialist, by skilled pedorthists in professional laboratories. Most professional laboratories employ podiatric consultants to assist them in providing a scientifically correct foot orthotic device (Figs 13.4–13.8).

Semirigid Orthotic Device Construction consists of cutting out a ⅛-inch thick piece of felt large enough to cover the plantar, medial and lateral aspects of the cast allowing for heel cupping and a toe crest. One piece is used for each cast. The felt is soaked in synthetic liquid latex, squeezed gently and then molded over the weightbearing surface of the cast. At this stage the technician may apply properly skived felt pads, wedges, etc. for accom-

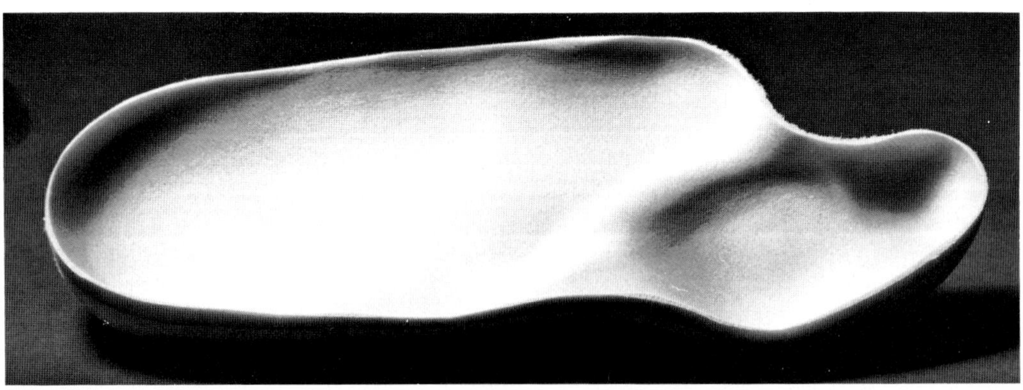

Figure 13.4. Orthotic device for traumatic arthritis. A traumatic arthritis of the first metatarsophalangeal articulation and the interphalangeal joint of the hallux may be adequately accommodated by an arthotic device of this type. (Courtesy of Foot Management, Inc.).

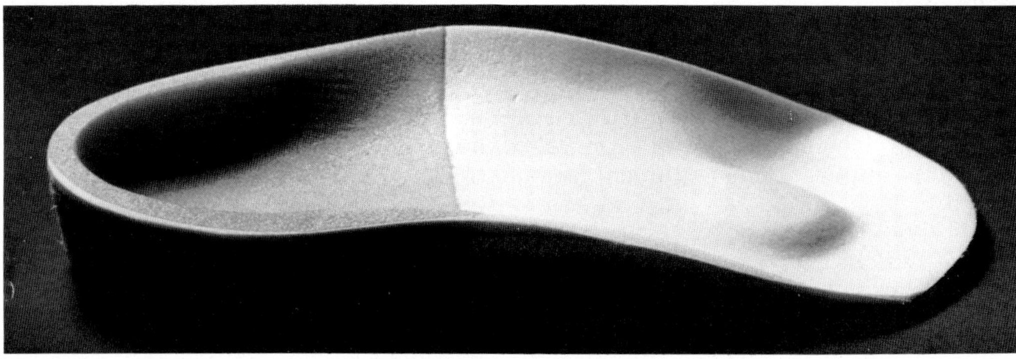

Figure 13.5. Soft comfortable orthoses. Note the soft comfortable heel seat and raise under the second metatarsophalangeal joint to relieve pressure in the presence of degenerative joint disease. Can be useful for loss of adipose under heel and metatarsal areas of the foot. (Courtesy of Foot Management, Inc.)

modation or control of the deformity in accordance with the doctor's studied design. By soaking these pads well in latex, they will become firm after application to the previously latexed felt. Smoothing out edges, using a rubber examining glove, will provide for a smooth, strong orthotic device when dry. Firmness can be added by using combinations of felt and adhering rubberized cork materials to the felt. A semirigid orthotic device may include a thin-gauge Celastic longitudinal strip be-

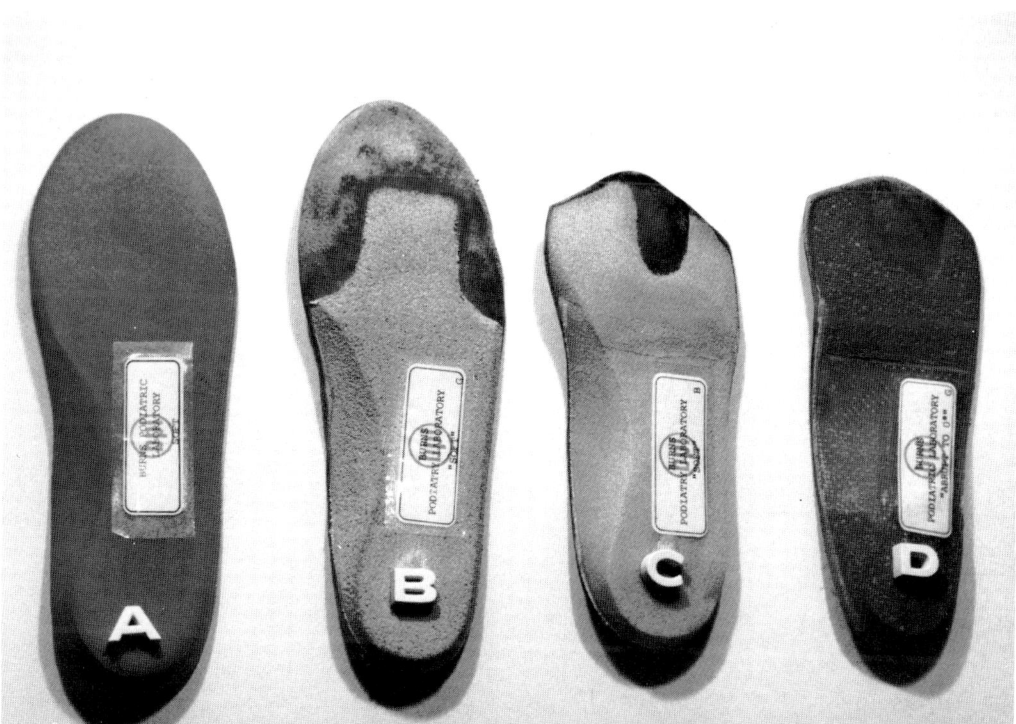

Figure 13.6. Accommodative orthotic devices. *A,* Soft orthotic insert for the diabetic, arteriosclerotic and arthritic with loss of plantar fat pad. Provides stability and shock absorption. *B,* Soft orthotic device with accommodation for first and fifth metatarsal heads to relieve pressure on prominent joints. *C,* A cutout depression for third metatarsophalangeal joint. *D,* A firmer orthotic device to remove gravitational stress from second, third, and fourth metatarsophalangeal joints. (Courtesy of Burns Podiatry Laboratory, McCook, NB.)

tween the heel seat and metatarsal necks. Use of cork and firm rubber compounds or a thin layer of fiberglass will maintain the semirigid construction of the device. Celastic or fiberglass when used is placed over the initial felt pattern for firmness prior to the application of additional latex soaked pads.

Rigid Orthotic Device These orthotic devices can be constructed of Rohadur, polyethylene, duraaluminum, steel, monel metal, steel springs, thick-gauge fiberglass or plastics. However, the author has never found these materials, used alone, to be totally satisfactory for most adult foot pathology. Experience dictates that patients require constant adjustments of any device they wear in order to maintain comfort. Joint changes that manifest as progressive deformity or exacerbations of an acute arthritic attack require subtle changes in an orthotic device. The author has found after many years of experience that rigid plastic orthoses prescribed for cavus foot conditions are, in the majority of instances, ineffective in relieving symptomatology. Semirigid foot orthoses incorporating a viscoelastic polymer for shock absorption are most desirable.

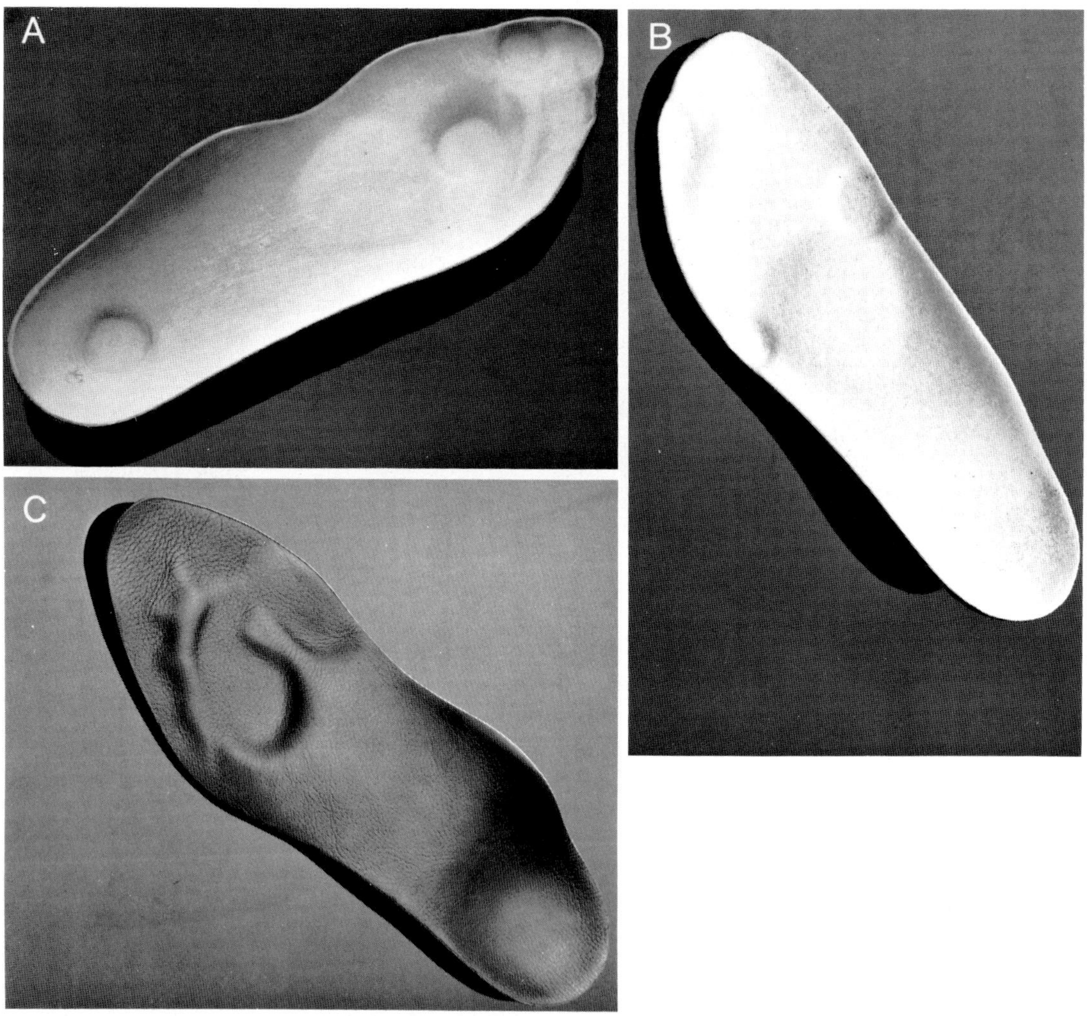

Figure 13.7. *A–C,* Accommodative orthoses. Typical orthoses constructed to a plaster cast of rheumatoid arthritic feet. Note depressions to accommodate prominent metatarsophalangeal joints, rheumatoid nodules and calcaneal spurs. (Courtesy of Levy and Rappel Laboratory, NY.)

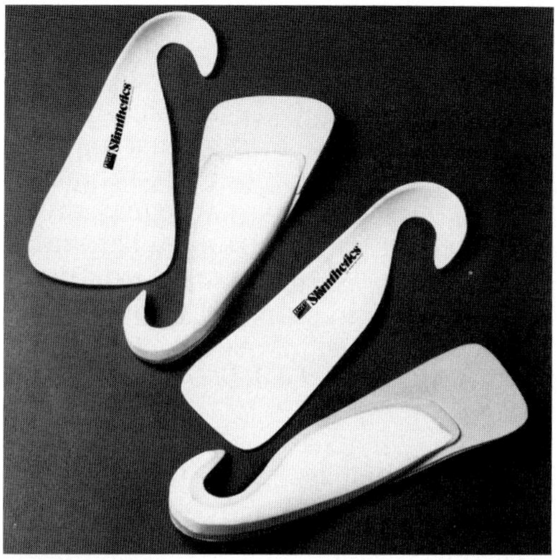

Figure 13.8. Slimthotics are specially designed to control foot function in shoes that will not accept full-size orthotic devices because of style, type or internal space limitations. (Courtesy of Langer Biomechanics Group.)

The following rigid orthotic device construction may be tried for functional control and accommodation.

1. A plaster cast impression is taken of the foot in a semi-weightbearing relaxed state.
2. When the plaster positive is dry a ⅛ inch thick felt foot pattern impregnated with latex is applied as previously described. (Rub well into contours of the plaster cast.)
3. When this is dry a #125–#130 piece of Celastic is cut to shape to include a medial and lateral longitudinal flange, and heel seat. The Celastic "shell" is extended forward to the metatarsal necks.
4. The Celastic is dipped in acetone or alcohol, allowed to dry for a few minutes until tacky and then molded into the previously latexed felt that is covered with rubber cement for adherence. When this is dry the doctor may apply additional Celastic or even a layer of fiberglass. The need for further rigidity or bulk must now be established. One layer of Celastic followed by felt impregnated with latex molded over the Celastic in a desirable longitudinal-metatarsal design, with or without cut-outs and elevations as needed, is most comfortable.
5. When the material is thoroughly dry it can be ground down to fit the shoe and adjusted by grinding for accommodation and/or functional control of the foot. The top is covered with leather or a suitable substitute. The bottom may or may not be covered depending on the preference of the doctor or the limitations of footgear.

Viscoelastic polymers (Sorbothane, Novalite), soft foam, PPT, rubber or synthetic compressible materials can be incorporated within the device. These materials are always applied to the bottom surface of the orthotic device.

Impression Techniques for Construction of Orthoses and Shoes

The most popular methods of taking impressions are done after indelible markings are placed on the skin over painful excrescences. Marked off helomas or tylomas will transfer their outlines from the skin to the negative cast on impression and then to the positive cast after the model is poured.

Slipper Cast Technique

Plaster of paris splints or bandages are dipped in water and molded about the affected foot off weightbearing. About three layers of the material are necessary for a strong slipper cast, which extends over the toes from the plantar surface, about the heel, under the malleoli and about the dorsomedial and dorsolateral aspects of the foot. For subtalar joint neutral control, the subtalar joint is stabilized, whereas the forefoot is abducted and everted as the cast dries.

Toe slipper casts are made in a similar way by marking off the deformity or excrescence and either pouring plaster around the toe using impression trays or applying wet strips of plaster of paris splints around the toe. Toe slipper casts are used for the construction of shields.

The entire foot or a single toe may be dipped in melted artist's wax after covering the part with a lubricant. The wax is cooled off by dipping the foot in cold water. This method is quite accurate for preparing study models in evaluating deformities of the foot. Pedi-Cast or dental impression compounds may be spatulated over the part to make a negative impression. A positive is poured, and the impression material is removed when the cast is dry.

Simplified Casting Technique for Orthoses and Molded Shoes

Miller (personal communication, 1973) uses the following technique for molded shoes. It can also be used for construction of orthotic devices.

Materials required include two polyfoam blocks measuring 1½ inches thick, 6 inches wide and 14 inches long and plaster of paris bandage splints, extra fast setting, sizes 8 × 14, 6 pieces, 5 × 15, 10 pieces. Separator material is optional. A tincture of green soap solution may be used as a separator. Absorbent paper towels and a basin of water are also necessary.

The polyfoam is covered with a paper towel. To cast the plantar area and heel, wet three pieces of the 8 × 14 inch splint and place on top of the towel. Immediately place the foot on top of the splints. Fold a piece of the 5 × 15 splint in half making it 5 × 7½, wet it and place it on the heel of the foot, bringing it well above the malleolus. To reinforce this edge, fold the splint back on itself at the malleoli. Bring the splint up around the heel and the inner and outer borders of the foot. Depress the foam rubber in front of the toes, and with your fingers push the splints up into the crest area. Now do the other foot. When you have completed the other foot, the first cast will be dry enough to work the upper impression.

To cast the upper impression, paint the separating medium on the edges of the heel and plantar splints (optional). Using the 5 × 15 splints folded in half, build up the upper cast by laying one piece over the toes and overlapping the plantar impression. Then place a splint across the top of the foot from the malleolus forward, one on each side overlapping on the dorsum. The fourth piece should be placed on top of the foot from the top of the ankle to the toe. To reinforce the edges at the malleoli, fold the splint back on itself leaving an overlap of the heel splint of approximately ¼ inch. Repeat this process on the other foot.

To remove the foot from the cast, loosen the edges that were reinforced at the malleoli and lift the front top piece upward. Pull gently away from the foot. Now lift the foot from the plantar and heel impression as gently as possible to prevent distortion. The upper and plantar negative casts are put together as a whole before sending them to the laboratory for processing.

Foot Impression Technique (FIT) (1–3) (Grease Method)

The grease compound impression technique first described by Adler and Babbitt (personal communication) has proved most successful in making plantar models of the feet (Fig. 13.9). The materials used are water pump grease, cup grease no. 3, two pans (each about 6 × 13 × 2 1/2 inches deep), two pieces of cloth (larger than the pans, the cloth should be similar to that used in a man's T-shirt, a cotton bed sheet or a smooth face towel), and a 3-inch metal spatula. Cover the bottom of the pans with one 1-inch layer of water pump grease. On top of the water pump grease place a 1 1/2-inch layer of cup grease no. 3. (This only has to be done the first time except when replenished because the same preparation is used over and over again after being smoothed out with the spatula.) Wring out the cloths in water and apply smoothly over the compound. Allow the patient to stand, with moderate weightbearing, in the compound and to flex the toes back and forth slightly. Then have the patient sit down with the foot and knee at right angles, and work the compound through the cloth under and around the foot, making the amount of correction you feel is necessary. After the foot is removed from the compound, further corrections, such as depressions for heel spurs, cysts or particularly sensitive bony prominences, may be made before pouring the plaster for the positive cast. No separating medium is required. The positive is easily removed, and if the impression was properly taken, the cast will be perfectly balanced and further correc-

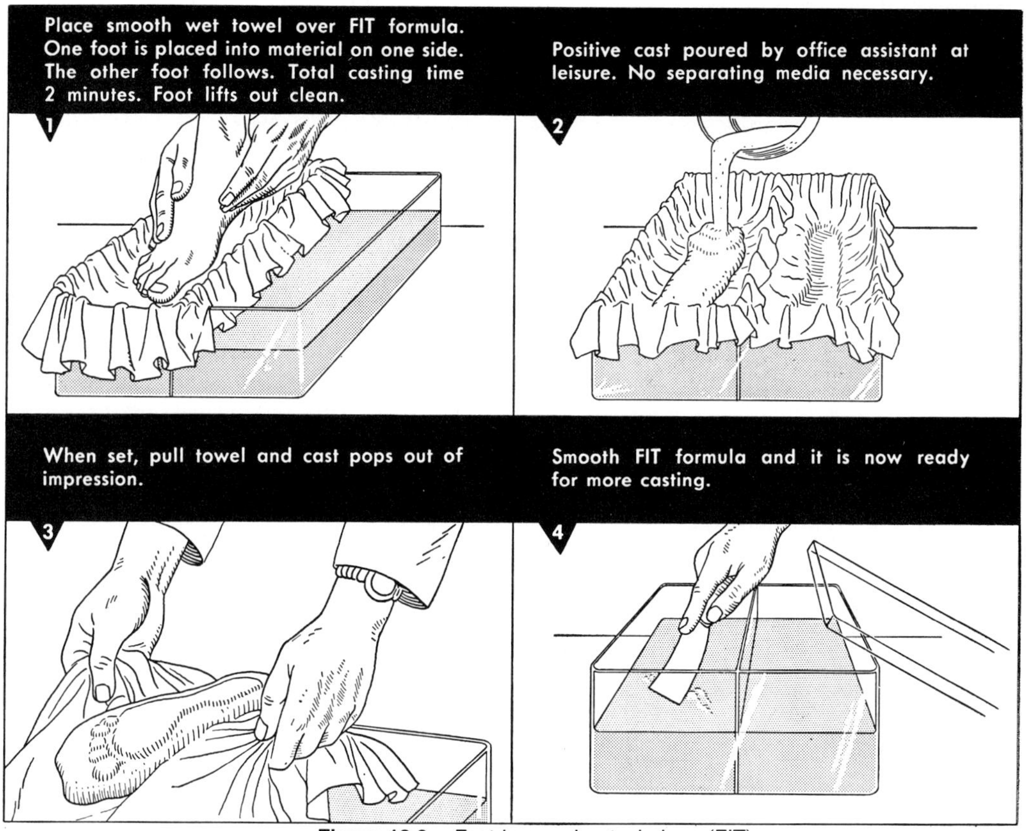

Figure 13.9. Foot impression technique (FIT).

tion on the positive is unnecessary. The procedure takes no more than 2 min of the podiatrist's time, is accurate and the patient's foot remains clean.

Remove the cloths, smooth out the compound with the spatula and it is now ready for another impression. Hundreds of casts may be taken with the same batch of compound. The author is using this technique today for 99% of patients' foot impressions (1–3). It is especially suitable for the Root techniques (4–6). Levine (7) described a similar technique and gives credit to Skliar and Schuster.

With careful analysis of the plaster casts of feet of patients suffering from biomechanical disturbances, a proper orthotic device can be designed. Corroborative weightbearing points, marked off excrescences and weightbearing radiographs are used to ensure accuracy in construction.

The use of the plaster slipper cast technique has been in disrepute until recent years. However, the evolution of biomechanical principles has revived many plaster slipper cast techniques. Heretofore, impression techniques were based on the doctor's ability to correct and balance the cast before designing the orthosis. As a result the orthosis frequently was subject to the errors produced by human inaccuracies and lack of standardization. Very little correction of the positive cast is necessary with modern impression techniques for the construction of foot orthoses.

Polyfoam Cast Technique (Bio-Foam Impression Technique System)

Another method widely used is the foot impression made in a solid tray of polyfoam. The foot is pressed carefully into the foam. When the foot is removed, a beautiful, clean negative impression is ready in seconds. The disadvantage to this method is that the solid tray of foam can only be used once and is discarded.

Shields

Dynamic or static shields may be constructed of felt, sponge, foam, gauze or any other resilient material, alone or in combination with moldable silicone putty, liquid latex or silicone gel bathtub caulk.

1. Dynamic shields (to foot or toe)
   a. Hallux
   b. Sesamoid
   c. Hammer toe
   d. Digiti quinti varus
   e. Crest pad
   f. Heloma
   g. Bursitis
   h. Tyloma
   i. Hyperkeratosis
   j. Other
2. Static shields (to plaster cast)
   a. Dip method
   b. Brush method
   c. Materials
      (1) Liquid latex
      (2) Silicone gel bathtub caulk
      (3) Sponge
      (4) Felt
      (5) Gauze

Dynamic Shields

Polyurethane Polyurethane in a block about 3 × 3 × 1 inch can be used for a customized orthodigital correction for overlapping or underlapping toes. Small holes are punched in the material for insertion of the second, third and fourth toes. A hole may be lower or higher for an individual toe, depending on the need to lower or raise the toe. The polyurethane is placed in a plastic bag with some liquid latex and squeezed repeatedly to allow for absorption of the liquid rubber. When the polyurethane is saturated the toes are placed through the previously cut holes. The entire mass is covered by a plastic bag and stocking. The foot is carefully placed in the shoe; the patient walks and shapes a flexible but firm forefoot mold over the deformed toes. This technique provides a polyurethane pad that will protect deformed toes and correct minor deformities where surgical correction is contraindicated. A plantar crest and dorsal pressure pad are formed to retain the parts in apposition.

Whitney (8, 9) described and illustrated urethane mold therapy. McGlamry and Kitting (10) later used these molds for postoperative retainers and rehabilitation. The methods used are essentially the same, and the finished product is limited only by the creative skill of the operator. Metal punches for the toe holes, urethane foam 1 and 2 inches thick, Vultex rubber (General Latex and Chemical Co), urethane mold coating (Vinyl) for finishing and a small sanding drum for Carborundum disks are all that are needed.

Moldable Podiatric Compound (Fig. 13.10) The ingenuity of the podiatrist is challenged by the possibilities embodied in the use of this product. The technique of activating the silicone putty compound is as follows:

1. A slight depression is made in the flattened putty, and the appropriate number of drops (depending on the amount of putty) of hardener catalyst is added.
2. The catalyst is kneaded well into the putty for 30 to 45 sec, and the mixture is rolled into a ball to eliminate any separations in the kneaded silicone.
3. The putty is now ready to be molded to the patient's foot, which has been cleansed with isopropyl alcohol.
4. It is placed within the toe sulcus and manipulated to the desired form, incorporating anchoring (usually first and/or fourth interspace) posts.
5. The device is then covered with a single wrap of plastic film to provide a smooth appearance as well as to prevent silicone putty from adhering to stockings.
6. The patient may then leave, wearing the custom-fitted device after being assured of its comfort. The plastic film is discarded at home after allowing several hours for curing.
7. The patient returns to the office within several days. The device may be smoothed on a grinding wheel. Additions may be made. Pads covered with silicone gel may be added.

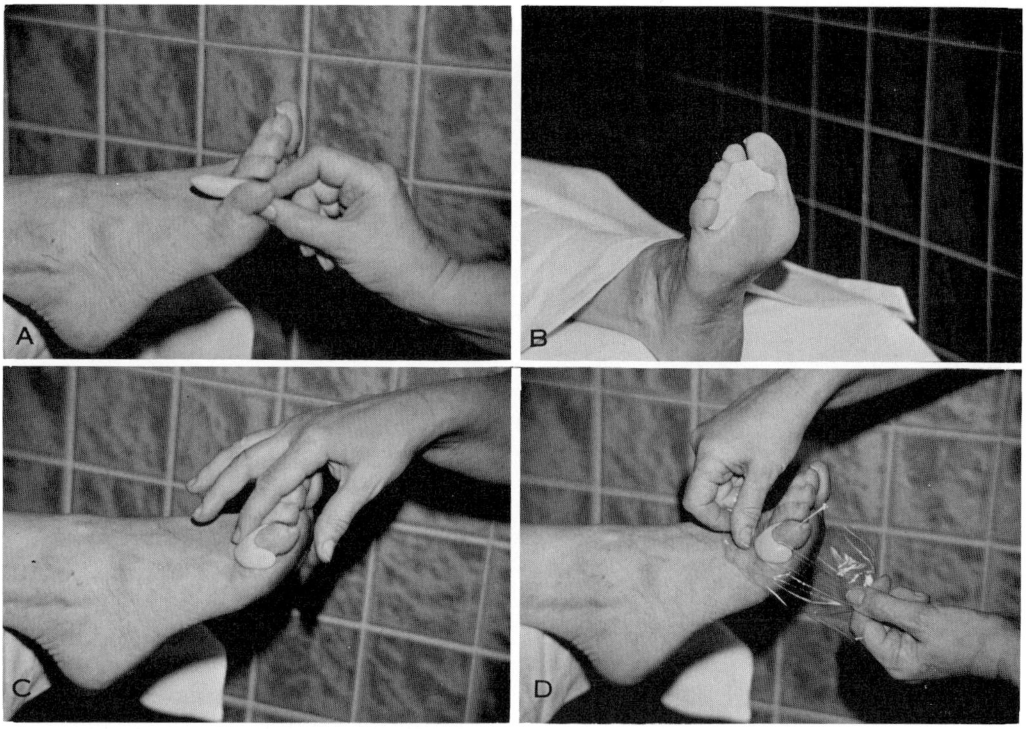

Figure 13.10. Construction of moldable podiatric compound shield. (Courtesy of RO Schuster.)

Cornstarch is applied daily between the device and the skin.

Static Shields

Fisher (11) described a technique of taking impressions of deformities of the toes using dental impression materials. This is followed by pouring a positive cast and the construction of a rubber and plastic orthodigital device under heat and pressure. The completed device can be ground down or increased in bulk to exert corrective forces on underlapping, varus and valgus of the toes, hammer toes, overriding toes, hallux valgus and a variety of forefoot deformities. The device is semirigid, durable and easily adjusted.

Latex Dip Method It is essential to use great care in taking the negative cast of a part. Impressions of deformed toes or other bony prominences on the foot are smoothed by fine sandpaper. The plaster cast is then dipped into natural latex several times and allowed to vulcanize and dry. A suitable foam, sponge or felt accommodative pad is adhered to the latex by rubber cement. The entire mass is then dipped into liquid latex two more times to cover the adhered pad. This mass is allowed to dry for 24 hr. The shield on the positive cast is powdered well, removed from the cast and trimmed to fit the casted toe. Podiatric laboratories are available for construction of latex shields to positive casts.

Tubegauze Brush Method (Fig. 13.11) The positive toe cast or affected toe is covered with rubber cement or silicone gel. Tubegauze is cut to provide a covering for the entire toe, with an overlap in back and forward of the toe. This is slipped on the toe or cast.

The bony prominences and excrescences are accommodated with sponge rubber, foam, felt or other suitable material adhered by cement or silicone gel over the tubegauze. The tubegauze is coated with natural liquid latex or silicone gel, and the distal overlapping tubegauze is turned back on itself to cover the shield. The entire shield is coated with more natural

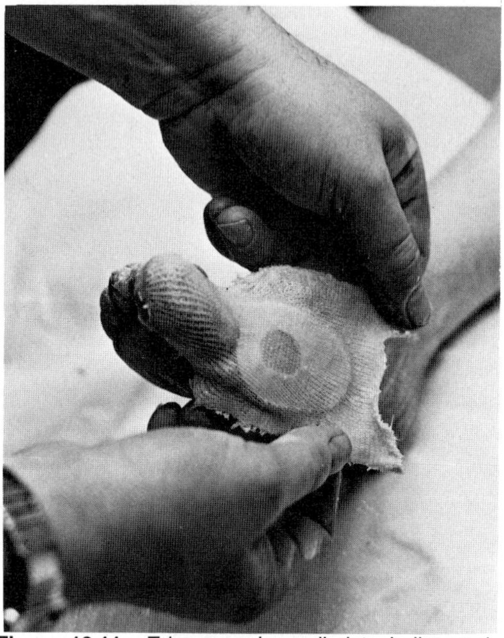

Figure 13.11. Tubegauze is applied to hallux and overlapping first metatarsophalangeal joint. Shield is adhered to protect bunion. Tubegauze is folded back and adhered with silicone gel. Entire shield is covered with silicone gel to construct permanent shield. Cover with plastic wrap. (Courtesy of S Rosoff.)

latex or silicone gel to a desired thickness and allowed to dry on the cast for 24 hr.

The prosthesis made on the toe is allowed to vulcanize on the toe as a dynamic shield or on the cast as a static shield. It is protected by household plastic wrap and covered with stocking and shoe. At the next visit the shield is removed from the positive cast or toe, trimmed, covered by more latex or silicone and dispensed as a replaceable shield.

Accommodative Techniques

Inside Shoe

Materials—Felt, foam combinations, molo, Aliplast, Celastic, Plastazote, moldable compounds, Spenco, PPT, cork, rubberized cork, etc.

1. Longitudinal skived pads ⅛, ¼ or ⅜ inch;
2. Pads for accommodating painful skin lesions, bone enlargements, spurs, osteophytes, etc. beneath the sesamoids and metatarsophalangeal joints (Fig. 13.12);
3. Special designs for relief of heel pain;
4. Extensions under first or fifth metatarsals properly skived and cut out to accommodate excrescences;
5. Celastic cut to Whitman design, combination longitudinal with lateral clip, cutouts and/or extensions; heel wedges, lifts, cutouts, protectives.

Custom Arthritic Footgear

Markell constructs the Improved Mobility Shoe. This shoe is extra light in weight, supersoft with foam on top, has bottom and sides constructed over an extra wide and deep last and has removable foam insoles for a variety of fittings. The sole is constructed of nonskid material, and the overall depth is ⅜ inch deeper than the average shoe. Fit adjustments are made easier for the arthritic by using a Velcro closure. This shoe is adaptable to the swollen, deformed and sensitive feet of the arthritic patient.

The ENERGaire sole (Mountain View, CA) replaces the existing sole of the patient's shoe. The doctor can design a custom air sole and heel to accommodate an existing deformity or painful site. The average inflatable air pressure is 4 lb, which can be adjusted up or down to facilitate comfort. Too much pressure may affect the mechanics of the foot, and too little may not provide the needed comfort. However, this unique sole can be altered by proper design to assist in the function and relief of plantar sites of discomfort in the arthritic foot. Varus, valgus, metatarsal shearing and pronatory forces can be markedly reduced.

The Extra Depth Shoes, molded shoes to plaster casts, postsurgical shoes and a variety of specialized footgear have been most beneficial as an adjunct to treatment of the arthritic foot. The Extra Depth Shoe (PH Minor and Son, Inc) and the molded shoe constructed to plaster casts prescribed by the foot specialist are now being constructed with a manufactured ¼ inch thick insole.

The Extra Depth Shoe insole can be removed, allowing for ¼ inch extra depth in the shoe to provide for the dorsiflexed toes of the rheumatoid or osteoarthritic patient. In the event that room is needed in the forefoot, the forepart of the insole can be ground down to remove the ¼ inch thickness while continuing to provide good heel control. Likewise, it is possible to remove material from the heel seat to control subtalar joint pronation or even relieve pressure from a painful heel spur or bursa. Additional padding may be placed on the bottom of these insoles to enhance the accommodations already cut or ground out.

Because extra depth is available upon removing the insole, the doctor prescribing orthotic devices finds it much easier to adapt the device to the shoe. The Blucher tie shoe or Velcro strap can provide the greatest leeway for swollen arthritic extremities. Elasticized laces that stretch as the foot enters the shoe even when using a shoe horn are available. A one-handed, self-tightening shoe lace fastener (Alimed, Inc) may be obtained.

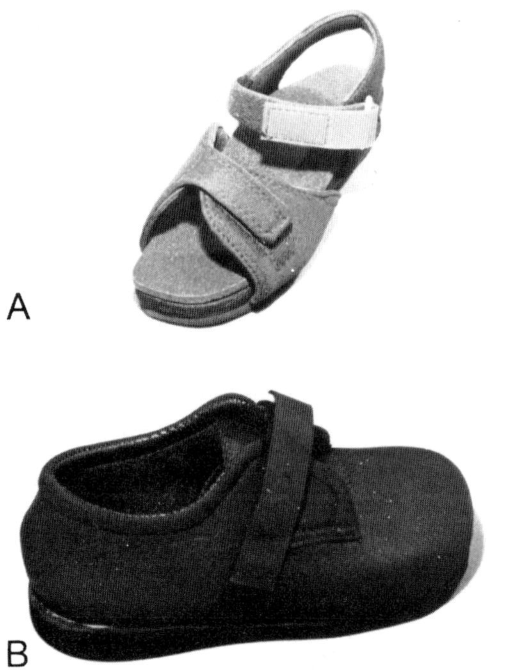

Figure 13.12. *A,* The Plastazote sandal provides comfort and style. (Courtesy of Ali-Med. Inc, Boston. *B,* The Plastazote extra-depth oxford shoe provides good stability, long wear and an acceptable look. It is one of the few shoes of this type with an internal heel counter. The vamp may be gently heated (via a heat gun) to soften the toe box and then easily stretched and molded to any prominence. Insoles can be heat-molded or they will mold dynamically to the foot through wear. (Courtesy of Ali-Med. Inc, Boston.)

Molded shoes constructed to plaster casts have special advantages. They are made over plaster cast models of the foot in a neutral position. The molding provides for foot and toe deformities (Fig. 13.13). The removable inlay is molded like any other orthotic device to conform to the affected foot. Such requirements as cutouts, elevations, posts and wedges can be utilized to relieve the painful foot. The expertise of the podiatrist and technicians can make these kinds of footgear a viable therapeutic approach to foot comfort.

The Jerry Miller molded shoe has introduced "Alpha Construction" for sensitive feet, including those of the arthritic patient. Each shoe weighs 6–9 oz., depending on its requirements. The use of extra soft leather inside and out, together with a lightweight, high-abrasion sole and removable Plastazote-molded insole, has proven helpful in treating arthritic foot deformity. Molded shoes can be constructed to accept external and internal braces using a channel braceplate.

Custom-molded shoes made by Tru-Mold, Shoes, Inc to plaster casts of patients' feet are constructed in a variety of styles and colors. "They are lightweight (6 oz) and can be constructed with a removable Plastazote in-sole, safety toe."

Most custom-molded shoes are made of the finest leathers and are fully leather lined. The construction of an accurate plaster cast of the foot is essential for a good fit. As in the prescription to a laboratory constructing foot orthotic devices, it is necessary to provide a brief clinical evaluation of the patient's problems to ensure a maximum degree of comfort.

A new concept in comfort footwear for both normal and deformed feet has been developed by Thermal-Moldable Shoes, Inc (Williamsville, NY). It is the Extra Depth Shoe that is completely lined with Plastazote and can be formed instantly to the deformed arthritic foot. A perforated Plastazote lining is laminated to the leather upper. The shoe is either placed in an oven or softened by a heat gun for spot adjustments to its "extra depth last." The

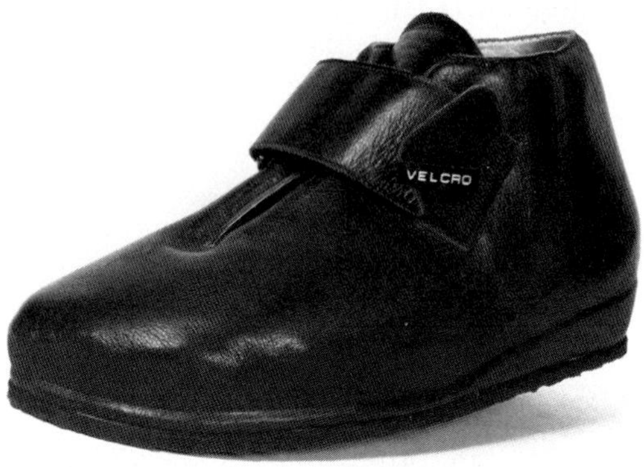

Figure 13.13. Custom-molded shoe. Note Velcro strap to facilitate closure of shoes when fingers deformed by arthritis cannot lace through eyelets. (Courtesy of Tru-Mold Shoes, Inc, Buffalo, NY.)

technician can provide for a three-dimensional fit. The doctor's prescription can be filled in the shoe store.

A commercial shoe called Super "D" has been developed by Alden Shoe with specific features that are conducive to accommodating deformed arthritic feet and other deforming states. It not only provides extra depth but also a Plastazote insole insert ⅝ inch thick that allows for firm rearfoot control. The pattern is designed with four conventional eyelets and a highly desirable backlace eyelet for firm fit over the dorsum of the foot. The high wall forepart of this blucher, soft upper, vamp-lined shoe allows for accommodating a variety of deforming states. Stretching and reshaping are easily performed by the foot specialist confronted with inoperable arthritic deformities. Skillful adjustment of the Plastazote insert can provide additional freedom, whereas compensatory additions may add to the comfort level of the suffering patient.

A molded shoe constructed to a plaster cast of the patient's foot allows for greater flexibility in accommodating inoperable arthritic foot deformities.

The *sheepskin comfort shoe* was originally conceived for the deformed feet of arthritic patients with edema. Because most of these moderately ambulatory patients did not wear shoes but at best wore cutout nonsupportive slippers, this shoe became a valuable asset. The shoe not only provided space for edema but also accommodated the arthritic deformity, and it kept the foot warm in the winter and cool in the summer. According to Citron (Veterans Administration Medical Center, Phoeniz, AZ), the shoe has been helpful in the treatment of ulcers and can be wedged and built up to accommodate a short limb or a poly/brace. It cannot be used for hiking, but together with a long firm counter it is suitable for long walks. A softer counter allows for ambulation in the more sedentary arthritic patients or for those confined to a wheelchair (Fig. 13.14). The sheepskin comfort shoe has also been beneficial for patients with multiple sclerosis and for those suffering foot deformity from spinal injury.

Other Podiatric Treatment Techniques

Fluid Silicone and Collagen Implantation of the Foot

Many years of independent investigation by Balkin indicate that fluid silicone is effective in the control of helomas, tylomas, scar tissue and healed neuropathic ulcers in the diabetic foot. Classified as a biomaterial device, the fluid simulates adipose tissue while remaining inert and remarkably stable, despite the enormous pressures of weightbearing. Following implantation, soft tissue is increased by histiocytic engulfment, encapsulation within thin-walled sacs, and the formation of new collagen fibers.

Silicone fluid is introduced into the subdermal tissue through a 25 gauge needle attached to a Luer-Lok three-ring control syringe. Serial injections, using only fractional amounts per injection, create a palpable synthetic cushion at the site of digital or plantar pressure.

Although the material has proven successful in 60–80% of injected cases for reducing transmitted forces at points of pressure, authorized multicentered studies under federal regulatory guidelines are required, as safety and efficacy have not been confirmed. Approval and proper use of this implant material can provide relief from painful weightbearing by this percutaneous silicone augmentation of plantar fat pads (Fig. 13.15).

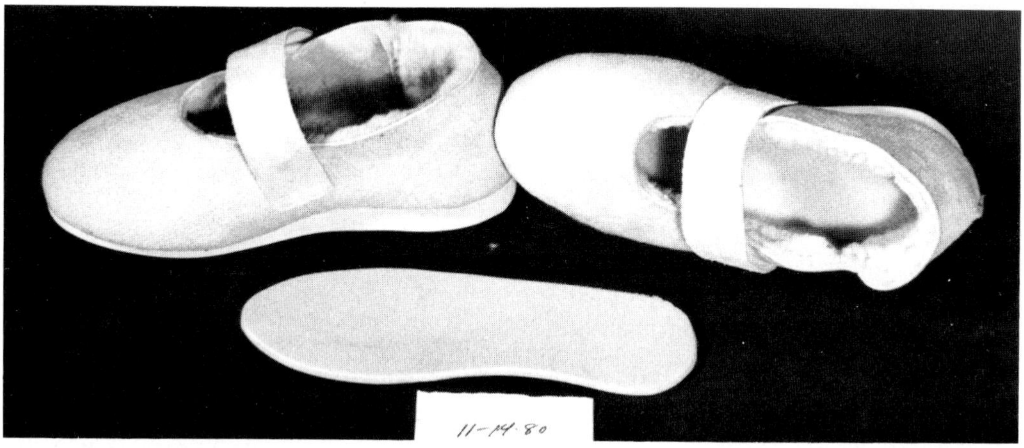

Figure 13.14. Sheepskin comfort shoe. This type of footgear is suitable for the feet of an arthritic patient who may be sedentary or only minimally mobile.

Keragen Implant is a homogeneous gel composed of highly purified bovine dermal collagen that is chemically crosslinked and suspended in physiologic saline containing 0.3% lidocaine. Clinical evaluation of Keragen Implant, which began in 1983, allowed for 20 investigators with a maximum of 500 treated patients.

Keragen Implant is indicated for subdermal injections beneath keratotic lesions of the foot arising from stresses between skin and underlying bone. By injecting Keragen Implant into the subdermal space, a "cushion" is formed between the lesion and the underlying bone. Formation of the cushion is intended to prevent the painful lesion from recurring at the same site. The site and extent of the lesion, the volume of Keragen Implant injected, the nature of the bony deformity and the degree of stress to which the site is subjected may affect the results.

Conditions amenable to treatment include lesions produced by enlarged phalangeal condyles, deformities of interphalangeal joints (such as hammer, mallet and claw toes), enlarged or displaced metatarsal heads, atrophied subcutaneous fat

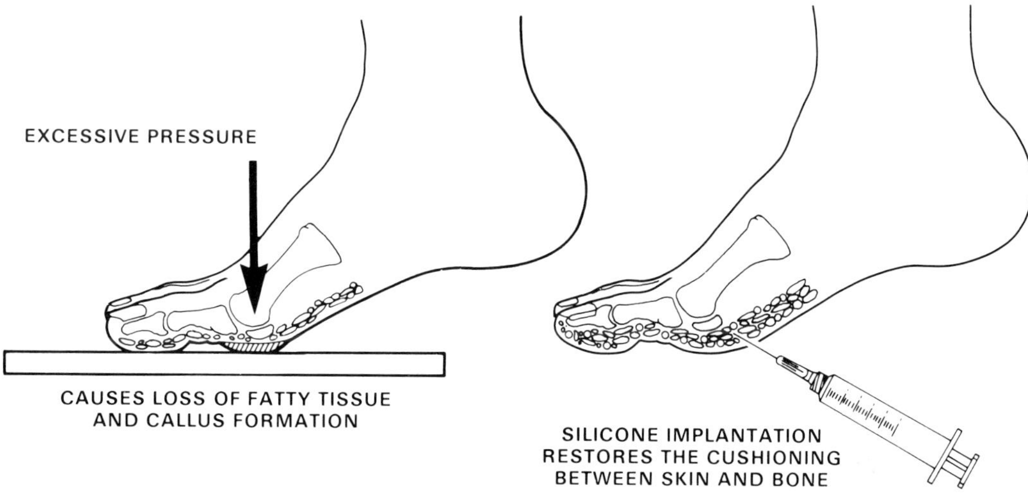

Figure 13.15. Fluid silicone implantation of an adipose-depleted metatarsal area is accomplished by a series of fractional injections placed between the skin and an underlying bony prominence. (Courtesy of SW Balkin, D.P.M.)

pads and scars. Treatment results may last from 6 to 12 months or longer and may be repeated when necessary.

Celastic in Shoes The author uses Celastic shells cut out to size in a Whitman brace design for maintaining the feet of children up to age 5, in a structurally acceptable position. The improvement of function generally relieves abnormal weight distribution through the rearfoot. The shell consists of a longitudinal medial flange with a lateral clip and cut-out heel. This approach to functional foot control serves the podiatrist well as a means for early treatment of those feet requiring rigid orthoses. Celastic extensions under the first or fifth segments and a variety of elevations may be placed in the shoe to control the malfunctioning foot.

The Celastic shell is dipped in acetone or alcohol and placed in the shoe. It is smoothed out with the gloved fingers, using a heavy-grade plastic glove to prevent finger irritation. The longitudinal area may be raised in subsequent visits by adding Celastic to the original shoe correction. The shoe is dried by a heat blower and powdered to relieve tackiness prior to wearing.

Felt Pads Cemented in Shoes There are many techniques for the construction of accommodative felt raises in shoes. These include the placement of ¼-inch precut and knife-skived felt pads in the shoe to limit subtalar pronation and compensatory forefoot problems in a manner conducive to relief of pain. Pads are adhered with rubber cement. The skived side is adhered to the inner sole, and the pad may be covered with cover leather. The design of felt pads for shoes must consider the biomechanical advantages.

Felt Pads Applied to Foot

A ¼-inch skived white felt longitudinal metatarsal (L and M) pad is utilized to change the direct line pull of the plantar fascia and plantar calcaneonavicular ligament to a curved line pull, by supinating the foot for relief of plantar fasciitis and medial longitudinal arch strain, respectively. A ¼-inch skived white felt metatarsal pad placed just proximal to the metatarsal heads is used to relieve metatarsophalangeal joint periarticular fibrocitis and take pressure off painful plantar metatarsal head lesions. These and other accommodative pads are incorporated into low or high Dye strappings over a thin layer of kling after the foot has been treated with pretape skin adherent and after appropriate injection and/or physical therapy has been performed.

Shoe Sole Modifications

The podiatrist provides relief from pain through accommodation of objective lesions in the foot. A plantar skin lesion, degenerative joint disease, a bony prominence, a malfunctioning forefoot, gravitational stress and many foot deformities have been relieved through adequate shielding, padding and wedging of the part. It has been proven time and again that duplicating foot therapy through construction of an accommodative or corrective orthosis is yet another treatment. Permanent shields of plastic, leather, latex and felt have served as excellent therapeutic agents for many chronic foot ailments. Another technique to accommodate foot pathology is described here.

A sturdy leather, rigid-shanked, firm or extended counter, straight last shoe is most desirable. This shoe must have a Ripple sole through which all accommodations are made. The shoe must fit well, allowing for freedom of the forefoot with a snug fit in the arch and heel.

A dorsoplantar and lateral radiograph is taken of the foot in the ripple sole shoe using a radiopaque material, such as zinc oxide paste, metallic tape or other metallic substance on a deformity or pressure point. Metal washers are very effective when adhered over a heloma, tyloma, or painful site before taking the foot radiograph.

The radiopaque material will show on the radiograph underlying one or more flexible ribs in the sole. Thus, the site of the painful lesion is localized and easily accommodated.

This technique promises excellent results in the treatment of a deep-seated tyloma or verruca. Bursae, degenerative joint disease, sesamoiditis and defor-

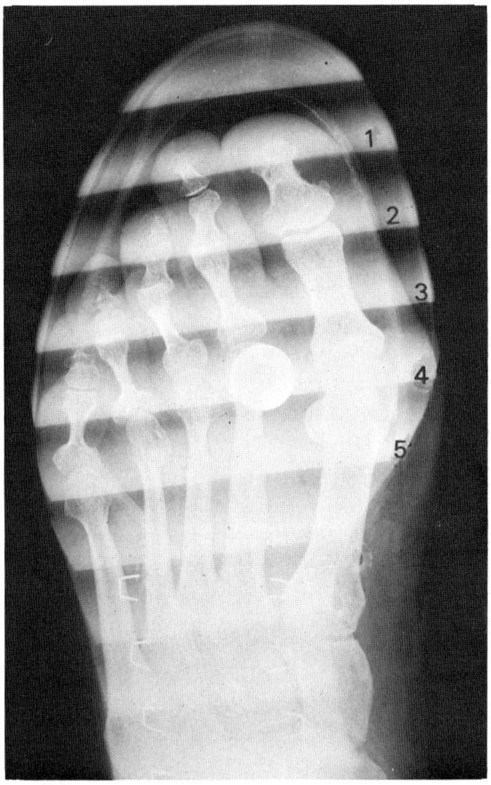

Figure 13.16. Locating lesions on foot for accommodation in ripple sole shoes.

mities of the toes may be accommodated. Calcaneal spurs, plantar heel bursa, hallux limitus and a variety of structural and functional disturbances can be treated with ease.

When the site of discomfort has been identified, a small section of a ripple or ripples in the sole is removed to accommodate the condition (Figs. 13.16 and 13.17). Thus, if a deep tyloma is noted directly below the seventh ripple under the first metatarsal head, a section of the seventh ripple is removed. This necessitates removal of only the section beneath the lesion at the medial side of the sole.

This same technique applies to lesions under any of the metatarsal heads, and it is possible to suspend all of the metatarsal heads between ripples if necessary. Helomas on the distal ends of toes seen in digiti flexus may be helped by removing a ripple. Similar cutouts can be used in alleviating pressure on the painful heel or under sesamoids.

There are many and varied shoe sole modifications to remove pressure from specific painful sites on the plantar surface of the foot. The Thomas heel is often used, in conjunction with an orthotic de-

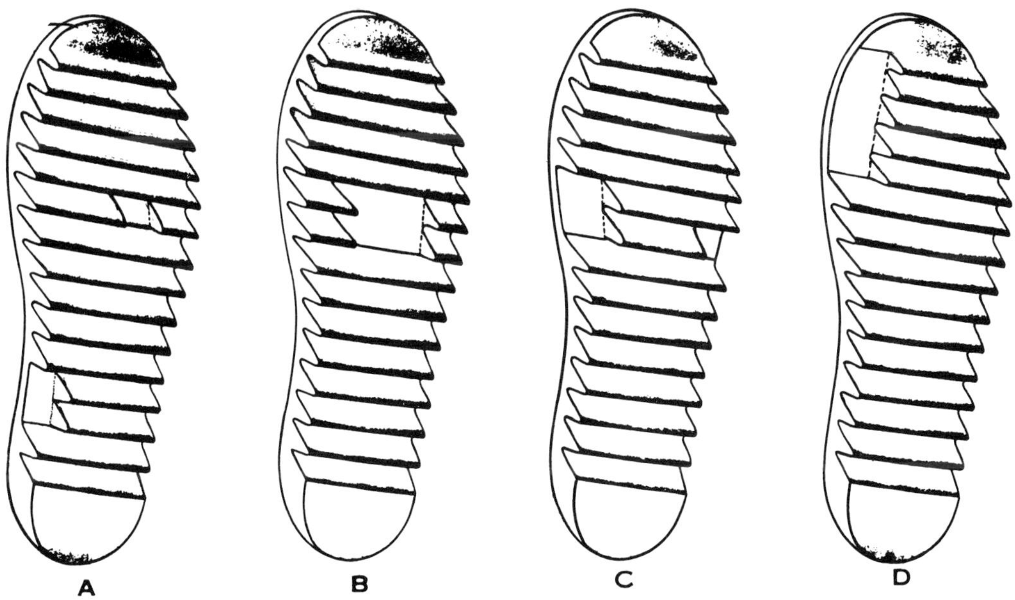

Figure 13.17. *A,* Removal of ripple under third metatarsal head and at spur site, medial tubercle, plantar surface calcaneus. *B,* Removal of ripple to accommodate second, third and fourth metatarsophalangeal joints. *C,* Cutout ripples for sesamoiditis and deep-seated tylomas, plantar surface, head of first and fifth metatarsal heads. *D,* Removal of ripples to relieve stress from hallux joint in hallux rigidus.

vice worn inside a shoe, to relieve stress on joints in the rearfoot. This heel is especially desirable where rearfoot valgus develops with destruction of articular cartilage and severe pronation. Heels may be extended medially or laterally with 1⁄16-inch wedges added to facilitate heel strike and foot function. A rubber heel is preferred.

The Thomas metatarsal bar, crescent-shaped bar, Mayo bar, and kidney-shaped bar are quite similar in their function. They are cemented to the sole of the shoe proximal to the forefoot treading surface to remove pressure and stress from arthritic metatarsophalangeal articulations.

An anterior heel is often effective in providing a broad distribution of weight. It consists of a leather raise skived to a feather edge extending from the front part of the shank where it meets the sole backward to half the distance of the shank, rising to the same height as the breast of the heel at its posterior margin.

Wedges can be used at the medial and lateral aspects of the shoe sole. They are placed between the outer sole and midsole, not on the outer sole.

A very effective accommodative shoe sole modification together with an in-shoe orthotic device is the first metatarsal head wedge. Here a wedge of leather is extended from the medial aspect of the breast of the heel, along the shank of the shoe forward along the outer sole beneath the first metatarsal shaft to just behind the sesamoids.

The shoe modifications described are but a few of many available to accommodate painful foot joints and secondary skin lesions.

Treatment of Arthritic Patients

The benefit of rest for a painful arthritic joint is apparent. In the treatment of the rheumatoid arthritic patient using good judgment is very important. In some rheumatoid and osteoarthritic syndromes, rest may hasten stiffness and limit function. The following procedures are recommended: (*a*) Relieve acute pain by combinations of analgesics and rest. (*b*) Shield and protect potential sites of trauma on the foot. (*c*) Improve function by active and passive movements of the affected limbs. (*d*) Use deep heat to relax tissues. (*e*) Provide currents to motor points in limbs to stimulate movement of affected joints. (*f*) Encourage mild, nonviolent exercise, daily walking, swimming and stretching by manual or mechanical traction.

Treatment of the rheumatoid arthritic by daily contrast foot baths, whirlpool at 105°F, infrared rays, short wave diathermy, hot packs and galvanic and sinusoidal currents followed by massage can be an important adjunct to systemic treatment by the rheumatologist. Injections of noncrystalline steroids or local anesthetics can be helpful. Medical relaxation and positive suggestion are of benefit in relief of spasms and pain.

The author has found the use of local anesthetic nerve block, field block, intra- and periarticular injection highly desirable in the treatment of acute painful arthritis of the foot joints (Table 13.1).

When a joint is limited in function, painful in motion, and tender to palpation it can be relieved by the injection of a local anesthetic in minimal doses intra-articularly under traction. If the pain is not relieved, a field block is indicated using 1–5 ml of an intermediate or long-acting local anesthetic, depending on the size of the joint. Applying traction to the joint intermittently, by hand or using weights and traction devices, may not only relieve pain, but also improve function. Manipulation should be performed with caution. If complete foot nerve blocks are used and motor function is compromised, the patient should be warned and assisted in stance and gait until sensation returns.

In a double-blind crossover study comparing Duranest (etidocaine 0.1%) with Sensorcaine (bupivacaine 0.5%), Dobbs et al (12) found etidocaine to have a more rapid onset and a longer duration than bupivacaine or a lidocaine-bupivacaine mixture.

Manipulation of rheumatoid arthritic joints must be based on careful clinical and radiographic evidence of minimal joint obstruction to manipulative thrusts. Acutely painful joints must not be manipulated until the etiology is established. However, manual movements of joints to their maximum capability can be beneficial. Acute exacerbations are given rest until the inflammation subsides.

Podiatrists are relieving the sequela of a high percentage of rheumatic disease sufferers by combining their biomechanical skills with surgical correction. Studied cases may require tendon repair, metatarsal osteotomy or ostectomy, synovectomy, adjustment by surgical shortening or lengthening of the small intrinsic muscles in the foot, metatarsophalangeal joint implants, stabilizing joints by arthrodesis and using a variety of surgical approaches to arthroplasty in the correction of toe deformities secondary to arthritis (see Chapter 11, Podiatric Surgery).

The bottom line in the treatment of stiff and painful arthritic articulations is skill

Table 13.1.
Local Anesthetic Review[a]

Agent (Common Name)	Onset	Duration of Action	Reappearance of Pain Sensation	Site of Metabolism	Maximum Single Dose	+EPI	Relative Potency	Comments
Ester compound	*min*	*min*	*min*		*mg*	*mg*		
Procaine (Novocaine)	7 ± 1	45–60	19 ± 3	Plasma	500 mg	600 mg	1	Indicated where history of malignant hyperpyrexia, very rapidly metabolized
Amide compound								
Lidocaine (Xylocaine)	5 ± 1	90–150	40 ± 3	Liver	300 mg	500 mg	4	Excellent spreading ability, local vasodilator, most popular local
Mepivacaine (Carbocaine)	4 ± 2	120–180	99 ± 6	Liver	300 mg	500 mg	4	Duration slightly longer than equal doses of lidocaine and blood levels not as sensitive to inclusion of adrenaline as lidocaine, thus may be useful if adrenaline not desired
Bupivacaine (Marcaine, Sensorcaine)	8 ± 3.2	180–600	415 ± 23	Liver	175 mg	250 mg	16	Lowest degree of placental transmission. Excellent for postoperative analgesic because of minimal motor block

[a] Dimidjian C: Review of Local Anesthetics, First Ray, Vol. X, No. 1, Oct. 1983

in and knowledge of "how to relieve a painful foot." The doctor must not only strive for this desirable situation but must also enhance the privilege of serving the patient by providing "tender loving care" and an interest in maintaining and improving his or her response to the patient's needs.

It is the author's opinion that all arthritic patients require foot orthoses properly constructed to alleviate stress on the articulations of the feet as they prevent further damage to diseased and pathological articulations.

The arthritis patient suffering discomfort when moving his/her pathological ankle is often provided with flexible castings or adhesive immobilization to relieve acute pain. Despite the damage to joint cartilage resulting in disability, the patient's pain is usually relieved by immobilization. This is especially true when the anterior talofibular, calcaneofibular, posterior talofibular and/or deltoid ligaments are torn, weakened or stretched. Following temporary relief the doctor may construct an Orthoplast ankle splint. This can provide partial immobilization of an arthritic joint. The construction of this splint depends on the ingenuity and design of the doctor and the skill of the assistant or brace maker. A paper pattern properly conceived is used to cut out the orthoplast which is ultimately heated and shaped to conform to the affected part.

The immobilization of an arthritic foot may be obtained with Scotch Cast, an improved fiberglass casting material. According to Albert (13), the tape used in this casting method is a "knitted fiberglass fabric impregnated with polyurethane resin which hardens upon exposure to water in a matter of minutes." Once hardened, "the tape is not significantly affected by additional exposures to water or moisture, and the cast is strong, lightweight, radiolucent and porous." The tape laminates well and is readily molded to body contours.

The use of this method of casting or flexible casting and adhesive immobilization may be necessary when a single anatomical part is affected by acute inflammation. Maintaining a part at rest by casting while the patient is mobilized may be highly desirable for some unilateral arthritic complaints.

The Aircast pneumatic ankle brace has been used effectively for relieving discomfort and swelling in arthritic ankle joints. Limitation of motion is necessary in the subacute or chronic arthritic ankle joint that has suffered acute trauma. The Aircast can provide compression of edematous periarticular soft tissues, limit articular effusion and provide sufficient immobilization to allow for articular cartilage and osseous repair. The application and adjustment of the Aircast pneumatic ankle brace should take only a few minutes. The airbags are inflated by blowing through a plastic tube. It is fully constructed and ready for use without requiring laboratory facilities or technical assistance (see Chapter 8, Arthritic and Other Inflammatory Disorders).

Physical Therapeutic Techniques

Active motion, passive motion, massage, manipulation, traction, hot and cold application, paraffin bath, short wave diathermy, ultrasound, infrared energy, high-voltage electrogalvanic stimulation, low-voltage galvanic stimulation, transcutaneous electrical nerve stimulation, iontophoresis, hypnosis, massage, controlled manipulation and whirlpool are discussed with reference to their application and reasons for use. Rest alone may be the judicious choice of treatment (see Chapter 12, Sports Medicine).

Active Exercise

Active exercise of an injured joint is used to engender confidence in the patient's ability to use the part. During the subacute and chronic stages of trauma and osteoarthritis affecting the foot, the patient should be asked to perform a select group of voluntary movements of the foot. These movements should include a variety of muscle and joint motions to ascertain functional capacity of the foot. This may require reinforcement by the doctor, the staff, and the patient's family. It is essential for proper function that the patient think of the movement required and pursue that movement with full control and concentration of mind and body. The motion initiated must be one that provides beneficial effects. Active motion may be assisted if contraction of the muscles does not move the affected joint. This must be pursued daily on a regular basis by skilled personnel. If the patient is homebound, a member of the family should be taught the routine.

Progressive resistive and manual resistive isotonic, isokinetic and isometric exercise increase muscle strength, endurance and tone. Active exercise programs are useful as a means of improving general health, following trauma or surgery, for weak and atrophied muscles and in treatment programs for the arthritic. Neuromuscular physiotherapeutic techniques are an adjunct to the treatment of paretic and paralyzed muscles.

Passive Exercise

Passive exercise is initiated by the doctor or a member of his or her staff, a family member, or other trained personnel. Here the doctor guides the toes, forefoot, rearfoot, or ankle joint into a movement range that provides a little more stretch at each treatment session. Notes are made of restrictions, immobility and complaints of discomfort. Limitations of certain joint movements are measured and recorded.

If the joint is hot and swollen, the best approach is to provide rest and appropriate internal medication until the part has "cooled down." However, if possible, contraction of the muscles involved to prevent atrophy is desirable. Continued muscle function is beneficial, especially when the patient is immobilized in a plaster cast or splint or is on crutches. Muscles unable to contract actively may be stimulated to do so by low- and high-voltage currents during rehabilitation. Passive exercise programs are indicated for prevention of contractures and joint adhesions, muscle paralysis or extreme paresis, decreased joint range of motion due to casting, mild muscle spasm or, secondary to trauma, in instances where the patient displays poor conscious and proprioceptive states, arthritic conditions, and amputation.

Traction

Traction is helpful in the relief of chronic pain by opening up the joint space and stretching the capsular and intra-articular ligaments. This results in improved mobility, less stiffness and a decrease in pain and provides an opportunity for the elimination of intra-articular material while increasing the supply of blood to nourish the damaged joint. Traction should not be used on an acutely inflamed joint.

Traction can be applied by hand to the small joints of the foot. When a joint is placed under traction, the opening of the articulation causes a dimpling of the overlying skin into the joint space. This dimpling also provides the site for intra-articular injections.

Painful limitation of motion in interphalangeal or metatarsophalangeal joints can be helped by daily home traction treatments.

Toe traction requires adhesive tape, an S hook and the rung of a chair. The toe can be prepared with a skin adherent or tincture of benzoin compound to prevent irritation and increase adherence of the tape.

This procedure should be performed at home for 8 min. twice a day. The patient will note a numbness of the toe in about 4 min. When numbness occurs, the loop should be released from the S hook for a minute of rest and rehooked again for 4 min when numbness disappears. The same technique is used again later in the day before retiring. The toe loses some of its stiffness and pain. Function gradually improves following several weeks of daily traction. Joint stretching devices can be used professionally for controlled traction.

Hot and Cold Application

Many arthritic, neuritic and overuse foot injuries are improved with the application of heat. Heating pads or the application of dry heat is not as effective as moist heat. The use of hot packs or foot soaks in hot water not over 105°F can be helpful in relieving pain and stillness. Stiffness is markedly improved while the part is being treated with moist or wet heat if the affected area is actively and passively exercised at the same time. Despite the relief one may obtain with wet heat, inflamed and swollen soft tissues and joints may do better when ice packs or cold water soaks are used alone or in combination with other physiotherapeutic measures.

Where small vessel circulation is impaired, the use of both hot and cold foot soaks in a synchronous manner is effective. The technique is to plunge the affected foot into hot water (99–105°F) for 2 min followed immediately by placing the foot in cold water for ½ min. This procedure should follow hot to cold for 15–20 min twice daily. The patient must move the affected part to tolerance while in the water. The temperature should be checked by a thermometer or by hand tolerance before foot immersion. Under no circumstance should direct heat be applied when the patient suffers from circulatory insufficiency.

The Hydrocolator Steam Pack (Chattanooga, TN) provides a convenient method of applying moist heat to the debilitated foot. This method of application of hot packs results in retention of heat for longer periods of time compared to hot foot soaks. Moist hot packs produce local analgesia, facilitate drainage, result in muscle sedation and increase local blood circulation. The application of moist heat is indicated for strains and spasms (48 hr postinjury), neuritis, fibrocitis, phlebitis, myositis, myalgia and cellulitis (14).

Cold applications for acute swelling, redness and pain can be beneficial. Col Pac (Chattanooga, TN) reusable compresses may be effective. This cold pack is moldable to fit the contours of the affected part. It is essentially dry and must be prescribed by the doctor. Cold pack application is indicated for reduction of edema and relief of pain caused by acute trauma or surgical procedure. It is essential to evaluate the circulatory status of the patient before administering either hot or cold applications.

Contrast baths may be helpful in breaking the pain cycle. The feet are first immersed in warm water (approximately 100°F) for 60 sec, followed by cold water (approximately 55°F) for 60 sec for a total of 6 min.

Vasodilatation for relief of pain may be obtained by soaking the forearms in warm to hot water for 15 min. This provides a reflex vasodilatation in the lower extremities. A warm water bag on the lower abdomen or lower back provides a similar reflex vascular response in the feet.

Paraffin Bath

Superficial heat from the paraffin bath is helpful in the treatment of rheumatoid and osteoarthritis, bursitis, fibrocitis and tenosynovitis. As with other forms of heat, arterial insufficiency and sensory impairment are contraindications. The foot is dipped in paraffin (approximately 125°F) and withdrawn. The paraffin is allowed to dry, and the process is repeated 5–10 times. The paraffin is left on the foot for 30 min and then removed.

Short Wave Diathermy

The use of short wave diathermy provides a unique approach to applying heat to the debilitated foot. The technique differs depending upon the type of electrodes or treatment leads being used. A space should exist between the active electrodes and the affected part. The electronic principles of dielectric hysteresis provide for energy being passed through the softer superficial tissues, into more dense structures, such as muscle, cartilage and bone. When energy passes through the deeper and heavier structures, the friction of its passage through a joint, for example, causes the part to become warm. It is absolutely essential that the patient be carefully observed to establish tolerance. Also, the patient's sensory perception must be good and circulation adequate to prevent deep burns. The machine is monitored closely. Some machines allow for treatment of two areas at the same time by being equipped with two independent induction treatment heads. An induction coil is used by wrapping it about the affected part. The part is covered by felt or toweling. Treatment may range from once a day to three times a week for 15–30 min sessions. Induction short wave diathermy is used for treating chronic arthritis, bursitis, neuritis, strains and sprains. Diathermy should not be used in the presence of acute injury, sensory or vascular deficit, joint or metal implants, malignancy, pacemakers, infection or in children or the elderly.

Ultrasound

Ultrasound has been used extensively for relieving pain, decreasing stiffness, improving tissue metabolism and delivering chemicals into the tissues.

Ultrasound is administered in a range of 0.5 and 2.5 watts/cm (1). Increased intensity is indicated over muscle and a lesser intensity over the bony areas of the foot and ankle. The greater the intensity, the greater the amount of energy absorbed and converted to heat (14). Cavitation, the alternate compression and rarefaction of the ultrasound exposed tissues, is produced by high-intensity ultrasound. This phenomenon results in dissolution of intermolecular bonds and is useful in treating adhesions, fibrosis and scar tissue. The heat produced by ultrasound causes localized hyperemia, thereby relieving the pain and inflammation associated with strains, sprains, neuritis, bursitis, tenosynovitis, periarticular fibrocitis, muscle spasm and joint adhesions. A coupling agent (gel, cream or ointment) must be used between the applicator head and the area of treatment. The applicator must be left in constant motion so as to avoid burns. If heat or discomfort is expericnccd, the intensity must de decreased. Phonophoresis, the cutaneous transport of medication, is accomplished by using a steroid, analgesic or other cream, ointment or gel, as the coupling agent. Underwater application is performed with the applicator head less that 1 inch from the treatment area. Ultrasound treatments may be utilized daily, several times a week, alone or in combination with other physical therapy modalities (e.g., massage, whirlpool, exercise, electrogalvanic stimulation, etc). Application time varies from 3–15 min depending on the size of the area being treated. Contraindications for use include sensory deficit, vascular insufficiency, pregnancy and malignancy, and it should not be applied over pacemakers, the spinal cord, epiphyses and metal or Silastic implants (14).

Infrared Energy

This is a convective dry heat form that can provide a mild heat to the affected part. The part should be watched closely for the possibility of burns from heat beyond the tolerance of the skin overlying the arthritic foot joint. It is often applied to the affected part along with an antiphlogistic cream to produce an erythematous skin reaction. Radiant heat penetrates skin to a depth of 2–3 mm (14). Infrared energy is used in short 5-min exposures, 2 ft away from the foot, for local vasodilatation, sedation, muscle relaxation and relief of pain. Dry heat may be beneficial in treating chronic arthritis, abrasions and superficial skin infections. Heat should not be used in patients with microangiopathy, neuropathy, malignancy, acute inflammation, nor over joint or metal implants, in children or in the elderly.

Direct (Galvanic) and Alternating (Sinewave and Faradic) Current

Direct galvanic current is either uninterrupted or interrupted. Direct current entering the body through a positive electrode elicits a warm, tingling sensation. Steady uninterrupted direct current has an anti-inflammatory action. Pulsed interrupted direct current stimulates skeletal muscle contraction, retarding atrophy, reducing edema and enhancing joint range of motion. Treatment duration is gradually increased from 3–15 min three times a week.

Alternating sinewave current is administered in frequencies between 1–1000 cycles/sec. Frequencies of 20 cycles sec and greater will cause muscle contraction (14). Alternating faradic current causes uncomfortable sensory effects and is rarely utilized (14). Alternating sinewave current is used to diminish inflammation and muscle atrophy, to increase muscle tone and to re-educate muscles in chronic arthritis, strains, sprains, muscle atrophy and after tendon transposition or transfer. Contraindications for direct and alternating current use include pregnancy, metal implants, pacemakers, neuroangiopathy, fracture, infection, skin pathology, malignancy and in children.

High-Voltage Electrogalvanic Stimulation

Currents have been refined and smoothed out to avoid the slight shocking pulsations delivered by earlier low-voltage equipment. The ideal equipment provides for applying electrodes to specific motor points over muscles, resulting in movement of the part or parts. The foot can be moved through a variety of incursions dependent on the structures receiving the current. The power of the impulse being delivered is controlled, and the ballistic impulse can be selected to deliver the desired number of strokes/min. Each impulse can also be coordinated with a sound to reinforce the muscle reaction to the current in accordance with the research of Pavlov. Individual toes can be flexed or extended by proper application of the electrodes. The foot can be moved through all of its normal functions by this current. This also includes involuntary flexion or extension of the foot at the ankle. Treatments are best given three times weekly for 5–12 min. The patient should be encouraged to move the part at the sound and feel of the impulse.

The effect of this stimulation is especially helpful to the arthritic patient. Peripheral nerves are stimulated to produce a muscle contraction that is controlled in intensity and frequency in accordance with the pathological requirements. When muscles move they cause the joints they control to flex or to extend. Spasms are readily relieved, and the muscular contractions improve the quality of venous return. Those suffering from acute and chronic traumatic arthritis, osteoarthritis and rheumatoid arthritis can benefit measurably when atrophic musculature assumes a more normal function.

The short sharp pulsation of these unidirectional modalities controls the limits of nerve stimulation and decreases sensory perception so prevalent in the use of low-voltage generators. Because the voltage is high it is able to penetrate body tissues without undue sensory disturbance. This lends itself to treatment of bone and joint disease and the secondary complications attendant with foot deformity and local metabolic dysfunction.

The induction of electrical impulses into the tissues may produce a tissue response from the muscles due to activation of the nerves supplying the muscles. These stimuli can be accurately calculated and controlled as to their effectiveness when used for diagnosis or treatment. The high-voltage, low-amperage generator is neither galvanic, faradic nor sinusoidal. It is a low-frequency, short-duration impulse generator suitable for stimulating nerves, contracting muscles and thus moving joints by passive electronic stimuli. Pain is often relieved, stiffness controlled and motion improved. Transmission of stimuli is believed to be through autonomic nervous system fibers. Improvement in circulatory status can be noted with evidence of an increase in microcirculation.

Iontophoresis

Drugs that are negatively or positively charged can be driven into the tissues by using galvanic current beneath the proper electrode. The medication or chemical of choice in solution is placed beneath an electrode of positive or negative current. The electrodes are checked carefully for proper connection to the galvanic generator. The solution-soaked electrode is placed over the part into which the solution is to be electronically induced. The solution might be magnesium sulfate, iodine, a local anesthetic, histamine or any other suitable medication. The indifferent electrode is placed a short distance from the active electrode. Following the principle of "like signs repel and unlike signs attract," a negative medication will be drawn into the tissue toward the positive electrode when the machine is turned on to a tolerable 4–6 mA. This type of treatment can be helpful for its sedating chemical effect on tissue.

Medications applied at the positive anode pole include copper sulphate for fungus infections, sodium chloride for bromhyperidrosis, zinc sulphate for ulcers, calcium chloride for muscle spasm, magnesium sulphate for analgesia, hydrocortisone and lidocaine(14). Medications applied at the negative cathode pole include salicylate for analgesia, iodine for fibrosis and acetic acid as an anti-inflammatory agent (14). Iontophoresis should not be used in the presence of sensory loss, metal implants or pacemakers. Treatment time may vary from 5–15 min.

Whirlpool (Hydrotherapy)

The same principles apply to the use of whirlpool as to the use of hot or cold water. Because the swirling of water is also a form of massage, the patient should not be placed in a whirlpool bath until the doctor ascertains that a phlebitis or thrombophlebitis does not exist to throw off emboli into the vascular system. Whirlpool treatment provides massage, muscle relaxation and debridement of necrotic tissue. This treatment is used postoperatively and after immobiliztion for joint stiffness, adhesions, pain and chronic inflammation. Treatment for burns and ulcerations is augmented by whirlpool therapy. All contraindications to this treatment must be cautiously observed. Treatment with this modality can be dangerous in the presence of endarteritis obliterans, fragility of the capillaries or in any microcirculatory disease that cannot cope with heat-induced metabolites. Other contraindications include noninflammatory edema, acute injury, sensory deficit and use in infants or in the elderly with chronic cardiac or respiratory disease. Prolonged treatment is not suggested. Treatment periods 10–20 min at 87–105°F are adequate.

Betadine, chlorophyll or other antiseptics may be used in the water. The patient is encouraged to flex, extend, invert and evert the foot while whirlpool treatment is proceeding in order to prevent dependent or congestive edema.

Massage

Massage performed for specific beneficial effects can be used successfully on the periarticular tissues and muscles that originate in the leg and foot and insert in the foot. The distant musculature performing movement in the foot may be restricted due to arthritic and other pathology and may show evidence of disuse atrophy. All atrophic muscles should be massaged to maintain their integrity when they are unable to perform their full range of activity. Exercises should be prescribed. All contraindications to massage must be observed. Gentle mobilization of a painful part has always been a source of comfort.

In previously reported investigations, Brantingham et al (15–17), using electromyographically measured muscle activity, show that in certain muscles of the leg a significant change in contraction intensity occurs with each slight change in the angular position of the foot with respect to the horizontal supporting surface. On the other hand, the electromyographic activity pattern remains relatively static in the absence of such slight angular changes of foot position, even though the surface may be soft.

Assuming that the efficiency of the venous pump mechanism, and thus that of peripheral circulation in general, is dependent upon phasic activity of muscles in juxtaposition to valved veins in the extremities, the author set out to make direct measurements on venous pump parameters during prolonged standing on softened flat surfaces of varied density. Two parameters were measured. First, venous pressure at the ankle level was directly measured and monitored. Second, thermographic studies of the posterior aspect of the calf were undertaken in order to ascertain the extent of venous flow in the superficial circulation. In addition to the research reported here on the effects of a variable terrain on the venous circulation, the author recognizes a basic incongruity between the osteologic configuration of the human forefoot and the unrelentingly flat substratum of a modern urban environment. It appears logical that a variable terrain should act to diminish physical stress on elements of the foot and ankle during weightbearing, thus alleviating many of the subclinical symptoms of foot discomfort prevalent today. In support of this conclusion, Brantingham et al. report dynamic studies undertaken to evaluate the subjective responses of hundreds of persons whose regular daily occupations demand that they stand for more than 2 hrs. daily. They also feel it is quite possible that many chronic pathological alterations of the structural integrity of the foot and ankle could be prevented by reducing physical stress during standing and walking. In addition to those people who must stand in their workplace, walkways involve the entire population. Studies lead the author to believe that better walkways will encourage walking. As with the standing workplace, the flat smooth walkway, a surface designed with the wheel in mind, appears to be the subject of complaint by patients. These complaints include foot and leg fatigue and discomfort, resulting in a limit to the desire to stand and walk.

Controlled Manipulation

The ability to control manipulation of foot joints depends on individual skills and familiarity with the human foot. A stiff joint may be put into a maximal position range of motion, and with a quick, short, gentle thrust, an additional joint force may be exerted, resulting in an opening of the joint space. This technique requires clinical skill and a thorough knowledge of the pathology existing in the specific joint being manipulated. The result of this thrust provides an influx of blood and tissue fluids into the joint space, forcing out the products of pathological joint metabolism: the tight articular, periarticular and capsular structures are stretched, and adhesions are often stretched or broken. A local hyperemia ensues. All of the joints in the foot are amenable to controlled manipulation. The doctor must be sure of the physical status of an arthritic joint before manipulative therapy is pursued. The danger of fracture in the hands of the unskilled is always present.

Manipulation increases mobility, relieves pain and provides a feeling of improvement in periarticular tissues.

Hypnosis (Medical Relaxation)

Every technique for relief of pain may be coupled with positive suggestion by the doctor. Every physician has seen the sign of dismay come over the face of a patient who has been informed that he or she has a condition known to the lay person as "incurable." The doctor must know and treat the emotional side of the patient, as well as the physical. Arthritis is one of those incurable diseases requiring both somatic and psychological treatment approaches.

The desirable approach to treatment is by positive suggestion. Explain briefly the physiological effects known about the treatment. With repetition and by evoking confidence the patient will not only accept the treatment but ultimately will develop the same positive philosophy. Some improvement can be expected from confidence alone and the patient's positive attitude toward the illness. The doctor must be honest at all times. With a positive attitude the patient will perform auto-suggestion to potentiate therapy and enable marked improvement of the foot problem.

Hypnosis and medical relaxation have been used by the author with good results in relieving pain, stiffness and muscle spasm. Hypnosis should be performed by the experienced hypnotherapist, psychiatrist or psychologist, who can augment the medical, podiatric or surgical approach to chronic foot pathology.

Hypnosis has resulted in relief of pain, limitation of joint stiffness due to protective spasm and relaxation of the musculature providing for improved joint motion.

Transcutaneous Electrical Nerve Stimulation (TENS)

TENS has proven to be a drugless method for relieving pain in a variety of chronic as well as acute disorders. The painful foot is a condition that may be helped by the use of TENS techniques. Special electrodes have been developed to fit the contours of the anatomical part. The technique is useful alone or when combined with non-narcotic pain-relieving drugs and other physical therapeutic measures.

It is imperative that a proper diagnosis be made before prescribing TENS therapy. Cardiac problems, pregnancy, malignancy, circulatory and local neurotrophic disorders must be approached with caution. Skin irritations under electrodes may be serious in diabetics with capillary fragility. As in most therapeutic regimens, the doctor is cautioned against psychological dependence. Treatment time varies from a few minutes to hours. An electrical nerve stimulator, Electro-Acuscope-80, provides the conventional mode of TENS with an additional "computer-controlled circuitry with all forms of feedback" (see Chapter 3, The Painful Foot).

PHARMACOLOGY (18, 19)

I. PRESCRIPTION WRITING

A. Prescription Writing

Name ______________________________ Chart No. ______________

Address ______________________________ Date ______________

RX Ampicillin 250 mg.
Disp #30 (xxx)
Sig ī Tab P.O. T.I.D./HR P.C.

DAW ________
LABEL ________
NR 1 2 3 PRN _____
DEA ______________________ ______________________ DPM

B. Prescription Coding

ad	To, up to
ad lib	When desired
ASIT BENE	Shake well
A.C.	Before meals
B.I.D.	Twice a day
Q.O.D.	Every other day
D.	A day
Dur. Dol.	While pain lasts
H.	An hour
H.S.	At bedtime
Int. CIB	Between meals
Int. Noct.	During the night
Noct.	At night
N.P.O.	Nothing by mouth
Q.D.	Every day
OMN. HOR.	Every hour

OMN. MAN.	Every morning
P.O.	By mouth
P.C.	After meals
P.R.N.	When necessary
Q.I.D.	Four times a day
q.	Every
Sig	Write or label
T.I.D.	Three times a day
Ut Dict	As directed
GTT	A drop
$\dot{\tau}$	One
$\overline{SS}$	½
$\bar{S}$	Without

$\bar{c}$	With
Q.S.	As much as is sufficient
gm	Gram
gr	Grain
1 ML	1 cc
Teaspoon	5 cc = 1 dram

3 teaspoons = 1 tablespoon = ½ fluid oz
1 grain = 60 mg
Ex. Tylenol #1 = 7.5 mg = ⅛ grain
Tylenol #2 = 15 mg = ¼ grain
Tylenol #3 = 30 mg = ½ grain
Tylenol #4 = 60 mg = 1 grain
250 mg tablet = 400,000 units of penicillin

Young's Rule—$\frac{\text{Age in years}}{\text{Age in years} + 12} \times$ adult dose = child's dose

Clark's Rule—$\frac{\text{Weight in lbs}}{150 \text{ lbs}} \times$ adult dose = child's dose

Fried's Rule—Infants up to 2 years = $\frac{\text{Age in months}}{150} \times$ adult dose

**Most accurate child dose = $\frac{\text{Body surface area of child in m}^2}{1.273 \text{ m}^2} \times$ adult dose

II. NON-NARCOTIC AND NARCOTIC ANALGESICS

A. Non-Narcotic Analgesics (Plain)

1. *Acetaminophen (Phenaphen, Tylenol, Datril)*
   Tabs: 325,500, 600 mg
   Caps: 325,500 mg
   Elixir: 120 mg/5 ml
   Suppository: 120, 125, 325, 600 mg
   Sig: $\dot{\tau}$ or $\dot{\tau}\dot{\tau}$ q 4–6 P.R.N.
   Toxic dose: Do not exceed more than (12) 325 mg tabs or caps/day
   Pediatric dose: Children 6–12 years, ½ to 1 TAB T.I.D. or Q.I.D.; under 6 years, use good judgment
2. *Acetylsalicylic Acid (ASA)*
   Tabs: 325,600 mg
   Caps: 325 mg
   Sig: $\dot{\tau}$ or $\dot{\tau}\dot{\tau}$ q. 4–6 H. P.R.N.
   Toxic dose: Do not exceed more than (12) 325 mg caps or tabs/day
   Pediatric dose: Suppository dose 65, 130 mg
3. *Ascriptin (Buffered Aspirin)*
   Tabs: 300 mg of aspirin, 150 mg Maalox
   Ascriptin ad 300 mg of aspirin, 300 mg Maalox
   Sig: $\dot{\tau}$ or $\dot{\tau}\dot{\tau}$ Tabs Q.I.D.
   Toxic dose: Do not exceed 12 tabs/day
   Not recommended for children under 12
4. *Pentazocine (Talwin)*
   Tabs: 50 mg
   IV, IM: 30 mg/ml/ampule
   Sig: $\dot{\tau}$ tab q. 3–4 H. P.R.N.
   Toxic dose: Do not exceed 600 mg/day
   Caution to patients predisposed to alcohol and drug abuse
5. *Propoxyphene Preparations (Darvon, Propoxyphene, Wygesic, Dolene)*
   Darvon: Caps: 32, 65 mg
   Sig. $\dot{\tau}$ or $\dot{\tau}\dot{\tau}$ caps q. 3–4 H. P.R.N.
   Darvon compound caps (with APC): 65 mg
   Sig: $\dot{\tau}$ or $\dot{\tau}\dot{\tau}$ caps q. 3–4 H. P.R.N. or T.I.D. or Q.I.D.
   Darvon-N Tabs: 100 mg
   Sig: $\dot{\tau}$ or $\dot{\tau}\dot{\tau}$ tabs q. 3–4 H. P.R.N.
   Darvocet-N Tabs: 50 mg propoxyphene and 325 mg acetaminophen
   Sig: $\dot{\tau}$ or $\dot{\tau}\dot{\tau}$ Tabs q. 4 H.
   Darvocet N 100: Tabs 100 mg propoxyphene and 325 mg acetaminophen
   Sig: $\dot{\tau}$ Tab q. 4 H.
   Darvon with ASA Caps: 65 mg propoxyphene and 325 mg ASA
   Sig: $\dot{\tau}$ or $\dot{\tau}\dot{\tau}$ caps q. 4 H.
   Darvon-N with ASA Tabs 100 mg propoxyphene and 325 mg ASA
   Sig: $\dot{\tau}$ Tab q. 4 H.
   Toxic dose: Do not exceed 390 mg/day of propoxyphene
   Pediatric dose: Only if recommended by physician
   Caution to patients predisposed to alcohol or drug abuse
   Propoxyphene is now a Class IV substance—need DEA#

B. Non-Narcotic Analgesics (Combos)

1. *ASA Compound*
   Tabs: 230 mg ASA and 32 mg caffeine
   Caps: 250 mg ASA and 32 mg caffeine
   Sig: ī or īī P.O. q. 4–6 H. P.R.N.
   Toxic dose: Do not exceed 12 tab/day
   Pediatric dose: Use good judgment
2. *Amytal and ASA*
   Caps: 50 mg amobarbitol and 325 mg ASA
   Sig: ī or īī cap q. 4 H. P.R.N.
   Toxic dose: Not more than 1 gm q. 6 H.
   Pediatric dose: Not recommended
3. *Fiorinol*
   Tabs: 50 mg butalbital and APC
   Caps: 50 mg butalbital and APC
   Sig: ī or īī q. 4 H. P.R.N.
   Toxic dose: Do not exceed 6 caps or tabs/day
   Pediatric dose: Not recommended
4. *A.P.C. Compound*
   Tabs: APC
   Caps: APC
   Sig: ī or īī B.I.D. or T.I.D.
   Toxic dose: Do not exceed 12 caps or tabs/day
   Pediatric dose: Not recommended
5. *Synalgos*
   Caps: 6.25 mg promethazine hydrochloride, 356.4 mg aspirin, 30 mg caffeine
   Sig: īī cap q. 4 H. P.R.N. pain
   Toxic dose: Do not exceed 12 caps/day
   Pediatric dose: Not recommended
6. *Talwin Compound*
   Caps: 12.5 mg pentazocine, 325 mg aspirin
   Sig: īī cap P.O. T.I.D. or Q.I.D.
   Toxic dose: Do not exceed 2.4 gm/day
   Pediatric dose: Not recommended unless specified by physician
   Pentazocine has about 1/50 the antagonistic activity of naloxone (Narcan).
7. *Pentazocine (Talwin)*
   Tabs: 50 mg
   Inj: 30 mg/ml
   Sig: ī Tab Q. 3–4 H. P.R.N.
   Toxic dose: 600 mg/day
   Pediatric dose: 60 mg/day
   Narcan (naloxone hydrochloride) is isused as an antidote in 0.1 mg/kg given IM, IV, Sub Q and may be repeated in 2–3 min intervals. If failure to obtain significant response after 2 or 3 doses reassess diagnosis.

C. Narcotic Analgesics (Plain)

1. *Codeine*
   Tabs: 15, 30, 60 mg
   IM, IV 30 mg/ml, 60 mg/ml
   Sig: Analgesic: 15–60 mg Q.I.D.
   Antitussive: 5–10 mg
   Toxic dose: Do not exceed 6 gr/day
   Pediatric dose: Use good judgment
2. *Fentanyl (Sublimaze)*
   Inj: 0.05 mg/ml only supplied in ampules of 2 ml and 5 ml
   IV, IM = ½ to 1 h preoperatively
   Sig: 0.05–0.1 mg preoperative dosage
   Pediatric dose: Children 2–12 years, 0.02 to 0.03/20–25 lb
   Toxic dose: Do not exceed recommended dosage
3. *Hydromorphone (Dilaudid)*
   Tabs: 1,2,3,4 mg tablets
   Inj: 1,2,3,4 mg/ml ampules
   Suppository 3 mg
   Sig: 2–4 mg q. 4–6 H. P.R.N.
   Pediatric dose: Not recommended for children under 12
   Toxic dose: Do not exceed 25 mg/day
4. *Meperidine (Demerol)*
   Tabs: 50, 100 mg
   Inj: 25, 50, 75, 100 mg/ml
   Syrup: 50 mg/5cc
   Sig: For pain: 50–100 mg q. 3–4 H. P.R.N.
   Preop 50–100 mg IM or Sub Q. 30–90 min prior to surgery
   Pediatric dose: 0.5–0.8 mg/lb P.O. q. 3–4 H. P.R.N.
   Preop—0.5–0.1 mg/lb 30–90 min prior
5. *Morphine Sulfate (Morphine)*
   Tabs: 10, 15, 30 mg
   Inj: 2–4 mg/ml
   Elixir: 10 mg/5 ml
   Sig: 5–10 mg q. 4 H.
   Pediatric dose: 0.1–0.2 mg/kg/dose
   Toxic dose: Do not exceed 120 mg/day

D. Narcotic Analgesics (Combo)

1. *APC with Codeine (Various)*
   Tabs: 227 mg aspirin, 162 mg phenacetin and 32 mg caffeine
   Caps: 227 mg aspirin, 162 mg phenacetin and 32 mg caffeine
   Tabs or Caps APC with ⅛ gr = 7.5 mg/codeine = #1
   ¼ gr = 0.15 mg/codeine = #2
   ½ gr = 0.30 mg/codeine = #3
   1 gr = 60 mg/codeine = #4
   Sig: ī or īī P.O. q. 4–6 H.
   Toxic dose: Do not exceed 600 mg/day
   Pediatric dose: Not recommended for children under 12; use good judgment
2. *Ascriptin with codeine*
   Tabs: #2 ¼ gr codeine and 325 mg ASA with 150 mg Maalox
   # 3 ½ gr codeine and 325 mg ASA with 150 mg Maalox
   Sig: ī or īī Tab q. 3–4 H. P.R.N. pain

Toxic dose: Do not exceed 600 mg/day or 12 tabs/day

3. *ASA and Codeine Compound (Empirin)*
   Tabs: #1, #2, #3, #4
   Sig: ī or īī tab q. 4–6 H. P.R.N. pain
   Toxic dose: Do not exceed 600 mg/day
   Pediatric dose: Not recommended for children under 12
4. *Fiorinol with Codeine*
   Caps: #1, #2,#3
   Sig: ī or īī Cap q. 4–6 H. P.R.N. pain
   Toxic dose: Do not exceed 600 mg/day
   Pediatric dose: Not recommended
5. *Mepergan Fortis*
   Caps: 50 mg meperidine and 25 mg promethazine (Phenergan)
   Sig: ī Tab P.O. q. 4–6 H. P.R.N. pain
   Toxic dose: Do not exceed 300 mg/day
   Pediatric dose: Not recommended for children over 12
6. *Percodan*
   Tabs: 4.5 mg oxycodone hydrochloride, 0.38 mg oxycodone terephthalate, 325 mg ASA
   Sig: ī tab q. 6 H. P.R.N. pain
   Toxic dose: Do not exceed 18 mg/day or 4 tabs/day
   Pediatric dose: Not recommended
7. *Percodan Demi*
   Tabs: 2.25 mg oxycodone, 0.19 mg oxycodone terephthalate, 325 mg ASA
   Sig: ī or īī Tab P.O. q. 6 H. P.R.N. pain
   Toxic dose: Do not exceed 18 mg/day
   Pediatric dose: Children 12 and older, ½ tab q. 6 H.
   Children 6–12, ¼ tab Q. 6 H.; not recommended for children under 6.
8. *Percocet-5*
   Tabs: 5 mg oxycodone hydrochloride and 325 mg acetaminophen
   Sig: ī tab P.O. q. 6 H. P.R.N. pain
   Toxic dose: Do not exceed 18 mg/day
   Pediatric dose: Should not be administered
9. *Acetaminophen with Codeine (Phenaphen, Tylenol)*
   Tabs: 325 mg acetaminophen and #1, #2, #3, #4 codeine
   Elixir: 12 mg codeine, 120 mg acetaminophen, 7% alcohol
   Sig: ī or īī tab q. 4–6 H. P.R.N.
   Toxic dose: Do not exceed 600 mg/day
   Pediatric dose: Children 7–12, īī Tsp T.I.D. or Q.I.D.
   Children 3–6, Sig: ī Tsp T.I.D. or Q.I.D.
10. *Synalgos DC*
    Caps: 16.0 mg dihydrocodeine, 6.25 promethazine hydrochloride, 356.4 mg ASA, 30 mg caffeine
    Sig: ī cap q. 4 H. P.R.N. pain
    Toxic dose: Do not exceed 6 caps/day
    *All products containing codeine or other narcotic analgesic can be habit-forming.

III. ANTIANXIETY

1. *Chlordiazepoxide (Librium)*
   Caps: 5, 10, 25 mg (Librium)
   Tabs: 5, 10, 25 mg (Libritabs)
   Inj: 2, 5 ml ampules
   Sig: 5 or 10 mg T.I.D. or Q.I.D., mild to moderate anxiety and tension
   20 or 25 mg T.I.D. or Q.I.D. severe anxiety and tension
   Preoperative inj: 50, 100 mg IM 1 H. preoperatively
   Pediatric dose: 6–12 years, 5 mg B.I.D., T.I.D., Q.I.D., dosage may be increased P.R.N.; under 6 not recommended
   Toxic dose: Do not exceed 100 mg/day
   *Librium may be used for relief of withdrawal symptoms of acute alcoholism. The parenteral form is usually used initially.
2. *Diazepam (Valium)*
   Tabs: 2, 5, 10 mg
   Inj: 2, 10 ml ampules
   Sig: 2–10 mg B.I.D. or Q.I.D.
   Preoperative dose 2, 5, 10 mg
   Pediatric dose: Children 6–12, 1–2.5 mg T.I.D. or Q.I.D.; children under 6, not recommended
   Toxic dose: Do not exceed 40 mg/day
   *Valium may be used for symptomatic relief in acute alcohol withdrawal.
3. *Meprobamate (Equanil, Miltown, Sk-Bamate)*
   Caps: 200, 400 mg
   Sig: Adults 300–400 mg T.I.D. or Q.I.D.
   Children 6–12 years of age, 100–200 mg B.I.D. or T.I.D.; children under 6 years of age not recommended
   Toxic dose: Do not exceed 2.4 gm/day
   Interactions with alcohol, other CNS depressors and other psychotropic prescriptions
4. *Tybamate*
   Caps: 250 mg, 350 mg
   Sig: 250–500 mg T.I.D. or Q.I.D.
   Children 6–12 years, 20–35 mg/kg/day in divided doses; children less than 6 years, not recommended
   Toxic dose: Do not exceed 3 gm/day
5. *Lorazepam* (Divan)

Tabs: 0.5, 1, 2 mg
Inj: 2 mg/ml, 4 mg/ml
Sig: 2–3 mg/day B.I.D. or T.I.D.
IM 0.05 mg/kg up to 4 mg
IV sedation 0.02 mg/lb 15–20 min before procedure

6. *Midazolam* (Versed)
   IV sedation pre- and intraoperatively
7. *Triazolam* (Halcion)
   Tabs: 0.25, 0.5 mg
   Sig: one 0.25 or 0.5 mg tab H.S.
   For night time sedation
8. *Chlorazepate Dipotassium (Tranxene, Tranxene SD, Tranxene SD half-strength)*
   Tabs: 3.75, 7.5, 15 mg
   Caps: 3.75, 7.5, 15 mg
   Tabs: SD 22.5 mg
   Tabs: SD half-strength 11.25 mg
   Sig: 15–60 mg/day usually daily dose 30 mg/day
   Maintenance dose: 22.5 mg (single dose)
   Toxic dose: Do not exceed 90 mg/day
9. *Hydroxyzine Hydrochloride (Atarax)*
   Tabs: 10, 25, 50, 100 mg
   Syrup: 10 mg/tsp
   Sig: Adults, 50, 100 mg Q.I.D.
   Children 6–12 years, 50–100 mg in divided doses; children under 6, 50 mg in divided doses
   Toxic dose: Do not exceed 400 mg/day

IV. ANTIBIOTICS

A. Penicillins—Bactericidal—Cell Wall Synthesis Inhibitor, Broad-Spectrum 250 mg Tabs = 400,000 Units

a. *Penicillin—G*
   IM, IV, PO, not penicillinase resistant
   Tabs: 100; 200; 250; 400; 500; 800,000 units
   Streptococcus: Mild-moderate: 200–250,000 units q. 6–8 H. × 10 days
   Moderate-severe: 400–500,000 units q. 8 H. × 10 days
   Staphylococcus: Mild: 200–500,000 units q. 6–8 H.
b. *Procaine Penicillin G*
   IM only (not as painful) long-acting
   Various, Wycillin 300,000 U/ml
   Wycillin 600,000 U/ml
   Streptococcus: 600,000 1 million U/day × 10 days minimum
   Staphylococcus: 600,000 1 million U/day × 10 days minimum
c. *Benzathine Penicillin G*
   IM, oral, long-acting (2–4 weeks)
   IM: Bicillin long-acting
   Streptococcus-A: URI 1 inj of 1,200,000 units
   Venereal disease: 2.4–4.8 million U in 1 dose
   Tabs: Bicillin 200,000 U
   Streptococcus, Staphylococcus pneumococcus: 400–600,000 U q. 4–6 H. × 10 days
d. *Penicillin V (Phenoxymethyl Penicillin)*
   Oral: (tabs, liquid and powder) not penicillinase resistant
   Various: Tabs 125, 250, 500 mg
   Pen-Vee Tabs: 300 mg
e. *Penicillin V—Potassium*
   Various, Pen-Vee K, V-Cillen K
   Tabs: 125, 250, 500 mg
   Streptococcus: 125–300 mg q. 6–8 H. × 10 days
   Staphylococcus: 250–300 mg q. 6–8 H.
f. *Amoxicillin (Larotid)*
   Caps: 400; 800,000 units
   Suspension: 200; 400,000 units

*Not recommended for *Staphylococcus aureus*

1. *Penicillinase Resistant Penicillins*
   a. *Methicillin Sodium*
      IM, IV: Acapen, Celbenin, Staphcillin, 1, 4, 6 mg vials
      IM: 1 gm q. 4–6 H. (infants 25 mg/kg q. 6 H.)
      IV: 1 gm q. 6 H.
   b. *Nafcillin Sodium*
      IM, IV, P.O.
      Unipen tabs 500 mg
      Sig: 250–50 mg q. 4–6 H.
      IM 500 mg q. 6 H.
      IV 500 mg q. 4 H.
   c. *Oxacillin Sodium*
      IM, IV, P.O.
      Prostaphlin, Bactocill caps 250, 500 mg
      Inj: 50 mg, 1, 2, 4 gm vials
      Oral: Mild-moderate: 500 mg q. 6 H. × 5 days minimum
      Severe: 1 gm q. 4–6 H.
      IM 250–500 mg q. 4–6 H.
   d. *Cloxacillin Sodium*
      Oral
      Tegopen, Cloxapen caps 250–500 mg
      Oral: Mild-moderate: 250 mg q. 6 H. 1–2 H. A.C.
      Severe: 500 mg Q. 6 H. 1–2 H. A.C.
   e. *Dicloxicillin Sodium*
      Oral
      Dynapen caps 125, 500 mg
      Dycill, Pathocil caps 250 mg
      Mild-moderate: 125 mg q. 6 H.
      Severe: 250–500 mg q. 6 H.
2. *Nonpenicillinase Resistant* (Acid Stable)
   a. *Ampicillin Sodium*

IM, IV, P.O.
Inj: 125, 250, 500 mg, 1 gr vials
Tabs: 125 mg SK-Ampicillin, Amcill, Polycillin
Caps: 250, 500 mg various, Amcill, Pen-A
Oral: 250 mg q. 6 H. (50 mg/kg/day)
IM 250 mg q. 6 H.

b. *Carbenicillin Disodium*
IM, IV, P.O.
Especially for Pseudomonas and Proteus
Oral Geocillin: 382 mg tabs
Sig: 382–764 mg Q.I.D.
Inj: Geopen, Pyopen 1; 2; 5; 10 gm vials
Sig: 1–2 gm q. 6 H.

c. *Piperacillin*
IM, IV
Inj: 1–2 gm vials: piperacillin
Sig: 1–2 gm q. 6 H.
*Indicated for *Proteus mirabilis*; not indicated for *Staphylococcus aureus.*

B. Other Protein Synthesis Inhibitors

1. *Erythromycin*
Oral tabs: 250, 333, 400, 500 mg, enteric-coated various, E-Mycin, Ilotycin, Robimycin, EES
250–500 mg (stearate): various Erythrocin
500 mg (estorate): Ilosone 500
125 mg (stearate): Erythromycin stearate
400 mg (ethylsuccinate): EES
Caps (estolate) 125, 250 mg: Ilosone
Sig: 250 mg q. 6 H.—may go to 4 gm/day (30–50 mg/kg)
IM 50 mg/vial: Erythrocin Ethyl Succinate IM
Sig: 100 mg q. 4–8 H. (5–8 mg/kg/day)
*E-Mycin for patients allergic to penicillins

2. *Vancomycin HCl*
Inj and power
Inj: 500 mg/vial: Vancocin
Sig: 500 mg q. 6 H. or 1 gm q. 12 H. (20 mg/lb/day in divided doses)

3. *Lincomycin HCl*
Oral caps: 250, 500 mg: Lincocin
Sig: 500 mg T.I.D.
Inj: 300 mg 1, 2 gm/vial
IM: 600 mg q. 24 H.

4. *Clindamycin*
Oral caps: 75, 150 mg: Cleocin HCl
Sig: 150–300 mg q. 6 H. (8–12 mg/kg/day)
Inj: 300, 600, 900 mg: Cleocin Phosphate
Sig: 600–1200 mg/day

5. *Chloramphenicol*
Oral caps: 50, 100, 250 mg: various Chloromycetin
Inj: 100, 500 mg
Suspension: 150 mg/tsp
Sig: 50 mg/kg/day in divided doses Q. 6 H.

C. Cephalosporins—Bactericidal, Cell Wall Synthesis Inhibitor, Broad Spectrum, Penicillinase Resistant

1. *Cephalothin Sodium*
IM, IV
Inj: 1, 2, 4 gm/vial: Keflin
Sig: 500 mg–1 gm q. 4–6 H.
Do not exceed 12 gm/day

2. *Cephalexin*
P.O.
Keflex—Tab 1 gm
Caps: 250, 500 mg
Sig: 250–500 mg q. 6 H.—adult dose 1–4 gm/day
Pediatric dose: 25–50 mg/kg/day
Do not exceed 12 gm/day

3. *Cefazolin Sodium*
IM, IV
Inj: 250, 500 gm, 1, 5, 10 gm/vial—Kefzol, Ancef
Sig: 250—500 mg q. 8–12 H.
Do not exceed 12 gm/day
*Caution should be taken with patients with renal failure.

4. *Cefamandole Nafate*
IM, IVInj: 500 mg, 1 g, 2 g vials; Mandol
Sig: 1–2 mg q. 6 H. (normal renal function)
½–1 mg q. 8 H. (impaired renal function)
50–100 mg/kg/day
Do not exceed 12 gm/day

5. *Cefotaxime Sodium*
IM, IV
Inj: 50 mg, 1–2 mg vials; Claforan
Sig: 1 g q. 6–8 H.
50–100 mg/kg/day
Do not exceed 12 mg/day

6. *Cefadroxil Monohydrate*
P.O.
500 mg caps: Duricef
1 gm tabs
Suspension: 125, 250 mg/tsp
Sig: 1 g B.I.D., 500 mg Q.I.D. 30 mg/kg/day

7. *Cefaclor*
P.O.
Caps: 250, 500 mg: Ceclor
Suspension: 125, 250 mg/tsp
Sig: 250 mg–1 g q. 8 H.
20 mg/kg/day

8. *Moxalactam Disodium*
IM, IV
Inj: 1–2 mg vials; Moxam
Sig: 1–2 gm q. 6 H.
*Third-generation cephalosporin

D. Tetracyclines

1. *Tetracycline HCl*
   Oral caps: 100, 125, 250, 500 mg (various, Achromycin, Sumycin, Panmycin)
   Tabs: 250, 500 mg (various, Panmycin, Sumycin)
   Sig: 1–2 gm/day in 2–4 doses for 48–72 hr after symptoms (25–50 mg/kg/day in 4 doses)
   IM: 100, 250 mg/vial (Achromycin, Panmycin)
   Sig: 250 mg once per day or 300 mg q. 8–12 H.
   IV: 250, 500/vial Achromycin, Panmycin
   Sig: 250–500 mg
   Do not exceed 500 mg q. 6 H.
2. *Minocycline HCl*
   Oral caps: 50, 100 mg: Minocin
   Sig: 200 mg initial then 100 mg q. 12 H. or 100–200 mg
   Initial and 50 mg Q.I.D. (4 mg/kg then 2 mg/kg q. 12 H.)
   IV: 100 mg/vial: Minocin IV
   Sig: 200 mg then 100 mg q. 12 H.
   Do not exceed 400 mg/day
3. *Doxycycline Hyclate*
   Oral: 50, 100 mg caps (various, Vibramycin)
   Sig: 100 mg q. 12 H. for 24 hr, then 100 mg/day in single or divided doses (2 mg/lb in 21 doses for 24 hr then 1 mg/day)
   100 mg tabs—enteric-coated—Vibra-Tabs

E. Aminoglycosides

1. *Neomycin Sulfate*
   Oral tabs: 500 mg various, Mycifradin Sulfate, Neobiotic Sulfate
   Sig: Hepatic coma, 4–12 mg/day in divided doses
   Infectious diarrhea, 50 mg/kg/day
   Prophylaxis in abdominal surgery, 40 mg/lb/day q. 4 H.
   *Used mainly as gut sterilizer
2. *Streptomycin Sulfate*
   Inj: 1; 5 gm vials various
   Sig: Tuberculosis 1 gm/day with 200–300 mg isoniazid/day and 5 gm Pas T.I.D.
   Subacute bacterial endocardititis 1 gm B.I.D. for 1 week then 0.5 gm B.I.D. for second week
3. *Kanamycin Sulfate*
   Oral: Caps 500 mg; Kantrex
   Sig: lowers intestinal bacteria 8–12 gm/day in divided doses
   Inj: 500 mg, 1 gm vials: Kantrex
   IM less then 25 mg/kg/q. 12 H.
   IV les than 15 mg/kg/day
4. *Gentamycin*
   IV, inj 40 mg/ml vials: Garamycin
   Sig: 5 mg/kg/day in divided doses
5. *Tobramycin Sulfate*
   Inj: 40 mg vials: Nebcin
   Sig: IM with normal kidney 5 mg/kg q. 8 H. loading dose; 3 mg/kg/day q. 8 H. maintenance dose
6. *Amakacin*
   Inj: 100 mg/2 ml vials, 500 mg/2 ml vial—Amikin
   Sig: IM, 7.5 mg/kg as an infusion; IV, 7.5/kg as an infusion
   *Reserved for serious gram-negative infections
   Pediatric dose: 15 mg/kg/day in divided doses

F. Sulfadiazine—Used for Urinary Tract Infections

1. *Sulfamethoxazole*
   Tabs: 500 mg: Gantanol, Gantanol DS (1 gm tabs)
   Sig: Adult dose 1 gm T.I.D.
   Pediatric dose 75 mg/kg/day
   Toxic dose: Do not exceed 8–10 gm/day
   Pediatric suspension: ½ gm/tsp
2. *Sulfisoxazole*
   Oral Tabs: 500 mg: Gantrisin
   Sig: 2–5 gm/day B.I.D., T.I.D. or Q.I.D.
   Toxic dose: 150 mg/kg/day
   Inj: 400 mg/ml: Gantrisin
   Sig: 100 mg/kg/24 hrs
   Toxic dose: Do not exceed 6 gm/day
   Pediatric dose: 2 months–12 years 60–75 mg/kg
3. *Sulfadiazine*
   Oral tabs: 325, 500 mg
   Sig: 2–4 gm/day in 3–6 divided doses
   Inj: Sulfadiazine Sodium 250 mg/ml
   Sig: 100 mg/kg/day
   *If toxic dose is exceeded, renal impairment may be seen as well as CNS dysfunction and blood dyscrasias

G. Sulfonamides (Combo)

1. *Septra, Bactrim, Septrads, Bactrim DS*
   DS = Double strength
   Oral tabs: 400 mg sulfisoxazole and 80 mg trimethoprim
   Sig: $\dot{\tau}$ or $\dot{\tau}\dot{\tau}$ tab B.I.D.
   Pediatric dose: 8 mg/kg trimethoprim and 40 mg sulfisoxazole/day in 2 divided doses q. 12 H.
   Trimethoprim
   Oral: Tab 100 mg
   Sig: $\dot{\tau}$ tab B.I.D.
   Toxic dose: No reason to exceed normal dosage
   Daily dose: Drug only used for initial uncomplicated urinary tract infection

V. ANTIFUNGALS

1. *Nystatin*
   Tabs: 500,000 units: Nilstat, Mycostatin
   Sig: 0.5–1 million units T.I.D. for intestinal *Candida* infection with tetracyclines
   Terrastatin caps 0.25 million units plus 250 mg oxytetracycline
   Sig: 1 Q.I.D.
   Tetrastatin caps: 0.25 million units plus 25 mg tetracycline
   Sig: 4–8 caps/day Q.I.D.
   Declostatin caps 0.25 million units plus 150 mg demeclocycline
   Sig: 1 Q.I.D. or 2 B.I.D.
   Tabs: 0.5 million units plus 300 mg demeclocycline
   Sig: 1 B.I.D.
   Children above 8 years of age, usually daily dose of 3–6 mg/lb (body weight/day)
2. *Amphotericin B*
   Used for serious systemic fungal infections
   Inj: 50 mg/vial: Fungizone IV
   Sig: 0.25 mg/kg/day
   Toxic dose: 1.5 mg/kg/day
   *Caution should be taken with patients with renal failure
3. *Griseofulvin*
   For tinea, *Trichophyton, Microsporum, Epidermophyton*
   Tabs: 125, 250, 500 mg: Fulvicin-U/F, Grifulvin V
   Grisactin: Caps 125, 250 mg, Tabs 500 mg
   Gris-PEG: Ultramicrosize tabs (equivalent to 250 mg): 125 mg
   Sig: 500 mg/day up to 1 gm/day (5 mg/lb/day)
   *Blood dyscrasias, nausea, vomiting, diarrhea, CNS effects (i.e., dizziness, fatigue, mental confusion)
   *Caution should be exercised with patients with known allergies to penicillin
5. *Ketoconazole* (Nizoral)
   Synthetic, broad-spectrum
   Antifungal
   For Candidiasis, chronic mucocutaneous candidiasis, oral thrush, candiduria, coccidioidomycosis, histoplasmosis, chromomycosis, paracoccidioidomycosis
   Sig: 200 mg (1 tab) in a single daily dose

VI. ANTIMALARIALS

1. *Quinine Sulfate*
   Caps: 3, 5 gr, various
   Sig: 20 gr/day for 7 days
2. *Quinacrine HCl*
   Tabs: 100 mg Atabrine HCl
   Sig: 200 mg q. 6 H. × 5 days, then 100 mg T.I.D. for suppression 100 mg/day

3.*Chloroquine PhosphateTabs:* 250 mg various
Sig: 1 gm then 500 mg 6–8 hr later, then 500 mg/day for suppression: 500 mg same day each week

VII. ANTITUBERCULOSIS

1. *Isoniazid* (isonicotinic acid hydrazine), INH
   Tabs: 50, 100, 300 mg, various
   100, 300 mg: Hyzyd
   Sig: 5 mg/kg/day (up to 300 mg)
2. *Streptomycin:* See Aminoglycosides
3. *Viomycin Sulfate:* Viocin
4. *Ethambutol HCl:* Myambutol
5. *Rifampin:* Rifadin, Rimactane

VIII. ANTIDIABETICS

Insulin Injection: Iletin 40, 80, 100 units/ml 15–30 min before meal
Longer Acting: Insulin zinc suspension: 40, 80, 100 units/ml Semilente Iletin insulin
Isophane Insulin Suspension (NPH): same, NPH Iletin, Isophane Insulin
Insulin Zinc Susp: Short- and long-acting Lente suspension
Globin Zinc Insulin: Short- and long-acting
Protamine Zinc Insulin: Suspension (PZI) short- and long-acting
Insulin-Zinc Suspension: Extended—short- and long-acting Ultralente Iletin insulin
Sulfonylureas: Timed release of endogenous insulin

A. *Tolbutamide:* Various and Orinase—500 mg tabs, intermediate-acting, given B.I.D. or T.I.D. 1–2 gm/day
B. *Acetohexamide:* Dymelor—250, 500 mg tabs—short-acting, 1 or 2 doses/day 250 mg–1.5 g/day
C. *Tolazamide:* Tolinase—100, 250, 500 mg tabs, intermediate-acting, 1–2 doses/day—100–500 mg/day

Chlorpropamide: Diabinase—100, 250 mg tabs, long-acting, 1 dose/day, 100–250 mg/day
Glipizide: Glucotrol 5, 10 mg tabs long-acting 1–2 doses/day, 5–40 mg/day

Insulin Onset-Duration Chart

Type	Onset	Peak Action	Duration
	hours	*hours*	*hours*
Regular	½–1	2–3	6
Globin Zinc	2	8–16	24
NPH (Isophane Insulin)	1–1½	8–12	24
Lente (Zinc Suspension)	1–1½	8–12	24
PZI (Protamine Zinc Insulin)	4–8	14–20	36
Semilente (Zinc Suspension)	½–1	5–7	12–16
Ultralente	4–8	16–18	36

IX. ANTIEMETICS

A. Phenothiazines

1. *Prochlorperazine*
   Oral tabs: 5, 10, 25 mg Compazine
   Caps (sustained release): 10, 15, 30, 75 mg spansule
   Sig: 5 or 10 mg tabs T.I.D. or Q.I.D.
   15 mg caps q. a.m. or 10 mg caps q. 12 H.
   Inj: 5 mg/ml
   Sig: 5–10 mg if necessary repeat q. 3–4 H.
   Do not exceed 40 mg/day
   Suppositories: 2.5, 5.0, 25 mg
   Sig: 25 mg B.I.D.
   Syrup: 5 mg/5 ml
   Pediatric dose: Not to be used in children less than 20 lb or 2 years old
   Children 20–29 lb: 2–5 mg Q.D. or B.I.D. (do not exceed 7.5 mg/day)
   Children 30–39 lb: 2.5 mg B.I.D. or T.I.D. (do not exceed 10 mg/day)
   Children 40–85 lb: 2.5 mg T.I.D. or 5 mg B.I.D. (do not exceed 15 mg/day)
2. *Promethazine*
   Oral tabs: 12.5, 25, 50 mg Phenergan
   Sig: 25 mg Q.I.D.
   Suppositories: 12.5, 25, 50 mg
   Syrup: 6.25 or 25 mg/5 ml
   Inj Sig: 12.5 or 25 mg q. 4–6 H.
   *For prophylaxis or nausea and vomiting during surgery
   Sig: 25 mg q. 4–6 H.
3. *Hydroxyzine*
   Oral caps: 25, 50, 100 mg: Vistaril
   Sig: 25–100 mg B.I.D. or T.I.D.
   Inj: 25, 50, 75, 100 mg/ml
   Sig: 25–100 mg IM q. 4–6 H.
   Pediatric dose: 0.5 mg/kg IM

B. Antihistamines

1. *Dimenhydrinate*
   Oral tabs: 50 mg Dramamine
   Sig: 50 mg stat + 50 mg q. 4 H.
   Usual dose 1–2 tabs q. 4–6 H.
   Do not exceed 8 tabs/24 hr
   *Should be taken ½ to 1 hr before starting activity
   Pediatric dose: Children 6–12, ½ tab q. 6–8 H., do not exceed 3 tabs/24 hr; children 2–6, up to ½ tab q. 6–8 H., do not exceed 1½ tab/24 hr

X. ANTIHISTAMINES

1. *Diphenhydramine HCl*
   Oral caps: 25, 50 mg, Benadryl
   Sig: 50 mg T.I.D. or Q.I.D. (5 mg/kg/day)
   Inj: 10, 50 mg/ml Benadryl
   Sig: 10–50 mg IV or deep IM
   Toxic dose: 400 mg/day
   Pediatric dose: Children 2–12 years, 25–50 mg B.I.D. or T.I.D.; children under 2 years, use good judgment
2. *Chlorpheniramine Maleate*
   Oral tabs: 4 mg Chlor-Trimeton
   Sustained-release tabs: 8, 12 mg Chlortrimeton Repetabs
   Sustained-release caps: 8, 12 mg *various*
   Sig: 4 mg T.I.D. or Q.I.D.
   Sustained-release, 8–12 mg H.S. or q. 8–10 H. during day
3. *Chlorpheniramine HCl*
   Inj: 10, 20, 100 mg/ml Histaspan
   Chlor-Trimeton 10, 10 mg/ml
   Used for (*a*) anaphylaxis—10–20 mg IV single dose; (*b*) allergic response–5–20 mg as single dose; (*c*) adjunct to epinephrine
4. *Brompheniramine Meleate*
   Oral tabs: 4 mg Dimetane
   Sustained-release tabs: 8, 12 mg: Dimetane
   Sig: 4–8 mg T.I.D. or Q.I.D.
   8–12 mg of sustained-release tabs q. 8–12 H.
   Inj: 10 mg/ml: Dimetane-10
   100 mg/ml: Diametane-100
   5–20 mg q. 3–12 H.
   Toxic dose: 40 mg/day
   Pediatric dose: Use good judgment

5. *Promethazine HCl*
   Oral tabs: 12.5, 25, 50 mg Phenergan
   Used for: (*a*) allergy 25 mg H.S. or 12.5 mg A.C. and H.S.; (*b*)sedation: 25–50 mg (12.5–25 mg); (*c*) preoperatively: 50 mg night before (12.5-25 mg); 50 mg with equal amount meperidine; (*d*) postoperatively: with analgesic: 25–50 mg (12.5–25 mg); (*e*) nausea and vomiting: 25 mg then 12.5-25 mg q. 4–6 H. P.R.N.
   Inj: 25, 50 mg/ml Phenergan
   Used for: (*a*) allergy 25 mg IM or IV, repeat within 2 H. P.R.N.; (*b*) Sedation: same as oral dose; (*c*) Preoperatively: same as oral dose; (*d*) postoperatively: with analgesic same as oral dose; (*e*) nausea and vomiting: same as oral dose
   Suppository: 12.5, 25, 50 mg
   Syrup: 6.25 mg/tsp
   Pediatric dose: Usually 12.5–25 mg single dose
6. *Dimenhydrinate*
   Oral tabs: 50 mg Dramamine
   Sig: 50–100 mg q. 4 H.
   Inj: 50 mg/ml Dramamine
   Sig: 50 mg P.R.N.
   Suppository: 100 mg Dramamine
   Sig: 100 mg q. 12–24 H.
7. *Terfenadine*
   Oral tabs: 60 mg Seldane
   Sig: 60 mg B.I.D.

XI. NONSTEROIDAL ANTI-INFLAMMATORIES

1. *Ibuprofen*
   Tabs: 300, 400, 600, 800 mg Motrin, Rufen (not in 800 mg)
   Sig: 300–800 T.I.D. or Q.I.D., varies with patient
   Toxic dose: Do not exceed 3200 mg/day
   If patient has gastrointestinal symptoms, take with meal, milk, or antacid of choice
2. *Fenoprofen*
   Caps: 200, 300 mg Nalfon
   Sig: 200–300 mg q. 4–6 H.
   Toxic dose: Do not exceed 3200 mg/day
   If patient has gastrointestinal symptoms, take with meal, milk, or antacid of choice
   *Indicated for acute gouty attacks
3. *Ketoprofen*
   Caps: 50, 75 mg Orudis
   Sig: 75 mg T.I.D. or 50 mg Q.I.D.
   Toxic dose: Do not exceed 300 mg/day
4. *Suprofen*
   Caps: 200 mg Suprol
   Sig: One cap q. 4–6 H. P.R.N.
5. *Naproxen*
   Tabs: 250, 375, 500 mg Naprosyn
   Sig: 250–500 mg B.I.D.
   Toxic dose: Do not exceed 1.2 g/day
6. *Tolmetin*
   Tabs: 200 mg Tolectin-Tolectin DS 400 mg
   Sig: 200 mg T.I.D.
   Toxic dose: Do not exceed 2000 mg/day
   If gastrointestinal symptoms occur, take with milk, meal, or antacid of choice
7. *Indomethacin*
   Caps: 25, 50, 75 mg Indocin
   Sig: 25–50 mg B.I.D. or T.I.D., 75 mg B.I.D.
   *Indicated for treatment of acute gout; 50 mg T.I.D. until pain is tolerable, then decrease dose
8. *Phenylbutazone*
   Tabs: 100 mg Butazolidin, Azolid
   Caps: 100 mg
   Sig: For arthritis, initial 300–600 mg T.I.D. or Q.I.D.
   Gout: initial 400 mg then 100 mg q. 4 H. until inflammation is down—do not exceed a week—not recommended
9. *Oxyphenbutazone*
   Tabs: 100 mg Tandearil, Oxalid
   Sig: Same as for phenylbutazone
10. *Sulindac*
    Tabs: 150, 200 mg: Clinoril
    Sig: For arthritis, tab B.I.D. with meal, milk, or antacid of choice
    Toxic dose: 400 mg/day
11. *Choline Magnesium Trisilicate*
    Tabs: 500, 750 mg: Trisilicate
    Sig: For arthritis, 500 mg–1 gm B.I.D.
    Toxic dose: 1.5 g/day
12. *Magnesium Salicylate*
    Tabs: 545 mg: Magan
    Sig: For arthritis, tab q. 4 H.
    *Caution: All should be taken with meal, milk, or antacid of choice to minimize gastrointestinal symptoms.
    *Pediatric dose: Consult physician
13. *Piroxicam*
    Caps: 10, 20 mg: Feldene
    Sig: 20 mg Q.D.
14. *Diflunisal*
    Tabs: 250, 500 mg: Dolobid
    Sig: 1 gm initially followed by 500 mg q. 12 H.
    Do not exceed 1500 mg/day
15. *Meclofenamate Sodium*
    Caps: 50, 100 mg: Meclomen
    Sig: 50–100 mg T.I.D. or Q.I.D.
    Toxic dose: Do not exceed 400 mg/day

COMPARISON CHART—NONSTEROIDAL ANTI-INFLAMMATORY AGENTS[a]

Drugs	Indications	Effective Dosage	Principal Side Effects	Half-Life	Comparison with Aspirin
1. Aspirin	RA, OA, JRA, Antipyresis, colds	OA—300—600 mg RA—3.5–6 reg dose	GI irritation, bleeding, anemia	20 min	
2. Disalcid	RA, OA and other rheumatic disorders	1 gm B.I.D. or T.I.D. (3000 mg/day)	Nausea, dyspepsia, heartburn	1 hr	Less anti-inflammatory effects, milder side effects
3. Meclomen	RA, OA (hip, knee, foot), gout	200–400 mg/day	GI irritation, rash	2–3 hr	Lower toxicity, but still not the primary drug of choice in arthritic condition
4. Clinoril	RA, OA, AS, gout	150–200 mg B.I.D.	GI irritation	7.8 hr	
5. Nalfon	RA, OA (acute and long term)	300–600 mg T.I.D. or Q.I.D.	GI irritation (mild)	3 hr	
6. Motrin	RA, OA	400–600 mg T.I.D. or Q.I.D.	GI irritation, headache, rash	1.8–2.0 hr	
7. Indocin and Indocin S.R.	RA, OA, AS, gout (acute)	25 mg B.I.D. (150–200 mg/day); gout 50 mg T.I.D.	GI toxicity (mild), rash, headache	4.5 hr	
8. Naprosyn	RA, musculoskeletal and soft tissue inflammation, primary dysmenorrhea, acute gout, JRA	250 mg–500 mg B.I.D.	GI irritation, skin eruptions	13 hr	Low incidence of side effects
9. Butazolidin	RA, AS, gout (acute) OA (hip, knees), painful shoulder	Use at smallest effective dose—about 400 mg/day	GI irritation, nausea, dyspepsia	8.4 hr	Much stronger—not recommended
10. Tolectin	RA, OA, JRA	400 mg T.I.D. (1200 mg/day)	GI irritation	1 hr	Better tolerated

[a] RA, rheumatoid arthritis; OA, osteoarthritis; AS, ankylosing spondylitis; JRA, juvenile rheumatoid arthritis; GI, gastrointestinal.

IDENTIFICATION TABLE FOR NONSTEROIDAL AGENTS

Brand Name	Generic Name	Appearance	Cost/Pill
1. Aspirin	Acetylsalicylic acid	Round white tablets	about 1¢
2. Disalcid	Salsalate	Round green tablets or green and pale green capsules 1 cap = 500 mg	±9¢
3. Meclomen	Meclofenamate sodium	50 mg—orange and peach capsules	50 mg—±39¢
		100 mg—orange and white capsules	100 mg—±55¢

Brand Name	Generic Name	Appearance	Cost/Pill
4. Clinoril	Sulindac	Yellow hexagonal tablets	150 mg—±70¢ 200 mg—±83¢
5. Nalfon	Fenoprofen calcium	200 mg—yellow and white capsules 300 mg—orange capsules 600 mg—orange oval tablets	200 mg—±39¢ 300 mg—±46¢ 600 mg—±62¢
6. Motrin	Ibuprofen	300 mg—white round tablets 400 mg—orange round tablets 600 mg—peach oval tablets	300 mg—±12¢ 400 mg—±23¢ 600 mg—±33¢ 800 mg—±43¢
7. Indocin	Indomethacin	Blue and white capsules	25 mg—±12¢ 50 mg—±65¢ 75 mg—±95¢
8. Naprosyn	Naproxen	250 mg—yellow round tablets 375 mg—peach oval tablets 500 mg—yellow oval tablets	250 mg—±78¢ 375 mg—±97¢ 500 mg—±$1.06
9. Butazolidin	Phenylbutazone	Round red tablets	100 mg—±46¢
10. Tolectin	Tolmetin sodium	200 mg—white round tablets 400 mg—red capsules	200 mg—±43¢ 400 mg—±70¢
11. Dolobid	Diflunisal	250 mg—peach tablets 500 mg—orange tablets	250 mg—±40¢ 500 mg—±51¢
12. Feldene	Piroxicam	10 mg—maroon and blue capsules 20 mg—maroon capsules	10 mg—±$1.07¢ 20 mg—±$1.75¢

DRUG RATING TABLE

Rating Scale: 1 = low toxicity
6 = highest toxicity

Drug	Effectiveness	Toxicity	Convenience	Drug Interaction	Total
1. Aspirin	1	3	3	2	9
2. Disalcid	1	2	3	1	7
3. Meclomen	1	2	1	1	5
4. Clinoril[a]	1	1	1	1	4
5. Nalfon	1	1	3	1	6
6. Motrin	1	2	2	1	6
7. Indocin	1	5	2	1	9
8. Naprosyn[a]	1	1	1	1	4
9. Butazolidin	1	6	2	3	12
10. Tolectin	1	1	2	1	5

[a]Most effective with least toxicity

Additional Comments

A. The mode of action of the nonsteroidal anti-inflammatory agents is still unknown. It is known that their action is *not* due to pituitary adrenal stimulation. All inhibit prostaglandin synthesis, and this is believed to be involved in the anti-inflammatory action.
B. None of the nonsteroidals alter the course of the underlying disease.
C. All cause reduction in joint swelling, pain and morning stiffness and improved functional capacity.

D. All are rapidly absorbed after oral administration. The primary route of excretion is via the kidney and in the urine.
E. Most of the side effects are the same, with gastrointestinal irritation being the most common one reported. Others include CNS effects, headache, dizziness, pruritus, tinnitus, edema, dyspnea, etc.
F. Nonsteroidals are not recommended for pregnant women, nursing mothers or children.
G. Most effect platelet aggregation and increase bleeding time.
H. All nonsteroidals have the same effectiveness against inflammation and pain, with Clinoril and Naprosyn having the low side effects. Nevertheless, close supervision is recommended in the patient with upper gastrointestinal disease.

XII. CORTICOSTEROIDS

1. *Cortisone*
   Tabs: 5, 25 mg: Cortisone Acetate (various)
   Cortone Acetate
   Inj: 24, 50 mg various, Cortone Acetate
   Sig: Chronic: 25–50 mg/day, may be altered
   Acute: 75–120 mg/day, may be altered
2. *Hydrocortisone*
   Tabs: 10, 20 mg: various, Cortef (also 5 mg), Hydrocortone
   Sig: Chronic: 20–40 mg/day, may alter
   Acute: 60–120 mg/day, may alter
   Inj: Various: 25, 50 mg/ml; Cortef: 50 mg/ml, IM only; Hydrocortone Phosphate: 50 mg/ml; Solu-Cortef (NA Succinate): 100, 250, 500, 1000 mg/vial
   Sig: ⅓–½ oral dose q. 12 H.
   Local inj: Hydrocortisone Acetate: various 25, 50 mg/ml; Cortef Acetate: 50 mg/ml
   Sig: Small joint: 10–25 mg
   Tendon: 5–12 mg
3. *Prednisone*
   Tabs: Various: 1, 2, 5, 20, 40 mg
   Deltasone: 2.5, 5, 10, 20, 50 mg
   Sig: 5–60 mg/day
4. *Prednisolone*
   Tabs: Various: 1, 2.5, 5 mg; Delta-Cortef: 5 mg
   Sig: 5–60 mg/day
   Local inj: As a phosphate: 20 mg/ml: various, Hydeltrasol
   Sig: Small joint: 4–5 mg and 4 mg/ml: Celestone Phosphate; Tendon sheath: 2–5 mg; Bursa: 10–15 mg
   As an acetate: various: 25, 50, 100 mg/ml
   Sig: Small joint: 5–12.5 mg; Tendon: 5–10 mg
5. *Triamcinolone*
   Tabs: 2, 4, 8 mg: Various, Aristocort
   Sig: Rheumatoid arthritis, dermatitis, and allergy: 8–12 mg; Systemic lupus erythematosus 20–32 mg
   Local inj: Triamcinolone acetonide: Kenalog-10 or 40 (10 or 40 mg/ml); Triamcinolone hexacetonide: Aristospan: 20 mg/ml
6. *Methylprednisolone*
   Tabs: 2, 4, 6 mg: Medrol: Medrol Dose Pack (contains 21 4 mg tabs)
   Caps: (sustained action): 2, 4 mg Medrol
   Sig: 4–48 mg/day
   Local inj (Acetate): 20, 40, 80 mg/ml: Depo-Medrol
   Sig: Small joints: 4–10 mg
7. *Dexamethasone*
   Tabs: 0.25, 0.5, 0.75, 1.5, 4 mg: various, Decadron, Hexadrol (does not come in 0.25 mg)
   Sig: 0.75–9 mg/day
   Local inj: Phosphate: 4 mg/ml: various, Decadron Phosphate, Hexadrol Phosphate
   Sig: Small joints: 0.8–1 mg; Tendon sheath: 0.4–1 mg
   Acetate: 8 mg/ml: Decadron-LA
   Sig: 0.8–4 mg
8. *Betamethasone*
   Tabs: 6 mg: Celestone
   Sig: 6–7.2 mg/day
   Local inj: 3 mg acetate and 3 mg phosphate/ml in 5-ml vials: Celestone Soluspan
   Sig: For the foot at 3 day to 1 week intervals: Bursitis: 0.5ml ± 0.25ml
   Periarticular fibrocitis: Approximately 0.5ml
   Gout: 0.5–1ml

XIII. DIURETICS

1. *Thiazide Diuretics*
   a. *Chlorothiazide*: Onset 2 hr; 6–12-hr duration
      Oral Tabs: 250, 500 mg various: Diuril
      Used for (*a*) Edema: 0.5–1 gm Q. D. or B.I.D. may be intermittent; (*b*) Hypertension (Hypt): 0.5 gm Q. 12 H.; (*c*) Congestive heart failure (CHF): consult internist
      Inj: Diuril: 500 mg/20ml vial
      Pediatric dose: 10 mg/lb/day in 2 doses
      Children 2–12 years, 375 mg–1 gm daily in 2 doses;
      Children 6 months–2 years, 125 mg daily in 2 doses;
      Children infant–6 months: 15 mg/kg/day in 2 doses

b. *Hydrochlorothiazide*: Onset 2 hrs, 6–12-hr duration
   Oral tabs: 25, 50, 100 mg: Esidrix, Thiuretic, Hydrodiuril
   Used for (*a*) Edema: 25–125 mg/day; (*b*) (Hypt): 75 mg/day; (*c*) (CFH): Consult physician
   Pediatric dose: Children 2–12 years, 37.5–100 mg in 2 doses; Children infant–2 years: 12.5–37.5 mg in 2 doses
c. *Cyclothiazide*: Onset 2 hr, 6–12-hr duration
   Oral tabs: 2 mg: Anhydron
   Sig: 2 mg/day
   Pediatric dose: Not indicated

2. *Acetazolamide (Carbonic Anhydrase Inhibitor)*
   Oral tabs: 125, 250 mg: Diamax
   Used for (*a*) Edema: 250–375 mg Q. D. for 1–2 days alternating with day of rest; (*b*) Hypt: Used as adjunct; (*c*) CHF
   Pediatric dose: Not indicated
3. *Furosemide* (Loop) – POTENT
   Oral tabs: 20, 40 mg: Lasix
   Sig: 20–80 mg Q. D. or B.I.D. or can be more if dosage not sufficient
   Toxic dose: 6 gm/day
   Pediatric dose: Infants: 2 mg/kg
   Inj: 10 mg/ml Lasix
   Sig: 20–40 mg ad or B.I.D. or more
   Oral solution: 10 mg/ml
4. *Methyclothiazide*: Onset 2 hr, 6–12-hr duration
   Oral tabs: 2.5, 5 mg: Eutron
   Sig: 2.5–10 mg Q.D.
   Used for (*a*) Edema: tab Q.D.; (*b*) CHF: tab Q.D.; (*c*) Hypt: used as adjunct 2.5–5 mg Q.D.
   Pediatric dose: Not indicated
5. *Metolazone*: Onset 2 hr, 6–12-hr duration
   Oral tabs: 2.5, 5, 10 mg: Zaroxolyn, Diulo
   Sig: Therapy should be individualized according to patient response
   Used for (*a*) Edema: individualized; (*b*) CHF: 2.5–10 mg Q.D.; (*c*) Hypt: 2.5–5 mg Q.D.; (*d*) Renal failure: 5–20 mg Q.D.
   Pediatric dose: Not indicated
6. *Ethacrynic Acid* (Loop)—POTENT
   Oral tabs: 25, 50 mg: Edecrin
   Sig: 50–100 mg/day (up to 200 mg) continuous or intermittent
   Used for (*a*) edema; (*b*) CHF; (*c*) Hypt
   IV: 5 mg/vial: Edecrin Q.D.
   Sig: 50 mg (0.5–1 mg/kg) or B.I.D.
7. *Spironolactone* (Distal Tubule, Competes with Aldosterone)
   Oral tabs: 25 mg: Aldactone
   Used for (*a*) Hypt: 50–100 mg/day in divided doses, may combo with thiazide; (*b*) Edema: 100 mg/day in divided doses
8. *Triameterene* (Distal Tubule, Does Not Compete with Aldosterone)
   Oral caps: 50, 100 mg: Dyrenium
   100 mg B.I.D. P.C. (not more than 300 mg/day)
9. *Mannitol Osmotic*
   Inj: 25% various
   5, 10, 15, 20% Mannitol IV, Osmitrol
   Sig: 50–200 mg/day
   Used for cerebral edema

A. Diuretics (Combo)

1. *Spironolactone Hydrochlorothiazide*
   Oral tabs: 25 mg spironolactone and 25 mg hydrochlorothiazide: *Aldactazide*
   Used for (*a*) Edema: 25 mg Q.I.D., may be more; (*b*) Hypt: 1–8tabs/day
   Pediatric dose: Edema: 0.75–1.5 mg/lb/day
   *Advantage—decreases potassium loss
2. *Triameterene Hydrochlorothiazide*
   Oral tabs: 25 mg triameterene and 25 mg hydrochlorothiazide: *Dyazide*
   Sig: $\bar{\text{i}}$ cap Q.D.
   Uses: See Aldactazide above
   Pediatric dose: Unknown
   *Advantage—decreases potassium loss

XIV. SYSTEMIC ENZYMES

1. *Ananase*: Bromelains Proteolytic Enzyme
   Oral tabs: 50 (50,000 units) and 100 (100,000 units)
   Sig: 100,000 units Q.I.D. maintenance: 100,000 units B.I.D.
   *Avoid using with patients allergic to pineapples
   *Anti-inflammatory enzyme

2. *Chymoral-100* Proteolytic Enzyme
   Oral tabs: 50,000 units trypsin, 100,000 units chymotrypsin
   Sig: 1 tab Q.I.D.
   Chymoral-100—100,000 armour units of enzymatic activity
   Chymoral—50,000 armour units of enzymatic activity
3. *Orenzyme Bitabs*
   Oral tabs: 100,000 units chymotrypsin, 8,000 units trypsin
   Sig: 1 tab Q.I.D.
4. *Papain Proteolytic Enzyme*
   Oral tabs: 100,000 Warner-Lambert units
   Sig: 2 tabs Q.I.D. × 4 days
   Used for (*a*) Digestive enzyme; (*b*) Anti-inflammatory agent

XV. MUSCLE RELAXANTS

1. *Curare*: Tubocurarine Chloride
   Nondepolarizing neuromuscular blockade —3 mg/ml
   Surgery: ½ unit/lb body weight
   Sig: 40–60 units (6–9) and 20–30 units 5 min later if required
   *May be used as a diagnostic agent for myasthenia gravis
2. *Gallamine Triethiodide* (Flexedil IV)
   Nondepolarizing neuromuscular blockade
   Inj: 20–100 mg/ml
   Sig: 1 mg/kg body weight
3. *Pancuronium BR* (Pavulon)
   Nondepolarizing neuromuscular blockade 5 times as potent as curare
   Inj: 2 mg/ml in 2-, 5-ml ampules
   1 mg/ml in 10-ml vials
   Sig: 0.04–0.1 mg/kg body weight
4. *Decamethonium BR* (Syncurine)
   Depolarizing neuromuscular blockade
   Inj: Initial IV; 2–2.5 mg
   1 mg/ml in 10-ml vials
5. *Succinylcholine* (Anectine, Sulostrin)
   Depolarizing neuromuscular blockade
   Inj: 20, 50, 100 mg/ml in 10-ml vials
   Sig: 25–75 mg IV
6. *Carisoprodol* (Rela, Soma)
   Oral tabs: 350 mg
   Sig: 350 mg Q.I.D.
   Toxic dose: 1.4 gm/day
   *Not recommended for children
7. *Chlorzoxazone* (Paraflex)
   Oral tabs: 250 mg
   250 mg T.I.D. or Q.I.D.
   Pediatric dose: 50–500 mg T.I.D. or Q.I.D.
8. *Orphenadrine Citrate* (Norflex, various)
   Inj: 30 mg/ml
   Sig: 60 mg IM or IV B.I.D.
   Oral tabs: 100 mg
   Sig: ī 100-mg tab B.I.D.
9. *Diazepam* (Valium)
   Oral tabs: 2, 5, 10 mg
   Inj: 5 mg/ml
   Adult: 2–10 mg T.I.D. or Q.I.D. oral dose
   Elderly: 2 mg 1–2/day oral dose
   Children: 1–2 mg T.I.D. or Q.I.D. oral dose
   IM or IV: 2–20 mg
10. *Methocarbamol* (Robaxin)
    Oral tabs: 500, 750 mg
    Sig: 1.5 gm T.I.D. or Q.I.D.
    Inj: 100 mg/ml
    Sig: 1 gm/day in divided doses
    Toxic dose: 3 gm/day for more than 3 days
11. *Cyclobenzaprine* (Flexeril)
    Oral tabs: 10 mg
    Sig: 20–40 mg/day in divided doses
    Toxic dose: Do not exceed 60 mg/day
12. *Quinamm*
    Oral tabs: 260 mg quinine sulfate
    Sig: 1 tab H.S. for nocturnal leg cramps
    *All medications in this category may cause dizziness, drowsiness, gastrointestinal upset, CNS depressant effects.

A. Muscle Relaxants (Combo)

1. *Parafon Forte*
   Oral tabs: 250 mg chlorzoxazone, 300 mg acetaminophen
   Sig: īī tab Q.I.D.
2. *Soma Compound*
   Oral tabs: 200 mg carisoprodol, 32 mg caffeine and 160 mg phenacetin
   Sig: ī or īī T.I.D. and at bedtime.
3. *Norgesic*
   Sig: ī or īī T.I.D. or Q.I.D.
4. *Norgesic Forte*
   Oral tabs: Double everything as in Norgesic above
   Sig: ½–1 tab T.I.D. or Q.I.D.
5. *Robaxisal*
   Oral tabs: 400 mg methocarbamol, 325 mg aspirin
   īī tab Q.I.D.

XVI. TOPICALS

A. Antihistamines: For itching; do not apply to raw, blistered or oozing wounds; if a burning sensation, discontinue use.

1. *Benadryl Cream*
   2% diphenhydramine HCl in 1 and 2 oz
2. *Caladryl Cream*
   1% diphenhydramine HCl with calamine in 1.05 oz
3. *Caladryl Lotion*
   1% diphenhydramine with calamine, camphor and 2% alcohol in 75ml and 6 oz
   All medications are available over-the-counter and should be applied T.I.D. or Q.I.D.

B. Antibiotics

1. *Clindamycin—Cleocin T*
   30; 60-ml bottle—topical solution
2. *Tetracycline:* Achromycin Ointment: 3% in ½ and 1 oz
3. *Chloramphenicol:* Chloromycetin Creme: 1% in 1 oz
4. *Erythromycin:* Ilotycin Ointment: 1% in ½, 1 and 16 oz; topical solution: 2% in 30 ml
5. *Gentamycin:* Garamycin or G-myticin ointment and creme: 1% sulfate in 15 gm
6. *Bacitracin Ointment:* Various: 500 U/gm in ½, 1, 4, 16 oz

7. *Neomycin Sulfate as ointment:* Various: 5 gm (0.5%), 1 gm in ½ and 1 oz
8. *Topicycline:* 2.2 mg/ml tetracycline HCl solution
   *All medications should be used B.I.D.

C. Combination Antibiotics

1. *Bacitracin-Neomycin Ointment:* Various: 500 U bacitracin and 5 mg neomycin/gm in ½ and 1 oz
2. *Neosporin-G Creme:* 10,000 U polymyxin B, 5 mg neomycin and 25 mg gramicidin/gm in 15 gm
3. *Polysporin Ointment:* 10,000 U polymyxin B, 500 U bacitracin 1 gm in ½ and 1 oz
4. *Neosporin Ointment:* 5,000 U polymyxin B, 5 mg neomycin and 400 U bacitracin/gm in ½ and 1 oz

D. Antibiotic Enzyme Combo

1. *Elase-Chloromycetin Ointment:* 10 mg chloromycetin, 1 U fibrinolysin and 6,666 U desoxyribonuclease/gm in 10 and 30 gm

E. Antifungals

1. *Calcium Undecylenate:* Antibacterial and antifungal
   Cruex: Powder 10%
   Squeeze bottle: 1.5 and 3 oz
2. *Undecylenic Acid:* Athlete's foot, ringworm, exclusive of hair and nails (over-the-counter)
   Onychomycetin—25%
   Desenex: Ointment 5% acid, 20% zinc: 0.9, 1.8 oz and 1 lb powder: 2% acid, 20% zinc: 1.5, 3 oz and 1 lb
   Solution: 10% acid: 1.5 oz
3. *Iodochlorhydroxyquin:* Ointment and creme for eczema, tinea pedis, etc., powder for wounds and ulcers
   Various: creme: 3%, 1, 4 oz and 1, 6 lb
   Ointment: 3%, 4 oz and 1, 6 lb
   Powder: ½, 4 oz
   Vioform Creme: 3%, 1 oz
   Ointment: 3%, 1 oz
   Powder: ½ oz
4. *Miconazole Nitrate: Trichophyton rubrum, Menagrophytes, Epidermophyton floccosum, Candida albicans*
   Micatin: Creme: 2%, 1 oz, 15 gm
   Lotion: 2%, 12 and 30ml
5. *Haloprogin:* Tineas: *Trichophyton, Microsporum, Epidermophyton floccosum*
   Halotex: Creme: 1%, 30 gm
   Solution: 1%, 10, 30ml
6. *Tolnaftate:* Tineas: *Trichophyton, Microsporum, E. floccosum*
   Tinactin: Cream: 1% in 15 gm
   Powder: 1% in 45 gm
   Aerosol: 1% in 5 oz (liquid or powder)
   Aftate: Gel: 1% in 0.5 oz
   Powder: 1% in 2.25 oz
   Aerosol: 1% in 5 oz (liquid or powder)
7. *Clotrimazole:* Tineas and *Candida albicans*
   Lotrimin: Creme: 1% in 15 and 30 gm
   Solution: 1% in 10 and 30 gm
   Mycelex: Creme: 1% in 15, 30 and 90 gm
   Solution: 1% in 10 and 30 gm
8. *Nystatin: Candida*
   Mycostatin: Ointment: 100,000 U/gm in 15 and 30 gm
   Creme: Same as ointment
   Powder: Same as ointment and creme, also 1 and 5 gm
   Nilstat: Ointment: 100,000 U/gm in 15 gm
   Creme: Same in 15 gm and ½ lb
9. *Amphotericin B: Candida*
   Fungizone: Creme: 30 mg/gm in 10 gm
   Lotion: 30 mg/ml in 30ml
   Ointment: 30 mg/gm in 20 mg
   All above Sig: 2–3 times/day
10. *Ketoconazole* (Nizoral): Tineas and *Candida:* Cream
11. *Ciclopirox olamine:* Tineas and *Candida*
    Loprox: Creme: 1% in in 15 and 30 gm

F. Antifungals (Combo)

1. *Clotrimazole,* Betamethasone diproplonate
   Lotrisone: Creme
   Sig: Apply to affected area B.I.D.
2. *Hydrocortisone, Iodochlorhydroxquin*
   Vioform HC: Creme: 3% iodo, 1% hydrocortisone
   Ointment: Same as creme
   Lotion: Same as creme
   Used as antifungal, antipruritic, for contact or atopic dermatitis, moniliasis, etc.
   Sig: Apply to affected area T.I.D. or Q.I.D.
   Also available in mild ointment and creme
3. *Onycho-Phytex:* 75 mg borotannic acid and 8 mg salicylic acid/ml in liquid form in 1 and 16 oz
   Sig: Apply to affected nails B.I.D. or T.I.D.
4. *Whitfield's Ointment:* 12% benzoic acid and 6% salicylic acid in 1 and 16 oz
   Sig: Apply to affected area B.I.D. or T.I.D.
5. *Castellani Paint:* basic fuchsin, phenol, resorcinol, acetone, alcohol
   Sig: Apply B.I.D.
6. *Fungoid Tincture:* cetyl pyridinium chloride, triacetin, chloroxylenol
   Sig: Apply to affected nails B.I.D.

G. Corticosteroids
Anti-Inflammatory, Antipruritic and Vasoconstrictor

1. *Hydrocortisone:* Ointment: Various; 0.25, 0.5, 1, 2, 2.5% in 1, 4, 8 oz and 1 lb
   Hytone: 0.5, 1, 2.5% in 1, 4 and 16 oz

Creme: Various; 0.25, 0.5, 1, 2.5% in ½, 1, 4 oz
Hytone: 0.5, 1, 2.5% in ½, 1, 4 oz
Lotion: Various: 0.25, 0.5, 1, 2.5% in 1 and 4 oz
Hytone: 0.5, 1% in 1 and 4 oz

2. *Betamethasone* Creme: Celestone
   A. Valerate: 1% ointment in 5, 15, 45 gm: Valisone
      1% creme in 5, 15, 45 mg: Valisone
      1% lotion in 20 and 60 ml: Valisone
   B. Diproprionate: 0.05% ointment in 15 and 45 gm: Diprosone, Diprolene
      0.05% creme in 15, 45 gm: Diprosone
      0.05% lotion in 20, 60ml: Diprosone
3. *Dexamethasone*
   Hexadrol: 0.4% creme in 10 and 30 gm
   D. Phosphate: Decadron Phosphate: 0.1% creme in 15 and 30 gm
4. *Fluocinolone Acetonide*
   Synalar: Ointment: 0.025% in 15, 60, and 425 gm
   Creme: 0.01% in 15, 45, 60, 120, 425 gm
   Synalar-HP: 0.2% creme in 5, 12 gm
   Solution: 0.01% in 20 and 60ml
   Do not exceed 2 gm/day
   Sig: Apply to affected area T.I.D. or Q.I.D.
5. *Fluocinonide*
   Lidex: 0.05% ointment in 15, 30, 60 gm
   Creme in 15, 30, 60 gm
   Topsyn: 0.05% gel in 15 and 60 gm
6. *Flurandrenolide*
   Cordan: Ointment: 0.025, .05% in 15, 30 and 60 gm
   Creme: 0.025, 0.05% in 15, 30 and 60 gm
   Lotion: 0.05% in 15 and 60ml
   Tape: μg/52 rolls of 24-inch and 80-inch length with 3 inches wide
7. *Halcinonide*
   Halog: 0.1% creme in 15, 60 gm and 8 oz
8. *Methylprednisolone Acetate*
   Medrol Acetate: 0.25, 1% in 7.5 and 30 gm and 1½ oz in a synthetic liquid base
9. *Triamcinolone Acetonide*
   Kenalog: Ointment: 0.025, 0.1, 0.5% in 15, 60, 80 gm
   Creme: 0.025, 0.1, 0.5% in 15, 60, 80 gm
   Lotion: 0.025, 0.1% in 15 and 60ml
   Aristocort: Ointment: 0.1, 15% in 15 gm
   Creme: 0.025, 0.1, 0.5% in 15 and 75 gm
10. *Prednisolone*
    Meti-Derm: 0.5% creme in 10 and 25 gm
11. *Desoximetasone*
    Topicort: 0.25% creme

H. Steroids (Combo)

Iodochlor compounds are antifungal, antibacterial and antiexczematous

1. *Pedi-Cort V*
   Creme: 1% hydrocortisone and 3% iodochlorhydroxyquin in 20 gm tube
2. *Hydrocortisone with Iodochlorhydroxyquin*
   Various: Creme: 0.5% hydroxycortisone, 3% iodochlor; 1%, 3% in 1 and 4 oz, 20 mg
   Ointment: 1%, 3% in 20 gm and 4 oz
3. *Vioform-Hydrocortisone* (Mild)
   Creme: 0.5, 3% in ½ and 1 oz
   1 and 3% in 5 and 20 gm
   Ointment: 0.5 and 3% in ½ and 1 oz
   1 and 3% in 5 and 20 gm
   Lotion: 1 and 3% in 15ml

I. Steroid-Antibiotic Combinations

1. *Neo-Hytone*
   Creme: 0.5% hydrocortisone and 0.5% neomycin sulfate in 1 oz
   1% hydrocortisone and 0.5% neomycin sulfate in 1 oz
2. Neo-Cortef
   Creme: 1% hydrocortisone and 0.5% neomycin in 20 gm
   2.5% hydrocortisone and 0.5% neomycin in 20 gm
   Ointment: 0.5% and 0.5% in ½ and 1 oz
   1% and 0.5% in 5, 20 gm and 4 oz
   2.5% and 0.5% in 5 and 20 gm
   Lotion: 1% and 0.5% in 15ml
3. *Mycolog*
   Creme: 1 mg triamcinolone, 2.5 mg neomycin, 0.25 mg gramicidin and 100,000 U nystatin/gm in 15, 30, 60 and 120 gm
   Ointment: 0.1%, 0.25%, 25%, 100,000 U/gm in 15, 30, 60, 120 gm
4. *Hydrocortisone-Neomycin*
   Various: Ointment: 0.5% and 0.5% in ½ and 1 oz
   1% and 0.5% in 5, 15, 20 gm and 4 oz
   2.5% and 0.5% in 5, 12, 20 gm

J. Burn Preparations

1. *Nitrofurazone*
   0.2% in soluble dressing, solution, ointment, creme
   Various: Furacin
   Apply to lesion or place on gauze
2. *Mafenide*
   Creme 85 mg/gm: Sulfamylon used for second- and third-degree burns
3. *Silver Sulfadiazine 1%*
   Creme: 10 mg/gm: Silvadene mostly used
4. *Silver Nitrate*
5. *Tannic Acid Compound*
   5% jelly: Amertan

K. Topical Tar Preparations: Antipruritic, Antieczematous and Keratoplastic for Psoriasis and Other Chronic Skin Diseases

1. Coal Tar Solution or Carbonic Detergents: 20% coal tar in 4 oz, 1 pt and 1 gal
2. *Estar Gel:* 5% coal tar in 3 oz
3. *Cotasol Creme:* 5% coal tar in 16 oz

L. Enzymes

1. *Biozyme Ointment*
   3.5 mg neomycin and 100,000 U trypsin-chymotrypsin
   ½ oz (15 gm) or 1 oz (30 gm)
   Biozyme C ointment—Collagenase: 250 collagenase U/gm used for: (*a*) removal of detritus; (*b*) debriding chronic dermal ulcers
   Sig: Apply Q.D.
2. *Elase, Elase Ointment*
   Fibrinolysin and desoxyribonuclease as ointment in 10 and 30 gm tubes and dry form
   Elase, Chloromycetin Ointment
   Fibrinolysin and desoxyribonuclease combined, with chloramphenicol ointment
   Broad-spectrum antibiotic used for debriding agent in a variety of inflammatory and infected lesions including (*a*) general surgical wounds, (*b*) ulcerative lesions, (*c*) second- and third-degree burns
   Sig: Dosage should be individualized but eschar must be debrided first
3. *Varidase*
   100,000 U streptokinase and 25,000 U streptodornase in vials
4. *Santyl Ointment*
   250 mg collagenase/gm in 25 gm jars inactivated by heavy metals (Domeboro) used for: (*a*) debriding chronic dermal ulcers, (*b*) severely burned areas
   Sig: Apply Q.D.
5. *Travase*
   Sutilains: ½ oz (14.2 gm) tubes with 82,000 casein units; 1 gm of hydrophylic ointment base inactivated by heavy metals (Domeboro) used for chemical debridement of second- and third-degree burns, decubitus ulcers
   Sig: Area must be cleansed thoroughly before application, repeat T.I.D. or Q.I.D.

XVII. URICOSURICS

Uricosurics: Also indomethacin, phenylbutazone and oxyphenbutazone: See under Anti-Inflammatories

1. *Probenecid:* Benemid
   Gout: Usually do not use until acute attack is over; chronic prophylaxis
   Sig: 0.25 gm B.I.D. for a week then 0.5 gm B.I.D.; may increase up to 2 gm/day with increased fluids and alkaline urine
   Penicillin therapy (general): 2 gm/day, divided
   Penicillin therapy for gonorrhea: Procaine penicillin G 4.8 million units with 1 gm probenecid 30 min prior; divided doses
2. *Sulfinpyrazone:* Anturane
   Oral caps: 100, 200 mg
   Sig: Initial 200–400 mg/day P.C. 1 week Maintenance: 400 mg B.I.D. up to 800 mg
3. *Probenecid-Colchicine Combo:* Colbenemid, Probenecid with Colchicine
   Oral tabs: 500 mg probenecid, 0.5 mg colchicine; after acute attack decrease to 1 tab/day for 1 week
4. *Aspirin Dosage:* 3–5 gm/day: uricosuric agent
   2–3 gm/day: uricoretentive

Other

1. *Allopurinol:* Zyloprim: Not uricosuric but is a xanthine oxidase inhibitor
   Oral tabs: 100, 300 mg
   Sig: Mild to moderate gout: 200–300 mg/day
   For severe, tophaceous gout: 400–600 mg/day B.I.D.
2. *Colchicine*
   Oral tabs: 0.3, 0.5, 0.6 mg: Abbott: 0.5-mg sugar-coated granules for acute gouty attack
   Sig: 1–1.5 mg then 0.5–0.6 mg q. 1 H. or 1–1.2 mg q. 2 H. until pain decreases or diarrhea occurs
   After initial dose: May take 0.5–0.6 mg q. 2–3 H.; 4–8 mg total may be needed
   Symptoms decrease within 12–24 hr

XVIII. MISCELLANEOUS

A. Vasodilators

1. *Tolazoline*
   Oral tabs: 25 mg: various and Priscoline
   Sig: 25 mg 4–6/day, may increase to 50 mg, 6 times/day if necessary
2. *Isoxsuprine*
   Oral tabs: 10 and 20 mg: Vasodilan, Rolisox
   Sig: 10–20 mg T.I.D. or Q.I.D.
3. *Nylidrin (B-Stim)*

Oral tabs: 6 mg: Arlidin
Sig: 3–12 mg T.I.D. or Q.I.D.

4. *Papaverine*
   Oral tabs: 30, 60, 100, 200 mg: various
   Timed-release caps: Dylate, Papacon, Pap-Kaps-150, Pavabid
   Sig: 100–300 mg 3–5 times/day or 150 mg q. 12H.
5. *Cyclandelate*
   Oral caps: 200 mg: Cyclospasmol
   Tabs: 100 mg: Cyclospasmol
   Sig: 1200–1600 mg/day in divided doses A.C. and H.S.
   Maintenance dose: 400–800 mg/day B.I.D. or Q.I.D.
6. *Nicotinic Acid*
   Oral tabs: 25, 50, 100 mg: Nyacin (Over-the-counter)
   500 mg (also available buffered): Various
   Timed-release caps: 125, 250, 400 mg: various
   Timed-release caps: 125, 250 mg: Nicobid
   Sig: 50–100 mg T.I.D. or Q.I.D., 1–2 gm/day
   Do not exceed 1–2 gm/day
7. *Pentoxifylline*
   Oral tabs: 400 mg: Trental
   Not a vasodilator—enhances erythrocyte flexibility
   Sig: 400 mg T.I.D. with meals

B. Wet Dressings and Soaks
Burow's Solution (Aluminum Acetate Solution)

1. Domeboro Tabs in 12's and 100's (Aluminum acetate, calcium acetate)
   Powder: 2.2 gm/packet—1–2 tabs or packets/pt water
   Have patient soak 15–20 min B.I.D. or T.I.D.
2. Bluboro or Pedi-Boro powder (Aluminum and Calcium Acetate)
   1–2 packets/pt water
   Have patient soak 15–20 min B.I.D. or T.I.D.
   Uses: (*a*) antimicrobial, (*b*) antipruritic, (*c*) astringent
   *Don't use with Santyl and Travase (topical); loses effectiveness with heavy metals
   *May use with Biozyme, Elase, Varidase
3. Acetic Acid 1%—for gram-negative *Pseudomonas* infections

C. Emolients—keeps evaporation to minimum

1. *Petroleum*—Vasilene, petroleum jelly
2. *Urea (Carbamide):* Promotes hydration and removal of excess keratin
3. *Aquacare 2%:* 2.5 oz; Lotion: 8 oz
   Aquacare H/P 10%: Creme: 2.5 oz; Lotion 8 oz
4. *Vitamin E*
5. *Vitamin A*
   Pedi-Vit A creme
6. *Vitamin A and D*
7. Carmol HC or Ureacin-10, 20
   Lotion: 10%: 6 oz
   Creme: 20%: 3 oz
   Calmurid Creme: 10%: 3.5 oz
   For lubrication, moisturizing, antipruritic
   Lubriderm Creme: 1.5, 4 oz
   Lubriderm Lotion: 4, 8, 16 oz
   Keri Lotion: 6.5, 13, 20 oz used for dryness
   Keri Creme: 2.5 oz
   Hydrisinol Creme: 4 oz, 1 lb
   Hydrisinol Lotion: 8 oz
   Dermassage Lotion: 6, 12, 16 oz
   Nutraderm Creme: 1.5 oz
   Nutraderm Lotion: 4, 8, 16 oz

D. Keratolytics

Salicylic Acid: Removes excess keratin in hyperkeratotic lesions, adjunct for verruca
Keralyt Gel 6%: Hydration prior to application enhances the effectiveness
Cantharidin: Cantharone: 7% Liquid usually used for warts: Apply and occlude
Ureacin-40: for diseased nails

References

1. Yale I: Foot impression technique. *Curr Podiatry*, 11–13, 1958.
2. Yale JF: An accurate foot impression technique on moderate weight bearing. *J Am Podiatry Students Assoc* 8:5–6, 1964.
3. Yale JF: Foot impression technique (F.I.T.): an accurate moderate weight bearing technique. *Arch Podiatr Med Foot Surg*, Annual Sports Medicine Edition May 1979, pp 117–119.
4. Root ML, Orien WP, Weed JW, Hughes RJ: *Biomechanical Examination of the Foot*. Los Angeles, Clinical Biomechanics, 1971.
5. Root ML, Orien WP, Weed JH: *Normal and Abnormal Function of the Foot*. Los Angeles, Clinical Biomechanics, 1971, vol I.
6. Root ML, Orien WP, Weed JH: *Normal and Abnormal Function of the Foot*. Los Angeles, Clinical Biomechanics, 1977, vol II.
7. Levine DP: An improved casting technique. In *Footprints*, Florida Podiatry Association, 1971.
8. Whitney AK: Urethane mould therapy. *N Engl J Podiatry* 42:17, 1963.
9. Whitney AK: Urethane moulds in podiatry. *Podiatry Q, Spring, 1965*.
10. McGlamry ED, Kitting RW: Postoperative urethane molds. *J Am Podiatry* Assoc 58:169, 1968.
11. Fisher C: A new technique in orthodigital correction and balance. *J Am Podiatry Assoc* 53:187–191, 1963.

12. Dobbs B, Esper R, Techner L, Hopkins W: A double-blind cross-over study comparing two doses of Duranest (etidocaine) 1% with a fixed dose of Sensorcaine (bupivacine) 0.5% utilizing infiltrating regional blocks of the fifth ray. *J Foot Surg* 23:467–469, 1984.
13. Albert SF: Scotch cast—an improved fiberglass casting material for use in podiatry. *J Am Podiatry Assoc* 71:338–340, 1981.
14. Finkelstein HB, Abraham MY, Crismal NC, Scherer RB, Tabak BA: *Basic Concepts of Physical Therapy for the Lower Extremity.* Chicago, M Facts, 1983.
15. Brantingham CR, Beekman BE, Moss CN, Gordon RB: Standing at the work place. presented at the section of Occupational Medicine. American Public Health Association, October 19, 1975.
16. Brantingham CR, Beekman BE, Moss CN, Gordon RB: Stress-reducing floor surface system at standing work places and walkways. Presented at the International Academy for Standing and Walking Fitness Meeting, in conjunction with the X International Congress on Podology, Copenhagen, Denmark, May 1982.
17. Brantingham CR, Beekman BE, Moss CN Gordon RB: A public health concern for walkways and work places. Podiatric Health Section, 110th Annual Meeting, American Public Health Association, Montreal, Canada, November, 1982.
18. Robbins, Jeffrey M., ed., Snyder, Stuart, contributor: Clinical Handbook of Podiatric Medicine - Pharmacology Section, OCPM, 1981.
19. Physician's Desk Reference, ed. 40, Oradell, NJ, Medical Economics, 1986.

Suggested Readings

Basmajian JV (ed): *Therapeutic Exercise,* ed 3. Baltimore, Williams & Wilkins, 1978.

Brown D, Smith C: Vacuum casting for foot orthoses. J Am Podiatry Assoc 66:582–587, 1976.

Bruno J, Helfand AE: Ultrasound and some podiatric considerations. *J Am Podiatry Assoc* 66:682–686, 1976.

Cadwallader DE: Drug interactions: some dangers of multiple drug use. *J Am Podiatry Assoc* 65:972–978, 1975.

Carleton FJ: *Shoes and Feet.* West Chester PA, Charles H Andress, 1940.

Coates IS: Silicone orthodigita and shielding, part I. *J Am Podiatry Assoc* 66:648–651, 1976.

Coates IS: Silicone orthodigita and shielding, part II. *J Am Podiatry Assoc* 66:706–711, 1976.

Coates IS: Silicone orthodigita and shielding, bunion shields, part V. *J Am Podiatry Assoc* 66:932–934, 1976

Coates IS: Silicone orthodigita and shielding, various other applications, part VI. *J Am Podiatry Assoc* 66:935–943, 1976.

Conn B (ed): *Current Diagnosis.* Philadelphia, WB Saunders, 1985.

Cutie MR, Cutie AJ: Podiatric drug reactions. *J Am Podiatry Assoc* 68:157–166, 1978.

Delaney JM: Chairside appliances of Plastazote. *Br J Chirop* 34:101, 1969.

Delaney JM: A simple Plastazote insole. *Br J Chirop* 35:77, 1970.

Gerbert J: The location of the terminal branching of the posterior nerve and its effect on administering a posterior tibial nerve block. *J Am Podiatry Assoc* 61:8–11, 1971.

Gilman AG, Goodman LS, Gilman A: *Goodman and Gilman's The Pharmacological Basis of Therapeutics,* ed 7. New York, Macmillin, 1985.

Griffen JE, Karselis: *Physical Agents for Physical Therapists.* Springfield, IL, Charles C Thomas, 1978.

Johnson M, Yale JF (eds): *A Monograph: Common Clinical Problems in Podiatric Medicine—A Synopsis of Diagnosis, Treatment, and Management for the Podiatric Physician.* Ansonia, CT, Yale Podiatry Group, P.C. 1984.

Kastrup E: *Facts and Comparisons.* Facts and Comparisons, 1981.

Kovacs R: *Electrotherapy and Light Therapy,* ed 3. Philadelphia, Lea & Febiger, 1938.

Krantz MK: Converting a commercial sandal into a molded sandal. *J Natl Assoc Chirop* 47:555, 1957.

Licht S: *Therapeutic Electricity and Ultraviolet Radiation,* ed 2. New Haven, CT, Licht, 1967.

Marderosian AH: Drug prescribing, therapy, or threat. *J Am Podiatry Assoc* 63:185–189, 1973.

Marr SJ: Toe buttressing for forefoot problems. *J Am Podiatry Assoc* 74:136–140, 1984.

McEntyre R: *Key Medications: A Practical Guide.* Philadelphia, WB Saunders, 1980.

McGlamry ED, Kitting RW: Postoperative urethane molds. *J Am Podiatry Assoc* 58:169–175, 1968.

Niehaus P: Sorbothotics soft tissue supplement orthoses. *J Am Podiatric Med Assoc* 75:46–47, 1985.

Physicians' Desk Reference for Nonprescription Drugs, ed 6. Oradell, NJ, Medical Economics, 1986.

Rosoff S: Contact podiatry. *J Podiatry* 10:30, 1953.

Rosoff S: The fabrication of contact appliances for use in conventional footwear. *J Am Podiatry Assoc* 51:189–194, 1961.

Rosoff S: Fabrication of orthotic devices with the use of silicone gel. *J Am Podiatry Assoc* 60:313–321, 1970.

Rosoff S: Further uses of orthotic gel devices. *Curr Podiatry,* Feb 1971.

Rossi CL: Drugs administered to 100 podiatry patients for office surgery. *J Am Podiatry Assoc* 66:310–312, 1976.

Sanders JT: Inducing hypnosis in the waking subject. *J Am Podiatry Assoc* 48:62, 1958.

Sivitz SC: A new approach to dynamic molding techniques. *J Natl Assoc Chirop* 46:21–26, 1956.

Stern J: Treatment standardization for iontophoresis. *J Natl Assoc Chirop* 45:39–40, 1955.

Stillman EG: A new dynamic foot mold. *J Am Podiatry Assoc* 48:144–147, 1958.

Tallarida RJ: *MPD 1985, Most Prescribed Drugs 1985.* Philadelphia, WB Saunders, 1985.

Weinstock RC: The wooden sole shoe in podiatry practice. *J Am Podiatry Assoc* 56:365–370, 1966.

Wright EW: Compensating and corrective appliances. *J Natl Assoc Chirop* 46:312–315, 1956.

Yale, I: A new therapeutic approach for accommodation of foot pathology. *J Am Podiatry Assoc* 48:477–480, 1958.

Index

Page numbers followed by "*t*" denote tables.